Ischemic Heart Disease

Giovanni Concistrè
Editor

Ischemic Heart Disease

From Diagnosis to Treatment

Springer

Editor
Giovanni Concistrè
Department of Adult Cardiac Surgery
Ospedale del cuore "G. Pasquinucci"
Massa, Italy

ISBN 978-3-031-25878-7 ISBN 978-3-031-25879-4 (eBook)
https://doi.org/10.1007/978-3-031-25879-4

This Springer imprint is published by the registered company Springer Nature Switzerland AG
The registered company address is: Gewerbestrasse 11, 6330 Cham, Switzerland

"To my family"

Foreword

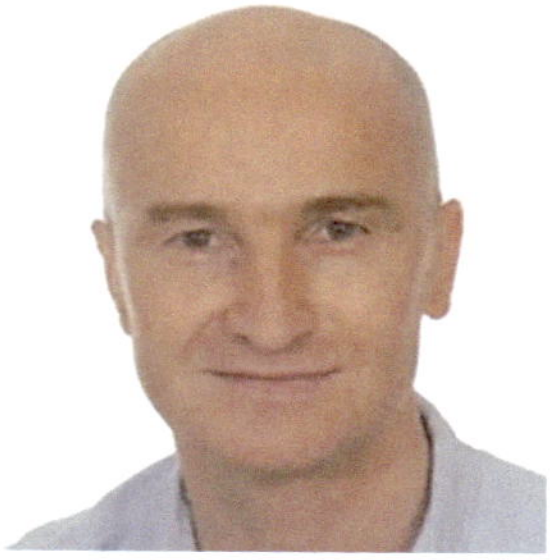

Cardiovascular disease remains the leading cause of death worldwide. According to the World Heart Federation, cardiovascular disease is responsible for 17.1 million deaths globally each year. Counterintuitively, 82% of these deaths actually occur in the developing world. Such numbers are often difficult to comprehend. The gravity of the situation is enhanced when portrayed as the following: Heart disease kills one person every 34 s in the USA alone, and 35 people under the age of 65 die prematurely in the UK every day due to cardiovascular disease (12,500 deaths per annum). Although still the leading killer, the incidence of cardiovascular disease has declined in recent years for several reasons: a better understanding of its pathology, implementation and enhancement of lipid-lowering therapy, new drug regimens including low-molecular-weight heparin and antiplatelet drugs such as glycoprotein IIb/IIIa receptor inhibitors, and acute surgical intervention.

The disease burden has a great financial impact on global healthcare systems and major economic consequences for world economies. Hospital care for patients with cardiovascular disease accounts for approximately 70% of the cost with 20% spent on pharmacological agents. However, the total cost should also include non-healthcare costs such as production losses in the workforce and informal care of people with the disease.

This text aims to elevate the current understanding and treatment of coronary artery disease at every level, and I particularly appreciate the multidisciplinary and international approach of the editors and authors. The authors are cardiologists, radiologists, pathologists, and cardiac surgeons who work in Europe, America, Asia, and Australia. The book is very comprehensive, covering all aspects of ischemic heart disease including anatomy, physiology, preoperative assessment by various techniques, and risk analysis that is especially relevant to an ever-increasing elderly population. The book then focuses on varied surgical procedures and newly emerging technologies, and its particular focus on modern innovations provides a very innovative slant.

While the book is primarily aimed at cardiology fellows in training, it will also appeal to a far wider audience including surgeons, cardiologists, imagers, interventionalists, as well as other clinicians and students involved in the diagnosis and treatment of ischemic heart disease. I believe that this book will help clarify daily questions regarding the clinical and surgical practice in ischemic heart disease, as well as induce inspiration and new insights into this field. For all these efforts and initiatives, the editors and authors deserve congratulations.

David P. Taggart
University of Oxford
Oxford, UK

Contents

Surgical Anatomy of Coronary Arteries: Morphogenesis, Normal and Pathological Anatomy

Alberto Aimo

Abbreviations

ALCAPA	Anomalous origin of the left coronary artery from the pulmonary artery
CA	Coronary artery
CAA	Coronary artery anomaly
CCTA	Cardiac computed tomography angiography
EPDC	Epicardium-derived cell
LA	Left atrium/atrial
LAD	Left anterior descending artery
LCA	Left coronary artery
LCX	Left circumflex artery
LMCA	Left main coronary artery
LV	Left ventricle/ventricular
MACE	Major adverse cardiac events
PDA	Posterior descending artery
RCA	Right coronary artery
RV	Right ventricle/ventricular
SCD	Sudden cardiac death

A. Aimo (✉)
Interdisciplinary Center for Health Sciences, Pisa, Italy

Cardiology and Cardiovascular Medicine Department, Fondazione Toscana Gabriele Monasterio, Pisa, Italy
e-mail: a.aimo@santannapisa.it; aimoalb@ftgm.it

G. Concistrè (ed.), *Ischemic Heart Disease*,
https://doi.org/10.1007/978-3-031-25879-4_1

The vessels that nourish the heart are called coronary arteries (CAs). An adequate blood flow at rest and during exercise is crucial to sustain cardiac function. Blood flow can be reduced by disorders affecting CAs or by congenital alterations in the origin and course of CAs. This chapter provides first an overview of the complex (and still incompletely understood) process of CA development. Normal CA anatomy and the main variants will then be presented. The last section of this chapter is devoted to congenital abnormalities.

1 Development of Coronary Blood Vessels

CAs in humans and other amniotic vertebrates join the systemic circulation at the aortic root. Until the late 1980s, CAs were thought to derive entirely from an outgrowth of the aortic root endothelium expanding to form an arterial bed, then a network of capillaries, and the venous system [1]. Several studies on avian models challenged this notion, showing that CAs do not stem from the aortic root. Indeed, at least part of the early arterial coronary vascular system forms through the coalescence of endothelial progenitor cells (or angioblasts) and subsequent fusion of endothelial cell clusters to form new blood vessels (vasculogenesis) [2]. These new vessels then gain access to the aortic lumen [3–6], possibly along a gradient of vascular endothelial growth factor C [7].

Larger CAs have an inner endothelial layer (intima), a medial wall formed by smooth muscle cells and elastic fibers (media), and an outer layer of fibrous tissue (adventitia). The coronary endothelium has a mesodermal nature. At least three different cellular sources of coronary endothelium have been proposed, i.e., the sinus venosus endocardium, the ventricular endocardium, and the epicardium. Although the relative importance of each source in mammalian coronary vascular development needs further evaluation [8], current evidence suggests that sinus venosus endocardium gives origin to venous endothelium, whereas endothelial cells from the ventricular endocardium and epicardium are the main contributors of the arterial components of the coronary tree [4–6, 9, 10]. The epicardium derives from the proepicardium, a cluster of coelomic cells located at the inflow of the developing heart during the fourth week of gestation in humans. Proepicardial cells spread over the surface of the embryonic myocardium, forming a monolayered epithelium (the primitive epicardium) over the myocardium. Some primitive epicardial cells immediately undergo an epithelial-to-mesenchymal transition [5, 10], producing a new population of highly invasive mesenchymal cells named epicardium-derived cells (EPDCs) [11]. EPDCs then migrate into the intimal, medial, and adventitial layers of developing coronary blood vessels.

EPDCs are also considered the source of smooth muscle cells forming the medial wall of CAs, although other sources such as the neural crest are not excluded [12, 13].

Fibroblasts are particularly abundant in the adventitial layer of large CAs. Coronary fibroblasts likely derive from the epicardium [14–16], although other origins such as the bone marrow cannot be excluded [17, 18].

Overall, animal studies (mostly murine and avian models) have allowed to understand that coronary blood vessels are a developmental mosaic, including cells derived from different embryonic sources [19]. Another quite established point is that CAs develop autonomously and then connect to the aortic root, instead of sprouting from the aortic root.

2 Normal Coronary Anatomy

2.1 Origins from the Sinuses of Valsalva

The aortic root is the portion of the left ventricular (LV) outflow tract that supports the leaflets of the aortic valve, delineated by the sinotubular junction superiorly and the bases of valve leaflets inferiorly [20]. The aortic root comprises the sinuses, the aortic valve leaflets, the commissures, and the interleaflet triangles. The sinuses of Valsalva are expanded portions of the aortic root, which are confined proximally by the attachments of the valve leaflets and distally by the sinotubular junction. Two sinuses are adjacent to the pulmonary root, and usually the major CAs originate from these sinuses. The remaining noncoronary sinus is usually the largest [20]. Coronary orifices are seldom positioned in the middle of the sinuses; they tend to be located just below, at, or just above the level of the sinotubular junction and are often not in the midline of the respective sinusal junctions [19].

2.2 Right Coronary Artery

Viewed from the frontal plane, the RCA arises at nearly 90° from the corresponding sinus. It enters the atrioventricular groove and descends anteriorly and inferiorly to the right border of the heart, issuing several branches [21]. In half of the subjects, the first branch is the infundibular (or conal) branch. In the other half, the infundibular artery arises directly from a second orifice within the right sinus [21]. The RCA supplies the infundibular musculature of the right ventricle (RV), often anastomosing with an infundibular branch of the anterior interventricular artery [22]. In three-fifths of the population, the RCA gives rise to the artery to the sinus node [23]. The largest branch of the RCA is the right marginal artery, which usually originates at least 1 cm proximal to the acute margin and travels to the apex of the heart [21]. The majority of hearts have right coronary dominance, **which means that** the posterior descending artery (PDA, also known as inferior interventricular artery) is supplied only by the RCA. This condition accounted for 81% of subjects in a large *postmortem* coronary angiogram study [24]. In subjects with right coronary dominance, the artery to the atrioventricular node arises from the RCA. In most cases of right coronary dominance, the artery itself continues beyond the crux and supplies branches to the infero-septal papillary muscle and the diaphragmatic wall of the LV.

2.3 Left Coronary Artery

The left main coronary artery (LMCA) originates from the left sinus and travels anteriorly and to the left towards the sternocostal surface of the heart, between the left atrial (LA) appendage and the pulmonary trunk [25]. It is very short (about 1–2 cm) and divides into the left anterior descending (LAD) artery (or anterior interventricular artery) and the circumflex artery [21]. In some individuals, the main stem gives rise to a third branch called intermediate artery. When present, it supplies the area normally covered by the diagonal and/or obtuse marginal arteries [23].

2.4 Left Anterior Descending Artery

The LAD is the direct anterior continuation of the LMCA. After curving around the pulmonary trunk, it enters the anterior interventricular groove and travels to the apex [21]. It then ascends within the inferior interventricular sulcus towards the crux, supplying branches to the apical parts of the inferior walls of both ventricles [21]. It terminates within the inferior interventricular groove adjacent to the inferior interventricular artery. The LAD gives rise to the diagonal arteries and the deep septal perforators, which both vary in their number and course. The diagonal arteries supply the LV free wall. The deep septal perforators branch at right angles to the interventricular artery and supply the anterior two-thirds of the muscular ventricular septum [23]. The most prominent branch is the left descending septal artery, which supplies the moderator band before terminating at the anterior papillary muscle. The LAD can also produce an infundibular or conal branch, which can anastomose in a circular pattern around the pulmonary infundibulum.

2.5 Left Circumflex Artery

The LCX branches at an angle perpendicular to the LMCA and enters the left atrioventricular groove [21]. In individuals who are right dominant, the LCX usually terminates as the left obtuse marginal artery [21]. Several branches supply the posterior and lateral walls of the LV and the superolateral papillary muscle [26]. Smaller unnamed branches arise from the LCX as it travels along the atrioventricular groove and supply the aortic root and ventricular myocardium adjacent to the groove [26]. In around 10% of individuals (9% in the *postmortem* study above) [24], the LCX reaches the cardiac crux and gives rise to the PDA. In this circumstance, the artery to the atrioventricular node derives from the circumflex artery (so-called balanced pattern) [21]. In other cases, there is no proper PDA, and the terminal branches of the RCA and LCX descend along the interventricular groove. This condition is known as codominance and was found in 10% of individuals in the *postmortem* study above [24].

3 Variants from Normal Coronary Anatomy

There is substantial interindividual variability in the origin, course, and branches of CAs. Normal variants differ from coronary artery anomalies (CAAs) because of their higher prevalence and benign nature [27–29]. Apart from the right or left dominance or codominance, we have already mentioned the variable perfusion of sinoatrial and atrioventricular nodes, the emergence of a conus branch from the right sinus, or an intermediate artery originating from a trifurcation of the LMCA [29, 30]. The absence of the LMCA, with a separate origin of the LAD and LCX, is found in up to 0.67% of subjects [28] and is regarded as a variant. Additionally, an origin with a more acute angle or a higher takeoff and an increased tortuosity is generally considered a benign variant, but may complicate percutaneous coronary interventions [31, 32].

4 Coronary Artery Anomalies

Although originally described in the eighteenth century, CAAs were first classified in 1969 [33]. The use of a heterogeneous nomenclature in historical reports may have led to underestimation of the real prevalence of CAAs. When assessing the prevalence of CAAs, other potential sources of bias should be considered: 1) *postmortem* examination of coronary arteries is more likely performed in young victims of sudden cardiac death (SCD) and 2) patients with suspected or known CAAs are more often referred to specialized angiographic centers [34]. The estimated prevalence of CAAs ranges from 0.2% to 5.8%, based on angiography, cardiac computed tomography angiography (CCTA), and autopsy databases [19]. The diffusion of CCTA is expected to advance our knowledge of the epidemiology of CAAs [35, 36], whose prevalence might be even higher (8% in a recent cohort of 1759 patients) [35].

CAAs with potential hemodynamic and clinical implications can be labelled as "malignant," whereas the others can be designated as "benign." Furthermore, CAAs may be encountered in otherwise normal hearts, but can also coexist with heart malformations such as tetralogy of Fallot, transposition, or bicuspid aortic valve, and may in some cases complicate their management [21]. Despite these considerations, the classification of CAAs relies merely on anatomical considerations. A classification system proposed by a position statement of the European Society of Cardiology identifies anomalies of CA connection (origin and course), anomalies of intrinsic CA anatomy, and anomalies of CA/myocardial interaction [19] (Table 1).

Table 1 Classification of coronary artery anomalies (CAAs)

Anomalies of CA connection

- To the pulmonary artery (PA)/pulmonary circulation
  - LCA to posterior facing sinus (ALCAPA)
  - LCX to posterior facing sinus
  - LAD to posterior facing sinus
  - RCA to anterior right facing sinus
  - Ectopic connection (outside facing sinuses) of any CA to PA left
  - Sinus, trunk, or branch
  - RV
- To the aorta/systemic circulation
  - Absent left main trunk (split LCA)
  - Anomalous CA ostium location within or near proper aortic sinus of:
  - Valsalva:
    High tubular aorta
    Low aorta
    Commissural (with acute angle)
  - Anomalous CA ostium location at improper aortic sinus—wrong sinus:
    RCA to left sinus
    LCA to right sinus
    LCX to RCA or sinus
    LAD to RCA or sinus
    RCA or LCA to posterior sinus with anomalous course: interarterial, prepulmonic, intraseptal, retroaortic, posterior atrioventricular groove or retrocardiac, posteroanterior interventricular groove
  - Single CA
  - Anomalous CA ostium location outside sinotubular aorta:
    LV
    Ascending aorta
    Aortic arch
    Others (innominate artery; right carotid artery; internal mammary artery; bronchial artery; subclavian artery; descending thoracic aorta)

Anomalies of intrinsic CA anatomy

- CA ostial stenosis or atresia
- CA ostial dimple
- CA ectasia or aneurysm
- Absent CA
- CA hypoplasia
- Anomalous CA ramification:
  - Anomalous origin of PD from LAD or septal penetrating branch
  - Split RCA
  - Split LAD
  - Ectopic origin of first septal branch (RCA, right sinus, diagonal, LCX)

Table 1 (continued)

Anomalous myocardial/CA interaction
- Intramural course ("myocardial bridge")
- Subendocardial course
- Fistulae from RCA, LCA, or infundibular artery to RV, RA, coronary sinus, superior vena cava, PA, PV, LA, LV, multiple
- Inadequate arteriolar/capillary ramifications

ALCAPA, anomalous origin of the left coronary artery from the pulmonary artery; LA, left atrium/atrial; LAD, left anterior descending artery; LCA, left coronary artery; LCX, left circumflex artery; LV, left ventricle/ventricular; MACE, major adverse cardiac events; PA, pulmonary artery; PDA, posterior descending artery; PV, pulmonary vein; RA, right atrium/atrial; RCA, right coronary artery; RV, right ventricle/ventricular. Adapted with permission from Pérez-Pomares et al. (2016) [19]

4.1 Anomalies of CA Connection

The *origin of CAs from the pulmonary artery* is one of the most serious CA anomalies, with an estimated prevalence of 1 in 300,000 live births and an established association with myocardial infarction and SCD. In the most common form, the LMCA connects to the pulmonary artery (anomalous origin of the left coronary artery from the pulmonary artery, ALCAPA), while the RCA connects normally to the aorta. Coronary steal may occur when the low blood pressure in the pulmonary artery causes blood from the LCA to flow towards the pulmonary artery instead of the heart, causing myocardial ischemia and promoting the formation of collateral vessels. The extent of the acquired collateral circulation between the two CAs is the major determinant of the degree of ischemia, severity of clinical presentation, and outcome. Thus, patients with well-established collateral vessels have the "adult type" of the disease, and those without or with few collaterals have the "infant type," with early onset of symptoms when pulmonary arterial pressure decreases [37]. The availability of less invasive diagnostic modalities, such as CCTA, has led to a more frequent identification of this condition in an older cohort [38]. The definitive treatment for ALCAPA is surgical intervention, with direct reimplantation of the anomalous CA into the aorta.

Anomalies in the *origins of CAs from the aorta* are more common. Estimates from observational studies are extremely heterogeneous, but their prevalence is at least 1 in 1000 individuals [29, 32, 39]. The origin of a CA from the opposite sinus is the most frequent and clinically relevant anomaly, while the origin from the noncoronary sinus is unusual [28, 39, 40]. The presence of these CAAs is usually not associated with other congenital abnormalities [41], whereas other rarer subtypes (e.g., single or inverted CAs) are often observed in the setting of complex congenital heart diseases [33, 40].

In the setting of anomalous connection of either the RCA to the left coronary sinus or the LCA to the right coronary sinus, the proximal portion of the anomalous CA may run before the pulmonary trunk (prepulmonic), behind the aorta (retroaortic), or between the pulmonary artery and the aorta (interarterial) (Fig. 1). Among them, only those with an interarterial (aorta–pulmonary) course are regarded as conditions at risk of ischemia and even SCD [42]. Several mechanisms of ischemia during exercise have been proposed, including (1) increased cardiac output and expansion of the great vessels, with compression of the anomalous vessel between the aorta and the pulmonary artery; (2) spasm or kinking of the anomalous vessel; and (3) a flap-like closure of the coronary ostium due to an acute angle takeoff and a further stretch during exercise [28, 42]. Anomalous LCA connection to the right sinus is considered more dangerous than RCA connection to the left sinus because of the larger amount of myocardium at risk of ischemia [43]. Anomalous connection of a CA to the noncoronary sinus is quite rare and exceptionally associated with SCD [43].

The *LCX starting from the RCA or the right sinus* is considered the most frequent CA anomaly with an angiographic incidence of up to 0.67% [44, 45]. The LCX has a retroaortic course and crosses the aortic-mitral fibrous continuity (Fig. 1). This anomaly is usually considered benign and a rare cause of myocardial ischemia and SCD [46].

A *single CA* is a very rare condition seen in 0.0024–0.044% of the population [47], where only one CA connects to the aorta through a single ostium. The single CA may take

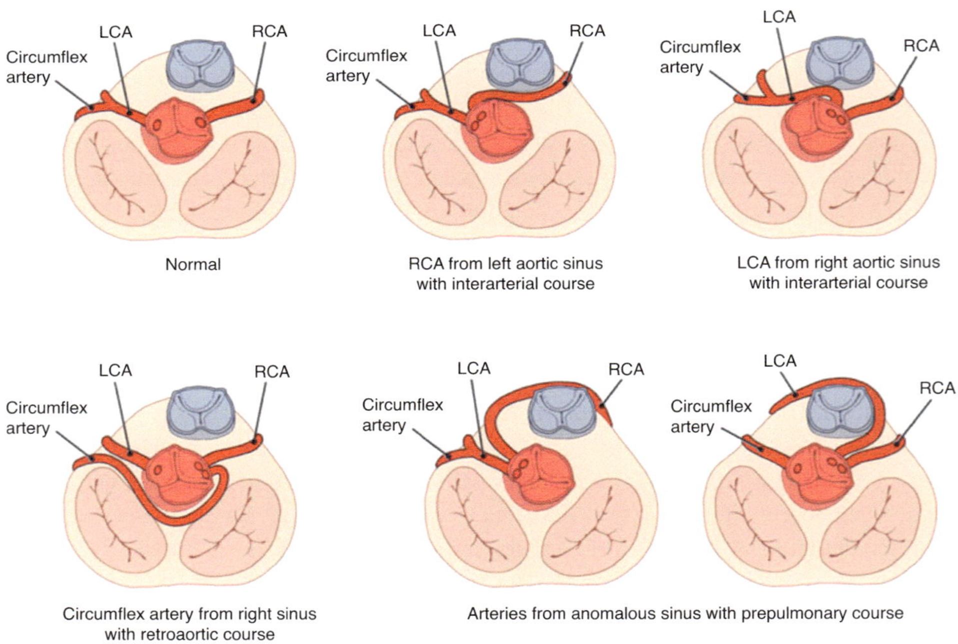

Fig. 1 Examples of anomalous origination of coronary ostia from the opposite aortic sinus. LCA, left coronary artery; RCA, right coronary artery

the course of either an RCA or an LCA and divide shortly from its origin into two or three of the main coronary branches [48]. A single CA may be compatible with a normal life expectancy, but acquired coronary stenosis is very dangerous because of the impossibility to develop proximal collateral branches, and there is a high risk of ischemia when a major CA branch courses between the pulmonary artery and the aorta [19].

4.2 Anomalies of Intrinsic CA Anatomy

Congenital atresia of the LMCA differs from LMCA absence in that a fibrous tract may hinder myocardial perfusion. There are few reports of congenital atresia of the LMCA in adults [49]. Absence or severe hypoplasia of the RCA or LCX is rare [29, 32].

An epicardial coronary artery, usually the LAD, may present an intramyocardial course. "*Myocardial bridges*" are much more common than other CAAs. The prevalence of myocardial bridges at angiography is lower than at autopsy (0.5–2.5% vs. 15–85%) since many bridges consist of thin loops of myocardium that do not affect coronary hemodynamics and then cannot be detected by angiography with the typical vessel constriction (so-called milking effect) [50]. Myocardial bridges are common in patients with hypertrophic cardiomyopathy, with a frequency of around 25% [51]. Exercise-induced ischemia has been attributed to tachycardia, which increases the myocardial oxygen requirement and reduces the time of diastole [52]. Beta-blockers are commonly used as first-line agents for patients with symptoms, because they reduce myocardial oxygen requirement and compression of the artery. Coronary stenting is not recommended [53]. The most common surgical approaches are coronary artery bypass grafting (CABG) and surgical myotomy. CABG seems to be most beneficial in long (>25 mm) or deep (>5 mm) myocardial bridges; in the other cases, surgical myotomy (with resection of the muscle fibers compressing the artery) should be considered [53, 54]. Myocardial bridges have been considered a possible cause of SCD; the existence of this cause-effect relationship, possibly mediated by ventricular arrhythmias elicited by myocardial ischemia, is still debated [46].

A *coronary aneurysm* is a focal dilatation of at least 1.5 times the normal coronary lumen, involving less than half of CA length, while ectasia is a dilation of more than half of CA length. Coronary aneurysms may be saccular (if the transverse diameter exceeds the longitudinal diameter) or fusiform (in the opposite case) [55]. Coronary aneurysms are usually acquired (e.g., atherosclerosis, syphilis, Kawasaki disease), while they are exceedingly rare as congenital anomalies [55, 56].

Coronary arteriovenous fistulas consist of the termination of a coronary artery into another vessel or a cardiac chamber. They are relatively common in the context of complex malformations, while they are rare in adults [57]. The most common site of drainage is the RV, followed by the right atrium and the pulmonary artery. Fistulae drain into the LA or LV in less than 10% of cases. The hemodynamic consequences depend on the site of drainage and the resistance to flow (which in turn depends on fistula diameter, length, and tortuosity). The blood flow from the CA to a venous structure or right-sided cardiac chamber occurs throughout the cardiac cycle. Large fistulae may cause a coronary steal during diastole, with ischemia symptoms, and a left-to-right shunt, with volume overload of both ventricles. When fistulae drain in the LA or a pulmonary vein, a left-to-left shunt with left-heart volume overload occurs. Small fistulae in asymptomatic children should be followed over time because of their tendency to grow with age. Symptomatic or asymptomatic patients with large, hemodynamically significant CA fistulae should be treated through surgical ligation, either isolated or in association with CA bypass grafting, and interventional closure with occlusion coils, umbrellas, vascular plugs, and covered stents [58].

5 Conclusion

A good knowledge of the normal coronary anatomy, including coronary variants, is crucial to recognize alterations in coronary anatomy caused by acquired disorders (such as atherosclerosis or Kawasaki disease) or abnormalities in CA development. The latter may be benign alterations that are discovered occasionally or *vice versa* may alter cardiac hemodynamics and increase the risk of myocardial ischemia and SCD, thus requiring a specific treatment.

Conflicts of Interest None.

References

1. Folkman J, Haudenschild C. Angiogenesis in vitro. Nature. 1980;288(5791):551–6.
2. Risau W, Flamme I. Vasculogenesis. Annu Rev Cell Dev Biol. 1995;11:73–91.
3. Bogers AJ, Gittenberger-de Groot AC, Poelmann RE, Péault BM, Huysmans HA. Development of the origin of the coronary arteries, a matter of ingrowth or outgrowth? Anat Embryol. 1989;180(5):437–41.
4. Mikawa T, Fischman DA. Retroviral analysis of cardiac morphogenesis: discontinuous formation of coronary vessels. Proc Natl Acad Sci U S A. 1992;89(20):9504–8.
5. Pérez-Pomares JM, Macías D, García-Garrido L, Muñoz-Chápuli R. The origin of the subepicardial mesenchyme in the avian embryo: an immunohistochemical and quail-chick chimera study. Dev Biol. 1998;200(1):57–68.
6. Männer J. Does the subepicardial mesenchyme contribute myocardioblasts to the myocardium of the chick embryo heart? A quail-chick chimera study tracing the fate of the epicardial primordium. Anat Rec. 1999;255(2):212–26.
7. Chen HI, Poduri A, Numi H, Kivela R, Saharinen P, McKay AS, et al. VEGF-C and aortic cardiomyocytes guide coronary artery stem development. J Clin Invest. 2014;124(11):4899–914.
8. Tian X, Pu WT, Zhou B. Cellular origin and developmental program of coronary angiogenesis. Circ Res. 2015;116(3):515–30.
9. Katz TC, Singh MK, Degenhardt K, Rivera-Feliciano J, Johnson RL, Epstein JA, et al. Distinct compartments of the proepicardial organ give rise to coronary vascular endothelial cells. Dev Cell. 2012;22(3):639–50.

10. Dettman RW, Denetclaw W Jr, Ordahl CP, Bristow J. Common epicardial origin of coronary vascular smooth muscle, perivascular fibroblasts, and intermyocardial fibroblasts in the avian heart. Dev Biol. 1998;193(2):169–81.
11. Pérez-Pomares JM, de la Pompa JL. Signaling during epicardium and coronary vessel development. Circ Res. 2011;109(12):1429–42.
12. Mellgren AM, Smith CL, Olsen GS, Eskiocak B, Zhou B, Kazi MN, et al. Platelet-derived growth factor receptor beta signaling is required for efficient epicardial cell migration and development of two distinct coronary vascular smooth muscle cell populations. Circ Res. 2008;103(12):1393–401.
13. Arima Y, Miyagawa-Tomita S, Maeda K, Asai R, Seya D, Minoux M, et al. Preotic neural crest cells contribute to coronary artery smooth muscle involving endothelin signalling. Nat Commun. 2012;3:1267.
14. Gittenberger-de Groot AC, Vrancken Peeters MP, Mentink MM, Gourdie RG, Poelmann RE. Epicardium-derived cells contribute a novel population to the myocardial wall and the atrioventricular cushions. Circ Res. 1998;82(10):1043–52.
15. Acharya A, Baek ST, Huang G, Eskiocak B, Goetsch S, Sung CY, et al. The bHLH transcription factor Tcf21 is required for lineage-specific EMT of cardiac fibroblast progenitors. Development. 2012;139(12):2139–49.
16. Ruiz-Villalba A, Ziogas A, Ehrbar M, Pérez-Pomares JM. Characterization of epicardial-derived cardiac interstitial cells: differentiation and mobilization of heart fibroblast progenitors. PLoS One. 2013;8(1):e53694.
17. Zhang N, Mustin D, Reardon W, Almeida AD, Mozdziak P, Mrug M, et al. Blood-borne stem cells differentiate into vascular and cardiac lineages during normal development. Stem Cells Dev. 2006;15(1):17–28.
18. Zeisberg EM, Kalluri R. Origins of cardiac fibroblasts. Circ Res. 2010;107(11):1304–12.
19. Pérez-Pomares JM, de la Pompa JL, Franco D, Henderson D, Ho SY, Houyel L, et al. Congenital coronary artery anomalies: a bridge from embryology to anatomy and pathophysiology—a position statement of the development, anatomy, and pathology ESC Working Group. Cardiovasc Res. 2016;109(2):204–16.
20. Underwood MJ, El Khoury G, Deronck D, Glineur D, Dion R. The aortic root: structure, function, and surgical reconstruction. Heart. 2000;83(4):376–80.
21. Loukas M, Sharma A, Blaak C, Sorenson E, Mian A. The clinical anatomy of the coronary arteries. J Cardiovasc Transl Res. 2013;6(2):197–207.
22. Loukas M, Clarke P, Tubbs RS, Kapos T. Raymond de Vieussens. Anat Sci Int. 2007;82(4):233–6.
23. Patel S. Normal and anomalous anatomy of the coronary arteries. Semin Roentgenol. 2008;43(2):100–12.
24. Knaapen M, Koch AH, Koch C, Koch KT, Li X, van Rooij PC, et al. Prevalence of left and balanced coronary arterial dominance decreases with increasing age of patients at autopsy. A postmortem coronary angiograms study. Cardiovascular pathology: the official journal of the Society for. Cardiovasc Pathol. 2013;22(1):49–53.
25. Zimmermann E, Schnapauff D, Dewey M. Cardiac and coronary anatomy in computed tomography. Semin Ultrasound CT MR. 2008;29(3):176–81.
26. Estes EH Jr, Entman ML, Dixon HB II, Hackel DB. The vascular supply of the left ventricular wall. Anatomic observations, plus a hypothesis regarding acute events in coronary artery disease. Am Heart J. 1966;71(1):58–67.
27. Angelini P. Normal and anomalous coronary arteries: definitions and classification. Am Heart J. 1989;117(2):418–34.
28. Angelini P. Coronary artery anomalies: an entity in search of an identity. Circulation. 2007;115(10):1296–305.

29. Villa AD, Sammut E, Nair A, Rajani R, Bonamini R, Chiribiri A. Coronary artery anomalies overview: The normal and the abnormal. World J Radiol. 2016;8(6):537–55.
30. Shriki JE, Shinbane JS, Rashid MA, Hindoyan A, Withey JG, DeFrance A, et al. Identifying, characterizing, and classifying congenital anomalies of the coronary arteries. RSNA. 2012;32(2):453–68.
31. Angelini P, Trujillo A, Sawaya F, Lee VV. "Acute takeoff" of the circumflex artery: a newly recognized coronary anatomic variant with potential clinical consequences. Tex Heart Inst J. 2008;35(1):28–31.
32. Yamanaka O, Hobbs RE. Coronary artery anomalies in 126,595 patients undergoing coronary arteriography. Catheter Cardiovasc Diagn. 1990;21(1):28–40.
33. Ogden JA. Congenital anomalies of the coronary arteries. Am J Cardiol. 1970;25(4):474–9.
34. Angelini P. Coronary artery anomalies—current clinical issues: definitions, classification, incidence, clinical relevance, and treatment guidelines. Tex Heart Inst J. 2002;29(4):271–8.
35. Ghadri JR, Kazakauskaite E, Braunschweig S, Burger IA, Frank M, Fiechter M, et al. Congenital coronary anomalies detected by coronary computed tomography compared to invasive coronary angiography. BMC Cardiovasc Disord. 2014;14:81.
36. Namgung J, Kim JA. The prevalence of coronary anomalies in a single center of Korea: origination, course, and termination anomalies of aberrant coronary arteries detected by ECG-gated cardiac MDCT. BMC Cardiovasc Disord. 2014;14:48.
37. Frommelt PC, Frommelt MA. Congenital coronary artery anomalies. Pediatr Clin N Am. 2004;51(5):1273–88.
38. Yau JM, Singh R, Halpern EJ, Fischman D. Anomalous origin of the left coronary artery from the pulmonary artery in adults: a comprehensive review of 151 adult cases and a new diagnosis in a 53-year-old woman. Clin Cardiol. 2011;34(4):204–10.
39. Cheezum MK, Liberthson RR, Shah NR, Villines TC, O'Gara PT, Landzberg MJ, et al. Anomalous Aortic Origin of a Coronary Artery From the Inappropriate Sinus of Valsalva. J Am Coll Cardiol. 2017;69(12):1592–608.
40. Dodge-Khatami A, Mavroudis C, Backer CL. Congenital Heart Surgery Nomenclature and Database Project: anomalies of the coronary arteries. Ann Thorac Surg. 2000;69(4 Suppl):S270–97.
41. Michalowska IM, Hryniewiecki T, Kwiatek P, Stoklosa P, Swoboda-Rydz U, Szymanski P. Coronary Artery Variants and Anomalies in Patients With Bicuspid Aortic Valve. J Thorac Imaging. 2016;31(3):156–62.
42. Basso C, Maron BJ, Corrado D, Thiene G. Clinical profile of congenital coronary artery anomalies with origin from the wrong aortic sinus leading to sudden death in young competitive athletes. J Am Coll Cardiol. 2000;35(6):1493–501.
43. Eckart RE, Scoville SL, Campbell CL, Shry EA, Stajduhar KC, Potter RN, et al. Sudden death in young adults: a 25-year review of autopsies in military recruits. Ann Intern Med. 2004;141(11):829–34.
44. Page HL Jr, Engel HJ, Campbell WB, Thomas CS Jr. Anomalous origin of the left circumflex coronary artery. Recognition, angiographic demonstration and clinical significance. Circulation. 1974;50(4):768–73.
45. Chaitman BR, Lespérance J, Saltiel J, Bourassa MG. Clinical, angiographic, and hemodynamic findings in patients with anomalous origin of the coronary arteries. Circulation. 1976;53(1):122–31.
46. Basso C, Burke M, Fornes P, Gallagher PJ, De Gouveia RH, Sheppard M, et al. Guidelines for autopsy investigation of sudden cardiac death. Pathologica. 2010;102(5):391–404.

47. Desmet W, Vanhaecke J, Vrolix M, Van de Werf F, Piessens J, Willems J, et al. Isolated single coronary artery: a review of 50,000 consecutive coronary angiographies. Eur Heart J. 1992;13(12):1637–40.
48. Smith JC. Review of single coronary artery with report of 2 cases. Circulation. 1950;1(5):1168–75.
49. Musiani A, Cernigliaro C, Sansa M, Maselli D, De Gasperis C. Left main coronary artery atresia: literature review and therapeutical considerations. Eur J Cardiothorac Surg. 1997;11(3):505–14.
50. Angelini P, Trivellato M, Donis J, Leachman RD. Myocardial bridges: a review. Prog Cardiovasc Dis. 1983;26(1):75–88.
51. Basso C, Thiene G, Mackey-Bojack S, Frigo AC, Corrado D, Maron BJ. Myocardial bridging, a frequent component of the hypertrophic cardiomyopathy phenotype, lacks systematic association with sudden cardiac death. Eur Heart J. 2009;30(13):1627–34.
52. Möhlenkamp S, Hort W, Ge J, Erbel R. Update on myocardial bridging. Circulation. 2002;106(20):2616–22.
53. Lee MS, Chen CH. Myocardial Bridging: An Up-to-Date Review. J Invasive Cardiol. 2015;27(11):521–8.
54. Corban MT, Hung OY, Eshtehardi P, Rasoul-Arzrumly E, McDaniel M, Mekonnen G, et al. Myocardial bridging: contemporary understanding of pathophysiology with implications for diagnostic and therapeutic strategies. J Am Coll Cardiol. 2014;63(22):2346–55.
55. Kawsara A, Nunez Gil IJ, Alqahtani F, Moreland J, Rihal CS, Alkhouli M. Management of Coronary Artery Aneurysms. JACC Cardiovasc Interv. 2018;11(13):1211–23.
56. Seabra-Gomes R, Somerville J, Ross DN, Emanuel R, Parker DJ, Wong M. Congenital coronary artery aneurysms. Br Heart J. 1974;36(4):329–35.
57. Yun G, Nam TH, Chun EJ. Coronary Artery Fistulas: Pathophysiology, Imaging Findings, and Management. RSNA. 2018;38(3):688–703.
58. Mangukia CV. Coronary artery fistula. Ann Thorac Surg. 2012;93(6):2084–92.

Pathogenesis of Atherosclerosis: A Multifactorial Process

L. Maximilian Buja

Abbreviations

(hs)-cTn	High-sensitivity cardiac troponin
ACS	Acute coronary syndromes
AMI	Acute myocardial infarction
CAD	Coronary artery disease
CHIP	Clonal hematopoiesis of indeterminate potential
CHIP	Clonal hematopoiesis of indeterminate potential
CMV	Cytomegalovirus
CRP	C-reactive protein
cTn	Cardiac troponin
DAMP	Danger-associated molecular patterns
EDRF	Endothelium-derived relaxing factor
FH	Familiar hypercholesterolemia
ICAM-1	Intercellular adhesion molecule
IHD	Ischemic heart disease
IL-18	Interleukin-18
IL-1β	Interleukin-1β
LD	Linkage disequilibrium
LDL	Low-density lipoprotein

L. M. Buja (✉)
Department of Pathology and Laboratory Medicine, McGovern Medical School,
The University of Texas Health Science Center at Houston (UTHealth), Houston, TX, USA

Texas Heart Institute, Houston, TX, USA
e-mail: l.maximilian.buja@uth.tm.edu

G. Concistrè (ed.), *Ischemic Heart Disease*,
https://doi.org/10.1007/978-3-031-25879-4_2

MR	Mendelian randomization
NF-κB	Nuclear factor-kappa B
NO	Nitric oxide
PAMP	Pathogen-associated molecular patterns
PDGF	Platelet-derived growth factor
PRP	Pattern recognition receptors
TNF	Tissue necrosis factor
UDMI	Universal definition of myocardial infarction
VCAM-1	Vascular cell adhesion molecule 1
VSMC	Vascular smooth muscle cell

1 Introduction

Atherosclerosis is a vascular disease that is characterized by the presence of fibrofatty raised lesions (plaques) involving the aorta and its main distributing branches—the coronary arteries, the carotid and cerebral arteries, and the iliofemoral arteries [1]. During the twentieth century, the fundamental pathobiology was determined for atherosclerosis and CAD, also designated as IHD [2]. In essence, atherosclerosis results from an inflammatory and immunologically driven response of the arterial wall to multifactorial and repetitive injury [1, 2]. This understanding of the pathogenesis of atherosclerosis has come from a convergence of evidence from multiple lines of investigation including epidemiology, population-based pathology, vascular cell and molecular biology, and pathology of lesions in humans and experimental animals (Table 1) [2].

In the last 20 years, major research advances have provided important new insights with new opportunities for more effective therapy. This chapter builds on fundamental knowledge presented in previous reviews and provides a synthesis of new information regarding the pathobiology of atherosclerosis and CAD/IHD [3–9].

Table 1 Major lines of evidence for the response to injury theory of atherosclerosis[a]

Epidemiology
Risk factor analysis
Seven Countries Study
Framingham Study
Population-based pathology
Korean Conflict Casualties
International Atherosclerosis Project/Geographic Pathology of Atherosclerosis Study (GPAS)
Bogalusa Heart Study
Pathological Determinants of Atherosclerosis in Youth (PDAY)
Experimental animal studies
Diet-induced models
Genetic-based models

Table 1 (continued)

Pathology of atherosclerotic lesions
Cytology and ultrastructure of lesions
Morphometrics of aorta and coronary arteries
Unstable/vulnerable plaque
Updated classification of atherosclerotic lesions and relationship to clinical events
Vascular cell biology
Endothelial cells and smooth muscle cells
Adhesion molecules and cytokines
Angiogenesis
Pathogenesis
Response to injury theory
Role of hemodynamics
Roles of inflammation and innate and acquired immunity
Monoclonal construct

[a]Lines of evidence discussed in Buja LM. Innovators in atherosclerosis research: A historical review. Int J Cardiol. 2020 May 15;307:8–14. https://doi.org/10.1016/j.ijcard.2020.02.016

2 Epidemiology, Natural History, and Risk Factors

Atherosclerosis and its complications constitute the leading cause of disability and death worldwide. There is a dichotomy between a decrease in atherosclerotic disease prevalence in the United States and other developed countries due to advances in prevention and treatment and increase in the prevalence of atherosclerosis-related diseases in developing countries in recent decades [10, 11].

The natural history of atherosclerosis involves a long clinically silent phase followed by the onset, often sudden, of symptomatic disease [1, 2] (Fig. 1). The clinical complications of atherosclerosis result from progressive growth of plaques and secondary changes in the plaques. Progression of atherosclerosis can lead to luminal stenosis, thrombosis, embolization, aneurysm formation, and vessel rupture. The resultant clinical manifestations include CAD/IHD, stroke, and peripheral vascular disease. Since progression of atherosclerosis increases over time, age is a significant risk factor for clinical expression of disease. Progression of atherosclerosis is also influenced by specific genetic defects, such as familial hypercholesterolemia, as well as more heterogeneous genetic factors which contribute to a positive family history of disease [12–18]. A large body of experimental, clinical, and epidemiological work has firmly established hypercholesterolemia and other forms of hyperlipidemia as the dominant risk factor in the development of atherosclerotic disease [12–19]. Epidemiological studies have also established that the four major risk-treatable factors for disease are hyperlipidemia, hypertension, cigarette smoking, and diabetes mellitus [1, 2, 19].

The metabolic syndrome is a clustering of hyperglycemia/insulin resistance, obesity, and dyslipidemia. It identifies patients who are at high risk of developing atherosclerotic cardiovascular disease and type 2 diabetes mellitus [20]. Obesity predisposes to the development of other components of the metabolic syndrome. However, a paradoxical inverse

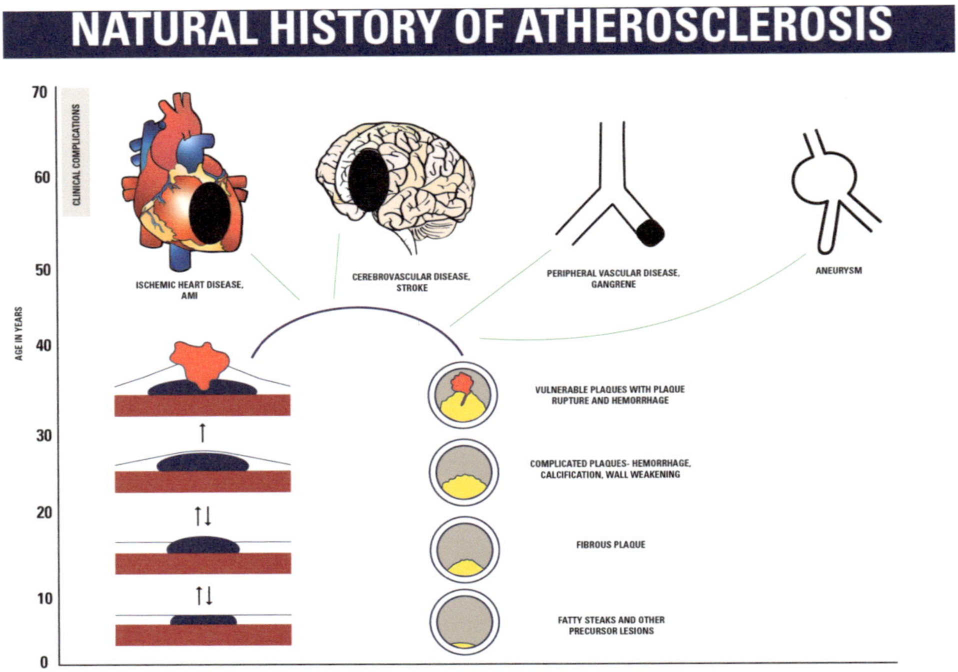

Fig. 1 Schematic depiction of the natural history of human atherosclerosis and atherosclerosis lesions based on population-based pathology studies with supportive evidence from epidemiological studies and experimental studies and with incorporation of the potential for regression of established atherosclerotic lesions and the potential for development of unstable/vulnerable plaques with associated thrombosis. Reproduced with permission from reference 2: Buja LM. Innovators in atherosclerosis research: A historical review. Int J Cardiol. 2020 May 15;307:8–14. https://doi.org/10.1016/j.ijcard.2020.02.016

correlation has been observed between body mass index and atherosclerosis of the aorta [21, 22].

Contemporary epidemiological and basic studies have focused attention on "nontraditional" risk factors, including CRP and other markers of inflammation, altered coagulation factors, increased blood level of homocysteine, and exposure to infectious organisms, particularly herpesviruses and Chlamydia [23]. These studies indicate that progression of atherosclerosis can be influenced by a broad array of metabolic, immunological, and inflammatory factors.

3 Vascular Lesions

Arteries consist of an adventitia of connective tissue, a muscular media containing smooth muscle cells, and an intima lined by endothelium [24]. The aorta is designated as an elastic artery based on the presence of numerous longitudinal elastic fibers as well as smooth muscle cells in the media, whereas the major aortic distributing vessels are designated as muscular arteries based on the media containing abundant smooth muscle cells without elastic fibers [24].

Diffuse intimal thickening occurs in both the aorta and the distributing arteries over time due to accumulation of smooth muscle cells and connective tissue matrix in the intima [25]. Early vascular lesions consist of focal alterations within the diffusely thickened intima [4, 25–27]. Gray gelatinous lesions are focal areas of excess fluid accumulation in the intima. Fatty streaks are foci of lipid accumulation within the intima. The lipid usually has a predominantly intracellular localization but may be partially or exclusively extracellular. The lipid-containing foam cells are macrophages derived from blood monocytes and smooth muscle cells derived from the vessel wall. Microthrombi, composed of platelets and fibrin, constitute another type of focal lesion along with gray gelatinous lesions and fatty streaks. There is a general similarity in the distribution of pre-atherosclerotic lesions and lesions in the initial stages of atherosclerosis with localization in and around branch points of the aorta and distributing branch arteries (Fig. 2).

The lesions of established atherosclerosis are atherosclerotic or fibrous plaques (Fig. 3). These are raised intimal lesions composed of variable combinations of lipid, cells, and connective tissue matrix, as characterized by light and electron microscopic study [25–27]. Further detail of the cellular pathology of atherosclerotic lesions has been provided by light and electron microscopic analysis of vascular lesions from subjects with homozygous familial hypercholesterolemia and the Watanabe heritable hyperlipidemic (WHHL) rabbit model (Fig. 4) [28–30]. The lipid composition of lesions has also been determined [31, 32].

The classical atherosclerotic lesion (plaque) was originally termed an atheroma and more recently has been designated as a fibroinflammatory lipid plaque [4]. However, atherosclerotic plaques exhibit heterogeneity in the proportions of fibrous and lipid components. The spectrum of established atherosclerotic lesions consists of pathological intimal

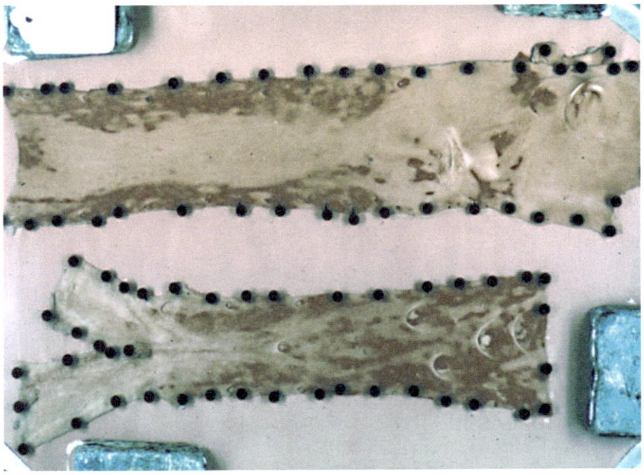

Fig. 2 Distribution of early atherosclerosis. Aorta of young accident victim stained with oil red O for demonstration of lipid deposition. Note the lipid deposition in atherosclerosis-prone areas adjacent to the ostia of the aortic arch branches and the intercostal arteries in the descending thoracic aorta and the more extensive deposition in the abdominal aorta

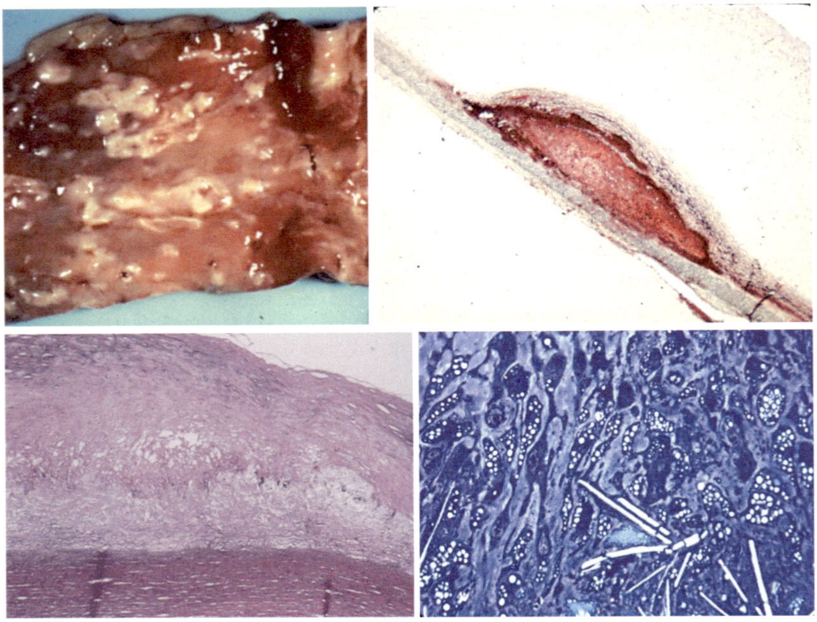

Fig. 3 Gross and histological features of an atherosclerotic plaque. Top left: Atherosclerotic plaques are yellow raised lesions. Top right: Low-magnification photomicrograph of section stained with oil red O demonstrates the lipid-rich core and fibrous cap of the plaque. Bottom left: Medium-magnification photomicrograph of histological section (hematoxylin and eosin stain) shows fibrous cap and lipid core at the edge of the plaque. Bottom right: High-magnification photomicrograph of thin section (toluidine blue stain) showing foam cells containing cholesterol ester-rich lipid droplets and enclosing free cholesterol crystals

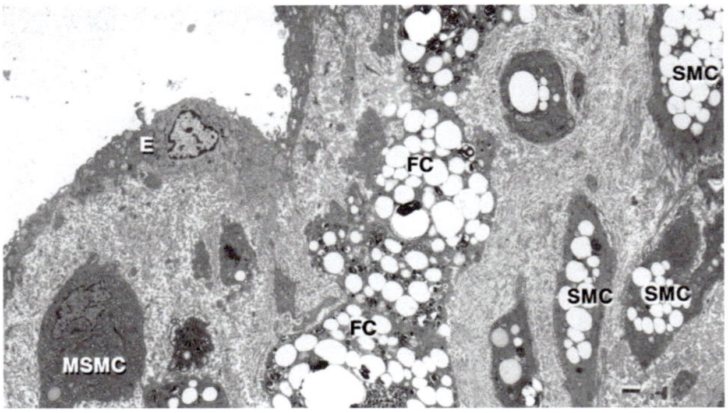

Fig. 4 Electron micrograph of an advanced intimal lesion from a 6-month-old WHHL rabbit. The lesion is lined by endothelium (E). The lesion contains numerous smooth muscle cells (SMCs) with lipid deposits, a modified smooth muscle cell (MSMC), and lipid-laden foam cells. Bar = 1 micrometer. Reproduced at the discretion of the author (https://www.ahajournals.org/permissions-rights) from reference 28: Buja LM, Kita T, Goldstein JL, Watanabe Y, Brown MS. Cellular pathology of progressive atherosclerosis in the WHHL rabbit. An animal model of familial hypercholesterolemia. Arteriosclerosis. 1983 Jan-Feb;3(1):87–101. https://doi.org/10.1161/01.atv.3.1.87

thickening, fibroatheroma, complicated fibroatheroma, and thin-cap fibroatheroma based on the lack or presence of a central lipid core and the thickness of the fibrous cap (Table 2) [33, 34]. So-called hard plaques are composed predominantly of fibrous tissue, soft plaques, or atheromas and have a core of necrotic, lipid-rich material covered by a fibrous cap. The central core contains necrotic debris, is rich in extracellular lipid, and often is vascularized by an ingrowth of vessels from the vasa vasorum. The fibrous cap of atheromatous plaques is completely or partially lined by endothelium and is composed of smooth muscle cells, collagen fibers, glycosaminoglycans, and a few elastic fibers. Peripheral and deep portions of the lesions are composed of similar tissue. Lipid-laden foam cells of macrophage and smooth muscle origin are present in the connective tissue matrix, especially adjacent to the central core. The lesions also contain T lymphocytes and macrophages derived from blood monocytes. The term complicated plaque is a histo-

Table 2 Contemporary classification of arterial lesions related to atherosclerosis[a]

Non-atherosclerotic intimal lesions	
Diffuse intimal thickening	Age-related accumulation of smooth muscle cells (SMCs) in the absence of extracellular lipid, macrophage foam cells, and thrombosis
Intimal fatty streak/xanthoma	Focal intimal accumulation of foam cells without necrosis or fibrosis; potential for regression
Progressive atherosclerotic lesions	
Pathological intimal thickening	Plaque rich in SMCs in a matrix rich in glycosaminoglycans; focal (PIT) accumulation of extracellular lipid; no necrosis
Fibroatheroma	Characteristic lesion of established atherosclerosis; lipid-rich necrotic core and overlying fibrous cap; foam cells derived from SMCs and macrophages and matrix produced by SMC; with or without calcification
Complicated fibroatheroma	Intraplaque hemorrhage or plaque fissure
Thin-cap fibroatheroma (TCFA)	Thin fibrous cap (<65 μm) infiltrated by macrophages and lymphocytes
Lesions with acute thrombi	
Ruptured plaque	TCFA with cap disruption. Thrombosis is present, can be mural or occlusive. Luminal thrombus communicates with the underlying necrotic core
Eroded plaque	Focal loss of endothelium and subendothelial disruption of a plaque. Can also occur on pathological intimal thickening. Thrombus is present, can be mural or occlusive. No communication of thrombus with underlying necrotic core
Calcified nodule	Nodule of calcium with an underlying fibrocalcific plaque with minimal or no necrosis. Thrombus is usually not occlusive
Healed lesions	Healed plaque rupture, plaque with superficial layer with features of organized thrombus
	Erosion or calcified nodule and/or new growth of fibrocellular tissue

[a]Based on the American Heart Association Classification modified by Virmani and colleagues [33, 34]

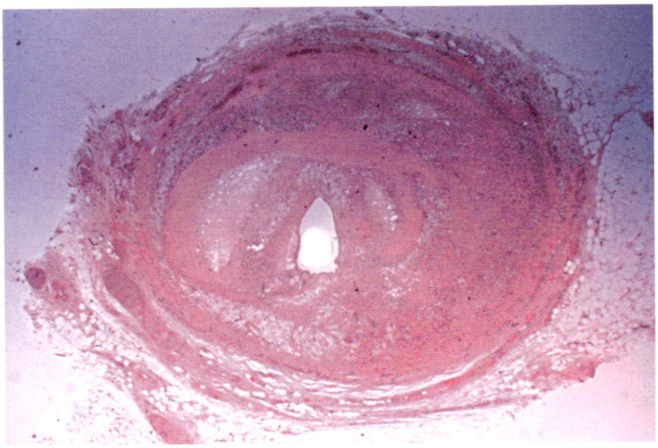

Fig. 5 Photomicrograph of cross section of the left main coronary artery from the explanted heart of a 6-year-old girl with homozygous familial hypercholesterolemia who underwent liver and heart transplantation. Reproduced with permission from reference 30: Buja LM, Clubb FJ Jr., Bilheimer DW, Willerson JT. Pathobiology of human familial hypercholesterolaemia and a related animal model, the Watanabe heritable hyperlipidaemic rabbit. Eur Heart J. 1990 Aug;11 Suppl E:41–52. https://doi.org/10.1093/eurheartj/11.suppl_e.41

pathological designation to describe advanced fibroinflammatory lipid plaque development with secondary changes, including intraplaque hemorrhage and plaque fissure, often associated with clinical disease. Advanced atherosclerotic plaques are associated with medial degeneration and weakening as well as adventitial fibrosis with lymphocytic infiltrates. Thus, advanced atherosclerosis lesions involve all three layers of the vessel wall (Fig. 5).

Detailed characterization of the cellular and chemical composition of vascular lesions has provided the basis for understanding the processes involved in formation and interrelationships of these lesions [35–38]. The early vascular lesions do not produce significant focal thickening, lack necrosis, and are reversible. In contrast, plaques produce focal intimal thickening, usually have necrotic cores, and are less easily reversible. In a population with prevalent risk factors, early lesions progress to intermediate fibrofatty lesions and then into atherosclerotic plaques [1, 2]. For both fatty streaks and atherosclerotic plaques, the intracellular lipid in foam cells consists of cholesterol esters, and the extracellular lipid is composed of free cholesterol, phospholipid, and intact lipoprotein. Both the intracellular and extracellular lipids are derived from plasma LDL, which undergoes modification and metabolism in the evolving lesions [36–40].

In the coronary arterial system, atheromatous lesions associated with coronary thrombosis are unstable or vulnerable plaques [41–43]. Most of these vulnerable plaques are thin-cap fibroatheromas, which are subject to plaque fissuring and rupture. Others are thick-cap fibroatheromas, which are subject to endothelial erosion and thrombosis (Table 2).

4 Response to Injury Theory

Atherogenesis involves complex interactions between the vessel wall and soluble and formed elements of the blood [1–4]. All three layers of the arterial wall, i.e., the adventitia, media, and intima, participate in the formation of lesions in the intima. Important factors in the initiation and growth of plaques in the intima are (1) endothelial injury and dysfunction; (2) monocyte/macrophage accumulation; (3) influx of T lymphocytes; (4) platelet aggregation and attachment; (5) VSMC migration from the media and phenotypic modulation, plasticity, and proliferation in the intima; (6) influx of plasma LDL; (7) oxidation of LDL; (8) progressive lipid accumulation in foam cells from uptake of oxidatively modified LDL and free cholesterol; (9) apoptotic death of foam cells; (10) extracellular lipid deposition; (11) modulation by the adventitia; and (12) modulation by hemodynamic influences related to blood pressure and pattern of blood flow.

The response to injury theory of atherogenesis is based on multiple lines of evidence and incorporates and expands on earlier theories (Table 1) [44–48]. The theory recognizes that atherogenesis is intrinsically linked to inflammation and activation of innate and acquired immune systems [49, 50] (Fig. 6). The theory also recognizes that atherosclerosis is a dynamic process with potential for both progression and stabilization, or even regression, when risk factors are aggressively managed [51–53].

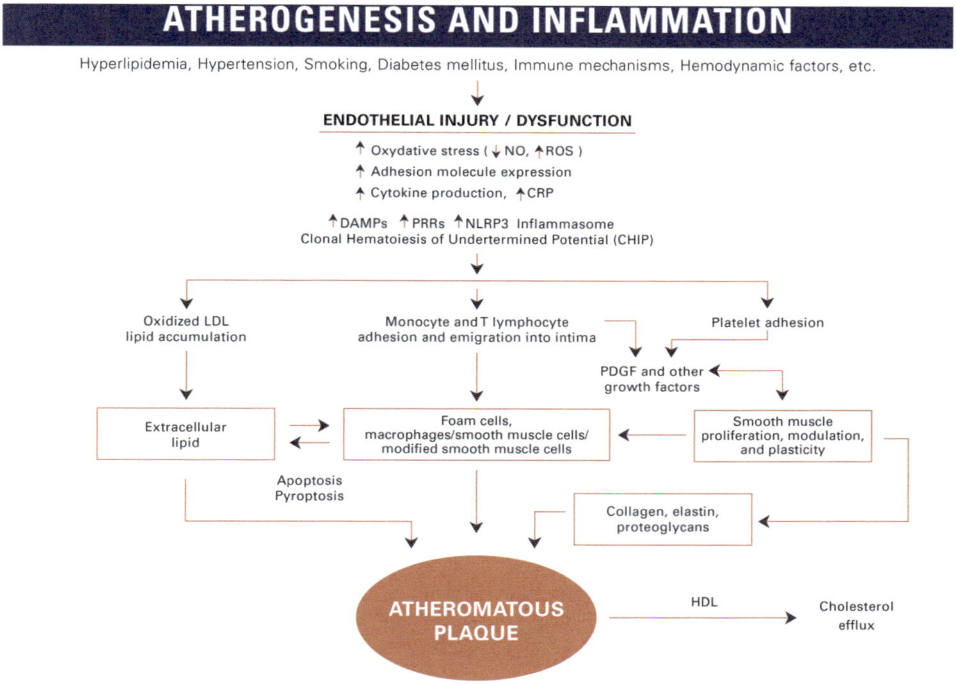

Fig. 6 Atherogenesis and inflammation. Mechanisms of atherogenesis mediated by inflammation

5 Role of Endothelium

Vascular integrity is critically dependent on the maintenance of homeostasis of the endothelium [54, 55]. The endothelium is a major source of humoral mediators, including antithrombotic as well as prothrombotic factors, cytokines, growth factors, and vasodilatory factors, including prostacyclin and EDRF, i.e., NO, as well as vasoconstrictors, including endothelin [3, 4, 35]. Normal endothelium is in a mode favoring vasodilation, antithrombosis, and fibrinolysis. Conversely, endothelial injury can shift the balance toward vasoconstriction and thrombosis. At the foci of endothelial injury, the thrombotic process is initiated by platelet aggregation with secondary activation of the coagulation cascade. Complex interactions between the endothelium, platelets, and coagulation factors then follow, including further platelet aggregation by activation of thrombin receptors.

Endothelial function is mediated through gene expression [3, 4, 35, 54, 55]. Activation of the transcription factor, NF-κB, is a key event in the subsequent activation of physiologically important genes and gene products, including those that regulate the interactions of endothelial cells and leukocytes. NO production is an important regulator of NF-κB activation. NO can inhibit the expression of adhesion molecules on the endothelial cell surface.

Early endothelial injury involves modulation of endothelial cell function without loss of cells. Chronic repetitive endothelial injury is important in lesion initiation and progression, with the endothelium participating in the activation of an inflammatory cascade that is instrumental in the process. Injurious factors can include hypertension; high circulating levels of LDL, lipoprotein (a), and other atherogenic lipids; components of cigarette smoke; high levels of homocysteine; immunologic mechanisms; and injury induced by herpesviruses and Chlamydia [23].

Endothelial dysfunction is related to oxidative stress with an excess production of reactive oxygen species and a decrease in NO [3, 4, 35, 54, 55]. An important early event in lesion development is the adhesion of blood monocytes and platelets to the endothelial surface and the entry of monocytes into the intima. Leukocyte recruitment involves the contributions of both adhesion and signaling molecules expressed on the surfaces of both the leukocytes and endothelial cells. Receptors called selectins mediate the transient adhesion of leukocytes to regionally activated endothelium. This is followed by activation of the loosely adherent leukocytes, with subsequent upregulation of other molecules known as integrins, which increase adhesion and mediate emigration.

6 Role of Smooth Muscle Cells

SMC involvement in the development of intimal lesions is another major component of the response to injury theory [44–48]. Heterogeneity of SMC in different vascular beds has been shown along with supportive evidence for the occurrence of SMC clones [56, 57]. SMCs migrate into the intima in response to molecular signals released by activated endothelial cells, leukocytes, and platelets. Simultaneously, SMCs undergo phenotypic modulation changing from contractile to synthetic phenotype. SMCs then proliferate in the growing atherosclerotic plaque. SMCs also exhibit plasticity and express markers for other cell types, including macrophages and fibroblasts, driven by cholesterol uptake triggering the unfolded protein response [58–62]. Recent studies utilizing lineage tracing analysis indicate that SMCs represent the major cell type of plaques. SMCs produce the collagen and matrix components of the plaque.

7 Role of the Adventitia

The adventitia, the outer layer of the blood vessel wall, has been found to be a dynamic microenvironment in which adventitial and perivascular adipose tissue cells initiate and regulate important vascular functions in disease, especially intimal hyperplasia and atherosclerosis [63, 64]. The adventitia has a profound influence on the population and function of intimal and medial endothelial, macrophage, and smooth muscle cells. Vascular injury and dysfunction of the perivascular adipose tissue promote expansion of the vasa vasorum, activation of fibroblasts, and differentiation of myofibroblasts. This regulates further biologic processes, including fibroblast and myofibroblast migration and proliferation, inflammation, immunity, stem cell activation and regulation, extracellular matrix remodeling, and angiogenesis. Ongoing work is aimed at determining as to whether the adventitia initiates disease or is just an important participant in atherogenesis.

8 Role of Hemodynamics

Initially, atherosclerosis is a focal disease. There is a predilection for the formation of atherosclerotic plaques adjacent to branch points in areas of low-velocity flow and low shear stress adjacent to areas of high shear stress [65–67]. Activation of leukocytes and platelets likely occurs in zones of high shear and turbulent flow, and the activated cells are primed to interact with endothelium in zones of low shear and flow.

Biomechanical forces generated by blood flow also act as important modulators of regional endothelial gene expression, phenotype, and function. Induction of the transcription factors KLF2 and Nrf2 by atheroprotective flow orchestrates a multifunctional genetic program, the net effects of which contribute to the maintenance of endothelial vasoprotective phenotypes. Statins, and potentially other yet-to-be-defined agents, through their induction of KLF2 can function as pharmacomimetics of atheroprotective flow [54, 55].

9 Plaque Growth

The growth of atherosclerotic plaques involves continued accumulation of macrophages and lymphocytes, proliferation of smooth muscle cells, and accumulation of lipid in the intima. Cytokines and growth factors mediate smooth muscle proliferation by paracrine and autocrine pathways. A key factor in local cellular lipid accumulation is the local formation of oxidized LDL and other forms of altered LDL [35–38, 48]. This altered LDL can be taken up progressively via the scavenger receptor pathway into vascular cells, leading to the formation of foam cells filled with numerous droplets of esterified cholesterol [39, 40]. This pathway is not subject to feedback inhibition as is the LDL pathway [39, 40].

Plaques develop a considerable content of collagen, glycosaminoglycans, and some elastin. These matrix components are synthesized by smooth muscle cells [1–4, 44–47]. Repetitive endothelial injury, including patchy endothelial denudation, is important in the growth of plaques. This, in turn, leads to platelet aggregation and attachment with release of PDGF and other platelet products and further smooth muscle proliferation [1–4].

Progressive intimal thickening leads to the development of hypoxia in the depths of the plaque in and around the intimal-medial junction [1–4]. Excess oxidative stress, products of the inflammatory process, and hypoxia likely serve as important initiating factors for apoptosis and necrosis of foam cells and release of their lipids. Local influence of vascular growth factors is also likely involved in the vascularization of plaques by the ingrowth of vessels from the vasa vasorum. Dystrophic calcification of the necrotic lipid frequently occurs. The vessels in the cores of the plaques are a source of petechial hemorrhages and leakage of plasma. These blood components contribute to lipid accumulation in the plaques.

10 Atherosclerosis as an Inflammatory Disease

Inflammation associated with the activation of innate and acquired immune mechanisms is intrinsic to the pathogenesis and clinical expression of atherosclerosis [48–50] (Fig. 6). Atherogenesis is linked to key features of the cellular and molecular biology of inflammation [68, 69]. Cellular responses in inflammation are mediated by the formation of inflammasomes, which are cytoplasmic multiprotein complexes that form in response to signals from damaged cells. Inflammasomes are multimeric protein complexes that typically comprise a sensor, an adaptor, and the zymogen procaspase-1 [70–73]. An inflammasome assembles in response to a diverse range of PAMPs and DAMPs. The DAMPs and PAMPs exert their effects by binding to PRPs, including toll-like receptors. The inflammasome platform leads to the activation of caspase-1 through proximity-induced self-cleavage, which further induces maturation of IL-1β and IL-18 through proteolytic cleavage of pro-IL-1β and pro-IL-18. Activated caspase-1 also cleaves gasdermin D, which leads to a particular form of cell death called pyroptosis.

NLRP3 inflammasomes trigger vascular wall inflammatory responses that lead to the progression of atherosclerosis [70–73]. NLRP3 inflammasomes have a specific activation pathway that involves numerous stimuli, including a wide range of DAMPs. NLRP3 inflammasomes are activated by various danger signals, such as cholesterol crystals, calcium phosphate crystals, and oxidized low-density lipoprotein in macrophages, to initiate inflammatory responses in the atherosclerotic lesion. NLRP3 inflammasomes regulate caspase-1 activation and subsequent processing of pro-IL-1β, trigger vascular wall inflammatory responses, and lead to progression of atherosclerosis [70–73]. Recent studies have further clarified the regulatory mechanisms and the potential therapeutic agents that target NLRP3 inflammasomes.

Altered endothelial cells in lesion-prone areas express a selective profile of adhesion molecules that lead to the recruitment, attachment, and transmigration of circulating platelets, monocytes, and T lymphocytes, but not neutrophils, and the transmigration of leukocytes into the vessel wall [1–4, 35]. The local environment within the intima leads to the transformation of leukocytes into activated macrophages and T lymphocytes and promotes the chemical signaling between the two cell types. Cytokines produced by the macrophages create a pro-inflammatory environment that facilitates the recruitment of more inflammatory cells. The production of other mediators, including PDGF-like molecules, leads to the recruitment and proliferation of vascular smooth muscle cells in the lesions.

Production of superoxide anion and other reactive oxygen species leads to oxidation of LDL [35–40]. Native LDL uptake into cells is mediated by LDL receptors, which initiate a regulated metabolic pathway with feedback inhibition of further LDL uptake. However, oxidized LDL uptake into cells is mediated by scavenger receptors, which initiate an unregulated pathway of continued uptake of oxidized LDL. The unregulated uptake of oxidized LDL by modified smooth muscle cells and macrophages via their scavenger receptors leads to the formation of foam cells. As the plaques grow, foam cells undergo cell death, and a central core of necrotic debris and extracellular lipid develops. Apoptosis of plaque cells contributes significantly to the development of the necrotic plaque core. Apoptosis can be mediated by TNF and other inflammatory mediators. Smooth muscle cells lay down the connective tissue matrix comprising the fibrous capsule of the plaque. The adventitia has a significant role in mediating and modulating these phenomena.

Macrophages produce collagenases and metalloproteinases that are important in the turnover of the connective tissue matrix. An excess of the degradative enzymes leads to degradation and thinning of the fibrous capsule [1–4, 33, 34]. Plaques prone to rupture and ruptured plaques exhibit an inflammatory profile characterized by prominent numbers of macrophages and lymphocytes adjacent to the plaque capsule, increased expression of inflammatory mediators, increased local concentration of metalloproteinases, and prominent apoptosis of plaque cells. Somatic mutations in myeloid precursors, termed CHIP, can lead to activation of pro-inflammatory pathways by selective expansion of inflammatory monocyte-macrophage lineages producing mediators such as IL-1 [74, 75].

11 Atherosclerosis and Coronary Artery Disease

Atherosclerosis is the substrate for the development of CAD also designated as IHD. Coronary atherosclerosis is the primary substrate for the development of ACS [76, 77]. Two key processes are basic mechanisms for the growth of advanced atherosclerotic plaques in the coronary arteries and other vascular beds: (1) positive remodeling with outward abluminal expansion of the arterial wall (the Glagov phenomenon) [78] and (2) subclinical plaque rupture of hemodynamically insignificant lesions, with incorporation of the mural thrombus into the lesion [79, 80]. Subsequently, a new plaque disruption can lead to occlusive thrombosis and sudden cardiac death or acute myocardial infarction. These thrombosis-prone lesions are vulnerable plaques. Most of these vulnerable plaques are thin-cap fibroatheromas, which are subject to plaque fissuring and rupture. Others are thick-cap fibroatheromas, which are subject to endothelial erosion and thrombosis (Table 2). The severity of CAD is best determined clinically by quantitative coronary arteriography and measurement of fractional flow reserve across coronary lesions [81].

The UDMI is a comprehensive system for the evaluation and classification of patients with cardiovascular symptomatology [77, 82, 83]. Based on biomarker analysis, specifically detection of myocardial injury is done by elevated serum cTn, with preference for (hs)-cTn. Clinicopathological studies have confirmed the pathological correlates of the UDMI classification of five types of AMI.

12 Genetics of Atherosclerosis and Coronary Artery Disease

A major advance in the twenty-first century has been the application of contemporary genetics (next-generation sequencing and whole-genome analysis) to determine the interaction of genetic determinants with environmental factors in cardiovascular risk (Table 3) [7, 15–18]. Single-gene mutations lead to premature CAD in some patients. FH is an autosomal dominant form of elevated cholesterol and premature CAD [12–14, 30]. A 5 kb deletion in *LDLR*, which encodes the low-density lipoprotein receptor, leads to impaired receptor-mediated hepatic LDL uptake, elevated levels of circulating cholesterol, and premature CAD [84]. Family-based studies subsequently identified mutations in *APOB*, which encodes apolipoprotein B, and gain-of-function mutations in *PCSK9*, which encodes proprotein convertase subtilisin/kexin type 9, which are additional causal genes for FH [85, 86]. Mutations in *APOB* prevent the binding of LDL particles to LDLRs for uptake. Gain-of-function mutations in *PCSK9* promote LDLR catabolism. In addition, autosomal recessive form of hypercholesterolemia has been linked to null mutations in *LDLRAP1*, which encodes the LDLR adaptor protein 1, and genes, encoding the ATP-binding cassette subfamily G member, *ABCG5* and *ABCG8* [87, 88].

In addition to rare monogenic forms, CAD has long been noted to cluster in families as a complex trait. In the Framingham Offspring Study, family history of premature CAD increases age-specific CAD incidence by >2-fold [89]. The Swedish Twin Registry, that followed 21,000 subjects for >35 years, estimated the heritability of fatal CAD to be approximately 40–60%, with heritability playing a greater role in males and younger individuals [90]. These seminal studies provide not only evidence that CAD is a complex trait but also the impetus for using genetic approaches to uncover novel biology of CAD. Recent technological advances, such as high-throughput whole-genome array, have enabled large-scale genome-wide association studies that has further propelled the understanding of the genetic architecture of CAD. The first CAD genomic locus identified by GWAS is a 53 kb

Table 3 Gene mutations impacting coronary artery disease (CAD)[a]

Gene	Carrier frequency	Intermediate phenotype	CAD risk
Inactivating mutations conferring increased risk			
LDLR	1 in 221 (0.5%)	Increased LDL cholesterol	320% Increase
LPL	1 in 249 (0.4%)	Increased triglyceride-rich lipoproteins	84% Increase
APOA5	1 in 216 (0.5%)	Increased triglyceride-rich lipoproteins	120% Increase
Inactivating mutations conferring decreased risk[b]			
PCSK9	1 in 50 (2%)[c]	Decreased LDL cholesterol	88% Decrease
NPC1L	1 in 650 (0.2%)	Decreased LDL cholesterol	53% Decrease
ASGR1	1 in 120 (0.8%)	Decreased LDL cholesterol Decreased triglyceride-rich lipoproteins	34% Decrease
APOC3	1 in 150 (0.7%)	Decreased triglyceride-rich lipoproteins	40% Decrease
ANGPTL4	1 in 360% (0.3%)	Decreased triglyceride-rich lipoproteins	53% Decrease
LPA	1 in 285 (0.4%)	Decreased lipoprotein(a)	24% Decrease

Abbreviations: ANGPTL4, angiopoietin-like 4; APO, apolipoprotein; ASGR1, asialoglycoprotein receptor; CAD, coronary artery disease; EMA, European Medicines Agency; FDA, US Food and Drug Administration; LDLR, low-density lipoprotein receptor; LPA, lipoprotein (a); LPL, lipoprotein lipase; NPC1L1, Niemann–Pick C1-like intracellular cholesterol transporter 1; PCSK9, proprotein convertase subtilisin/kexin type 9

[a] Damaging mutations in at least nine genes have been robustly associated with the risk of coronary artery disease; in each case, identified genes disrupt pathways related to low-density lipoprotein (LDL) cholesterol, triglyceride-rich lipoproteins, or lipoprotein (a) metabolism. Data summarized in Khera AV, Kathiresan S. Genetics of coronary artery disease: discovery, biology and clinical translation. Nat Rev. Genet. 2017 Jun;18(6):331–344. https://doi.org/10.1038/nrg.2016.160

[b] Pharmacological therapies are in current use or development to mimic the protective variants for five of the six genes in which inhibition of the related protein would be predicted to reduce risk

[c] Prevalence estimate for PCSK9 mutation based on individuals of African ancestry. Carrier frequency substantially lower in other racial and ethnic groups

LD block at the chromosome 9q21.3 locus among Europeans [91–93]. At an allele frequency of 0.48, the risk allele confers a 30% increase in CAD risk. Since the discovery of the 9p21 locus, progressively larger sample sizes have led to the identification of additional loci of smaller effect size with genome-wide significance (p-value $<5 \times 10^{-8}$). GWAS meta-analysis has further increased the number of distinct genetic loci associated with CAD at genome-wide significance to greater than 160 [7, 15–18]. These include genes with known function in lipoprotein metabolism, hypertension, and other CAD-associated phenotypes. Genomic loci located outside of protein-coding regions or harboring genes of no known relevance to atherosclerosis and plaque rupture have also been identified. Less than 25% of the significant loci are related to known CAD risk factors, highlighting the importance of novel factors contributing to CAD [7, 15–18]. While the majority of GWAS for CAD have been performed in Europeans, many of the GWAS loci have been replicated in East and South Asians. In contrast, most of the CAD loci have failed to replicate in black populations, as a result of differences in haplotype structure and greater genetic diversity among Africans. Future GWAS targeting different populations may lead to the identification of additional genomic loci or biological pathways for CAD.

Approaches in genetics can be utilized to prioritize drug targets by providing confidence that the drug target is causal in the pathophysiology of CAD. MR is based on the principle that if a biomarker has a causal association with disease, the genetic determinants of the biomarker will associate with disease risk. Using this approach, biomarkers, such as lipoprotein (a), LDL-C, and triglycerides, were shown to have a causal association with CAD and therefore drug targets [7, 15–18, 94, 95].

13 Atherosclerosis and CAD/ICD: From Theory to Clinical Practice

The inflammatory nature of atherosclerosis is manifest by the correlation of increased blood levels of inflammatory markers, especially high-sensitivity CRP and subsequent development of atherosclerotic disease [23]. CRP is known to be an acute-phase reactant produced by the liver in inflammatory states. It is not certain whether the inflammation in the vessel wall leads to systemic CRP elevation or whether both the CRP elevation and the vessel wall inflammation are in response to various initiators of the atherosclerotic process. Nevertheless, CRP is now known to be a mediator as well as a marker of vessel wall inflammation. In response to stimulation by inflammatory cytokines, especially interleukin-1 beta and interleukin-6, human coronary artery smooth muscle cells produce CRP. In turn, CRP can induce human endothelial cells to express VCAM-1, ICAM-1, and E-selectin. These molecules are important in the adhesion and recruitment of leukocytes into the vascular wall. The clinically beneficial effects of the HMG-CoA reductase inhibitors, the statins, are mediated by their pleiotropic effects as suppressors of inflammation in addition to their lipid-lowering properties [19, 23].

Infectious agents have been postulated as the cause of vascular inflammation leading to atherosclerosis [23]. Particular attention has been directed to CMV in the Herpesviridae family and *Chlamydia pneumoniae*. The infection theory is based on the identification of the organisms or components of organisms at high frequency in atherosclerotic lesions and serologic evidence of an association between high titers of antibodies to the organism and atherosclerotic disease. However, clinical trials with antibiotics have not reduced recurrent cardiovascular events, nor have vaccination strategies yet achieved clinical translation. While these clinical trials provide strong evidence against a primary role for microorganisms in the pathogenesis of atherosclerosis, it is possible that infectious processes and products of the endogenous microbiome might modulate atherosclerosis and its complications either directly or indirectly by eliciting local and systemic responses that potentiate disease expression.

Important confirmatory evidence for the role of inflammation in atherogenesis has come from the CANTOS clinical trial [75]. Results of this clinical trial showed significant reduction in clinical cardiovascular events in patients treated with the interleukin1β inhibitor, canakinumab. Other clinical trials have shown positive results from therapy with the anti-inflammatory agent, colchicine. These results represent a major outcome from the symbiosis of translational research and clinical trials confirming the importance of inflammation in atherogenesis in man and leading to new avenues for prevention and treatment of atherosclerotic diseases.

Mutations in genes that encode inflammasome components are associated with many inflammatory disorders, and studies in the past decade have highlighted the importance of appropriate activation of the inflammasome in homeostasis and disease pathogenesis. Therefore, much attention is being paid to uncover the modulators of inflammasome activation. The combination of CANTOS with the recent colchicine trials firmly establishes inflammation in atherosclerosis as both a theory and a clinical reality. Ongoing research is exploring modulation of other cytokines other than IL-1 as therapeutics for atherothrombosis.

Recently, a link has been discovered between clonal hematopoiesis and increased cardiovascular risk [74, 75]. The expansion of myeloid cell clones in geriatric bone marrow (so-called clonal hematopoiesis of indeterminate potential or CHIP) has been correlated not only with an increased risk of hematologic malignancy but also with atherosclerotic disease risk. This discovery provides a new and previously unsuspected link between systemic inflammation and aggravation of atherosclerosis. The observation shows that individuals with CHIP have elevated cardiovascular risk that appears to result at least in part from activation of pro-inflammatory pathways. The relationship may be mediated by the selective expansion in inflammatory monocyte-macrophage lineages producing mediators such as IL-1. This provides another opportunity for therapy.

14 Summary

Atherosclerosis is an inflammatory response of the vessel wall to chronic injury related to multiple risk factors, including aging, hyperlipidemia, hypertension, cigarette smoking, and diabetes mellitus. An inflammatory cascade involves endothelial cell dysfunction, increased oxidative stress, production of inflammatory cytokines, expression of adhesion molecules, and accumulation of oxidized low-density lipoprotein. Atherosclerotic plaques form as a result of endothelial damage, proliferation of modified smooth muscle cells, influx of monocytes and T lymphocytes, unregulated lipid uptake, foam cell formation, and connective tissue deposition. Inflammation is also important in the erosion or rupture of vulnerable plaques leading to clinical complications of atherosclerosis. Genetic studies are uncovering multiple gene loci with the potential for targeted therapy.

References

1. Libby P, Buring JE, Badimon L, Hansson GK, Deanfield J, Bittencourt MS, Tokgözoğlu L, Lewis EF. Atherosclerosis Nat Rev Dis Primers. 2019 Aug 16;5(1):56. https://doi.org/10.1038/s41572-019-0106-z.

2. Buja LM. Innovators in atherosclerosis research: A historical review. Int J Cardiol. 2020 May;15(307):8–14. https://doi.org/10.1016/j.ijcard.2020.02.016.
3. Buja LM, McAllister HA Jr. Atherosclerosis: pathological anatomy and pathogenesis. In: Willerson JT, Cohn JN, Wellens HJJ, Homes Jr DR, editors. Cardiovascular Medicine, third edition. London: Springer-Verlag; 2005. p. 1581–91.
4. Xu S, Bendeck M, Gotlieb AI. Vascular pathobiology: atherosclerosis and large vessel disease. In: Buja LM, Butany J, editors. Cardiovascular Pathology, 4th edition. Amsterdam: Elsevier/Academic Press, 2016, pp. 85–124. Cardiovascular Pathology, 5th edition. Amsterdam: Elsevier/Academic Press, 2022., In press.
5. Buja LM, McAllister HA Jr. Coronary artery disease: pathological anatomy and pathogenesis. In: Willerson JT, Cohn JN, Wellens HJJ, Homes Jr DR, editors. Cardiovascular Medicine. 3rd ed. London: Springer-Verlag; 2005. p. 593–610.
6. Buja LM. Coronary artery disease: pathological anatomy and pathogenesis. In: Willerson JT, Holmes Jr DR, editors. Coronary Artery Disease, Cardiovascular Medicine. London: Springer-Verlag; 2015. p. 1–20.
7. Fishbein GA, Fishbein MC, Wang JJ, Buja LM. Myocardial ischemia and its consequences. In: Buja LM, Butany J, editors. Cardiovascular Pathology, 4th edition. Amsterdam: Elsevier/Academic Press, 2016, pp. 239–270. Cardiovascular Pathology, 5th edition. Amsterdam: Elsevier/Academic Press, 2022., In press.
8. Buja LM, Vander Heide RS. Pathobiology of Ischemic Heart Disease: Past, Present and Future. Cardiovasc Pathol. 2016;May–Jun;25(3):214–20. https://doi.org/10.1016/j.carpath.2016.01.007.
9. Buja LM, Ottaviani G, Mitchell RN. Pathobiology of cardiovascular diseases: an update. Cardiovasc Pathol. 2019;Sep–Oct;42:44–53. https://doi.org/10.1016/j.carpath.2019.06.002.
10. Barquera S, Pedroza-Tobías A, Medina C, Hernández-Barrera L, Bibbins-Domingo K, Lozano R, Moran AE. Global Overview of the Epidemiology of Atherosclerotic Cardiovascular Disease. Arch Med Res. 2015;Jul;46(5):328–38. https://doi.org/10.1016/j.arcmed.2015.06.006.
11. Herrington W, Lacey B, Sherliker P, Armitage J, Lewington S. Epidemiology of Atherosclerosis and the Potential to Reduce the Global Burden of Atherothrombotic Disease. Circ Res. 2016 Feb 19;118(4):535–46. https://doi.org/10.1161/CIRCRESAHA.115.307611.
12. Goldstein JL, Brown MS. Atherosclerosis: the low-density lipoprotein receptor hypothesis. Metabolism. 1977;26:1257–75. https://doi.org/10.1016/0026-0495(77)90119-6.
13. Goldstein JL, Brown MS. The LDL receptor. Arterioscler Thromb Vasc Biol. 2009 Apr;29(4):431–8. https://doi.org/10.1161/ATVBAHA.108.179564.
14. Goldstein JL, Brown MS. A century of cholesterol and coronaries: from plaques to genes to statins. Cell. 2015 Mar 26;161(1):161–72. https://doi.org/10.1016/j.cell.2015.01.036.
15. Musunuru K, Kathiresan S. Surprises From Genetic Analyses of Lipid Risk Factors for Atherosclerosis. Circ Res. 2016 Feb 19;118(4):579–85. https://doi.org/10.1161/CIRCRESAHA.115.306398.
16. Nordestgaard BG. Triglyceride-Rich Lipoproteins and Atherosclerotic Cardiovascular Disease: New Insights From Epidemiology, Genetics, and Biology. Circ Res. 2016 Feb 19;118(4):547–63. https://doi.org/10.1161/CIRCRESAHA.115.306249.
17. Kessler T, Vilne B, Schunkert H. The impact of genome-wide association studies on the pathophysiology and therapy of cardiovascular disease. EMBO Mol Med. 2016 Jul 1;8(7):688–701. https://doi.org/10.15252/emmm.201506174.
18. Khera AV, Kathiresan S. Genetics of coronary artery disease: discovery, biology and clinical translation. Nat Rev Genet. 2017;Jun;18(6):331–44. https://doi.org/10.1038/nrg.2016.160.
19. Steinberg D. Thematic review series: the pathogenesis of atherosclerosis. An interpretive history of the cholesterol controversy, part V: the discovery of the statins and the end of the controversy. J Lipid Res. 2006;Jul;47(7):1339–51. https://doi.org/10.1194/jlr.R600009-JLR200.

20. Huang PL. A comprehensive definition for metabolic syndrome. Dis Model Mech. 2009;May–Jun;2(5–6):231–7. https://doi.org/10.1242/dmm.001180.
21. Brodsky SV, Barth RF, Mo X, Yildiz V, Allenby P, Ivanov I, Moore S, Hitchcock CL, Smith S, Sachak T, Yao K, Ball M, Rosborough K, Olson Z, Kiehl M, Muni N, Virmani R. An obesity paradox: an inverse correlation between body mass index and atherosclerosis of the aorta. Cardiovasc Pathol. 2016 Nov–Dec;25(6):515–20. https://doi.org/10.1016/j.carpath.2016.09.002.
22. Qaisar S, Brodsky LD, Barth RF, Leier C, Buja LM, Yildiz V, Mo X, Allenby P, Moore S, Ivanov I, Chen W, Thomas D, Rivera AC, Gamble D, Hartage R, Mao G, Sheldon J, Sinclair D, Vazzano J, Zehr B, Patton A, Brodsky SV. An unexpected paradox: wall shear stress in the aorta is less in patients with severe atherosclerosis regardless of obesity. Cardiovasc Pathol. 2021;Mar-Apr;51:107313. https://doi.org/10.1016/j.carpath.2020.107313.
23. Libby P, Loscalzo J, Ridker PM, Farkouh ME, Hsue PY, Fuster V, Hasan AA, Amar S. Inflammation, Immunity, and Infection in Atherothrombosis: JACC Review Topic of the Week. J Am Coll Cardiol. 2018 Oct 23;72(17):2071–81. https://doi.org/10.1016/j.jacc.2018.08.1043.
24. Maleszewski JJ, Lai CK, Veinot JP. Anatomic considerations and examination of cardiovascular specimens (excluding devices). In: Buja LM, Butany J, editors. Cardiovascular Pathology, 4th edition. Amsterdam: Elsevier/Academic Press, 2016, pp.1–56. Cardiovascular Pathology, 5th edition. Amsterdam: Elsevier/Academic Press, 2022, In press.
25. Haust MD. The morphogenesis and fate of potential and early atherosclerotic lesions in man. Hum Pathol 1971 Mar;2(1):1–29. https://doi.org/10.1016/s0046-8177(71)80019-9. PMID: 4937772.
26. Haust MD. The genesis of atherosclerosis in pediatric age-group. Pediatr Pathol. 1990;10(1–2):253–71. https://doi.org/10.3109/15513819009067112.
27. Haust MD. Atherosclerosis—lesions and sequelae. In: Silver MD, editor. Cardiovascular Pathology. 1st ed. New York; Churchill Livingstone; 1983. p. 191–315.
28. Buja LM, Kita T, Goldstein JL, Watanabe Y, Brown MS. Cellular pathology of progressive atherosclerosis in the WHHL rabbit. An animal model of familial hypercholesterolemia. Arteriosclerosis 1983 Jan–Feb;3(1):87–101. https://doi.org/10.1161/01.atv.3.1.87.
29. Buja LM, Kovanen PT, Bilheimer DW. Cellular pathology of homozygous familial hypercholesterolemia. Am J Pathol. 1979;Nov;97(2):327–57.
30. Buja LM, Clubb FJ Jr, Bilheimer DW, Willerson JT. Pathobiology of human familial hypercholesterolaemia and a related animal model, the Watanabe heritable hyperlipidaemic rabbit. Eur Heart J. 1990;Aug;11(Suppl E):41–52. https://doi.org/10.1093/eurheartj/11.suppl_e.41.
31. Lundberg B. Chemical composition and physical state of lipid deposits in atherosclerosis. Atherosclerosis. 1985;Jul;56(1):93–110. https://doi.org/10.1016/0021-9150(85)90087-5.
32. Stegemann C, Drozdov I, Shalhoub J, Humphries J, Ladroue C, Didangelos A, Baumert M, Allen M, Davies AH, Monaco C, Smith A, Xu Q, Mayr M. Comparative lipidomics profiling of human atherosclerotic plaques. Circ Cardiovasc Genet. 2011;Jun;4(3):232–42. https://doi.org/10.1161/CIRCGENETICS.110.959098.
33. Virmani R, Kolodgie FD, Burke AP, Farb A, Schwartz SM. Lessons from sudden coronary death: a comprehensive morphological classification scheme for atherosclerotic lesions. Arterioscler Thromb Vasc Biol. 2000;20(5):1262–75. https://doi.org/10.1161/01.atv.20.5.1262.
34. Yahagi K, Kolodgie FD, Otsuka F, Finn AV, Davis HR, Joner M, Virmani R. Pathophysiology of native coronary, vein graft, and in-stent atherosclerosis. Nat Rev Cardiol. 2016;Feb;13(2):79–98. https://doi.org/10.1038/nrcardio.2015.164.
35. Libby P, Schoen FJ. Vascular lesion formation. Cardiovasc Pathol. 1993;Sept; 2(3, Suppl):43–52. https://doi.org/10.1016/1054-8807(93)90046-5.

36. Williams KJ, Tabas I. The response-to-retention hypothesis of atherogenesis reinforced. Curr Opin Lipidol. 1998;Oct;9(5):471–4. https://doi.org/10.1097/00041433-199810000-00012.
37. Williams KJ, Tabas I. Lipoprotein retention—and clues for atheroma regression. Arterioscler Thromb Vasc Biol. 2005;Aug;25(8):1536–40. https://doi.org/10.1161/01.ATV.0000174795.62387.d3.
38. Maguire EM, Pearce SWA, Xiao Q. Foam cell formation: A new target for fighting atherosclerosis and cardiovascular disease. Vasc Pharmacol. 2019;Jan;112:54–71. https://doi.org/10.1016/j.vph.2018.08.002.
39. Park YM. CD36, a scavenger receptor implicated in atherosclerosis. Exp Mol Med. 2014;46(e99) https://doi.org/10.1038/emm.2014.38.
40. Mineo C. Lipoprotein receptor signaling in atherosclerosis. Cardiovasc Res. 2020;116:1254–74. https://doi.org/10.1093/cvr/cvz338.
41. Aikawa M, Libby P. The vulnerable plaque: pathogenesis and therapeutic approach. Cardiovasc Pathol. 2004;May-Jun;13(3):125–38. https://doi.org/10.1016/S1054-8807(04)00004-3.
42. Finn AV, Nakano M, Narula J, Kolodgie FD, Virmani R. Concept of vulnerable/unstable plaque. Arterioscler Thromb Vasc Biol. 2010;30(7):1282–92. https://doi.org/10.1161/ATVBAHA.108.179739.
43. Bentzon JF, Otsuka F, Virmani R, Falk E. Mechanisms of plaque formation and rupture. Circ Res 2014 Jun 6;114(12):1852–1866. https://doi.org/10.1161/CIRCRESAHA.114.302721. PMID: 24902970.
44. Ross R. The pathogenesis of atherosclerosis—an update. N Engl J Med. 1986;314:488–500.
45. Ross R. The pathogenesis of atherosclerosis: a perspective for the 1990s. Nature. 1993;362:801809.
46. Ross R. Atherosclerosis: an inflammatory disease. N Engl J Med. 1999;340:115–26.
47. Furie MB, Mitchell RN. Plaque attack: one hundred years of atherosclerosis in The American Journal of Pathology. Am J Pathol. 2012;Jun;180(6):2184–7. https://doi.org/10.1016/j.ajpath.2012.04.003.
48. Libby P, Hansson GK. From focal lipid storage to systemic inflammation: JACC review topic of the week. J Am Coll Cardiol. 2019 Sept 24;74(12):1594–607. https://doi.org/10.1016/j.jacc.2019.07.061.
49. Hansson GK, Libby P, Schönbeck U, Yan Z-Q. Innate and adaptive immunity in the pathogenesis of atherosclerosis. Circ Res. 2002;91:281–91. https://doi.org/10.1161/01.res.0000029784.15893.10.
50. Ketelhuth DF, Hansson GK. Adaptive Response of T and B Cells in Atherosclerosis. Circ Res. 2016 Feb 19;118(4):668–78. https://doi.org/10.1161/CIRCRESAHA.115.306427.
51. Wissler RW, Vesselinovitch D. Studies of regression of advanced atherosclerosis in experimental animals and man. Ann N Y Acad Sci. 1976;275:363–78. https://doi.org/10.1111/j.1749-6632.1976.tb43368.x.
52. Sdringola S, Loghin C, Boccalandro F, Gould KL. Mechanisms of progression and regression of coronary artery disease by PET related to treatment intensity and clinical events at long-term follow-up. J Nucl Med. 2006;Jan;47(1):59–67.
53. Daida H, Dohi T, Fukushima Y, Ohmura H, Miyauchi K. The Goal of Achieving Atherosclerotic Plaque Regression with Lipid-Lowering Therapy: Insights from IVUS Trials. J Atheroscler Thromb. 2019 Jul 1;26(7):592–600. https://doi.org/10.5551/jat.48603.
54. Gimbrone MA Jr, García-Cardeña G. Vascular endothelium, hemodynamics, and the pathobiology of atherosclerosis. Cardiovasc Pathol. 2013;Jan-Feb;22(1):9–15. https://doi.org/10.1016/j.carpath.2012.06.006.
55. Gimbrone MA Jr, García-Cardeña G. Endothelial Cell Dysfunction and the Pathobiology of Atherosclerosis. Circ Res. 2016 Feb 19;118(4):620–36. https://doi.org/10.1161/CIRCRESAHA.115.306301.

56. Roostalu U, Wong JK. Arterial smooth muscle dynamics in development and repair. Dev Biol. 2018 Mar 15;435(2):109–21. https://doi.org/10.1016/j.ydbio.2018.01.018.
57. Schwartz SM, Virmani R, Majesky MW. An update on clonality: what smooth muscle cell type makes up the atherosclerotic plaque? F1000Res. 2018 Dec 21;7:F1000 Faculty Rev-1969. https://doi.org/10.12688/f1000research.15994.1.
58. Wirka RC, Wagh D, Paik DT, Pjanic M, Nguyen T, Miller CL, Kundu R, Nagao M, Coller J, Koyano TK, Fong R, Woo YJ, Liu B, Montgomery SB, Wu JC, Zhu K, Chang R, Alamprese M, Tallquist MD, Kim JB, Quertermous T. Atheroprotective roles of smooth muscle cell phenotypic modulation and the TCF21 disease gene as revealed by single-cell analysis. Nat Med. 2019 Aug;25(8):1280–9. https://doi.org/10.1038/s41591-019-0512-5.
59. Basatemur GL, Jørgensen HF, Clarke MCH, Bennett MR, Mallat Z. Vascular smooth muscle cells in atherosclerosis. Nat Rev Cardiol. 2019;Dec;16(12):727–44. https://doi.org/10.1038/s41569-019-0227-9.
60. Chattopadhyay A, Kwartler CS, Kaw K, Li Y, Kaw A, Chen J, LeMaire SA, Shen YH, Milewicz DM. Cholesterol-Induced Phenotypic Modulation of Smooth Muscle Cells to Macrophage/Fibroblast-like Cells Is Driven by an Unfolded Protein Response. Arterioscler Thromb Vasc Biol. 2021;Jan;41(1):302–16. https://doi.org/10.1161/ATVBAHA.120.315164.
61. Chattopadhyay A, Guan P, Majumder S, Kaw K, Zhou Z, Prakash SK, Anita Kaw A, Buja LM, Kwartler CS, Milewicz DM. Perk-dependent signaling in vascular smooth muscle cells drives phenotypic modulation and atherosclerotic plaque formation. In submission.
62. Varghese DS, Ali BR. Pathological Crosstalk Between Oxidized LDL and ER Stress in Human Diseases: A Comprehensive Review. Front Cell Dev Biol. 2021;May 26(9):674103. https://doi.org/10.3389/fcell.2021.674103.
63 Vela D, Buja LM, Madjid M, Burke A, Naghavi M, Willerson JT, Casscells SW, Litovsky S. The role of periadventitial fat in atherosclerosis. Arch Pathol Lab Med. 2007;Mar;131(3):481–7. https://doi.org/10.5858/2007-131-481-TROPFI.
64. Tinajero MG, Gotlieb AI. Recent Developments in Vascular Adventitial Pathobiology: The Dynamic Adventitia as a Complex Regulator of Vascular Disease. Am J Pathol. 2020;Mar;190(3):520–34. https://doi.org/10.1016/j.ajpath.2019.10.021.
65. Glagov S, Zarins C, Giddens DP, Ku DN. Hemodynamics and atherosclerosis. Insight and perspectives gained from studies of human arteries. Arch Pathol Lab Med. 1988;112:1018–31.
66. VanderLaan PA, Reardon CA, Getz GS. Site specificity of atherosclerosis: site-selective responses to atherosclerotic modulators. Arterioscler Thromb Vasc Biol. 2004;24:12–22.
67. Cunningham KS, Gotlieb AI. The role of shear stress in the pathogenesis of atherosclerosis. Lab Investig. 2005;Jan;85(1):9–23. https://doi.org/10.1038/labinvest.3700215.
68. Weavers H, Martin P. The cell biology of inflammation: From common traits to remarkable immunological adaptations. J Cell Biol. 2020 Jul 6;219(7):e202004003. https://doi.org/10.1083/jcb.202004003.
69. Buja LM. The cell theory and cellular pathology: Discovery, refinements and applications fundamental to advances in biology and medicine. Exp Mol Pathol. 2021 Jun;8(121):104660. https://doi.org/10.1016/j.yexmp.2021.104660.
70. Zindel J, Kubes P. DAMPs, PAMPs, and LAMPs in Immunity and Sterile Inflammation. Annu Rev Pathol. 2020 Jan;24(15):493–518. https://doi.org/10.1146/annurev-pathmechdis-012419-032847.
71. Malik A, Kanneganti TD. Inflammasome activation and assembly at a glance. J Cell Sci. 2017 Dec 1;130(23):3955–63. https://doi.org/10.1242/jcs.207365.
72. Poznyak AV, Melnichenko AA, Wetzker R, Gerasimova EV, Orekhov AN. NLPR3 Inflammasomes and Their Significance for Atherosclerosis. Biomedicine. 2020 Jul 10;8(7):205. https://doi.org/10.3390/biomedicines8070205.

73. Karasawa T, Takahashi M. Role of NLRP3 Inflammasomes in Atherosclerosis. J Atheroscler Thromb. 2017 May 1;24(5):443–51. https://doi.org/10.5551/jat.RV17001.
74. Jaiswal S, Natarajan P, Silver AJ, Gibson CJ, Bick AG, Shvartz E, McConkey M, Gupta N, Gabriel S, Ardissino D, Baber U, Mehran R, Fuster V, Danesh J, Frossard P, Saleheen D, Melander O, Sukhova GK, Neuberg D, Libby P, Kathiresan S, Ebert BL. Clonal Hematopoiesis and Risk of Atherosclerotic Cardiovascular Disease. N Engl J Med 2017 Jul 13;377(2):111–121. https://doi.org/10.1056/NEJMoa1701719. Epub 2017 Jun 21.
75. Libby P. Inflammation in Atherosclerosis-No Longer a Theory. Clin Chem. 2021 Jan 8;67(1):131–42. https://doi.org/10.1093/clinchem/hvaa275.
76. Crossman D. Acute coronary syndromes. Clin Med (Lond). 2001;May-Jun;1(3):206–13. https://doi.org/10.7861/clinmedicine.1-3-206.
77. Kotecha T, Rakhit RD. Acute coronary syndromes. Clin Med (Lond). 2016 Dec;16(Suppl 6):s43–8. https://doi.org/10.7861/clinmedicine.16-6-s43.
78. Glagov S, Weisenberg E, Zarins CK, Stankunavicius R, Kolettis GJ. Compensatory enlargement of human atherosclerotic coronary arteries. N Engl J Med. 1987 May 28;316(22):1371–5.
79. Libby P. Mechanisms of acute coronary syndromes and their implications for therapy. N Engl J Med. 2013;368(21):2004–13. https://doi.org/10.1056/NEJMra1216063.
80. Libby P, Pasterkamp G, Crea F, Jang IK. Reassessing the Mechanisms of Acute Coronary Syndromes. Circ Res. 2019;124(1):150–60. https://doi.org/10.1161/CIRCRESAHA.118.311098.
81. Elgendy IY, Conti CR, Bavry AA. Fractional flow reserve: an updated review. Clin Cardiol. 2014 Jun;37(6):371–80. https://doi.org/10.1002/clc.22273.
82. Buja LM, Zehr B, Lelenwa L, Ogechukwu E, Zhao B, Dasgupta A, Barth RF. Clinicopathological complexity in the application of the universal definition of myocardial infarction. Cardiovasc Pathol. 2020;Jan-Feb;44:107153. https://doi.org/10.1016/j.carpath.2019.107153.
83. Michaud K, Basso C, d'Amati G, Giordano C, Kholová I, Preston SD, Rizzo S, Sabatasso S, Sheppard MN, Vink A, van der Wal AC; Association for European Cardiovascular Pathology (AECVP). Diagnosis of myocardial infarction at autopsy: AECVP reappraisal in the light of the current clinical classification. Virchows Arch 2020 Feb;476(2):179–194. https://doi.org/10.1007/s00428-019-02662-1.
84. Lehrman M, Schneider W, Sudhof T, Brown M, Goldstein J, Russell D. Mutation in LDL receptor: Alu-Alu recombination deletes exons encoding transmembrane and cytoplasmic domains. Science (80–) 1985;227:140–6. https://doi.org/10.1126/science.3155573.
85. Soria LF, Ludwig EH, Clarke HR, Vega GL, Grundy SM, McCarthy BJ. Association between a specific apolipoprotein B mutation and familial defective apolipoprotein B-100. Proc Natl Acad Sci. 1989;86:587–91. https://doi.org/10.1073/pnas.86.2.587.
86. Abifadel M, Varret M, Rabès J-P, Allard D, Ouguerram K, Devillers M, et al. Mutations in PCSK9 cause autosomal dominant hypercholesterolemia. Nat Genet. 2003;34:154–6. https://doi.org/10.1038/ng1161.
87. Garcia CK. Autosomal Recessive Hypercholesterolemia Caused by Mutations in a Putative LDL Receptor Adaptor Protein. Science (80–) 2001;292:1394–8. https://doi.org/10.1126/science.1060458.
88. Berge KE. Accumulation of Dietary Cholesterol in Sitosterolemia Caused by Mutations in Adjacent ABC Transporters. Science (80–) 2000;290:1771–5. https://doi.org/10.1126/science.290.5497.1771.
89. Lloyd-Jones DM, Nam B-H, D'Agostino RB Sr, Levy D, Murabito JM, Wang TJ, et al. Parental Cardiovascular Disease as a Risk Factor for Cardiovascular Disease in Middle-aged Adults. JAMA. 2004;291:2204. https://doi.org/10.1001/jama.291.18.2204.

90. Zdravkovic S, Wienke A, Pedersen NL, Marenberg ME, Yashin AI, De Faire U. Heritability of death from coronary heart disease: a 36-year follow-up of 20 966 Swedish twins. J Intern Med. 2002;252:247–54. https://doi.org/10.1046/j.1365-2796.2002.01029.x.
91. McPherson R, Pertsemlidis A, Kavaslar N, Stewart A, Roberts R, Cox DR, et al. A Common Allele on Chromosome 9 Associated with Coronary Heart Disease. Science (80–) 2007;316:1488–91. https://doi.org/10.1126/science.1142447.
92. Helgadottir A, Thorleifsson G, Manolescu A, Gretarsdottir S, Blondal T, Jonasdottir A, et al. A Common Variant on Chromosome 9p21 Affects the Risk of Myocardial Infarction. Science (80–) 2007;316:1491–3. https://doi.org/10.1126/science.1142842.
93 Samani NJ, Erdmann J, Hall AS, Hengstenberg C, Mangino M, Mayer B, et al. Genomewide Association Analysis of Coronary Artery Disease. N Engl J Med. 2007;357:443–53. https://doi.org/10.1056/NEJMoa072366.
94. Clarke R, Peden JF, Hopewell JC, Kyriakou T, Goel A, Heath SC, et al. Genetic Variants Associated with Lp(a) Lipoprotein Level and Coronary Disease. N Engl J Med 2009;361:2518–2528. https://doi.org/10.1056/NEJMoa0902604, https://doi.org/10.1016/j.jacc.2012.09.017.
95. Nordestgaard BG, Varbo A. Triglycerides and cardiovascular disease. Lancet. 2014;384:626–35. https://doi.org/10.1016/S0140-6736(14)61177-6.

Prevention of Coronary Atherosclerosis

Gemma A. Figtree, Katharine A. Kott, and Stephen T. Vernon

1 Introduction

Ischaemic heart disease is the primary cause of cardiovascular disease mortality in men and women worldwide [1, 2]. The personal and socio-economic burden is immense. Despite atherosclerotic plaque developing over years, many people have no warning symptoms prior to a MI or sudden cardiac death. The key roles of hypertension, dyslipidaemia, diabetes mellitus, and cigarette smoking in driving atherosclerotic coronary disease are well recognised at a population level and have been the target of our primary prevention strategies for over 50 years, resulting in a substantial reduction in the morbidity and mortality associated with coronary artery disease. Strategies targeting these traditional risk factors remain essential, with a need for ongoing improvements in education, screen-

G. A. Figtree (✉)
Cardiothoracic and Vascular Health, Kolling Institute of Medical Research, Sydney, Australia

Department of Cardiology, Royal North Shore Hospital, Northern Sydney Local Health District, Sydney, Australia

Northern Clinical School, Faculty of Medicine and Health, University of Sydney, Sydney, Australia

Charles Perkins Centre, University of Sydney, Sydney, Australia
e-mail: gemma.figtree@sydney.edu.au

K. A. Kott · S. T. Vernon
Cardiothoracic and Vascular Health, Kolling Institute of Medical Research, Sydney, Australia

Department of Cardiology, Royal North Shore Hospital, Northern Sydney Local Health District, Sydney, Australia

Northern Clinical School, Faculty of Medicine and Health, University of Sydney, Sydney, Australia

G. Concistrè (ed.), *Ischemic Heart Disease*,
https://doi.org/10.1007/978-3-031-25879-4_3

ing, and equitable access to effective preventative therapies. However, risk stratification strategies used to date have struggled with how to manage the substantial group of people that are assessed to be at intermediate risk, resulting in both overall higher costs through overtreatment of some individuals as well as undertreatment and failure to prevent events in others. This issue is highlighted by the substantial proportion of MI patients (15–25%) that present with life-threatening MI but are apparently from a low-risk group, with none of the standard modifiable risk factors explaining the development of their CAD [3–5]. The drivers of individual susceptibility to develop atherosclerosis in response to particular risk factors are poorly understood. Clearly, new solutions are required. Here, we discuss established and emerging approaches at both a community and an individual level, focussing on traditional risk factors, as well as opportunities for earlier detection of CAD in its subclinical phase to allow more personalised administration of effective therapies and prevention of heart attack. Figure 1 provides a schematic overview.

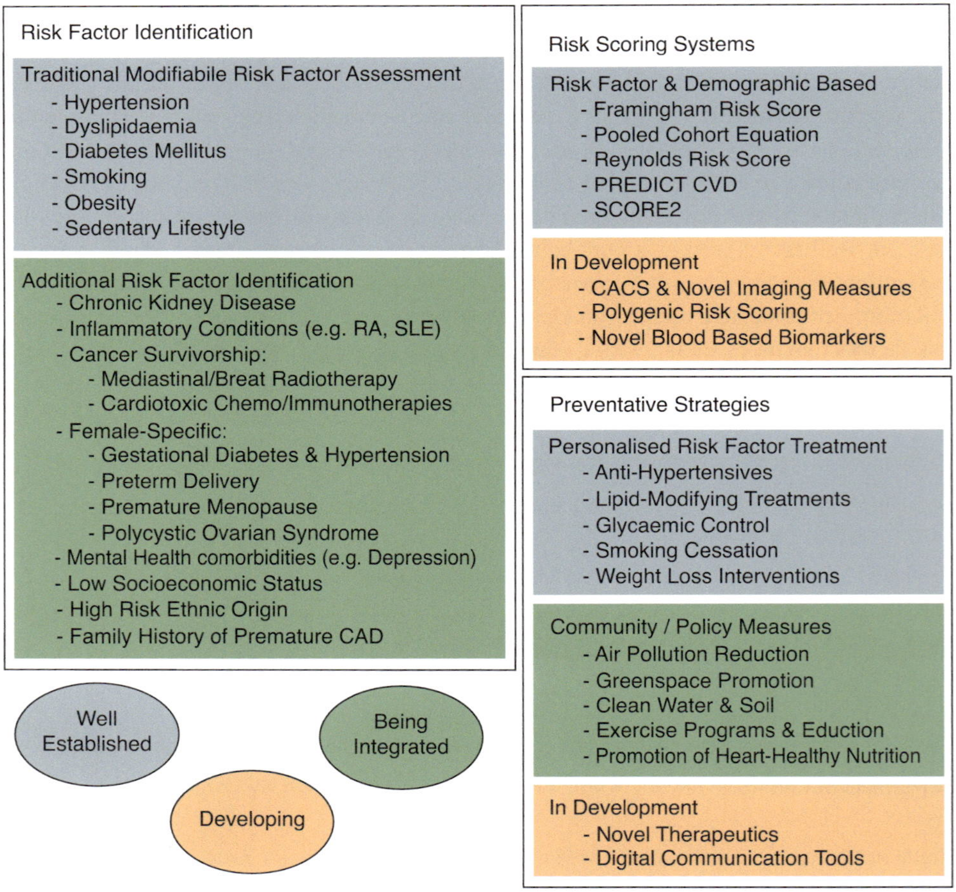

Fig. 1 Schematic overview of the established and emerging approaches to prevention of coronary artery disease

2 Public Health Approaches to Screening and Treating Traditional Modifiable Risk Factors

Over recent decades, improved management of ACS using clinically proven interventions and pharmacotherapy has increased survival. This has led to a dramatic rise in the number of people living with CVD and subsequent reduced quality of life. Further efforts are required to improve primary and secondary prevention. The most important way to prevent CAD is to promote a healthy lifestyle throughout all of life, particularly by not smoking [6]. The coupling of this with screening for and treatment of well-established modifiable risk factors has been effective and is now available at greater global scale for more equitable access with generic drugs available at low costs [6], including in "polypill" formulas [7]. Additionally. at a community level, strategies, including town planning approaches such as incorporating green spaces to encourage physical activity and clean air, are important.

2.1 Hypertension

Hypertension is the leading risk factor for ischaemic heart disease globally [8]. This appears to be more tightly associated with women, who have a higher risk of acute MI associated with the prevalence of hypertension than men [9]. There is a linear relationship between blood pressure measures, including within the normal range, and risk of death from either coronary artery disease or stroke [6]. Additionally, evidence from the SPRINT trial demonstrated that aggressive management of systolic blood pressure to ranges below 120 mmHg protects against major cardiovascular events and death [10]. Thus, individual absolute risk and patient tolerance are major factors in decisions guiding initiation of pharmacotherapy and blood pressure targets. Lifestyle changes including salt-reduced diets, weight loss, and exercise are effective, but are challenging to maintain over long periods. There are a wide variety of antihypertensive agents, many now available off patent, and they are accessible as "generics" globally. Whilst there are theoretical benefits above and beyond the antihypertensive effect of the aldosterone-angiotensin signalling pathway relating to reduction in angiotensin II and NADPH oxidase activity, little difference has been observed between the various classes if target blood pressure is achieved [11–13]. Pragmatically, this results in physicians and patients working together to achieve target with minimum side effects. Additionally, there is a wide body of research showing that when escalation of therapy is required, using two or more agents, rather than maximal dose of a single agent, is both more effective and better tolerated from a side effect perspective [7, 14, 15].

2.2 Dyslipidaemia

The causal role of elevated cholesterol, particularly LDL cholesterol, has been cemented by observational [9] and interventional studies [16], as well as genetic and Mendelian randomisation studies [17, 18]. Lipid-modifying treatment using statins which inhibit HMG-CoA reductase reduces both cardiovascular events and mortality in individuals with established coronary artery disease (secondary prevention) [19, 20]. In a primary prevention setting, evidence-based thresholds for commencing statins vary according to overall risk for the individual, with the absolute benefit of lowering LDL-C depending on the absolute risk of CVD [20, 21]. Whilst other agents such as ezetimibe have been effective in lowering LDL [22] by inhibiting cholesterol uptake in the small intestine, via the Niemann-Pick C1-like 1 protein, their benefits on cardiovascular events have been less compelling, with controversy as to whether ezetimibe therapy confers additional reduction in cardiovascular risk above a statin, even in an individual with persistently elevated LDL-C levels. It was not until the IMPROVE-IT study published in 2015 that we have seen randomised control trial evidence that ezetimibe conferred a protective effect against major cardiovascular events when used in addition to a statin in high-risk patients [23]. Its role in primary prevention is less clear. However, there has been an acceptance of its role in individuals who are intolerant of statins to achieve target LDL-C levels [24].

In the past 5 years, the emergence of monoclonal antibody PCSK9 inhibitor has demonstrated powerful effects on LDL cholesterol, with a reduction in major adverse cardiovascular events in those with established CAD [25, 26]. Whilst equitable access to expensive monoclonal antibody approaches is an important limitation, emerging small interfering RNA (siRNA) strategies, such as inclisiran which targets PCSK9, may have advantages related to scalability of production as has been witnessed with the RNA technology tackling COVID-19. In addition, the need for only twice-yearly injections is attractive to both patients and healthcare providers. However, whilst randomised controlled trials have been completed and confirm substantial reductions in LDL-C in patients with atherosclerotic disease with persistently elevated LDL on a statin [27], the effect of inclisiran on cardiovascular morbidity and mortality has not yet been determined and is the focus of an ongoing cardiovascular outcome trial. Despite this, the impressive results have resulted in FDA approval as an add-on therapy in high-risk individuals.

2.3 Diabetes Mellitus

The rising prevalence of diabetes mellitus is driven by type 2 diabetes mellitus and is closely related to increases in obesity, unhealthy diets, and sedentary lifestyles. Both type 1 and type 2 diabetes are independent risk factors for atherosclerotic cardiovascular disease, increasing the risk of an event by approximately two times. However, the risk appears to be more significant in females. Data from >800,000 patients across 64 studies found that the risk for incident coronary heart disease was 44% higher in women with diabetes than in men with diabetes [28]. Similarly, data from the UK Biobank showed ~29% higher risk of MI in association with diabetes in women compared with that in men [29]. Important aspects of prevention strategies require multidisciplinary efforts at both a population and an individual level to enhance diet, reduce body mass index, increase exercise, and reduce sedentary behaviours. Whilst earlier pharmacotherapies such as metformin or insulin which are successful in improving glycaemic control had disappointing benefits on atherosclerotic and cardiovascular events [30], there is increasing evidence for the cardioprotective effects of new therapies targeting SGLT2 [31–33] and GLP1 [34]. In the case of SGLT2 inhibitors, the most profound effect has been protection against heart failure events, with minimal effect versus MI only seen in very large meta-analyses [35]. Whilst international guidelines have acted rapidly to include SGLT2 inhibitors as recommended prevention strategies against heart failure in patients with diabetes [36], they are not specifically recommended to prevent atherosclerotic events.

2.4 Smoking

Cigarette smoking is responsible for 50% of all avoidable deaths in smokers, with half of these resulting from atherosclerotic cardiovascular disease [37]. Astonishingly, the CVD risk in young smokers (<50 years) is fivefold higher than in non-smokers, with even higher risk in women versus men [38]. Mechanisms include endothelial dysfunction, with reduced nitric oxide bioavailability, increased platelet and macrophage activation, and a pro-inflammatory vascular environment that drives tissue remodelling [39]. Preventative strategies need to include prevention of smoking initiation, public messaging, policy approaches including taxing and packaging rules, as well as laws preventing smoking at indoor public locations. New Zealand has taken a particularly strict stance, making it illegal to buy cigarettes or tobacco for "the next generation" (current and all future minors) throughout their lifetime [40]. However, whilst smoking cessation is the most effective measure for reversing vascular injury and preventing associated events, the addictive nature makes success rates low even with nicotine replacement or anti-addiction pharmacotherapies such as bupropion [41]. As such, working, in parallel with cessation efforts, to optimise overall cardiovascular health in smokers, including other risk factors, is a pragmatic approach.

2.5 Obesity

Obesity is a burgeoning health challenge across the globe, which increases CVD risk via its association with major conventional risk factors above, as well as through additional mechanisms. Treatments range from diet and lifestyle interventions, through to pharmacological (e.g. phentermine, liraglutide) [42] and bariatric surgical approaches. The high failure rate of diet and lifestyle interventions had led to a paucity of evidence that targeting obesity with non-invasive approaches improves cardiovascular outcomes. However, recently, bariatric surgery has been found to reduce the incidence of major adverse cardiac events in several matched cohort studies [43–45].

3 Community Measures to Optimise Cardiovascular Health

In addition to education, screening, and risk factor management, communities may benefit from policy decisions that influence the environment for the broader population. This may include efforts to reduce air pollution, promote incidental exercise and activity, and improve the quality of food options. Such factors may be particularly important to developing countries and communities with a lower socio-economic status.

1. **Environment**

   Air pollution is thought to be the most important environmental CVD risk factor, and fine particulate matter <2.5 μm, nitrogen dioxide, and ozone gas are some of the major determinants [46]. Exposure to air pollution has been associated with increased risk of stroke and CAD, even at levels lower than currently allowable by public health policies [47]. Additional environmental factors which should be considered in policy include extreme temperature events, adequate greenspace proximity in the form of civic foliage and public parks, and monitoring of waterways and soils for toxins such as heavy metals [48].
2. **Exercise**

   Maintaining physical fitness is a key component to optimising cardiovascular health in both primary and secondary prevention of atherosclerosis. Meta-analysis of studies investigating physical activity in the general population has shown 14–20% lower risk of coronary heart disease in those who exercised 150–300 min per week at a moderate intensity level [49]. The benefits of exercise-based cardiac rehabilitation in patients with existing CVD are also significant, with reduction seen in mortality, lipid levels, blood pressure, and smoking rates [50].
3. **Diet**

   Diet has a profound effect on health and affects all the major cardiovascular risk factors but is largely impacted by cultural and socio-economic situation. Though it is a difficult area to study conclusively, several studies have demonstrated that changes in diet could alter CVD risk. Diets high in saturated and trans-fats create a more atherogenic lipid profile, and it is estimated that a 2% increase in calories from trans-fats results in a 23% increase in the incidence of CVD[51]. The "Western diet"—high in processed food, sugars, saturated fats, and red meat—has been associated with increased obesity and type 2 diabetes [51]. A heart-healthy diet is currently thought to consist of vegetables, fruits, whole grains, lean protein with minimal red meat intake, and low levels of saturated and trans-fats [48], though further research is required to fully understand the impact of diet on cardiovascular health.

4 Risk Scores

Estimation of CVD risk provides information for tailored intervention on an individual level, in apparently healthy subjects, but also in older individuals or those with comorbidities such as diabetes mellitus. This allows for shared decision-making and individualised treatment. Multiple risk scores have been developed and refined in recent decades using multivariate models in large population studies. However, only a proportion have been adopted in clinical practice. Key factors that determine whether a risk calculator is adopted include the ease of use, the applicability to specific patient populations, and professional society recommendations. Some of the more widely adopted absolute cardiovascular risk scores are summarised below:

1. Framingham Risk Score 2008 (FRS): The most recent iteration of the FRS includes the following predictor variables: age, gender, total cholesterol (mg/dL), HDL cholesterol (mg/dL), systolic blood pressure (mmHg), blood pressure treatment (yes/no), diabetes mellitus (yes/no), and current smoking (yes/no). This iteration assesses additional end points not included in earlier iterations including stroke, transient ischaemic attack, claudication, and heart failure. The estimated risk is thus higher than in scores that predict only coronary heart disease events [52]. The Framingham risk scores have been derived from a largely White American population; however, with recalibration, they have been demonstrated to perform well in multiple ethnic groups [53].
2. Pooled Cohort Equation (PCE): The American College of Cardiology/American Heart Association-endorsed Pooled Cohort Equation was the first model to include data from large populations of both White and Black Americans. The model includes the same predictor variables as the 2008 FRS, but includes only hard end points (fatal and non-fatal MI and stroke) [54].
3. Reynolds Risk Score: The sex-specific Reynolds Risk Score was developed in a large prospective cohort of non-diabetic North Americans. The main differences between the Reynolds Risk Score and many of the other risk equations are the inclusion of hs-CRP and premature family history of MI as predictor variables [55, 56]. The end points assessed include cardiovascular death, non-fatal MI, non-fatal stroke, and coronary revascularisation.
4. PREDICT CVD risk predictor (2018): The PREDICT CVD risk calculator was developed in a massive cohort of over 400,000 New Zealanders with no prior history of cardiovascular or renal disease. The end points assessed include cardiovascular death (including MI, stroke, or atherosclerotic aneurysm), non-fatal MI, coronary artery revascularisation, non-fatal stroke, transient ischaemic attack, peripheral vascular disease including revascularisation procedures, heart failure, and cardiomyopathy (unless specified as non-ischaemic in origin). PREDICT CVD estimates 5-year rather than 10-year or lifetime risk. PREDICT CVD highlights the importance of having a risk score that is calibrated to the population it will be used in, with PREDICT CVD performing substantially better in a New Zealand population than the Pooled Cohort

Equation, which was found to overestimate risk by as much as 60% in the New Zealand context [57].

5. SCORE2: SCORE2 uses risk prediction models derived using 45 cohorts in 13 European countries and is recommended by the European Society of Cardiology. Given that the estimated absolute risk for a given age and combination of risk factors differed substantially across regions within Europe, SCORE2 includes four separate models calibrated for the four risk regions in Europe, incorporating region-specific CVD mortality and risk factor distributions. The outcomes assessed in SCORE2 include the combined outcome of fatal and non-fatal CVD events. Compared with the earlier iteration, SCORE2 better estimates the total burden of CVD, particularly in younger individuals, and has improved risk discrimination [58].

Whilst initial scores focussed on 5- or 10-year absolute cardiovascular risk which is heavily influenced by age, there is an increasing recognition of the importance of lifetime CVD risk estimates. This is in response to the recognised failure of 10-year risk algorithms, consistently underestimating risk in younger individuals who may have important modifiable risk factors that would be best addressed early [59]. Adopting a lifelong perspective may allow for improved decisions of individual patients around smoking cessation, blood pressure lowering, and metabolic optimisation [6].

5 Atypical Risk Factors

A number of under-recognised risk factors for CAD are increasingly appreciated, including psychological, social, economic, and cultural issues, particularly in women. These factors incorporate mental health disorders, socio-economic status, intimate partner violence, and sociocultural roles. The strong association between mental health conditions and cardiovascular health and disease in both men and women has been increasingly recognised [60]. Conditions specific to women that are now recognised to have risk factors for cardiovascular disease include gestational hypertension, gestational diabetes, preterm delivery, giving birth to a small-for-gestational-age infant, premature menopause, and polycystic ovary syndrome [61]. Chronic kidney disease and systemic autoimmune inflammatory disease [62] are also important factors when considering overall risk in an individual, in addition to cancer survivorship and exposure to mediastinal or breast radiation, or specific chemo- or immuno-therapies [63]. Elevated lipoprotein (a) may occur independently of elevated LDL and is associated with high burden of atherosclerosis [64]. Emerging RNA technology may help target this otherwise challenging non-traditional factor [65]. Whilst many of these additional risk factors are not modifiable, increasing awareness by both physicians and the community is important to guide decisions about screening and thresholds for commencing additional preventive strategies. Future risk scoring systems should consider addition of these non-traditional factors into their algorithms, which may particularly increase accurate prediction of the development of CAD in females.

6 A Need for New Solutions

Despite a common perception that CVD is well understood and managed, it remains a leading global killer and current screening programmes are missing patients at risk. Major advances were made decades ago in the identification and treatment of modifiable risk factors for CAD in the community as discussed above [66]. However, until recently, these risk factors have been all that clinicians and patients had to predict CVD events and guide early preventative strategies. Whilst these population measures are helpful to determine the risk in demographic groups, it is not uncommon for patients to present with extensive atherosclerosis and life-threatening heart attacks who have no personal risk factors for CAD. Patients without any of the standard modifiable cardiovascular risk factors (SMuRFs) who present with STEMI comprise 15–25% of initial STEMI presentations and have a surprisingly higher (>50%) mortality rate compared to those with one or more risk factors, a difference that is more pronounced in women [4, 5, 67].

The SMuRFless STEMI group highlights that whilst the existing risk scoring systems are beneficial on a population level, they still have failings at the level of the individual. When one of these patients inevitably asks, "why me?", it is hard to give them a satisfactory answer. Improved systems to detect early CAD in patients with and without SMuRFs are urgently required and will likely take the form of a combination of risk factor screening, non-invasive imaging measures, and blood-based biomarker testing.

6.1 CT Coronary Calcium Score

The strong association between CAC and atherosclerotic burden was first reported by Rumberger and colleagues in 1995 [68]. This directly reflects the pathophysiological process in the artery, with deposition of calcium phosphate hydroxyapatite crystals in the extra-cellular matrix of the intima being a common and typical feature of atherosclerosis [69]. Standardised measures of CAC have been developed utilising a non-contrast ECG-gated CT acquisition and a protocol to quantify CAC to establish the Agatston score. This involves quantifying the amount of calcium at each focus, scaled by an attenuation factor and added to produce an overall score [70]. The rigour and leadership amongst the field, particularly working together on a harmonised protocol, have allowed for a large body of evidence to grow and for the tool to be available to guide the management of an individual. The resulting CAC score, which is our only non-invasive marker of coronary atherosclerosis itself, is the most successful single marker of subsequent coronary events [71, 72]. Several studies have demonstrated the ability for the CAC score to correctly reclassify patients from intermediate-risk groups based on traditional risk scores into a high- or low-risk group [71, 73, 74]. International guideline bodies therefore recommend using CAC score for screening in individuals at intermediate risk, where findings are considered likely to influence therapy. However, given the unmet need of individuals who develop atherosclerosis despite a calculated low absolute risk score, there have been calls for its use in this group also. Early identification of plaque in this group would allow for effective therapy to prevent progression and heart attack that they would otherwise not be able to access, with statins shown to benefit patients with established CAD even with "low" cholesterol [20]. However, this approach remains controversial, and dedicated prospective implementation studies are required if this is to be considered in future.

6.2 Polygenic Risk Score as an Aid to Improve Risk Identification

PRS for CAD has been developed from large populations and clinical biobanks such as the UK Biobank and integrates the number of risk variant alleles for an individual weighted by the impact of each allele on disease risk. PRS for CAD has expanded from a few SNPs [75] to millions of variants [76], and advances in molecular profiling and data analytics provide powerful new tools to improve risk identification. Inouye and colleagues led a large international collaboration to apply a meta-analytic approach that combines large-scale, genome-wide, and targeted genetic association data to develop a new "meta" PRS consisting of 1.7 million genetic variants [77]. The metaGRS stratified individuals with those in the top 20% of risk having a hazard ratio of 4.17 compared with those in the bottom 20% [77]. The PRS has been validated in American [78] and Canadian cohorts of European descent [79]. Botta and colleagues have expanded this further, showing that additional SNPs have residual predictive power in combination [80]. However, there is an urgent need to test this potentially powerful tool in prospective studies, evaluating the feasibility, patient experience, impact on risk assessment and management, and health economic potential, as outlined in our recently published expert perspective [81].

These PRSs have improved predictive performance over conventional risk factors in observational studies and have the potential advantage that they can be determined at any time in the lifespan, indeed, many years prior to the development of CAD. However, there is currently no clear evidence regarding what proportion of patients that are currently "missed" by traditional risk scores could be identified using a PRS, and little information regarding how well a PRS could be implemented into clinical pathways, or at what cost and with what value to patients and providers. Prospective studies need to also consider challenges in communicating results of PRS to primary care physicians and patients and should provide clear guidelines regarding how this would be integrated with traditional risk factor scores to optimise preventative strategies and inspire behaviour modification.

6.3 Unmet Need for Blood-Based Biomarker of Atherosclerosis Itself

Whilst many of the risk factors discussed above are mechanistically involved in the initiation and progression of atherosclerosis, there is a large degree of variation in the "host" arterial response [82]. This can be best appreciated in the more extreme examples of patients suffering from MI secondary to coronary atherosclerosis in the absence of traditional risk factors [3, 83], or in the more resilient individuals, who may have a whole suite of risk factors, but live healthy lives, and be found to have angiographically normal coronary arteries [84]. High-throughput multi-omic platforms, paired with advanced coronary imaging and machine learning in large cohorts, provide us with the opportunity to hunt for the "holy grail": a blood-based biomarker of coronary atherosclerosis burden and/or activity which can be used to guide personalised approaches to CAD and MI prevention [85–87]. Collaborative platforms to prospectively test emerging biomarkers will be required to demonstrate efficacy in improving outcomes.

7 Integration of Technology: Community Education and Novel Approaches to Shared Decision-Making

A decision to modify lifestyle or commence on effective preventative medication has lifelong implications, and motivation may be difficult to achieve when individuals are treating themselves based on the probability of developing disease, rather than having the disease itself. To improve joint decision-making, communication is key and should focus on calculated risk and demonstrating anticipated risk reduction with various treatment approaches. The approach to this communication needs to be tailored to the individual's preference, as well as their education status and numeracy [6]. Numerous digital communication tools have been developed, with evidence showing that visual aids improve the understanding of disease risk. Botta and colleagues have developed an interactive app available on devices or as a web-based interface to communicate risk incorporating polygenic risk scores and modifiable factors [80]. In addition, studies have demonstrated that visualising personal plaque burden—for example by seeing one's own coronary calcium score results—enhances adherence with preventative therapies and success in achieving recommended targets [88]. Future efforts to integrate technology into risk factor reduction by allowing patients to track their own individual results and progress in an application may promote adherence to therapy and lifestyle efforts by "gamifying" the process, to the benefit of all involved.

8 Summary and Conclusion

Atherosclerotic cardiovascular disease remains a massive burden to the people and economies of the world; however, we have made great gains in the last 50 years. The identification of the major—now "traditional"—standard modifiable cardiovascular risk factors or SMuRFs prompted the development of treatment strategies which have truly reduced morbidity and mortality for a large number of patients over the intervening decades. Effective therapies for hypertension, dyslipidaemia, diabetes, obesity, and smoking cessation are in our current medical repertoire and are used to benefit millions of patients at risk for CAD daily. Education programmes have been developed to promote heart-healthy diets and exercise regimens, which promote better lifestyle choices at the community level.

However, despite these achievements, much work remains to be done. There is still an outstanding and urgent need for improved risk scoring systems that can identify individuals who are missed by current screening systems—those that end up being "SMuRFless STEMIs" because of unidentified atherosclerotic risk. Integration of traditional risk matrices with atypical risk factors, genetic risk scoring, new imaging measures, and novel biomarkers may prove to be an effective mix that identifies CAD risk in all patients, but this remains to be proven in long-term clinical studies. There is also an ongoing need for discovery work that will result in novel therapeutics and adjuncts to care, which improve compliance with medications and lifestyle changes, as well as continued advocacy for population measures that will improve the outcomes of cardiovascular patients on the community level.

References

1. Roth GA, Mensah GA, Johnson CO, Addolorato G, Ammirati E, Baddour LM, Barengo NC, Beaton AZ, Benjamin EJ, Benziger CP, Bonny A, Brauer M, Brodmann M, Cahill TJ, Carapetis J, Catapano AL, Chugh SS, Cooper LT, Coresh J, Criqui M, DeCleene N, Eagle KA, Emmons-Bell S, Feigin VL, Fernandez-Sola J, Fowkes G, Gakidou E, Grundy SM, He FJ, Howard G, Hu F, Inker L, Karthikeyan G, Kassebaum N, Koroshetz W, Lavie C, Lloyd-Jones D, Lu HS, Mirijello A, Temesgen AM, Mokdad A, Moran AE, Muntner P, Narula J, Neal B, Ntsekhe M, Moraes de Oliveira G, Otto C, Owolabi M, Pratt M, Rajagopalan S, Reitsma M, ALP R, Rigotti N, Rodgers A, Sable C, Shakil S, Sliwa-Hahnle K, Stark B, Sundstrom J, Timpel P, Tleyjeh IM, Valgimigli M, Vos T, Whelton PK, Yacoub M, Zuhlke L, Murray C, Fuster V, Group G-N-JGBoCDW. Global Burden of Cardiovascular Diseases and Risk Factors, 1990–2019: Update From the GBD 2019 Study. J Am Coll Cardiol. 2020(76):2982–3021.
2. Vogel B, Acevedo M, Appelman Y, Bairey Merz CN, Chieffo A, Figtree GA, Guerrero M, Kunadian V, Lam CSP, Maas A, Mihailidou AS, Olszanecka A, Poole JE, Saldarriaga C, Saw J, Zuhlke L, Mehran R. The Lancet women and cardiovascular disease Commission: reducing the global burden by 2030. Lancet. 2021;397:2385–438.
3. Figtree GA, Vernon ST, Hadziosmanovic N, Sundstrom J, Alfredsoo J, Arnott C, Delatour V, Leodottir M and Hagstrom E. Mortality in STEMI patients without standard modifiable risk factors: a sex disaggregated analysis from the SWEDEHEART registry. Lancet 2021;S0140–6736:272–5.
4. Vernon ST, Coffey S, Bhindi R, Soo Hoo SY, Nelson GI, Ward MR, Hansen PS, Asrress KN, Chow CK, Celermajer DS, O'Sullivan JF, Figtree GA. Increasing proportion of ST elevation myocardial infarction patients with coronary atherosclerosis poorly explained by standard modifiable risk factors. Eur J Prev Cardiol. 2017;24:1824–30.
5. Vernon ST, Coffey S, D'Souza M, Chow CK, Kilian J, Hyun K, Shaw JA, Adams M, Roberts-Thomson P, Brieger D, Figtree GA. ST-Segment-Elevation Myocardial Infarction (STEMI) Patients Without Standard Modifiable Cardiovascular Risk Factors-How Common Are They, and What Are Their Outcomes? J Am Heart Assoc. 2019;8:e013296.
6. Visseren FLJ, Mach F, Smulders YM, Carballo D, Koskinas KC, Back M, Benetos A, Biffi A, Boavida JM, Capodanno D, Cosyns B, Crawford C, Davos CH, Desormais I, Di Angelantonio E, Franco OH, Halvorsen S, FDR H, Hollander M, Jankowska EA, Michal M, Sacco S, Sattar

N, Tokgozoglu L, Tonstad S, Tsioufis KP, van Dis I, van Gelder IC, Wanner C, Williams B, Societies ESCNC and Group ESCSD. ESC Guidelines on cardiovascular disease prevention in clinical practice. Eur Heart J. 2021;2021(42):3227–337.
7. Chow CK, Atkins ER, Hillis GS, Nelson MR, Reid CM, Schlaich MP, Hay P, Rogers K, Billot L, Burke M, Chalmers J, Neal B, Patel A, Usherwood T, Webster R, Rodgers A. Initial treatment with a single pill containing quadruple combination of quarter doses of blood pressure medicines versus standard dose monotherapy in patients with hypertension (QUARTET): a phase 3, randomised, double-blind, active-controlled trial. Lancet. 2021;398:1043–52.
8. Lim SS, Vos T, Flaxman AD, Danaei G, Shibuya K, Adair-Rohani H, Amann M, Anderson HR, Andrews KG, Aryee M, Atkinson C, Bacchus LJ, Bahalim AN, Balakrishnan K, Balmes J, Barker-Collo S, Baxter A, Bell ML, Blore JD, Blyth F, Bonner C, Borges G, Bourne R, Boussinesq M, Brauer M, Brooks P, Bruce NG, Brunekreef B, Bryan-Hancock C, Bucello C, Buchbinder R, Bull F, Burnett RT, Byers TE, Calabria B, Carapetis J, Carnahan E, Chafe Z, Charlson F, Chen H, Chen JS, Cheng AT, Child JC, Cohen A, Colson KE, Cowie BC, Darby S, Darling S, Davis A, Degenhardt L, Dentener F, Des Jarlais DC, Devries K, Dherani M, Ding EL, Dorsey ER, Driscoll T, Edmond K, Ali SE, Engell RE, Erwin PJ, Fahimi S, Falder G, Farzadfar F, Ferrari A, Finucane MM, Flaxman S, Fowkes FG, Freedman G, Freeman MK, Gakidou E, Ghosh S, Giovannucci E, Gmel G, Graham K, Grainger R, Grant B, Gunnell D, Gutierrez HR, Hall W, Hoek HW, Hogan A, Hosgood HD 3rd, Hoy D, Hu H, Hubbell BJ, Hutchings SJ, Ibeanusi SE, Jacklyn GL, Jasrasaria R, Jonas JB, Kan H, Kanis JA, Kassebaum N, Kawakami N, Khang YH, Khatibzadeh S, Khoo JP, Kok C, Laden F, Lalloo R, Lan Q, Lathlean T, Leasher JL, Leigh J, Li Y, Lin JK, Lipshultz SE, London S, Lozano R, Lu Y, Mak J, Malekzadeh R, Mallinger L, Marcenes W, March L, Marks R, Martin R, McGale P, McGrath J, Mehta S, Mensah GA, Merriman TR, Micha R, Michaud C, Mishra V, Mohd Hanafiah K, Mokdad AA, Morawska L, Mozaffarian D, Murphy T, Naghavi M, Neal B, Nelson PK, Nolla JM, Norman R, Olives C, Omer SB, Orchard J, Osborne R, Ostro B, Page A, Pandey KD, Parry CD, Passmore E, Patra J, Pearce N, Pelizzari PM, Petzold M, Phillips MR, Pope D, Pope CA 3rd, Powles J, Rao M, Razavi H, Rehfuess EA, Rehm JT, Ritz B, Rivara FP, Roberts T, Robinson C, Rodriguez-Portales JA, Romieu I, Room R, Rosenfeld LC, Roy A, Rushton L, Salomon JA, Sampson U, Sanchez-Riera L, Sanman E, Sapkota A, Seedat S, Shi P, Shield K, Shivakoti R, Singh GM, Sleet DA, Smith E, Smith KR, Stapelberg NJ, Steenland K, Stockl H, Stovner LJ, Straif K, Straney L, Thurston GD, Tran JH, Van Dingenen R, van Donkelaar A, Veerman JL, Vijayakumar L, Weintraub R, Weissman MM, White RA, Whiteford H, Wiersma ST, Wilkinson JD, Williams HC, Williams W, Wilson N, Woolf AD, Yip P, Zielinski JM, Lopez AD, Murray CJ, Ezzati M, AlMazroa MA, Memish ZA. A comparative risk assessment of burden of disease and injury attributable to 67 risk factors and risk factor clusters in 21 regions, 1990–2010: a systematic analysis for the Global Burden of Disease Study 2010. Lancet. 2012;380:2224–60.
9. Yusuf S, Hawken S, Ounpuu S, Dans T, Avezum A, Lanas F, McQueen M, Budaj A, Pais P, Varigos J, Lisheng L, Investigators IS. Effect of potentially modifiable risk factors associated with myocardial infarction in 52 countries (the INTERHEART study): case-control study. Lancet. 2004;364:937–52.
10. Group SR, Wright JT Jr, Williamson JD, Whelton PK, Snyder JK, Sink KM, Rocco MV, Reboussin DM, Rahman M, Oparil S, Lewis CE, Kimmel PL, Johnson KC, Goff DC Jr, Fine LJ, Cutler JA, Cushman WC, Cheung AK, Ambrosius WT. A Randomized Trial of Intensive versus Standard Blood-Pressure Control. N Engl J Med. 2015;373:2103–16.
11. Turnbull F, Neal B, Ninomiya T, Algert C, Arima H, Barzi F, Bulpitt C, Chalmers J, Fagard R, Gleason A, Heritier S, Li N, Perkovic V, Woodward M, MacMahon S. Effects of different regimens to lower blood pressure on major cardiovascular events in older and younger adults: meta-analysis of randomised trials. BMJ. 2008;336:1121–3.

12. Law MR, Morris JK, Wald NJ. Use of blood pressure lowering drugs in the prevention of cardiovascular disease: meta-analysis of 147 randomised trials in the context of expectations from prospective epidemiological studies. BMJ. 2009;338:b1665.
13. Materson BJ, Reda DJ, Cushman WC, Massie BM, Freis ED, Kochar MS, Hamburger RJ, Fye C, Lakshman R, Gottdiener J, et al. Single-drug therapy for hypertension in men. A comparison of six antihypertensive agents with placebo. The Department of Veterans Affairs Cooperative Study Group on Antihypertensive Agents. N Engl J Med. 1993;328:914–21.
14. Dickerson JE, Hingorani AD, Ashby MJ, Palmer CR, Brown MJ. Optimisation of antihypertensive treatment by crossover rotation of four major classes. Lancet. 1999;353:2008–13.
15. Epstein M, Bakris G. Newer approaches to antihypertensive therapy. Use of fixed-dose combination therapy. Arch Intern Med. 1996;156:1969–78.
16. Cholesterol Treatment Trialists C, Baigent C, Blackwell L, Emberson J, Holland LE, Reith C, Bhala N, Peto R, Barnes EH, Keech A, Simes J, Collins R. Efficacy and safety of more intensive lowering of LDL cholesterol: a meta-analysis of data from 170,000 participants in 26 randomised trials. Lancet. 2010;376:1670–81.
17. Ference BA, Ginsberg HN, Graham I, Ray KK, Packard CJ, Bruckert E, Hegele RA, Krauss RM, Raal FJ, Schunkert H, Watts GF, Boren J, Fazio S, Horton JD, Masana L, Nicholls SJ, Nordestgaard BG, van de Sluis B, Taskinen MR, Tokgozoglu L, Landmesser U, Laufs U, Wiklund O, Stock JK, Chapman MJ, Catapano AL. Low-density lipoproteins cause atherosclerotic cardiovascular disease. 1. Evidence from genetic, epidemiologic, and clinical studies. A consensus statement from the European Atherosclerosis Society Consensus Panel. Eur Heart J. 2017;38:2459–72.
18. Ference BA, Robinson JG, Brook RD, Catapano AL, Chapman MJ, Neff DR, Voros S, Giugliano RP, Davey Smith G, Fazio S, Sabatine MS. Variation in PCSK9 and HMGCR and Risk of Cardiovascular Disease and Diabetes. N Engl J Med. 2016;375:2144–53.
19. Shepherd J. The West of Scotland Coronary Prevention Study: a trial of cholesterol reduction in Scottish men. Am J Cardiol. 1995;76:113C–7C.
20. Cholesterol Treatment Trialists C, Mihaylova B, Emberson J, Blackwell L, Keech A, Simes J, Barnes EH, Voysey M, Gray A, Collins R, Baigent C. The effects of lowering LDL cholesterol with statin therapy in people at low risk of vascular disease: meta-analysis of individual data from 27 randomised trials. Lancet. 2012;380:581–90.
21. Heart Protection Study Collaborative Group. MRC/BHF Heart Protection Study of antioxidant vitamin supplementation in 20,536 high-risk individuals: a randomised placebo-controlled trial. Lancet. 2002;360:23–33.
22. Ballantyne CM, Houri J, Notarbartolo A, Melani L, Lipka LJ, Suresh R, Sun S, AP LB, Sager PT, Veltri EP, Ezetimibe Study G. Effect of ezetimibe coadministered with atorvastatin in 628 patients with primary hypercholesterolemia: a prospective, randomized, double-blind trial. Circulation. 2003;107:2409–15.
23. Cannon CP, Blazing MA, Giugliano RP, McCagg A, White JA, Theroux P, Darius H, Lewis BS, Ophuis TO, Jukema JW, De Ferrari GM, Ruzyllo W, De Lucca P, Im K, Bohula EA, Reist C, Wiviott SD, Tershakovec AM, Musliner TA, Braunwald E, Califf RM, Investigators I-I. Ezetimibe Added to Statin Therapy after Acute Coronary Syndromes. N Engl J Med. 2015;372:2387–97.
24. Serban MC, Banach M, Mikhailidis DP. Clinical implications of the IMPROVE-IT trial in the light of current and future lipid-lowering treatment options. Expert Opin Pharmacother. 2016;17:369–80.
25. Sabatine MS, Giugliano RP, Pedersen TR. Evolocumab in Patients with Cardiovascular Disease. N Engl J Med. 2017;377:787–8.
26. Schwartz GG, Steg PG, Szarek M, Bhatt DL, Bittner VA, Diaz R, Edelberg JM, Goodman SG, Hanotin C, Harrington RA, Jukema JW, Lecorps G, Mahaffey KW, Moryusef A, Pordy R,

Quintero K, Roe MT, Sasiela WJ, Tamby JF, Tricoci P, White HD, Zeiher AM. Committees OO and Investigators. Alirocumab and Cardiovascular Outcomes after Acute Coronary Syndrome. N Engl J Med. 2018;379:2097–107.

27. Ray KK, Wright RS, Kallend D, Koenig W, Leiter LA, Raal FJ, Bisch JA, Richardson T, Jaros M, Wijngaard PLJ, Kastelein JJP, Orion and Investigators O-. Two Phase 3 Trials of Inclisiran in Patients with Elevated LDL Cholesterol. N Engl J Med. 2020;382:1507–19.
28. Peters SA, Huxley RR, Woodward M. Diabetes as risk factor for incident coronary heart disease in women compared with men: a systematic review and meta-analysis of 64 cohorts including 858,507 individuals and 28,203 coronary events. Diabetologia. 2014;57:1542–51.
29. de Jong M, Woodward M, Peters SAE. Diabetes, Glycated Hemoglobin, and the Risk of Myocardial Infarction in Women and Men: A Prospective Cohort Study of the UK Biobank. Diabetes Care. 2020;43:2050–9.
30. Carbone S, Dixon DL, Buckley LF, Abbate A. Glucose-Lowering Therapies for Cardiovascular Risk Reduction in Type 2 Diabetes Mellitus: State-of-the-Art Review. Mayo Clin Proc. 2018;93:1629–47.
31. Zinman B, Wanner C, Lachin JM, Fitchett D, Bluhmki E, Hantel S, Mattheus M, Devins T, Johansen OE, Woerle HJ, Broedl UC, Inzucchi SE, Investigators E-RO. Empagliflozin, Cardiovascular Outcomes, and Mortality in Type 2 Diabetes. N Engl J Med. 2015;373:2117–28.
32. Neal B, Perkovic V, Mahaffey KW, de Zeeuw D, Fulcher G, Erondu N, Shaw W, Law G, Desai M, Matthews DR, Group CPC. Canagliflozin and Cardiovascular and Renal Events in Type 2 Diabetes. N Engl J Med. 2017;377:644–57.
33. Teo YH, Teo YN, Syn NL, Kow CS, Yoong CSY, Tan BYQ, Yeo TC, Lee CH, Lin W, Sia CH. Effects of Sodium/Glucose Cotransporter 2 (SGLT2) Inhibitors on Cardiovascular and Metabolic Outcomes in Patients Without Diabetes Mellitus: A Systematic Review and Meta-Analysis of Randomized-Controlled Trials. J Am Heart Assoc. 2021;10:e019463.
34. Sheahan KH, Wahlberg EA, Gilbert MP. An overview of GLP-1 agonists and recent cardiovascular outcomes trials. Postgrad Med J. 2020;96:156–61.
35. Arnott C, Li Q, Kang A, Neuen BL, Bompoint S, Lam CSP, Rodgers A, Mahaffey KW, Cannon CP, Perkovic V, Jardine MJ, Neal B. Sodium-Glucose Cotransporter 2 Inhibition for the Prevention of Cardiovascular Events in Patients With Type 2 Diabetes Mellitus: A Systematic Review and Meta-Analysis. J Am Heart Assoc. 2020;9:e014908.
36. McDonagh TA, Metra M, Adamo M, Gardner RS, Baumbach A, Bohm M, Burri H, Butler J, Celutkiene J, Chioncel O, JGF C, AJS C, Crespo-Leiro MG, Farmakis D, Gilard M, Heymans S, Hoes AW, Jaarsma T, Jankowska EA, Lainscak M, CSP L, Lyon AR, JJV MM, Mebazaa A, Mindham R, Muneretto C, Francesco Piepoli M, Price S, GMC R, Ruschitzka F, Kathrine Skibelund A, Group ESCSD. ESC Guidelines for the diagnosis and treatment of acute and chronic heart failure. Eur Heart J. 2021;2021(42):3599–726.
37. Doll R, Peto R, Boreham J, Sutherland I. Mortality in relation to smoking: 50 years' observations on male British doctors. BMJ. 2004;328:1519.
38. Prescott E, Hippe M, Schnohr P, Hein HO, Vestbo J. Smoking and risk of myocardial infarction in women and men: longitudinal population study. BMJ. 1998;316:1043–7.
39. Messner B, Bernhard D. Smoking and cardiovascular disease: mechanisms of endothelial dysfunction and early atherogenesis. Arterioscler Thromb Vasc Biol. 2014;34:509–15.
40. Dyer O. New Zealand plans to outlaw tobacco sales to citizens born after 2008. BMJ. 2021;375:n3057.
41. Piper ME, Smith SS, Schlam TR, Fiore MC, Jorenby DE, Fraser D, Baker TB. A randomized placebo-controlled clinical trial of 5 smoking cessation pharmacotherapies. Arch Gen Psychiatry. 2009;66:1253–62.

42. Srivastava G, Apovian CM. Current pharmacotherapy for obesity. Nat Rev Endocrinol. 2018;14:12–24.
43. Doumouras AG, Wong JA, Paterson JM, Lee Y, Sivapathasundaram B, Tarride JE, Thabane L, Hong D, Yusuf S and Anvari M. Bariatric Surgery and Cardiovascular Outcomes in Patients With Obesity and Cardiovascular Disease: A Population-Based Retrospective Cohort Study. Circulation 2021;143:1468–1480.
44. Singh P, Subramanian A, Adderley N, Gokhale K, Singhal R, Bellary S, Nirantharakumar K, Tahrani AA. Impact of bariatric surgery on cardiovascular outcomes and mortality: a population-based cohort study. Br J Surg. 2020;107:432–42.
45. Moussa O, Ardissino M, Heaton T, Tang A, Khan O, Ziprin P, Darzi A, Collins P, Purkayastha S. Effect of bariatric surgery on long-term cardiovascular outcomes: a nationwide nested cohort study. Eur Heart J. 2020;41:2660–7.
46. Al-Kindi SG, Brook RD, Biswal S, Rajagopalan S. Environmental determinants of cardiovascular disease: lessons learned from air pollution. Nat Rev Cardiol. 2020;17:656–72.
47. Wolf K, Hoffmann B, Andersen ZJ, Atkinson RW, Bauwelinck M, Bellander T, Brandt J, Brunekreef B, Cesaroni G, Chen J, de Faire U, de Hoogh K, Fecht D, Forastiere F, Gulliver J, Hertel O, Hvidtfeldt UA, Janssen NAH, Jørgensen JT, Katsouyanni K, Ketzel M, Klompmaker JO, Lager A, Liu S, MacDonald CJ, Magnusson PKE, Mehta AJ, Nagel G, Oftedal B, Pedersen NL, Pershagen G, Raaschou-Nielsen O, Renzi M, Rizzuto D, Rodopoulou S, Samoli E, van der Schouw YT, Schramm S, Schwarze P, Sigsgaard T, Sørensen M, Stafoggia M, Strak M, Tjønneland A, Verschuren WMM, Vienneau D, Weinmayr G, Hoek G, Peters A, Ljungman PLS. Long-term exposure to low-level ambient air pollution and incidence of stroke and coronary heart disease: a pooled analysis of six European cohorts within the ELAPSE project. Lancet Planet Health. 2021;5:e620–32.
48. Bhatnagar A. Environmental Determinants of Cardiovascular Disease. Circ Res. 2017;121:162–80.
49. Sattelmair J, Pertman J, Ding EL, Kohl HW, Haskell W, Lee I-M. Dose Response Between Physical Activity and Risk of Coronary Heart Disease. Circulation. 2011;124:789–95.
50. Taylor RS, Brown A, Ebrahim S, Jolliffe J, Noorani H, Rees K, Skidmore B, Stone JA, Thompson DR, Oldridge N. Exercise-based rehabilitation for patients with coronary heart disease: systematic review and meta-analysis of randomized controlled trials. Am J Med. 2004;116:682–92.
51. van Dam RM, Rimm EB, Willett WC, Stampfer MJ, Hu FB. Dietary Patterns and Risk for Type 2 Diabetes Mellitus in U.S. Men. Ann Intern Med. 2002;136:201–9.
52. D'Agostino RB Sr, Vasan RS, Pencina MJ, Wolf PA, Cobain M, Massaro JM, Kannel WB. General cardiovascular risk profile for use in primary care: the Framingham Heart Study. Circulation. 2008;117:743–53.
53. D'Agostino RB Sr, Grundy S, Sullivan LM, Wilson P. Validation of the Framingham coronary heart disease prediction scores: results of a multiple ethnic groups investigation. JAMA. 2001;286:180–7.
54. Goff DC Jr, Lloyd-Jones DM, Bennett G, Coady S, D'Agostino RB, Gibbons R, Greenland P, Lackland DT, Levy D, O'Donnell CJ, Robinson JG, Schwartz JS, Shero ST, Smith SC Jr, Sorlie P, Stone NJ, Wilson PW, Jordan HS, Nevo L, Wnek J, Anderson JL, Halperin JL, Albert NM, Bozkurt B, Brindis RG, Curtis LH, DeMets D, Hochman JS, Kovacs RJ, Ohman EM, Pressler SJ, Sellke FW, Shen WK, Smith SC Jr, Tomaselli GF. 2013 ACC/AHA guideline on the assessment of cardiovascular risk: a report of the American College of Cardiology/American Heart Association Task Force on Practice Guidelines. Circulation. 2014;129:S49–73.
55. Ridker PM, Buring JE, Rifai N, Cook NR. Development and validation of improved algorithms for the assessment of global cardiovascular risk in women: the Reynolds Risk Score. JAMA. 2007;297:611–9.

56. Ridker PM, Paynter NP, Rifai N, Gaziano JM and Cook NR. C-reactive protein and parental history improve global cardiovascular risk prediction: the Reynolds Risk Score for men. *Circulation*. 2008;118:2243–51, 4p following 2251.
57. Pylypchuk R, Wells S, Kerr A, Poppe K, Riddell T, Harwood M, Exeter D, Mehta S, Grey C, Wu BP, Metcalf P, Warren J, Harrison J, Marshall R, Jackson R. Cardiovascular disease risk prediction equations in 400 000 primary care patients in New Zealand: a derivation and validation study. Lancet. 2018;391:1897–907.
58. group Sw and collaboration ESCCr. SCORE2 risk prediction algorithms: new models to estimate 10-year risk of cardiovascular disease in Europe. Eur Heart J. 2021;42:2439–54.
59. DeFilippis AP, Young R, Carrubba CJ, McEvoy JW, Budoff MJ, Blumenthal RS, Kronmal RA, McClelland RL, Nasir K, Blaha MJ. An analysis of calibration and discrimination among multiple cardiovascular risk scores in a modern multiethnic cohort. Ann Intern Med. 2015;162:266–75.
60. Rajan S, McKee M, Rangarajan S, Bangdiwala S, Rosengren A, Gupta R, Kutty VR, Wielgosz A, Lear S, AlHabib KF, Co HU, Lopez-Jaramillo P, Avezum A, Seron P, Oguz A, Kruger IM, Diaz R, Nafiza M-N, Chifamba J, Yeates K, Kelishadi R, Sharief WM, Szuba A, Khatib R, Rahman O, Iqbal R, Bo H, Yibing Z, Wei L, Yusuf S, for the Prospective Urban Rural Epidemiology Study I. Association of Symptoms of Depression With Cardiovascular Disease and Mortality in Low-, Middle-, and High-Income Countries. JAMA Psychiat. 2020;77:1052–63.
61. Garcia M, Mulvagh SL, Merz CNB, Buring JE, Manson JE. Cardiovascular Disease in Women: Clinical Perspectives. Circ Res. 2016;118:1273–93.
62. Durante A, Bronzato S. The increased cardiovascular risk in patients affected by autoimmune diseases: review of the various manifestations. J Clin Med Res. 2015;7:379–84.
63. Alexandre J, Cautela J, Ederhy S, Damaj GL, Salem JE, Barlesi F, Farnault L, Charbonnier A, Mirabel M, Champiat S, Cohen-Solal A, Cohen A, Dolladille C and Thuny F. Cardiovascular Toxicity Related to Cancer Treatment: A Pragmatic Approach to the American and European Cardio-Oncology Guidelines. J Am Heart Assoc 2020;9:e018403.
64. Enas EA, Varkey B, Dharmarajan TS, Pare G, Bahl VK. Lipoprotein(a): An independent, genetic, and causal factor for cardiovascular disease and acute myocardial infarction. Indian Heart J. 2019;71:99–112.
65. Tsimikas S, Moriarty PM, Stroes ES. Emerging RNA Therapeutics to Lower Blood Levels of Lp(a). J Am Coll Cardiol. 2021;77:1576–89.
66. Mahmood SS, Levy D, Vasan RS, Wang TJ. The Framingham Heart Study and the epidemiology of cardiovascular disease: a historical perspective. Lancet. 2014;383:999–1008.
67. Figtree GA, Vernon ST, Hadziosmanovic N, Sundström J, Alfredsson J, Arnott C, Delatour V, Leósdóttir M, Hagström E. Mortality in STEMI patients without standard modifiable risk factors: a sex-disaggregated analysis of SWEDEHEART registry data. Lancet. 2021;397:1085–94.
68. Rumberger JA, Schwartz RS, Simons DB, Sheedy PF 3rd, Edwards WD, Fitzpatrick LA. Relation of coronary calcium determined by electron beam computed tomography and lumen narrowing determined by autopsy. Am J Cardiol. 1994;73:1169–73.
69. Otsuka F, Sakakura K, Yahagi K, Joner M, Virmani R. Has our understanding of calcification in human coronary atherosclerosis progressed? Arterioscler Thromb Vasc Biol. 2014;34:724–36.
70. Agatston AS, Janowitz WR, Hildner FJ, Zusmer NR, Viamonte M Jr, Detrano R. Quantification of coronary artery calcium using ultrafast computed tomography. J Am Coll Cardiol. 1990;15:827–32.
71. Mohlenkamp S, Lehmann N, Moebus S, Schmermund A, Dragano N, Stang A, Siegrist J, Mann K, Jockel KH, Erbel R, Heinz Nixdorf Recall Study I. Quantification of coronary atherosclerosis and inflammation to predict coronary events and all-cause mortality. J Am Coll Cardiol. 2011;57:1455–64.

72. Yeboah J, Young R, McClelland RL, Delaney JC, Polonsky TS, Dawood FZ, Blaha MJ, Miedema MD, Sibley CT, Carr JJ, Burke GL, Goff DC Jr, Psaty BM, Greenland P, Herrington DM. Utility of Nontraditional Risk Markers in Atherosclerotic Cardiovascular Disease Risk Assessment. J Am Coll Cardiol. 2016;67:139–47.
73. Kondos GT, Hoff JA, Sevrukov A, Daviglus ML, Garside DB, Devries SS, Chomka EV, Liu K. Electron-beam tomography coronary artery calcium and cardiac events: a 37-month follow-up of 5635 initially asymptomatic low- to intermediate-risk adults. Circulation. 2003;107:2571–6.
74. Kelkar AA, Schultz WM, Khosa F, Schulman-Marcus J, O'Hartaigh BW, Gransar H, Blaha MJ, Knapper JT, Berman DS, Quyyumi A, Budoff MJ, Callister TQ, Min JK, Shaw LJ. Long-Term Prognosis After Coronary Artery Calcium Scoring Among Low-Intermediate Risk Women and Men. Circ Cardiovasc Imaging. 2016;9:e003742.
75. Ripatti S, Tikkanen E, Orho-Melander M, Havulinna AS, Silander K, Sharma A, Guiducci C, Perola M, Jula A, Sinisalo J, Lokki ML, Nieminen MS, Melander O, Salomaa V, Peltonen L, Kathiresan S. A multilocus genetic risk score for coronary heart disease: case-control and prospective cohort analyses. Lancet. 2010;376:1393–400.
76. Khera AV, Chaffin M, Aragam KG, Haas ME, Roselli C, Choi SH, Natarajan P, Lander ES, Lubitz SA, Ellinor PT, Kathiresan S. Genome-wide polygenic scores for common diseases identify individuals with risk equivalent to monogenic mutations. Nat Genet. 2018;50:1219–24.
77. Abraham G, Havulinna AS, Bhalala OG, Byars SG, De Livera AM, Yetukuri L, Tikkanen E, Perola M, Schunkert H, Sijbrands EJ, Palotie A, Samani NJ, Salomaa V, Ripatti S, Inouye M. Genomic prediction of coronary heart disease. Eur Heart J. 2016;37:3267–78.
78. Dikilitas O, He B, Bailey K, Kullo I. Association of Polygenic Risk Scores with Premature Coronary Heart Disease: A Comparative Study. J Am Coll Cardiol. 2019:73.
79. Wunnemann F, Sin Lo K, Langford-Avelar A, Busseuil D, Dube MP, Tardif JC, Lettre G. Validation of Genome-Wide Polygenic Risk Scores for Coronary Artery Disease in French Canadians. Circ Genom Precis Med. 2019;12:e002481.
80. Bolli A, Di Domenico P, Botta G. Software as a service for the genomic prediction of complex diseases. bioRxiv. 2019; https://doi.org/10.1101/763722.
81. Nicholls SJ, Vernon S and Figtree GA. Taking the next steps to implement polygenic risk scoring for improved risk stratification and primary prevention of coronary artery disease. *European Journal of Preventive Cardiology*. 2020;In press (accepted July 2020: https://doi.org/10.1093/eurjpc/zwaa030).
82. Figtree GA, Vernon ST. Coronary artery disease patients without standard modifiable risk factors (SMuRFs)—a forgotten group calling out for new discoveries. Cardiovasc Res. 2021;117:e76–8.
83. Mazhar J, Figtree GA, Vernon S, Galougahi KK, Carlo J, Nissen SE, Nicholls SJ. Progression of coronary atherosclerosis in patients without standard modifiable risk factors. Am J Prev Cardiol. 2020;4:100116.
84. Vernon ST, Hansen T, Kott KA, Yang JY, O'Sullivan JF, Figtree GA. Utilizing state-of-the-art "omics" technology and bioinformatics to identify new biological mechanisms and biomarkers for coronary artery disease. Microcirculation. 2019;26:e12488.
85. Vernon ST, Tang O, Kim T, Chan AS, Kott KA, Park J, Hansen T, Koay YC, Grieve SM, O'Sullivan JF, Yang JY, Figtree GA. Metabolic Signatures in Coronary Artery Disease: Results from the BioHEART-CT Study. Cell. 2021:10.
86. Kott KA, Vernon S, Hansen T, de Dreau M, Das S, Fazekas B, Di Bartolo BA, McGuire HM and Figtree GA. Single-cell immune profiling in coronary artery disease: the role of state-of-the-art immunophenotyping with mass cytometry in the diagnosis of atherosclerosis. *J Am Heart Assoc*. 2020;In press (accepted October 2020).

87. Kott KA, Vernon ST, Hansen T, Yu C, Bubb KJ, Coffey S, Sullivan D, Yang J, O'Sullivan J, Chow C, Patel S, Chong J, Celermajer DS, Kritharides L, Grieve SM, Figtree GA. Biobanking for discovery of novel cardiovascular biomarkers using imaging-quantified disease burden: protocol for the longitudinal, prospective, BioHEART-CT cohort study. BMJ Open. 2019;9:e028649.
88. Mamudu H, Paul T, Veeranki SP, Budoff M. The effects of coronary artery calcium screening on behavioral modification, risk perception, and medication adherence among asymptomatic adults: A systematic review. Atherosclerosis. 2014;236:338–50.

History of Ischemic Heart Disease

Giovanni Concistrè

1 Introduction

Is heart attack a modern plague or does it come down from antiquity? Who first described the clinical picture and who first tied it to disease of the coronary arteries? When and by whom was the connection established between atherosclerosis or fatty arteries, and thrombosis and the syndromes of angina pectoris and myocardial infarction? What accounts for the long delay in recognizing the phenomenon of infarction with survival? Where and when did the idea about the potential of preventing heart attack arise?

John Hunter, a brilliant English physician of the eighteenth century, was probably the first in Western medicine to paint the clinical picture of chest pain, called angina pectoris, and sudden death. Noting that his own symptoms were aggravated by anger, he complained that his life was "in the hands of any rascal who chose to annoy or tease" him. He proved the case by dying abruptly after an argument with—we know not whether a rascal—a fellow member of his St. George's Hospital board (Liebowitz 1970, 102).

The history of coronary syndromes and sudden death, and apoplexy or stroke, goes back to antiquity and has been thoroughly treated by historians and experts from many disciplines. By the beginning of the twentieth century, a heart attack with myocardial infarction was well known to cause death, but comprehension of it as a syndrome that one might survive was much delayed. When that awareness finally came and diffused into the practicing community in the 1920s and after, it had a major effect on the recognition of coronary disease as an epidemic after World War II, which, in turn, gave preamble and

G. Concistrè (✉)
Adult Cardiac Surgery Unit, Ospedale del cuore "G. Pasquinucci", Fondazione Toscana G. Monasterio CNR—Regione Toscana, Massa, Italy

G. Concistrè (ed.), *Ischemic Heart Disease*,
https://doi.org/10.1007/978-3-031-25879-4_4

impetus to CVD epidemiology and preventive cardiology. Because coronary disease was newly epidemic, it was reasoned by a few pioneers that its causes, and conceivably its preventives, must therefore lie in changed environment.

2 Ancient Egypt

At the 2009 American Heart Association meeting in Florida, researchers presented study results showing that Egyptian mummies, some 3500 years old, had evidence of cardiovascular disease—specifically atherosclerosis (which narrows the arteries) in different arteries of the body. Pharaoh Merenptah, who died in the year 1203 BCE, was plagued by atherosclerosis. Of the other mummies studied, 9 of the 16 also had probable-to-definite evidence of the disease. How could this be possible? Researchers theorized that diet could be involved. High-status Egyptians may have eaten a lot of fatty meats from cattle, ducks, and geese. Beyond that, the study brought up some interesting questions and has prompted scientists to continue their work to fully understand the condition. "The findings suggest that we may have to look beyond modern risk factors to fully understand the disease," said co-principal investigator on the study, clinical professor of cardiology Dr. Gregory Thomas.

3 Arabia

There is also an accurate but incidental description of angina pectoris in old Arabic love literature revealed in a poem written by Qais ibn Al-Mulawah. It comes from the love story Majnoon Lila. The story is famous in Arabic literature as well as in Arab folk stories. A madman in Arabic is called "Majnoon," so Majnoon Lila means "Crazy about Lila." The poet's name is Qais who lived in the seventh century. In a nutshell, Majnoon Lila is about a young poet, Qais ibn Al-Mulawah, who fell in love with a girl named Lila. The father of Lila refused to consent to their marriage even though Lila also loved Qais [1]. Lila was forced to marry another man and moved out of town. Qais ran away to live in the desert, alone, losing interest in family, friends, and society. He was considered sick with "love madness." He wrote poems about his love to Lila. In his poems, he described his tears, sleeplessness, lack of appetite, racing heartbeats or palpitations, and fainting episodes when Lila left [2].

He died immediately after writing a poem to his beloved Lila saying:

"My heart is firmly seized By a bird's claws;
My heart is tightly squeezed, When Lila's name flows.
My body is tightly bound, My body is tightly bound,
Is like a finger ring around." [2]

An Arab cardiologist, Dr. H. A. Hajar Albinali, the author of an Arabic book Majnoon Lila: Between Medicine and Literature, translated the above poem into English. He claimed that it was the first clear and best description of angina in the history of medicine. He concluded in his book from that poem and other symptoms that the poet had CAD and died with myocardial infarction [2].

4 Seventeenth–Nineteenth-Century Europe

In Europe, it is customary to reference angina pectoris to William Heberden, but he was not the first to describe atherosclerosis. The medical literature is replete with narratives of the first descriptions of a particular disease by different physicians.

Among the first to describe atherosclerosis was Leonardo da Vinci, who reportedly stated that "vessels in the elderly restrict the transit of blood through thickening of the tunics" [3]. Leonardo was not a physician, but he was a great artist and leading intellectual of the Italian Renaissance; he is known as the embodiment of a "Renaissance man." He believed that studying science made him a better artist. He is renowned for painting the Mona Lisa. Leonardo's experiments, anatomical drawings, and notes (often in mirror writing) provide early descriptions of the structure and function of the heart and circulation. His interest in anatomy was inspired by the anatomist Marcantonio della Torre (1473–1511) who was a professor of anatomy in Pisa and then Padua and who commissioned da Vinci to provide the illustrations for his text on anatomy based on dissection [4].

It was, however, William Heberden who brought angina pectoris to the attention of the medical profession when he presented his paper, "Some Account of a Disorder of the Breast," at the Royal College of Physicians in London in 1768 [5]. Many aspects of his description are true to this day. He describes both typical exertional angina and variant angina, which affected a patient only when he/she was in bed and was relieved by sitting up. He also points out the influence of mental stress. Although it is a classic, it is not the first description of angina. Heberden wrote:

"Those who are afflicted with it are seized, while they are walking, and more particularly when they walk soon after eating, with a painful and most disagreeable sensation in the breast, which seems as if it would take their life away, if it were to increase or to continue: The moment they stand still, all this uneasiness vanishes" [3].

Heberden coined the term "angina pectoris" from Greek ankhonē which means "strangling" and Latin pectoris, meaning "chest." That historical term—"angina pectoris"—is still used in this modern era of medicine.

Of interest, John Hunter, the eighteenth-century Scottish surgeon and anatomist, suffered from angina pectoris and he was the first in Europe to mention the effect of emotions in precipitating an attack of angina. Hunter unintentionally proved that when he suddenly collapsed after a dispute with a colleague and died. Marked atheroma (presumably in his coronary) was found on autopsy [6]. John Hunter's death occurred during a period of emerging understanding of the relation between angina pectoris and CAD. However, physicians continued to describe the coronary lesions on pathology specimens without correlating them to clinical signs.

In 1761, the Italian anatomist Giovanni Morgagni described the lesions as "hardening of the arteries" for the first time. Edward Jenner (1729–1823), a British physician and pioneer of smallpox vaccine, and his contemporary colleague, Caleb Parry (1755–1822), linked the excruciating "disorder of the breast" to the "hardening of the arteries." However, the disease was looked on, as still, only with pathologic interest.

In 1856, Rudolf Virchow, the "father of pathology," defined the physiological elements in thrombosis within the vascular system and the risk factors that predispose arteries and veins to thrombus formation. Virchow's concepts on thrombosis remained relevant to the current medicine, especially in cardiology [7]. Only after Virchow postulated the features of thrombosis did scientists begin to consider the clinical implications of coronary heart disease seriously.

Near the end of the nineteenth century, cardiovascular physiologists noted that occlusion of a coronary artery in the dog caused "quivering" of the ventricle which was rapidly fatal. In 1879, the pathologist Ludvig Hektoen concluded that myocardial infarction is caused by coronary thrombosis "secondary to sclerotic changes in the coronaries." In 1910, two Russian clinicians described five patients with the clinical picture of acute myocardial infarction, which was confirmed at postmortem examination. Two years later, James Herrick established the importance of bed rest and used electrocardiography to diagnose the condition [8]. In 1628, in his work De Motu Cordis, William Harvey described the circulation and the function of the heart [8]. These milestones stimulated physicians in successive centuries to explore and put forth theories on the pathogenesis of coronary heart disease, and in the process, they made discoveries on how to improve diagnostic accuracy and treatment.

In the nineteenth century, Claude Bernard catheterized animals, measuring the pressures in the great vessels and cardiac chambers. Werner Forssmann, in 1929, performed cardiac catheterization on himself which led to the exploration of cardiac hemodynamics by Andre Frederic Cournand and Dickinson Richards. These three investigators were awarded the Nobel Prize in Physiology or Medicine in 1956 [8].

5 Coronary Arteriography

The coronary arteriogram truly revolutionized our understanding and management of cardiac patients. Dr. Mason Sones of Cleveland Clinic introduced the selective injection of contrast media into the coronary arteries in 1958 [1]. In the catheterization laboratory in Cleveland Clinic that day, a 26-year-old patient was being evaluated for rheumatic mitral and aortic valve disease when the catheter whiplashed into the ostium of the right coronary artery. Sones was reportedly in the catheterization laboratory at the time and reportedly exclaimed, "we've killed him!" [1].

However, there was no fatal ventricular arrhythmia; the monitor showed only prolonged asystole after sinus arrest that promptly responded to repeated deep coughs. Two days later, Sones proceeded to a planned selective injection of the coronary arteries [1]. The expected ventricular arrhythmias failed to occur, and the technique of selective coronary arteriography was born. The traditional thinking before the introduction of the technique was that if you injected dye into one coronary artery at a time, the resultant asymmetrical hypoxia of the coronary circulation would create an electrical imbalance and fatal ventricular arrhythmia would ensue [1].

The images of the coronary arteries obtained with arteriography provided objective evidence to support or refute the clinical diagnosis of angina pectoris.

Two radiologists, Drs. Judkins and Amplatz, designed catheters and used the Seldinger percutaneous technique to gain access to the femoral artery and engaged the ostia of either the left or the right coronary artery. Their technique required less training than the Sones' technique, which facilitated the widespread use of coronary angiography in cardiology as a diagnostic technique.

The coronary angiogram continues to play an integral role in the diagnosis, management, and planning of future treatment of CAD. It was the first reliable in vivo marker for the presence of obstructing coronary lesions. It provided objective evidence to support or refute the clinical diagnosis of angina pectoris. It became the standard diagnostic tool for defining vessel anatomy and led to the first studies of the natural history of patients with CAD. It also led to studies confirming the benefit of CABG over medical treatment in subsets of patients. It was instrumental in the introduction of percutaneous transluminal coronary angioplasty and delineation of restenosis. It has the ability to compare PCI versus CABG for revascularization outcomes [1].

6 The Treatment of Coronary Artery Disease

In our time, much progress has been learned about the pathogenesis and treatment of ischemic heart disease. Once CAD is diagnosed, the findings from coronary angiography guide the strategy for the best treatment. The options of medical therapy, angioplasty, stenting, or CABG depend largely on the severity of disease.

In general, at present, patients with coronary narrowing that does not limit coronary artery blood flow receive medications and lifestyle modification to help prevent progression. If a patient has coronary atherosclerosis that limits blood flow in the coronary arteries, balloon angioplasty and stenting can be offered. In patients with multiple areas of coronary artery narrowing or blockage, CABG surgery is generally recommended.

Below is a brief summary of the modern advances in the therapy of CAD and AMI.

6.1 Coronary Care Unit

Before 1961, patients with AMI were placed in nonmonitored beds in the hospital and far away from nurses' stations, so the patients would not be disturbed. Patients were found dead in their beds. The risk of death occurring in the hospital was approximately 30% [8]. Development of the CCU [9] took place in 1961. Establishment of the CCU provided continuous ECG monitoring of the patient, closed chest cardiac resuscitation, external defibrillation, and reduced in-hospital mortality by half among patients admitted with AMI. Other influences that reduced mortality were prompt and early diagnosis with sensitive and specific biomarkers [7] and development of surgical methods for revascularization.

6.2 Surgery

The coronary arteriogram provided the foundation for surgical treatment of CAD by means of coronary revascularization. The development and refinement of CABG for the treatment of CAD required close collaborations among surgeons, engineers, cardiologists, anesthesiologists, and hematologists. The heart–lung machine developed by Gibbon [10] was originally introduced into cardiac surgery for the repair of intracardiac defects but was soon adopted by cardiac surgeons for adult coronary revascularizations because of its ability to create a motionless, bloodless operative field. Tens of millions of patients benefitted from coronary revascularization on cardiopulmonary bypass.

6.3 Drug Therapy

There have been many advances in the medical therapy of CAD and AMI. Since the 1970s, large-scale trials have shown that the risk of death is lowered with aspirin, cholesterol-lowering drugs, β-blockers, and angiotensin-converting enzyme inhibitors. However, life-threatening heart failure still occurs late in patients with large infarcts. Prognosis in such patients has been improved with an implantable defibrillator, cardiac resynchronization therapy, pacemakers, and left ventricular assist devices.

Fibrinolytic therapy has been a major advance in the treatment of AMI, leading to improved early survival, less heart failure, less ventricular remodeling, and fewer arrhythmias [11]. SK was the first thrombolytic drug to be used in myocardial infarction. Researchers have known for some time of SK's ability to dissolve clots. Fibrinolysis induced by SK resulted in the breakdown of fibrin. SK was used initially for fibrinous pleural exudates, hemothorax, and tuberculous meningitis. Some researchers started using SK in patients with AMI, offering hope that CAD could be "cured." Experimental intracoronary infusion of SK produced conflicting results initially. Hence, the Italian Group for the Study of Streptokinase in Myocardial Infarction (Gruppo Italiano per la Sperimentazione della Streptochinasi nell'Infarto Miocardico) (GISSI) trial in 1986 addressed this issue by recruiting more than 10,000 patients and proved that SK reduced early mortality in patients with AMI [12].

The thrombolytic era was found on a fundamental concept that most cases of AMI are the result of sudden obstruction of an epicardial coronary artery by intracoronary thrombus superimposed on a ruptured or fissured atherosclerotic plaque. The GISSI study validated SK as an effective therapeutic method, and therefore fixed protocols for its use in AMI were established. SK has been supplanted by tissue plasminogen activator in developed nations, but SK remains essential to the management of AMI in developing nations. The Second International Study of Infarct Survival showed that the addition of aspirin (an antiplatelet drug) led to further reductions in mortality [13].

6.4 Angioplasty

In the recent years, PCI treatment (introduced by the German radiologist Andreas Gruentzig in 1977) for CAD is oftentimes preferred over CABG because the comparative effects of these two revascularization methods on long-term mortality are still unclear. PCI is also less invasive. However, the journal *JAMA* Inter Med [14] in 2014 published a meta-analysis of randomized clinical trials comparing CABG versus PCI. The study found that in patients with multivessel coronary disease, CABG leads to an unequivocal reduction in long-term mortality and myocardial infarctions and to reductions in repeat revascularizations, regardless of whether patients are diabetic or not [14].

Coronary angioplasty and stenting together with newer, more potent platelet inhibitors such as P2Y and glycoprotein IIb/IIIa platelet receptor blockers further reduced in-hospital mortality from AMI to about 7% [8]. The efficacy of these treatments depends on a short interval between the onset of symptoms and the patient arrival at the hospital.

7 Conclusion

CAD and AMI have been with us since antiquity. We understand now that coronary ischemia and AMI are the result of a sudden obstruction of a coronary artery by intracoronary thrombus superimposed on a ruptured atherosclerotic plaque. Advances in modern therapy are based on this concept. However, the clinical problem of CAD and AMI is still being actively investigated in an effort to refine management and hopefully find a cure.

References

1. Ryan TJ. The coronary angiogram and its seminal contributions to cardiovascular medicine over five decades. Circulation. 2002;106:752–6.
2. Hajar HA. Majnoon Lila Chairman's reflections Heart Views. 2003;4:127–33.
3. Slijkhuis W, Mali W, Appelman Y. A historical perspective towards a non-invasive treatment for patients with atherosclerosis. Neth Heart J. 2009;17:140–4.
4. Davies MK, Eollman A. Leonardo da Vinci (1452–1519). Heart. 1996;76:464.
5. van Tellingen C. Chest pain and angina pectoris-Or the ugly swan and the beautiful duckling. Neth Heart J. 2010;18:561–4.

6. Leach A. History of Angina. Res Medica 1967, Special Issue. Lauder Brunton Centenary Symposium on Angina Pectoris. 1967.
7. Hajar R. Evolution of myocardial infarction and its biomarkers: A historical perspective. Heart Views. 2016;17:167–72.
8. Nabel EG, Braunwald E. A tale of coronary artery disease and myocardial infarction. N Engl J Med. 2012;366:54–63.
9. Julian DG. Treatment of cardiac arrest in acute myocardial ischaemia and infarction. Lancet. 1961;2:840–4.
10. Gibbon JH. Jr Application of a mechanical heart and lung apparatus to cardiac surgery. Minn Med. 1954;37:171–85.
11. Yusuf S, Collins R, Peto R, Furberg C, Stampfer MJ, Goldhaber SZ, et al. Intravenous and intracoronary fibrinolytic therapy in acute myocardial infarction: Overview of results on mortality, reinfarction and side-effects from 33 randomized controlled trials. Eur Heart J. 1985;6:556–85.
12. Sikri N, Bardia A. A history of streptokinase use in acute myocardial infarction. Tex Heart Inst J. 2007;34:318–27.
13. Randomised trial of intravenous streptokinase, oral aspirin, both, or neither among 17,187 cases of suspected acute myocardial infarction: ISIS-2. ISIS-2 (Second International Study of Infarct Survival) Collaborative Group. Lancet. 1988;2:349–60.
14. Sipahi I, Akay MH, Dagdelen S, Blitz A, Alhan C. Coronary artery bypass grafting vs. percutaneous coronary intervention and long-term mortality and morbidity in multivessel disease: Meta-analysis of randomized clinical trials of the arterial grafting and stenting era. JAMA Intern Med. 2014;174:223–30.

Pathophysiology of Ischemic Syndromes in Coronary Artery Disease

Avinash V. Sharma and John A. Ambrose

1 Introduction

Heart disease remains the leading cause of death globally accounting for about 18.6 million deaths in 2019. In the USA, CVD was listed as the cause of death in 868,000+ cases in 2017. Coronary heart disease is responsible for over 40% of these deaths and, by far, is the leading contributor to the mortality of CVD. According to statistics from the American Heart Association, CAD accounted for 365,744 deaths in 2018. Approximately every 39 seconds, an American in the USA will have a heart attack [1]. Although the annual death rate related to coronary disease has been declining over the past decade, the burden of disease remains high and the direct and indirect costs of heart disease are in the hundreds of billions of dollars.

2 Pathophysiology of Ischemic Coronary Syndromes

Symptomatic CAD can manifest as stable angina, acute coronary syndromes including sudden coronary death, congestive heart failure, tachy- or brady-arrhythmias, and syncope. This chapter primarily considers the ischemic syndromes of stable angina and acute coronary syndromes including sudden cardiac death. In a majority of cases with the exception of some patients with either type 2 myocardial infarction by the Universal Definition of Myocardial Infarction or coronary microvascular dysfunction,

A. V. Sharma · J. A. Ambrose (✉)
UCSF, Fresno, CA, USA
e-mail: Avinash.sharma@UCSF.edu; john.ambrose@ucsf.edu

G. Concistrè (ed.), *Ischemic Heart Disease*,
https://doi.org/10.1007/978-3-031-25879-4_5

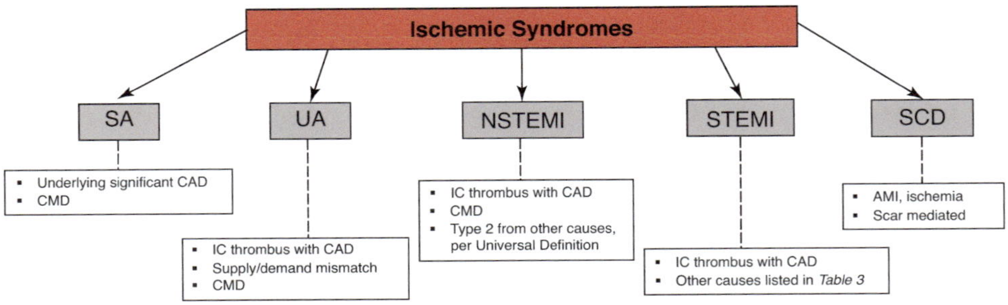

Fig. 1 Ischemic syndromes in coronary artery disease with associated etiologies and pathogenic mechanisms. *AMI* acute myocardial infarction, *CAD* coronary artery disease, *CMD* coronary microvascular dysfunction, *IC* intracoronary, *NSTEMI* non-ST-elevation myocardial infarction, *SA* stable angina, *SCD* sudden cardiac death, *STEMI* ST-elevation myocardial infarction, *UA* unstable angina

their pathophysiology typically involves epicardial coronary artery atherosclerosis (Fig. 1). For clarification, the Universal Definition of Myocardial Infarction is included in Table 1 [2].

Atherosclerosis is accelerated by known cardiovascular risk factors and can progress slowly or rapidly through plaque hemorrhage or intracoronary thrombosis. Common to all syndromes but not necessarily considered in most reviews is the concept of a relative or absolute perturbation in myocardial blood supply relative to myocardial oxygen demand ratio as the cause of all myocardial ischemia/necrosis. Whether one speaks about stable angina, acute syndromes such as myocardial infarction type 1 or 2, or even sudden death, there is an alteration in the supply/demand (S/D) ratio leading to symptoms, which may be extrinsic or intrinsic to the coronary bed. In MI with epicardial coronary artery thrombosis, the supply to the affected territory is usually completely absent at its onset. In type 2 MI, the perturbation in the S/D ratio is extrinsic to the coronary vascular bed caused by either a decreased supply or increased demand. There are other examples of a S/D mismatch intrinsic to the coronary bed. These might include either epicardial or microvascular spasm, microembolization to the distal vasculature bed, and coronary dissection. In stable angina, ischemia occurs when oxygen demands outstrip supply as occurs during exercise or other causes of stress.

Table 1 Fourth Universal Definition for Myocardial Infarction (MI), 2018 [2]. *cTn* cardiac specific troponin, *ECG* electrocardiogram, *MI* myocardial infarction, *RWMA* regional wall motion abnormality, *VF* ventricular fibrillation. *There is still great debate in the literature concerning the amount of troponin rise following percutaneous coronary intervention (PCI) to define the presence of post-PCI MI

Type of Myocardial Infarction	Definition	Notes
Type 1	Rise and/or fall of cTn with at least one value above the 99th percentile and with at least one of the following: • Symptoms of acute myocardial ischemia • New ischemic ECG changes • Development of pathologic Q weaves • Imaging evidence of new loss of viable myocardium or new RWMA in a pattern consistent with an ischemic etiology • Identification of a coronary thrombus by angiography including intracoronary imaging or by autopsy	This is in the setting og plaque rupture or erosion from an existing atherosclerotic plaque
Type 2	Rise and/or fall of cTn with at least one value above the 99th percentile and an imbalance between myocardial oxygen supply and demand unrelated to coronary thrombosis, with at least one of the following: • Symptoms of acute myocardial ischemia • New ischemic ECG changes • Development of pathological Q waves • Imaging evidence of new loss of viable myocardium, or new RWMA in a pattern consistent with an ischemic etiology	Can be secondary to another process (e.g. severe anemia, shock, tachy or brady-arrythmia, severe hypertension) or non-atherothrombotic event (e.g. spontaneous coronary artery dissection, vasospasm, coronary microvascular dysfunction)
Type 3	Cardiac death, with symptoms suggestive of myocardial ischemia with presumed new ischemic ECG changes or VF, but die before serum biomarkers can be obtained, or before increases in cardiac biomarkers can be identified, or MI is detected on autopsy.	
Type 4a	Coronary intervention-related MI, defined by elevation of cTn > 5 times the 99th percentile in patients with normal baseline values. In patients with elevated pre-procedure cTn in whom the cTn level are stable (≤ 20% variation) or falling, the post procedure cTn must rise by > 20%. The absolute post-procedural value must still be ≥ 5 times the 99th percentile with one of the following*: • Symptoms of actue myocardial ischemia • New ischemic ECG changes • Development of pathlogical Q waves • Imageing evidence of new loss of viable myocardium, or new RWMA in a pattern consistent with an ischemic etiology • Angiographic findings consistent with a procedural flow-limiting complication such as coronary dissection, occlusion of a major epicardial artery or a side brance occlusion/thrombus, disruption of collateral flow, or distal embolization	
Type 4b	MI as defined above, and it due to stent/scaffold thrombosis. Noted by timing ad below: • Acute if 0 to 24 hours after • Subacute 24 hours to 30 days • Late 30 days to 1 year • Very late > 1 year after stent/scaffold implantation	
Type 4c	MI as defined above, and it due to in-stent restenosis (ISR). ISR is usually noted focal or diffuse, or complex associated with elevated cTn consistent with above definition for MI	
Type 5	Elevation of cTn>10 times the 99th percentile in patients with normal baseline values. In patients with elevated pre-procedure cTn in whome the cTn level are stable (<20% variation) or falling, the post procedure cTn must rise by > 20%. The absolute post-procedural value must still be > 10 times 99th percentile with one of the following: • Development of new pathological Q waves • Angiographically documented new graft occlusion or new native coronary artery occlusion • Imaging evidence of nwe loss of viable myocardium or new RWMA in a pattern consistent with an ischemic etiology	Post-procedure MI in setting of coronary artery bypass graft surgery

3 Stable Angina

Classically, stable angina is either chest discomfort or atypical symptoms that occur with activity or emotional stress that is, as mentioned above, due to an imbalance in the supply/demand ratio. Most patients have significant coronary atherosclerosis, and symptoms/ischemia occur when the demand outstrips the blood supply. It is predictable and reproducible based on the amount of exercise. In some cases, there can be a variable threshold or even silent ischemia, but the symptoms/ischemia by definition are not changing over time. Variable threshold angina may be due to variations in resting coronary artery tone or different exercise thresholds to the onset of symptoms, but a constant rate pressure product is usually present (peak heart rate X blood pressure) to the onset of ischemia [3].

In patients with a stable angina syndrome and the presence of a single severe lesion on angiography, percutaneous intervention on the affected lesion eliminates symptoms and the patient is followed up with guideline-directed medical therapy. In other cases, in spite of a successful intervention and no other significant obstructive disease, there is still evidence for ongoing ischemia during stress. In those patients, microvascular dysfunction is likely contributing to the symptoms.

4 Coronary Microvasculature Dysfunction

Symptoms of stable angina can occur without the evidence of significant obstructive disease. Over the past several years, there has been an increasingly recognized patient population with symptoms of stable angina, but without evidence of significant obstructive coronary artery disease. Recently, clinical and research interest has grown to characterize this condition, which bears the name ischemia with nonobstructive coronary artery disease (INOCA). Patients experience typical anginal symptoms with objective evidence of ischemia, usually by noninvasive stress testing, and undergo angiography for an assessment of their coronary anatomy. The pathophysiology is usually not due to epicardial stenoses but in the arterioles, invisible on angiography. It is referred to as CMD. Angiography reveals nonobstructive CAD, <50% stenosis of epicardial coronary arteries including no recognizable angiographic stenosis in these patients. Varying population data and studies have reported that this entity may be present in approximately 50–70% of women and 30–50% of men who undergo clinically indicated angiography for evaluation of coronary ischemia [4, 5]. CMD not only is seen in stable angina, but may also present as unstable angina or NSTEMI.

The pathophysiology behind INOCA is believed to be multifactorial, and this chapter will not address the plaque-related causes, such as plaque rupture of small epicardial plaques [6]. Two specific processes may represent a majority of these cases. These include CMD and coronary vasospasm. The latter can exist both in the epicardial arteries occasionally and coronary microcirculation (e.g., arterioles and capillaries). These two may exist independently, but may also overlap such as in microvascular angina—clinical symptoms of ischemia with established CMD. Other causes for INOCA include coronary artery anomalies, valvular heart disease (e.g., severe aortic stenosis), increased platelet aggregability, and occasionally myocardial bridging [7]. Previously, myocardial bridging was thought to be highly prevalent, with up to 86% on older autopsy data [8]. However, more recent coronary CT angiography data estimates approximately 25–30% [9], still higher compared to angiography studies [8], but most of these patients are asymptomatic.

The coronary circuit can be divided into three compartments, as outlined by Del Buono et al. [10]. These include epicardial vessels (0.5–5 mm in diameter), pre-arteriolar vessels (100–500 μm), and intramural arterioles (<100 μm). The pre-arteriolar compartment is responsible for a large portion of vascular resistance to coronary blood flow and is sensitive to pressure changes across the system. Being the last and smallest compartment, intramural arterioles have a main role to match myocardial blood supply with tissue oxygen consumption and demand. CMD is characterized by cardiovascular symptoms and myocardial ischemia due to abnormalities in the coronary microcirculation, defined by the arterioles and capillaries (typically <500 μm in diameter). A variety of mechanisms have been proposed to contribute to the physiology behind CMD. These include structural, molecular, and functional abnormalities [11].

Normal endothelium in the microcirculation plays a role in modulating vascular tone in response to normal stimuli (e.g., physical stress and exercise) and biochemical signals (e.g., acetylcholine) as well as producing vasodilatory substances (e.g., nitric oxide). Alterations in the normal physiology and function of the endothelium that contribute to CMD are generally referred to as an endothelial dysfunction. Changes in the actual structure of the microvascular bed can also contribute to CMD. Structural changes include intimal thickening, smooth muscle proliferation, vascular wall infiltration (i.e., amyloidosis or Fabry disease), fibrosis, luminal obstruction, or rarely extrinsic compression (e.g., hypertrophy). While these structural changes do not include epicardial atherosclerotic disease, its presence can exacerbate CMD [12].

On the other hand, functional abnormalities and biochemical/molecular mechanisms can play a role in the physiology of CMD. Inflammation from known cardiovascular risk factors and the subsequent cascade produces inflammatory markers like reactive oxygen species (ROS) and vasoconstrictive substances, such as endothelin-1, which contribute to endothelial dysfunction and CMD [10, 11]. Functional alterations in the normal physiology of vasodilation are also responsible for CMD. Impaired vasodilation can be either endothelial dependent or independent. As mentioned above, normal endothelium modulates vascular tone via several mechanisms including a balanced production and degradation of vasoactive substances, such as nitric oxide. Disruption in this balance with endothelial dysfunction can result in an abnormal vascular response to physiologic stimuli. This includes impaired vasodilation but with a paradoxical vasoconstriction in large vessels upstream [10, 11]. Invasive assessment with intracoronary vasoreactivity testing, using acetylcholine, can help to identify endothelium-dependent pathways for CMD in this setting [4, 10, 13].

As mentioned above, CMD may be linked to other chronic conditions that have similar pathophysiology including chronic inflammation. This includes the process of atherosclerosis itself, as well as aging (increased arterial stiffness and medial thickening), hypertension (remodeling and arteriolar constriction), metabolic syndrome, smoking, chronic kidney disease, diabetes mellitus, elevated lipids, and both ischemic and nonischemic cardiomyopathies (myocardial stiffness resulting in decreased compliance limiting the microcirculation's ability to meet the increased demand for oxygen consumption) [4, 10, 11]. CMD can also play a role in clinical syndromes, such as stress-induced cardiomyopathy and acute coronary syndrome, among several others. See Fig. 2.

Growing awareness and standardization for CMD have been advocated, particularly since its presence is higher in females who were previously thought to have no pathology and managed without any standard medical therapy. The large prospective WISE study

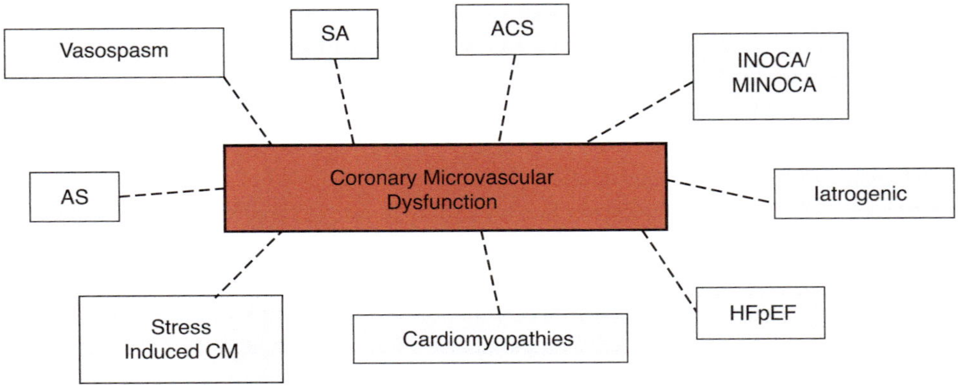

Fig. 2 Diagram highlighting different clinical entities where coronary microvascular dysfunction may play a role in the pathophysiology of ischemia. Modeled after del Buono et al. [10]. Iatrogenic disease may occur after percutaneous coronary intervention or surgical revascularization. *ACS* acute coronary syndromes, *AS* aortic stenosis, *CM* cardiomyopathy, *HFpEF* heart failure with preserved ejection fraction, *INOCA* ischemia with nonobstructive coronary artery disease, *MINOCA* myocardial infarction in nonobstructive coronary artery disease, *SA* stable angina

(Women's Ischemic Syndrome Evaluation) found that up to 47% of women with angina and nonobstructive CAD had CMD by invasive testing using CFR [14]. The increasing recognition of CMD, especially in INOCA, has led to steps for the standardization of defining and managing this clinical syndrome. The Coronary Vasomotion Disorders International Study Group (COVADIS) sought to standardize MVA, i.e., anginal symptoms in patients with CMD. These criteria include 1) presence of symptoms suggestive of myocardial ischemia; 2) objective documentation of myocardial ischemia; 3) absence of obstructive coronary artery disease (<50% coronary artery diameter and/or fractional flow reserve >0.80); and 4) confirmation of reduced coronary blood flow reserve and/or inducible microvascular spasm [15].

Previously less understood and recognized, INOCA and CMD were believed to be benign or less adverse than traditional obstructive CAD. As mentioned here, the interplay of these syndromes is complex and highly related to atherosclerotic disease. Five-year data from the prospective WISE study showed that patients with CMD have increased major adverse cardiovascular events, especially women, as compared to their counterparts with normal CFR and no CMD [16]. This is observed in other studies as well [17]. Different therapeutic options have been observed to improve patient symptoms and outcomes depending on the mechanism behind CMD; see Table 2. These are primarily based on observational and retrospective data, with limited randomized clinical trials. In order to identify the pathogenic mechanism (e.g., endothelial dependence, vasospasm), there are several proposed diagnostic workflows [4, 10, 13]. These are typically done using invasive coronary angiography with specialized diagnostic guidewires that measures CFR, index of IMR, and FFR. Several intracoronary medications are administered including adenosine,

Table 2 Proposed therapeutic options based off the believed pathogenic mechanism for coronary microvascular dysfunction, primarily from observational data with limited clinical trial evidence. ACEi - angiotensin converting enzyme inhibitor; ARB - angiotensin II receptor blocker; PDE-5i - phosphodiesterase 5 inhibitor

Endothelial Dependent
ACEi
ARB
Cardiac Eshabilitation
Enhanced External Counterpulsation
L-Arginine
Statins
Endothelial Independent
ACEi
Beta-Blocker
Ranolazine
PDE-5i
Vasospasm
Calcium Channel Blocker
Nitrates

acetylcholine, and nitroglycerin. After medication administration, any variation in these hemodynamic markers is measured in conjunction with changes in the coronary artery diameter.

It is recognized that patients can experience significant disability from INOCA, which can markedly impact their quality of life. However, continued research efforts are still needed in this arena. Future directions include large, prospective studies with an in-depth analysis using detailed hemodynamic profiling, standardized assessment of patient symptoms (e.g., Seattle Angina Questionnaire), and randomized clinical trials to help tailor management options to INOCA phenotype in order to improve patient outcomes.

5 Acute Coronary Syndromes

Acute coronary syndromes include the diagnoses of unstable angina and non-ST-elevation and ST-elevation myocardial infarction as well as sudden coronary death related to acute coronary occlusion. To best consider their pathogenesis, one should first explain the importance and history of the role of coronary thrombosis as the cause of acute MI.

Until the 1970s, the cause of acute myocardial infarction and the role of thrombosis were disputed throughout the twentieth century by cardiac pathologists. Was thrombus necessary and, if so, was it the cause of or the effect of slow flow in the coronary arteries? In an NIH-sponsored workshop in 1973 attended by leading cardiac pathologists, clinicians, and hematologists, it was finally concluded that coronary thrombosis was the primary cause of transmural MI but not subendocardial (non-transmural) MI [18]. These pathologic definitions roughly equate to the present-day designation of ST-elevation and non-ST-elevation MI, respectively. This conference was groundbreaking, but it only represented those patients who succumbed and had autopsies. What about the living patient?

This question concerning the primacy of coronary thrombosis as the cause of transmural MI was unequivocally answered by DeWood et al. in 1980 [19]. In 322 patients admitted to the hospital within 24 h of the onset of transmural infarction, coronary angiography noted acute coronary occlusion in 87% of those admitted within 4 h of symptom onset (n=126). Its incidence dropped to 65% when patients were studied 12–24 h after the onset of symptoms (n=57). Among 59 patients with angiographic features of coronary thrombosis at the time of open-heart surgery, the thrombus was retrieved by Fogarty catheter in 52 (88%). This discovery was paramount in changing the therapy for acute MI. One could now use agents to open the occluded artery and preserve myocardium. Initially, intravenous thrombolytic therapy and appropriate antithrombotic and anticoagulant regimens were the treatments of choice, and now, primary percutaneous intervention is preferred if available with the insertion of a drug-eluting stent at the site of coronary occlusion.

6 Pathogenesis of Coronary Thrombosis and ST-Elevation Myocardial Infarction

While thrombosis may be the cause of MI, how did it get there? This question was addressed by Chapman in 1965 and Constantinides in 1966 [20, 21]. Both showed that thrombus formed on a defect on the surface of an atherosclerotic plaque and essentially described the pathologic entity of plaque disruption as the primary mechanism for coronary thrombus formation in acute STEMI. Since then, there have been innumerable articles published on the pathogenesis of coronary thrombosis. In about 2/3 of cases of STEMI, thrombus formation is due to plaque rupture of a so-called thin-capped fibroatheroma or TCFA. Blood comes into contact with the undersurface of the torn or disrupted fibrous cap, and platelet deposition is followed by tissue factor activation leading to a platelet, fibrin, and red cell thrombus with the head being platelet rich and the tail red cell/fibrin rich and occlusive. These TCFAs contain a necrotic core of lipid and cellular debris, which overlies a thin fibrous cap devoid of collagen and smooth muscle cells and infiltrated by macrophages and T-lymphocytes. They are typically large plaques but due to positive remodeling are not occlusive on angiography in the weeks to months prior to the STEMI [22].

The second most common mechanism for thrombus formation is plaque erosion, and in this situation, thrombus forms on a defect in the endothelial lining covering the fibrous cap. These plaques are typically not TCFAs, and their caps are not usually thin. The predominant plaque type in some studies is proteoglycan rich, and lipid may not be an important component [23]. These pathologic observations have been corroborated by in vivo OCT, which has been utilized to investigate the pathogenesis of coronary thrombus during primary PCI for STEMI [24]. Over a guidewire, an OCT catheter is passed to the site of coronary occlusion and with its axial resolution of 10–15 microns, one can, with the proper

Table 3 Causes of STEMI Without Presence of Intracoronary Plaque Related Thrombus

Causes of ATEMI Without Presence of Intracoronary Plaque Related Thrombus
Coronary Emboli
Coronary Vasospasm
Spontaneous Coronary Artery or Aortic Dissection
Vasculitis
Blunt Traumatic Injury
Anomalous Origin of Coronaty Arteries

preparation and technique, interrogate the site and determine in most cases the pathogenesis of thrombus formation.

While these processes are responsible for the vast majority of patients presenting with STEMI, there are potentially other causes of STEMI. A potential list is given in Table 3. In most instances, even if thrombus is not the primary cause, slow or no flow can lead to secondary thrombus formation. Furthermore, every primary coronary thrombus does not necessarily lead to acute myocardial infarction. Asymptomatic thrombus formation may contribute to progression of atherosclerosis as the thrombus becomes incorporated into the wall of the artery [25].

7 Pathophysiology of Unstable Angina and Non-ST-Elevation Myocardial Infarction

7.1 Unstable Angina

The term unstable angina was coined in separate publications by Conti and Fowler to describe a syndrome in between that of stable angina and an acute MI [26, 27]. Patients had progressive angina and/or rest discomfort without an elevation of cardiac enzymes. The pathophysiology was unclear although some small studies suggested that intracoronary thrombus was present [28, 29] while other publications indicated no differences in coronary anatomy between stable and unstable patients at angiography [30, 31]. Given the different clinical presentations in unstable angina from that of stable angina, Ambrose et al. theorized that the angiographic lesions might qualitatively look different in unstable angina. In 1985, they published data indicating that in unstable angina with a patent angina-producing artery, the lesion responsible was eccentric and irregular (later called a complex plaque) while stable lesions usually did not have these characteristics [32]. Based

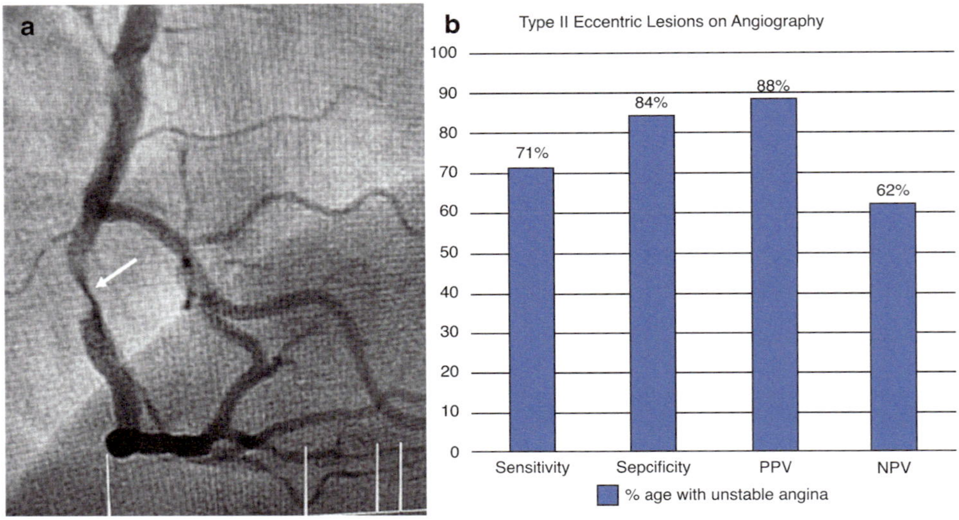

Fig. 3 (**a**) Invasive coronary angiography depicting typical example of a type II eccentric lesion (complex plaque)—white arrow. (**b**) Ambrose et al.'s study [32] on the qualitative assessment of the morphologic appearance of coronary arteries in patients presenting with unstable angina. Specifically, the relationship and diagnostic accuracy of having type II eccentric lesions in this ischemic syndrome outlined in bar graph on 3B

on a postmortem angiographic study of Levin and Fallon [33], our group suggested that these unstable lesions represented plaque disruption and/or intracoronary thrombus and they were seen in 71% of unstable patients but only in 16% of stable patients (Fig. 3).

As the preferred enzyme in the 1980s to exclude an infarct was CK-MB, today the more sensitive troponin is used. Thus, many of the early studies including ours contained patients that today might be classified as NSTEMI given the fact that troponin would likely have been elevated. In fact, unstable angina by the classic Braunwald definition [34] has become less frequent than in the past due to troponin as the preferred biomarker [35].

7.2 Non-ST-Elevation Myocardial Infarction

The pathogenesis of NSTEMI is complex as there are multiple potential causes. As troponin assays became more sensitive, the incidence of an elevated troponin increased. Were all these elevations indicative of an MI? In 2007, the First Universal Definition of MI was published [36], and it helped clarify the etiology of the troponin increase. It defined an MI as a rise of and/or fall of troponin above the upper reference level and clinical evidence of ischemia from either new ischemic symptoms, ischemic ECG changes, or wall motion abnormalities. If the troponin elevation did not meet the criteria for an MI, it was classified as myocardial injury. An infarction was subclassified into five groups, but for the purposes of our discussion, we will consider types 1 and 2 NSTEMI with which the clinician will most often be confronted. Type 1 MI is the MI related to atherothrombosis and is the one we have so far been considering in this chapter. On the other hand, type 2 MI meets the criteria for an MI but it is due to a supply/demand mismatch in the absence of atherothrombosis. The mismatch is usually extrinsic to the coronary bed and could be related to changes in blood pressure or pulse (in both instances, either too high or too low), hypoxia, or other less common causes as coronary spasm, coronary embolism, or dissection.

The pathophysiology of a type 1 NSTEMI is variable and comes in a variety of anatomical shapes and forms. One might find either a patent vessel with a new significant lesion due to plaque rupture or a plaque erosion with intermittent total occlusion or embolization of thrombotic material to the distal vascular bed, total occlusion of a major epicardial vessel with collaterals, or a new total occlusion of a branch vessel. There can be one-vessel or multivessel disease, and in about 40–50% of cases, a culprit lesion may not be apparent [37]. Finally, as discussed earlier, there may be insignificant or no angiographic coronary artery disease and no apparent S/D mismatch to explain the syndrome [38].

While type 2 MI has helped to clarify the etiology of troponin elevation, there are significant problems with this diagnosis. The incidence of a type 2 MI varies widely in the literature from a little over 1% to as high as 75% [38, 39]. We believe that a significant reason for this variability is related to the imprecision in the diagnostic criteria. The S/D mismatch is not standardized and variably interpreted as does its incidence. Also, symptoms may be either typical or atypical. Atypical symptoms such as dyspnea without ischemic ECG change will certainly lead to an inflated incidence of a type 2 MI in a patient with an exacerbation of congestive heart failure and an elevated troponin. We have shown that the diagnosis can also be missed even in patients with extreme prespecified criteria for the S/D mismatch and typical ischemic symptoms that would fit all criteria for an unequivocal type 2 MI [40]. This might explain the low incidence of a type 2 MI reported in some studies. While patients with a type 2 MI may have significant underlying coronary disease, we believe that more specific criteria should be developed for diagnosis.

8 Sudden Cardiac Death

SCD has been traditionally defined as unexpected, natural death from a cardiac etiology that occurs within 1 h from symptom onset [41]. Most information and research on this subject matter have been derived from patients who initially present to medical care as an OHCA. The risk of SCD increases with age, and the majority of cases in the adult population are due to CAD [42–44]. This is especially true in adults over 35 years old in industrialized countries. SCD from CAD in the setting of an AMI can present with arrythmias, such as PMVT and VF. SCD can also be the result of structural changes to the myocardium after an AMI that result in remodeling and scar, which can cause monomorphic VT and

VF. Other non-CAD mechanisms in SCD include pulmonary embolism, hypoxia, metabolic derangements, and channelopathies, among several others.

Within the context of CAD, there are several mechanisms that play a role in SCD. These include acute thrombotic events, such as an AMI, chronic transient ischemia in patients with established CAD, as well as scar from a prior ischemic insult with long-term remodeling. Autopsy data of patients with SCD suggest that active or acute changes in coronary atherosclerotic plaque can be seen in up to 57% of SCD cases [43]. These changes were defined as disrupted coronary plaques, thrombus, or both. There is also evidence that women, particularly younger females, presenting with SCD more frequently have plaque erosion with late-stage thrombus, as compared to men [23].

Chronic, stable CAD also plays a role in the development of arrythmias, which can cause SCD. With already limited blood flow to distal myocardium from an atherosclerotic lesion, this supply/demand relationship may be strained under certain circumstances. This includes hemodynamic changes in blood pressure, changes in pH, hypoxemia, electrolyte disturbances (hypokalemia and hypomagnesemia), and toxins (drugs or alcohol) [45]. This concept of transient ischemia and reperfusion can alter cell membrane physiology including potassium channel conductance and provide a nidus for the arrythmias responsible for SCD [46].

Convalescent remodeling after an AMI or in the setting of chronic ischemia from CAD can result in adaptive changes to the myocardium that put patients at an increased for SCD. This can initially be in the form of fibrosis and ultimately result in ventricular dilation with reduced systolic function. Reduced LVEF is independently associated with an increased risk for SCD [47, 48]. The common arrythmia that precedes SCD in this patient population is MMVT, which can further degenerate into VF. Recent advanced imaging studies with CMR show the extent of infarct and scar surface area along with the amount of mass, ventricular volumes, fibrosis, and edema correlating with an increased risk of MMVT and SCD [49, 50]. The cellular changes that occur in this setting create an environment of electrical dispersion, which translates to mechanical changes, as assessed on multi-modality imaging techniques including strain echocardiography and CMR [51, 52]. This provides a reentrant substrate for tachyarrhythmias, such as MMVT, and has been observed in patients with ventricular remodeling post-AMI.

The decreased incidence in SCD over the last several decades is believed to be due to multiple factors, including improved post-resuscitation care, early intervention in SCD with STEMI and prompt revascularization, increased uptake of bystander cardiopulmonary resuscitation, changes to the advanced cardiovascular life support algorithm, and implantable cardioverter defibrillators. There has also been a decrease in mortality due to CAD, which has been attributed to the advancement in medical care. This includes modern revascularization techniques along with evidence-based medical therapy [52]. Similarly, SCD after an AMI has also decreased over time [53, 54]. However, SCD still remains the initial presentation of underlying CAD in at least 30% of events [54]. Therefore, continued efforts are needed to identify high-risk individuals. This underscores the importance of understanding the pathophysiology of CAD in SCD and continually improving primary, secondary, and tertiary care.

9 Conclusion

Coronary artery disease can present as various clinical syndromes, each with a varied prognosis. Over the last 50 years, our understanding of their pathogenesis has resulted in various therapies that have vastly improved clinical outcomes. However, as still the leading cause of mortality worldwide, more effective preventive strategies and therapeutic options are still required.

References

1. Virani S, Alonso A, Aparicio HJ, et al. Heart Disease and Stroke Statistics—2021 Update. Circulation. 2021;143:e254–743.
2. Thygesen K, Alpert JS, Joseph S, et al. Fourth universal definition of myocardial infarction. Circulation. 2018;138:e618–51.
3. Clausen JP, Trap-Jensen J. Heart rate and arterial blood pressure during exercise in patients with angina pectoris. Effects of training and of nitroglycerin. Circulation. 1976;53(3):436–42.
4. Kunadian V, Chieffo A, Camici PG, et al. An EAPCI Expert Consensus Document on Ischaemia with Non-Obstructive Coronary Arteries in Collaboration with European Society of Cardiology Working Group on Coronary Pathophysiology & Microcirculation Endorsed by Coronary Vasomotor Disorders International Study Group. *European Heart Journal*. 2020;41(37):3504–20.
5. Shaw LJ, Leslee J, Merz NB, et al. Impact of ethnicity and gender differences on angiographic coronary artery disease prevalence and in-hospital mortality in the American College of Cardiology–National Cardiovascular Data Registry. Circulation. 2008;117:1787–801.
6. Reynolds HR, Srichai MB, Iqbal SN, et al. Mechanisms of Myocardial Infarction in Women without Angiographically Obstructive Coronary Artery Disease. Circulation. 2011;124(13):1414–25.
7. Pepine CJ. Multiple causes for ischemia without obstructive coronary artery disease. Circulation. 2015;131:1044–6.
8. Möhlenkamp S, Hort W, Ge J, et al. Update on myocardial bridging. Circulation. 2002;106:2616–22.
9. Konen E, Goitein O, Sternik L, et al. The prevalence and anatomical patterns of intramuscular coronary arteries: a coronary computed tomography angiographic study. Journal of the American College of Cardiology. 2007;49(5):587–93.
10. Del Buono M, Montone RA, Camilli M, et al. Coronary Microvascular Dysfunction across the Spectrum of Cardiovascular Diseases: JACC State-of-the-Art Review. Journal of the American College of Cardiology. 2021;78(13):352–1371.
11. Taqueti VR, Di Carli MF. Coronary Microvascular Disease Pathogenic Mechanisms and Therapeutic Options: JACC State-of-the-Art Review. Journal of the American College of Cardiology. 2018;72(21):2625–41.
12. Egashira K, Inou T, Hirooka Y, et al. Impaired coronary blood flow response to acetylcholine in patients with coronary risk factors and proximal atherosclerotic lesions. Journal of Clinal Investigation. 1993;91(1):29–37.
13. Tjoe B, Barsky L, Wei J, et al. Coronary Microvascular Dysfunction: Considerations for diagnosis and treatment. Cleveland Clinic Journal of Medicine. 2021;88(10):561–71.
14. Reis SE, Holubkov R, Conrad Smith AJ, et al. Coronary microvascular dysfunction is highly prevalent in women with chest pain in the absence of coronary artery disease: results from the NHLBI WISE study. American Heart Journal. 2001;141(5):735–41.

15. Ong P, Camici PG, Beltrame JF, et al. Coronary Vasomotion Disorders International Study Group. International standardization of diagnostic criteria for microvascular angina. International Journal of Cardiology. 2018;250:16–20.
16. Pepine CJ, Anderson RD, Sharaf BL, et al. Coronary microvascular reactivity to adenosine predicts adverse outcome in women evaluated for suspected ischemia: Results from the National Heart, Lung and Blood Institute Wise (Women's Ischemia Syndrome Evaluation) study. Journal of the American College of Cardiology. 2010;55(25):2825–32.
17. Merz NB, Pepine CJ, Walsh MN, et al. Ischemia and no obstructive coronary artery disease (INOCA). Circulation. 2017;135:1072–92.
18. Chandler AB, Chapman I, Erhardt L, et al. Coronary thrombosis in myocardial infarction. Report of a workshop on the role of coronary thrombosis in the pathogenesis of acute myocardial infarction. The American Journal of Cardiology. 1974;34(7):823–33.
19. DeWood MA, Spores J, Notske R, et al. Prevalence of total coronary occlusion during the early hours of transmural myocardial infarction. New England Journal of Medicine. 1980;303:897–902.
20. Chapman I. Morphogenesis of Occluding Coronary Artery Thrombosis. Archives of Pathology and Laboratory Medicine. 1965;80:256–61.
21. Constantinides P. Plaque fissures in human coronary thrombosis. Journal of Atherosclerosis Research. 1966;6(1):1–17.
22. Moreno PR. The high-risk thin-cap fibroatheroma. Circulation: Cardiovascular Interventions. 2009;2(6):500–2.
23. Farb A, Burke AP, Tang AL, et al. Coronary plaque erosion without rupture into a lipid core. A frequent cause of coronary thrombosis in sudden coronary death. Circulation. 1996;93(7):1354–63.
24. Kolte D, Yonetsu T, Ye JC, et al. Optical coherence tomography of plaque erosion. Journal of the American College of Cardiology. 2021;78(12):1266–74.
25. Bentzon JF, Otsuka F, Virmani R, et al. Mechanisms of plaque formation and rupture. Circulation Research. 2014;114(12):1852–66. https://doi.org/10.1161/circresaha.114.302721.
26. Conti CR, Greene B, Pitt B, et al. Coronary artery surgery on unstable angina pectoris. Circulation. 1971;44(Suppl 2):154.
27. Fowler NO. Preinfarctional Angina. Circulation. 1971;44(5):755–8.
28. Holmes DR, Hartzler GO, Smith HC, et al. Coronary artery thrombosis in patients with unstable angina. British Heart Journal. 1981;45(4):411–6.
29. Vetrovec GW, Cowley MJ, Overton H, et al. Intracoronary thrombus in syndromes of unstable myocardial ischemia. American Heart Journal. 1981;102(6):1202–8.
30. Alison HW, Russell RO, Mantle JA, et al. Coronary anatomy and arteriography in patients with unstable angina pectoris. The American Journal of Cardiology. 1978;41(2):204–9.
31. Fuster V, Frye RL, Connolly DC, et al. Arteriographic patterns early in the onset of the coronary syndromes. British Heart Journal. 1975;37(12):1250–5.
32. Ambrose JA, Winters SL, Stern A, et al. Angiographic morphology and the pathogenesis of unstable angina pectoris. Journal of the American College of Cardiology. 1985;5(3):609–16.
33. Levin DC, Fallon JT. Significance of the angiographic morphology of localized coronary stenoses: histopathologic correlations. Circulation. 1982;66(2):316–20.
34. Braunwald E. Unstable angina. A classification. Circulation. 1989;80(2):410–4.
35. Braunwald E, Morrow DA. Unstable angina: is it time for a requiem? Circulation. 2013;127(24):2452–7.
36. Thygesen K, Alpert JS, White HD. Universal definition of myocardial infarction. Circulation. 2007;116(22):2634–53.
37. Ambrose JA, Loures-Vale A, Javed U, et al. Angiographic correlates in type 1 and 2 MI by the universal definition. JACC: Cardiovascular Imaging. 2012;5(4):463–4.

38. Sandoval Y, Jaffe AS. Type 2 myocardial infarction. Journal of the American College of Cardiology. 2019;73(14):1846–60.
39. DeFilippis AP, Chapman AR, Mills NL, et al. Assessment and treatment of patients with type 2 myocardial infarction and acute nonischemic myocardial injury. Circulation. 2019;140(20):1661–78.
40. Saleh MA, Ambrose JA, Poosti K, et al. Misdiagnosis of type II myocardial infarction. Journal of the American College of Cardiology. 2019;74(13):1732–3.
41. Myerburg R, Castellanos A. Braunwald's Heart Disease. A Textbook of Cardiovascular Medicine. 2007;8:933–74.
42. Thomas AC, Knapman PA, Krikler DM, et al. Community study of the causes of "natural" sudden death. British Medical Journal. 1998;297:1453–6.
43. Farb A, Tang AL, Burke AP, et al. Sudden Coronary Death. Frequency of Active Coronary Lesions, Inactive Coronary Lesions, and Myocardial Infarction. Circulation. 1995;92:1701–9.
44. Myerburg RJ. Sudden Cardiac Death: Exploring the Limits of Our Knowledge. Journal of Cardiovascular Electrophysiology. 2001;12:369–81.
45. Zipes DP, Wellens HJJ. Sudden cardiac death. Circulation. 1998;98:2334–51.
46. Furukawa T, Bassett AL, Furukawa N, et al. The ionic mechanism of reperfusion-induced early afterdepolarizations in feline left ventricular hypertrophy. The Journal of Clinical Investigation. 1993;91(4):1521–31.
47. Solomon SD, Zelenkofske S, McMurray JV, et al. Sudden Death in Patients with Myocardial Infarction and Left Ventricular Dysfunction, Heart Failure, or Both. New England Journal of Medicine. 2005;352:2581–8.
48. Greenberg H, Case RB, Moss AJ, et al. Analysis of mortality events in the Multicenter Automatic Defibrillator Implantation Trial (MADIT-II). Journal of the American College of Cardiology. 2004;43(8):1459–65.
49. Bello D, Fieno DS, Kim RJ, et al. Infarct morphology identifies patients with substrate for sustained ventricular tachycardia. Journal of the American College of Cardiology. 2005;45(7):1104–8.
50. Al Jaroudi WA, Flamm SD, Saliba W, et al. Role of CMR imaging in risk stratification for sudden cardiac death. JACC: Cardiovascular Imaging. 2013;6(3):392–406.
51. Haugaa KH, Smedsrud MK, Steen T, et al. Mechanical dispersion assessed by myocardial strain in patients after myocardial infarction for risk prediction of ventricular arrhythmia. JACC: Cardiovascular Imaging. 2010;3(3):247–56.
52. Ford ES, Ajani UA, Croft JB, et al. Explaining the Decrease in U.S. Deaths from Coronary Disease, 1980–2000. New England Journal of Medicine. 2007;356:2388–98.
53. Adabag AS, Therneau TM, Gersh BJ, et al. Sudden death after myocardial infarction. The Journal of the American Medical Association. 2008;300(17):2022–9.
54. Myerburg RJ, Junttila MJ. Sudden Cardiac Death Caused by Coronary Heart Disease. Circulation. 2012;125:1043–52.

Epidemiology of Ischemic Heart Disease

Muhammad Jawad Hashim

1 Introduction

IHD is, at the same time, common and fatal, and yet preventable and treatable. In the current era, it remains the most common cause of deaths worldwide, easily surpassing any cancer or infectious disease.

The epidemiology of IHD is of relevance to clinicians as well as public health experts. Among clinicians, all specialties are involved. Cardiologists, cardiac surgeons, emergency medicine physicians, internists, and family physicians/general practitioners need to know pretest probabilities and high-risk groups. Public health officials need to plan for the rising burden of IHD due to population aging.

2 Risk Factors

Risk factors for IHD are divided into two categories: traditional and emerging risk factors (Table 1). Epidemiologically established risk factors include male sex, increasing age, diabetes mellitus, previously diagnosed atherosclerotic disease (such as peripheral arterial disease), chronic renal impairment, and family history of premature IHD [1]. Family history in this context is defined as an initial cardiac ischemic event in a first-degree relative (parent or sibling) of age less than 55 years (male relative) or 65 years (female relative). Hypertension and cigarette smoking contribute the largest proportion of risk among all IHD risk factors. Hypercholesterolemia has a strong dose-response relationship with

M. J. Hashim (✉)
Family Medicine, College of Medicine and Health Sciences, United Arab Emirates University, Al Ain, UAE
e-mail: jhashim@uaeu.ac.ae

G. Concistrè (ed.), *Ischemic Heart Disease*,
https://doi.org/10.1007/978-3-031-25879-4_6

Table 1 Risk factors for IHD

Traditional/established risk factors	Emerging risk factors
Modifiable	*Metabolic*
Cigarette smoking	Obesity
Hypertension	Overweight or elevated BMI
Diabetes mellitus	Elevated blood glucose
Hypercholesterolemia	Physical inactivity
Non-modifiable	Increased waist circumference
Male sex	Metabolic syndrome
Increasing age	Familial hypercholesterolemia
Family history of premature IHD	*Dietary*
	Meat and poultry consumption
	Saturated fat intake (animal fat and butter)
	Low intake of fish
	Low intake of legumes (beans, lentils)
	Dietary salt
	Processed meat
	Trans-fatty acids
	High sugar beverages
	Vitamin E and omega-3 fatty acids
	Alcohol intake
	Emerging associations
	Inflammatory conditions such as psoriasis
	Chronic kidney disease
	HIV/AIDS
	Nonalcoholic fatty liver disease
	Erectile dysfunction in men
	Microalbuminuria
	Remnant lipoproteins
	Hemostatic factors (fibrin, D-dimer)
	Periodontitis
	Radiation exposure to chest
	Passive exposure to tobacco smoke
	Waterpipe *shisha* smoking
	Screen time (television, smartphones)
	Urban residence
	Psychosocial and work stress
	Sleep deprivation
	Prolonged sitting
	Air pollution

IHD. Regrettably, cigarette smoking rates are rising among women, young adults, and men living in low- and middle-income countries [2].

Unhealthful diets are associated with IHD in observational studies [3]. Consuming fish appears to provide a protective effect [3]. A reduced intake of saturated fatty acids (meat, poultry, and dairy), substituted by polyunsaturated fatty acids (vegetable oils), may decrease the risk of IHD [4]. Animal fat including dairy products such as butter are sources of saturated fatty acids in human diet. Recently, the role of saturated fatty acids and calorie restriction has been re-evaluated in nutritional research. In particular, previous dietary recommendations to limit saturated fat while consuming more carbohydrates were misguided [4]. Dietary nuts and legumes (lentils, beans) are associated with a reduction in IHD events [5]. Intermittent fasting has been linked to cardiometabolic health in some studies [6].

In terms of general cardiovascular health, the overall effect of alcohol consumption is harmful. Alcoholic drinks increase the risk of IHD at moderate to high intake. Evidence for a potential protective effect of low daily intake comes from observational studies comparing average consumption across regions. Polyphenol flavonoids in nonalcoholic grape juice have a comparable cardioprotective effect [7–10]. Given the potential for escalation to moderate- and high-volume drinking, harmful effects of alcohol on other body systems [11], and psychosocial consequences, it is difficult to recommend alcohol consumption to prevent heart disease.

A variety of emerging risk predictors for IHD are being reported in epidemiological research (Table 1) [6]. These include pro-inflammatory conditions such as HIV/AIDS, psoriasis, chronic liver disease, as well as hemostatic biomarkers such as fibrin, D-dimer, and tPA [12]. These predictive variables are, in turn, associated with lifestyle factors such as smoking, alcoholism, obesity, and sedentariness. It is difficult to isolate and quantify the effect of individual risk factors from observational studies. Causal relationships cannot be proven in such studies [13].

In clinical settings, male patients older than 70 years with diabetes mellitus are more likely to have an ACS secondary to IHD [1]. However, the absence of these risk factors should not rule out IHD in a patient with chest pain or other signs and symptoms suggestive of ACS. For the diagnosis of ACS, clinical features are more important than risk factors. Nevertheless, 90% of patients with an ischemic cardiac event have at least one risk factor [14].

Online calculators are available to estimate the 10-year risk of a major cardiac event in an individual [15]. An individual with a risk estimate of 20% or more is considered to be at high risk [16]. Such individuals are typically stratified to "aggressive" treatment such as high-dose statins and coronary revascularization. Persons with a risk estimate between 5 and 20% are considered intermediate risk and usually considered for optimal medical therapy. A 10-year risk of less than 5% is considered low risk, and preventive interventions are advised to reduce modifiable risk factors. Risk stratification is superior to previously used rules of thumb such as counting the number of risk factors or using LDL cholesterol cutoff levels to guide clinical decision-making.

3 Disease Burden

An estimated 4% of adults (20+ years) worldwide have IHD [17]. Men are affected more than women (on average 1.3:1). Onset starts at around 30 years but is usually clinically manifested after 50 years of age (Fig. 1). Prevalence increases rapidly with aging. Among

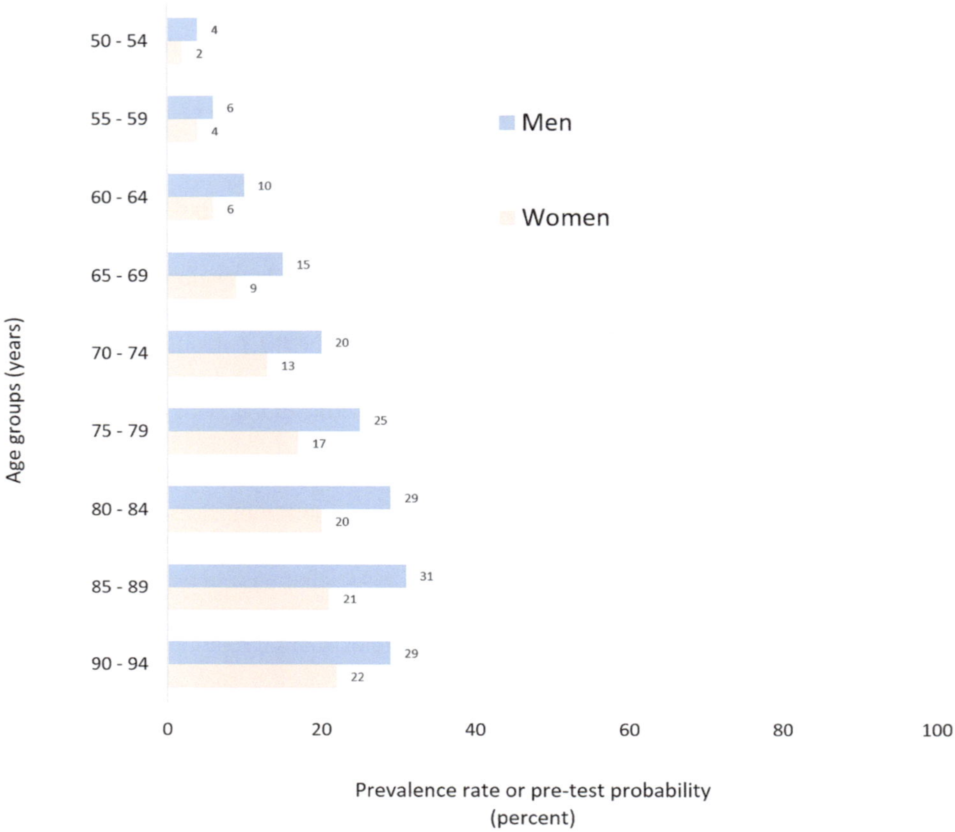

Fig. 1 Prevalence of ischemic heart disease in different age groups

the elderly (70+ years), the prevalence is 20%. This further increases to 24% among persons more than 80 years of age.

Globally, about 200 million persons have IHD. This translates to a prevalence rate of 3820 cases per 100,000 population worldwide. In a community of 100,000 adults, over 400 new cases can be expected every year (global average). This incidence rate is mostly due to first AMI.

Men are at a higher risk for IHD compared to women. The lifetime risk of IHD is about 50% among men and 33% in women, at age 40 years [14]. The gender differential decreases with advancing age. AMI and sudden cardiac death are rare in premenopausal women. Men tend to present with an initial AMI, while uncomplicated angina is more likely among women. Women tend to be underdiagnosed and undertreated leading to worse outcomes such as higher reinfarction rates and all-cause mortality [18]. Among women, IHD causes far more deaths than cancer including breast cancer.

Over nine million people die from IHD every year. This far exceeds deaths due to any other illness (lung cancer, the most common fatal malignancy, causes two million deaths per year). Overall, cardiovascular diseases cause almost twice the number of deaths compared to all cancer deaths combined. IHD is the number one cause of deaths worldwide.

Disability-adjusted life year (DALY) rates paint a truer picture of human suffering. In contrast to prevalence or mortality rates, DALY captures the reduced quality of life due to disability among survivors as well as the loss of life from premature deaths. IHD ranks first among all diseases as a cause of human suffering (DALY rates) among adults. If all ages are considered, IHD ranks second, after neonatal disorders, and is followed by stroke [17].

The economic burden of IHD is substantial. In the USA alone, the direct and indirect costs of IHD and stroke care exceed US$ 350 billion per year [19]. These expenditures are rising every year. Among patients with type 2 diabetes, IHD costs contribute 20–49% of total direct healthcare expenditures [20]. In lower middle-income countries, the cost of a single episode of IHD care exceeds several times the average annual health expenditure per person [21].

4 Regional Patterns

IHD is more common in developed regions. These regions include North America, western Europe, Australia, as well as rapidly developing nations in the Middle East and Asia Pacific. In particular, central and eastern European countries such as Estonia and Latvia stand out with the highest prevalence rates. IHD is relatively less common in South Asia and sub-Saharan Africa. The most widely accepted explanation is the adoption of Western lifestyle leading to obesity and diabetes [22].

In terms of total number of cases, countries with the largest populations have the greatest burden. China, India, and the USA sustain the largest number of individuals with IHD. India, for instance, has 37.5 million persons with IHD and can expect an addition of 4.7 million new cases every year. Russia, Iran, Pakistan, Bangladesh, and Egypt also rank in the top ten, mostly likely due to unhealthy dietary and lifestyle patterns. Health systems in these countries are under severe stress due to the failure of primary prevention coupled with a widespread shortage of cardiac tertiary care.

Heart failure is a major endpoint for IHD and other cardiovascular diseases. In developed countries, heart failure is most commonly due to coronary atherosclerosis. In developing countries such as those in sub-Saharan Africa, uncontrolled hypertension, cardiomyopathies, rheumatic heart disease, and congenital heart defects are more likely to be implicated [23].

5 Epidemiological Trends

IHD rates are decreasing in certain regions including North America and Europe (Fig. 2A). This is most likely due to greater public awareness of healthy living in the postindustrial societies. Contributing factors include a decline in cigarette smoking [24]. However, it is premature to declare this a global health success. The reversal has not been observed in less developed regions.

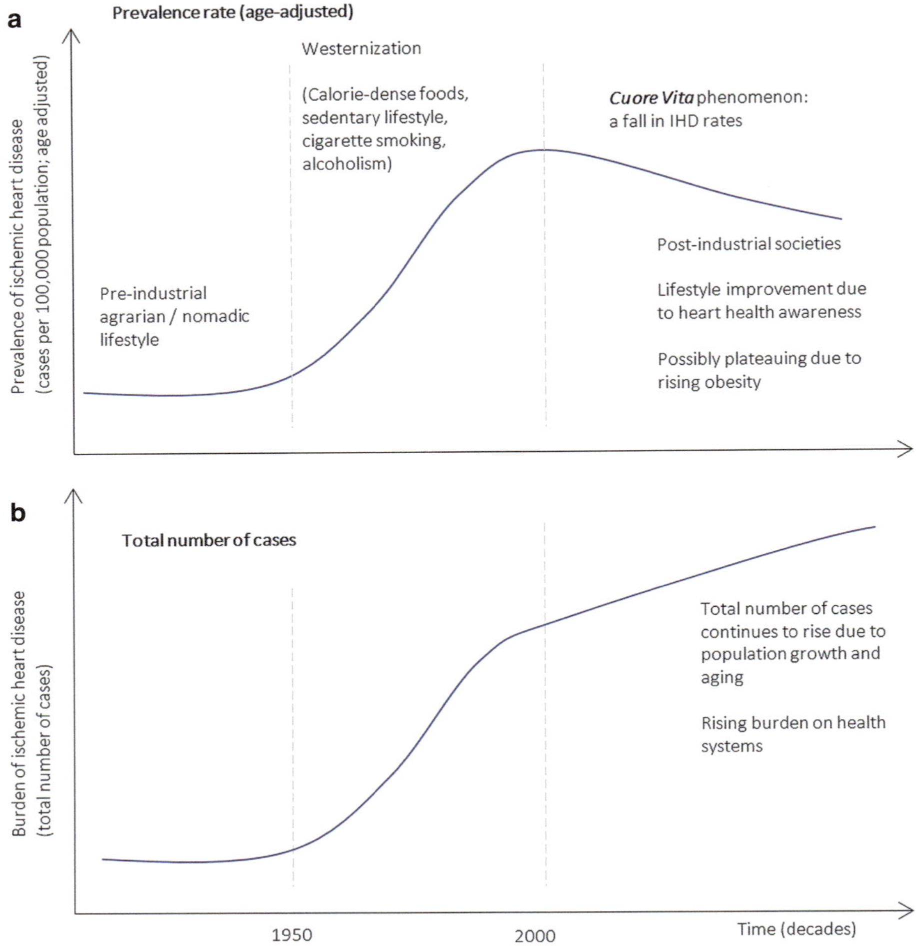

Fig. 2 Changing burden of ischemic heart disease with sociodemographic transition comparing (**a**) prevalence rate, and (**b**) total number of cases globally

5.1 Prevalence

Age-adjusted prevalence rates have dropped measurably in North America and Europe since 1990 [17]. Age-adjusted rates are useful for analyzing time trends across regions. These rates are adjusted for changes in underlying population structure due to aging and migration. For instance, in Italy, the age-adjusted prevalence dropped from 2274 cases in 1990 to 2032 cases per 100,000 population in 2019. However, low and low-middle developed regions have experienced a rise in prevalence rates. For example, in Pakistan, the rates rose from 3784 cases in 1990 to 4116 cases per 100,000 in 2019.

On the other hand, unadjusted prevalence rates are continuing to increase worldwide, in all regions (Fig. 2B). These unadjusted rates incorporate population growth and aging. Thus, the overall burden of IHD is increasing in all societies. Health systems need to plan for this absolute increase in the number of patients presenting with ACS and chronic IHD every year. This massive burden can overwhelm system capacity leading to delays in care, excessive waiting times, preventable premature deaths, and avoidable human suffering. IHD could be considered a global health system emergency.

5.2 Mortality

Death rates have fallen dramatically. Over the last few decades, from 1990 to present, the global age-adjusted mortality rate has decreased from 170 deaths to 118 deaths per 100,000 population [17]. The drop is even greater for several Western nations. For example, in Italy, age-adjusted mortality rates decreased from 121 deaths in 1990 to 55 per 100,000 population in 2019. In the UK, the rate fell from 198 deaths to 67 deaths per 100,000 annually. In certain countries such as Japan, Korea, Singapore, and Taiwan, due to the declining rates of IHD, cancers have become the number one cause of death [25].

This is a remarkable phenomenon and a global achievement in clinical medicine and public health. A new term is introduced in this book to describe this phenomenon: *Cuore Vita* (Italian for heart life). Public awareness of heart health has considerably increased due to media campaigns and clinical preventive counseling. Health promotion efforts towards healthy nutrition and physical activity, combined with more public spaces for outdoor activities and restrictions on cigarette smoking, have most likely contributed to this decline in IHD incidence (Box 1).

Box 1. Cuore Vita

Cuore Vita—a new term defined as public awareness and community action that results in a decline in heart disease.

However, the total number of deaths continues to rise due to population growth and aging. Unadjusted death rates as well as the total number of deaths are continuing to increase worldwide. Most of these deaths occur in the prime of productivity: during the fifth and sixth decades of life. More than 1.7 million people in the age group 60–69 years die from IHD every year. This number is expected to continue increasing in the foreseeable future. Personal and family tragedies unfold daily as fathers and mothers die leaving children and grandparents dependent and unsecure. This human face of IHD is all too familiar to cardiologists and other clinicians.

The rising epidemic of obesity, diabetes, and digital screen time may eclipse the *Cuore Vita* phenomenon. Renewed and sustained efforts are needed in preventive cardiology, public health promotion, and enhanced primary care. Community health activities, urban redesign (parks, bicycle lanes, decentralization), and reducing access to video games and processed foods (high in refined sugars) may be even more important.

The discovery of sensitive biomarkers such as troponin may have increased the diagnosis of acute myocardial infarction. These changes in diagnostic criteria, access to care, and community awareness can affect epidemiological estimates. Widespread and indiscriminate recording of cause of death as "cardiac arrest" may have inflated IHD rates. Documenting the proper underlying cause of death in death certificates is vitally important [26].

6 Clinical and Public Health Policy Implications

IHD is the foremost cause of premature death and disability worldwide. Unfortunately, most patients do not receive or adhere to optimal medical therapy. Regional variations in care indicate that clinicians often do not implement best practices. These factors lead to unnecessary and avoidable suffering and premature deaths. Thus, a large gap exists between research knowledge and its translation into clinical implementation. Several IHD interventions are low cost (Box 2). Healthy nutrition, exercise, and smoking cessation are less expensive than medical treatment. Control of blood pressure, cardioprotection with aspirin, and control of serum lipids and glucose can be managed at the primary care level. Shortage of tertiary care in a region should not necessarily lead to poor IHD care or outcomes. Public health interventions to reduce obesity and cigarette smoking while promoting an active, healthy lifestyle are cost effective. Alongside preventive approaches, regional health systems with large aging populations should plan for a rising burden of IHD.

Box 2. Key recommendations for heart health

1. *Active lifestyle*—avoid prolonged sitting and screen time; stay active with household and outdoor activities; make daily walks and exercise a priority; avoid labor-saving devices.
2. *Healthy nutrition*—avoid meat and dairy products; enjoy fresh fruits, vegetables, nuts, and lentils/beans; limit salt intake; reduce (but not eliminate) carbohydrates such as white bread, rice, refined sugars, bakery products, and sweetened beverages.
3. *Periodic checks* for high blood pressure, blood glucose, and serum cholesterol.
4. Avoid cigarette smoking and alcoholic drinks.

References

1. Barstow C, Rice MS, McDivitt JD. Acute Coronary Syndrome: Diagnostic Evaluation. Am Fam Physician. 2017 Feb 1;95(3):170–7.
2. Didkowska J, Wojciechowska U, Mańczuk M, Łobaszewski J. Lung cancer epidemiology: contemporary and future challenges worldwide. Ann Transl Med 2016 Apr;4(8):150. PMCID: PMC4860480.

3. Sekhar A, Kuttan A, Borges JC, Rajachandran M. Food for Thought or Feeding a Dogma? Diet and Coronary Artery Disease: a Clinician's Perspective. Curr Cardiol Rep. 2021 Jul 19;23(9):127.
4. Temple NJ. Fat, Sugar, Whole Grains and Heart Disease: 50 Years of Confusion. Nutrients 2018 Jan 4;10(1):E39. PMCID: PMC5793267.
5. Afshin A, Micha R, Khatibzadeh S, Mozaffarian D. Consumption of nuts and legumes and risk of incident ischemic heart disease, stroke, and diabetes: a systematic review and meta-analysis1234. Am J Clin Nutr 2014 Jul;100(1):278–288. PMCID: PMC4144102.
6. Lechner K, von Schacky C, McKenzie AL, Worm N, Nixdorff U, Lechner B, Kränkel N, Halle M, Krauss RM, Scherr J. Lifestyle factors and high-risk atherosclerosis: Pathways and mechanisms beyond traditional risk factors. Eur J Prev Cardiol 2020 Mar;27(4):394–406. PMCID: PMC7065445.
7. Islam SU, Ahmed MB, Ahsan H, Lee Y-S. Recent Molecular Mechanisms and Beneficial Effects of Phytochemicals and Plant-Based Whole Foods in Reducing LDL-C and Preventing Cardiovascular Disease. Antioxid Basel Switz 2021 May 15;10(5):784. PMCID: PMC8157003.
8. Blumberg JB, Vita JA, Chen C-YO. Concord Grape Juice Polyphenols and Cardiovascular Risk Factors: Dose-Response Relationships. Nutrients 2015 Dec 2;7(12):10032–10052. PMCID: PMC4690071.
9. Yousefi R, Parandoosh M, Khorsandi H, Hosseinzadeh N, Madani Tonekaboni M, Saidpour A, Babaei H, Ghorbani A. Grape seed extract supplementation along with a restricted-calorie diet improves cardiovascular risk factors in obese or overweight adult individuals: A randomized, placebo-controlled trial. Phytother Res PTR 2021 Feb;35(2):987–995. PMID: 33044768.
10. D'Elia L, Dinu M, Sofi F, Volpe M, Strazzullo P, SINU Working Group, Endorsed by SIPREC. 100% Fruit juice intake and cardiovascular risk: a systematic review and meta-analysis of prospective and randomised controlled studies. Eur J Nutr 2021 Aug;60(5):2449–2467. PMCID: PMC8275541.
11. Tasnim S, Tang C, Musini VM, Wright JM. Effect of alcohol on blood pressure. Cochrane Database Syst Rev 2020 Jul 1;7:CD012787. PMCID: PMC8130994.
12. Yarnell JWG, Sweetnam PM, Rumley A, Lowe GDO. Lifestyle and Hemostatic Risk Factors for Ischemic Heart Disease. Arterioscler Thromb Vasc Biol. Am Heart Assoc. 2000 Jan 1;20(1):271–9.
13. Sekhar A, Kuttan A, Borges JC, Rajachandran M. Food for Thought or Feeding a Dogma? Diet and Coronary Artery Disease: a Clinician's Perspective. Curr Cardiol Rep 2021 Jul 19;23(9):127. PMID: 34279741.
14. Mack M, Gopal A. Epidemiology, Traditional and Novel Risk Factors in Coronary Artery Disease. Cardiol Clin. 2014 Aug;32(3):323–32.
15. McCormack J, Pfiffner P. The Absolute CVD Risk/Benefit Calculator [Internet]. 2017. Available from: https://cvdcalculator.com/
16. Wong ND. Cardiovascular risk assessment: The foundation of preventive cardiology. Am J Prev Cardiol 2020 Mar;1:100008. PMCID: PMC8315480.
17. Institute of Health Metrics and Evaluation, University of Washington, Seattle. Global Burden of Disease [Internet]. Available from: http://ghdx.healthdata.org/gbd-results-tool.
18. Shah T, Palaskas N, Ahmed A. An Update on Gender Disparities in Coronary Heart Disease Care. Curr Atheroscler Rep 2016 May;18(5):28. PMID: 27029220.
19. Benjamin EJ, Muntner P, Alonso A, Bittencourt MS, Callaway CW, Carson AP, Chamberlain AM, Chang AR, Cheng S, Das SR, Delling FN, Djousse L, Elkind MSV, Ferguson JF, Fornage M, Jordan LC, Khan SS, Kissela BM, Knutson KL, Kwan TW, Lackland DT, Lewis TT, Lichtman JH, Longenecker CT, Loop MS, Lutsey PL, Martin SS, Matsushita K, Moran AE, Mussolino ME, O'Flaherty M, Pandey A, Perak AM, Rosamond WD, Roth GA, Sampson UKA, Satou GM, Schroeder EB, Shah SH, Spartano NL, Stokes A, Tirschwell DL, Tsao CW,

Turakhia MP, VanWagner LB, Wilkins JT, Wong SS, Virani SS, null. Heart Disease and Stroke Statistics—2019 Update: A Report From the American Heart Association Circulation. Am Heart Assoc. 2019 Mar 5;139(10):e56–e528.
20. Einarson TR, Acs A, Ludwig C, Panton UH. Economic Burden of Cardiovascular Disease in Type 2 Diabetes: A Systematic Review. Value Health J Int Soc Pharmacoeconomics Outcomes Res 2018 Jul;21(7):881–890. PMID: 30005761.
21. Gheorghe A, Griffiths U, Murphy A, Legido-Quigley H, Lamptey P, Perel P. The economic burden of cardiovascular disease and hypertension in low- and middle-income countries: a systematic review. BMC Public Health 2018 Aug 6;18(1):975. PMCID: PMC6090747.
22. Odegaard AO, Koh WP, Yuan J-M, Gross MD, Pereira MA. Western-style fast food intake and cardiometabolic risk in an Eastern country. Circulation 2012 Jul 10;126(2):182–188. PMCID: PMC4059207.
23. Yuyun MF, Sliwa K, Kengne AP, Mocumbi AO, Bukhman G. Cardiovascular Diseases in Sub-Saharan Africa Compared to High-Income Countries: An Epidemiological Perspective. Glob Heart 2020 Feb 12;15(1):15. PMCID: PMC7218780.
24. Barrington-Trimis JL, Braymiller JL, Unger JB, McConnell R, Stokes A, Leventhal AM, Sargent JD, Samet JM, Goodwin RD. Trends in the Age of Cigarette Smoking Initiation Among Young Adults in the US From 2002 to 2018. JAMA Netw Open 2020 Oct 1;3(10):e2019022. PMCID: PMC7539122.
25. Kim HC. Epidemiology of cardiovascular disease and its risk factors in Korea. Glob Health Med 2021 Jun 30;3(3):134–141. PMCID: PMC8239378.
26. Mieno MN, Tanaka N, Arai T, Kawahara T, Kuchiba A, Ishikawa S, Sawabe M. Accuracy of Death Certificates and Assessment of Factors for Misclassification of Underlying Cause of Death. J Epidemiol 2016;26(4):191–198. PMCID: PMC4808686.

Non-atherosclerotic Coronary Artery Disease

Rohit Samuel and Jacqueline Saw

When considering symptomatic myocardial ischemia, there is a predominant focus on the presence of obstructive coronary artery disease as the primary pathological process. However, in many cases, there is minimal or even no discernible obstructive plaque even when invasive coronary angiography is utilized. It is important to recognize the potential underlying pathologies in such scenarios as this can have a significant impact on the diagnosis, management, and overall patient outcomes. In this chapter, we will discuss processes within the coronary vasculature that can manifest through the full spectrum of acute and chronic coronary syndromes, collectively termed NACAD (Table 1).

Table 1 Causes of coronary artery disease

Atherosclerotic coronary artery disease
• Plaque rupture/erosion
• Imbalance of oxygen supply/demand
Non-atherosclerotic coronary artery disease
• Spontaneous coronary artery dissection
• Coronary vasospasm
• Coronary embolism
• Myocardial bridge
• Coronary vasculitis (e.g., Kawasaki disease)
• Coronary ectasia/aneurysm
• Congenital anomaly

R. Samuel · J. Saw (✉)
Division of Cardiology, Vancouver General Hospital, University of British Columbia, Vancouver, BC, Canada
e-mail: jsaw@mail.ubc.ca

G. Concistrè (ed.), *Ischemic Heart Disease*,
https://doi.org/10.1007/978-3-031-25879-4_7

1 Definitions

To identify the presence of NACAD, it is first important to define the presence of obstructive and potentially clinically relevant atherosclerotic disease. Obstructive coronary disease has previously been defined as a luminal stenosis of greater than or equal to 50%; however, values of up to 70% have been used [1]. It is important to recognize that atherosclerotic lesions causing less than 50% luminal stenosis may still have clinical relevance, and long-term follow-up data has shown an increase in MACE compared with those who have no identifiable coronary artery disease. Furthermore, although coronary angiography is considered the gold standard, it is still subject to significant interobserver variability [2]. These differences are particularly stark when lesions are of moderate severity. In these situations, the use of invasive physiological testing may be particularly beneficial to identify obstructive ischemia given the large evidence base for both hyperemic and non-hyperemic pressure ratios [3, 4].

NACAD pathologies can present through the full spectrum of coronary syndromes, from stable angina to STEMI. When there is evidence of myocardial injury, the term MINOCA is used [5]. This particular entity comprises a clinical presentation consistent with AMI based on clinical presentation and elevated cardiac biomarkers, but an absence of obstructive coronary disease (stenosis <50%) and no other direct clinical cause for the presentation. It is important to note that MINOCA is a descriptive term, and not a diagnosis in and of itself. If MINOCA is suspected based on accepted criteria, a thorough diagnostic evaluation should be performed with particular attention given to the pathologies outlined in the remainder of this chapter.

2 Spontaneous Coronary Artery Dissection

SCAD is an important cause of AMI, particularly in young women with minimal atherosclerotic risk factors [6]. It is defined as a spontaneous separation of the coronary artery wall that is not iatrogenic or related to trauma. SCAD is an important differential diagnosis in patients presenting with potential NACAD. Dissection may occur in small, branching vessels or in the distal termination of larger vascular beds. This can lead to missed diagnoses unless there is a high index of suspicion, and appropriate care is taken when interpreting the angiogram.

3 Epidemiology

The true prevalence of SCAD is unclear due to underdiagnosis, but it is increasingly recognized as a cause of AMI, especially in young women without traditional coronary risk factors [7]. It is estimated that SCAD is implicated in 0.1–4% of ACS overall, based on registry data and case series [8–10]. Women make up between 87 and 95% of SCAD presentations with a mean age between 44 and 53 years at the time of event [11]. Although rare, SCAD can still occur in men with approximately 10% of cases occurring in males [12]. Men presenting with SCAD tend to be younger than women and are more likely to present with a physical exertion trigger.

There is a large variability in physician comfort in assessing and managing SCAD patients, given this relative rarity [13]. The prevalence of SCAD is much greater when considering ACS in young women, ranging from 24 to 35% in two retrospective datasets [14, 15]. Pregnant women are at particularly high risk for SCAD [16]. SCAD is the most common cause of AMI in pregnancy, occurring in 15–43% in some series [17, 18]. P-SCAD can occur in the antepartum period, any time during pregnancy, or up to 24 months postpartum [19]; however, it is most common in the first postpartum month, and particularly in the first week [20].

SCAD can affect any section of the coronary vasculature but is most commonly observed in the LAD artery, where it can occur in up to 46% of cases [7]. The circumflex, obtuse marginal, and ramus intermedius territories are the next most commonly affected, followed by the RCA and its branches. De novo LM SCAD is relatively rare in most series, occurring in between 1.5 and 4% of cases. However, involvement of the LM is a high-risk feature with poor long-term outcomes [21].

SCAD has a high risk of recurrence, with a rate of 10.4% over a median follow-up of 3.1 years in one series, emphasizing the need for prompt diagnosis, appropriate management, and careful long-term follow-up of these patients [22].

4 Pathophysiology

The pathognomonic feature of SCAD is the presence of a false lumen containing intramural hematoma as demonstrated histologically [7]. The underlying mechanism of SCAD is not fully understood; however, two theories have been proposed (Fig. 1) [23]. The first

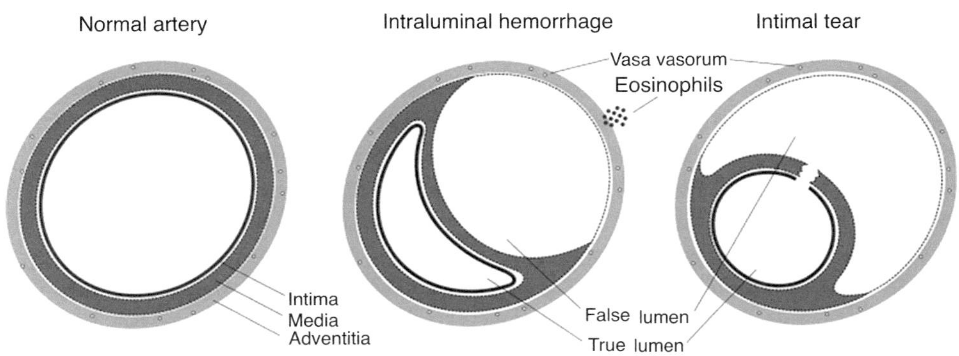

Fig. 1 Schematic diagram of the mechanisms of spontaneous coronary artery dissection. Reproduced with permission from Elsevier [23]

involves the formation of an intimal tear leading to the passage of endoluminal blood into the intimal space, leading to the formation of a false lumen. A second theory suggests that the rupture of vasa vasorum with subsequent intramural hemorrhage is the precipitating event for the formation of the false lumen. In both cases, there is a pressure-driven expansion of the false lumen by enlarging hematoma, which can lead to significant luminal narrowing with secondary myocardial ischemia and potentially infarction. Thrombus does not usually play a significant role in the obstruction of coronary flow in SCAD based on angiographic and OCT series [24–26].

Histological changes suggestive of periadventitial inflammation have been described previously. These "periarteritis"-like changes include an eosinophilic infiltrate, which have been described in multiple series [27]. It is unclear if the presence of this inflammatory milieu of cells contributes or predisposes to the formation of dissection through breakdown of the medial-adventitial interface. It is more likely that these findings are a reaction to the vascular injury as opposed to a causative factor. Cystic medial necrosis has been described in some older SCAD series, but the significance of this finding is uncertain and has not been described in more contemporary studies [7].

The female predominance for SCAD may suggest a genetic or hormonal component for the development of the condition [28]. As previously mentioned, there is a clear increased risk during pregnancy and the postpartum period, which may reflect the rapidly changing hormonal state. Elevated progesterone levels during pregnancy can weaken the arterial media through its effect on elastic fibers, collagen synthesis, and induction of cystic medial necrosis with disruption of the vasa vasorum [6, 29, 30]. For this reason, women who have had an episode of SCAD are advised to avoid exogenous hormonal therapies although this requires further investigation. The hemodynamic changes of pregnancy may also contribute to SCAD predisposition. The increase in cardiac output and state of relative volume retention have been shown to increase arterial shear stress, which can impact the aorta and further extend into the coronary arteries [31].

4.1 Predisposing and Precipitating Factors

A number of factors may play a role in the development of SCAD, such that the underlying etiologies are likely multifactorial. This is further suggested by the unusual demographics and lack of traditional cardiac risk factors found within the SCAD population [7]. Multiple studies have found associations between SCAD and arteriopathies, genetic factors, circulating hormones, and environmental stressors to precipitate SCAD.

One of the earliest described associations was the presence of FMD in patients with SCAD, first identified in 2005 and confirmed in multiple subsequent case series [32–35]. FMD is a non-atherosclerotic, non-inflammatory disease of the systemic vasculature that has a range of manifestations from tortuosity to aneurysm and dissection [36]. It is radiographically defined as alternating areas of stenosis and dilatation, resulting in a so-called

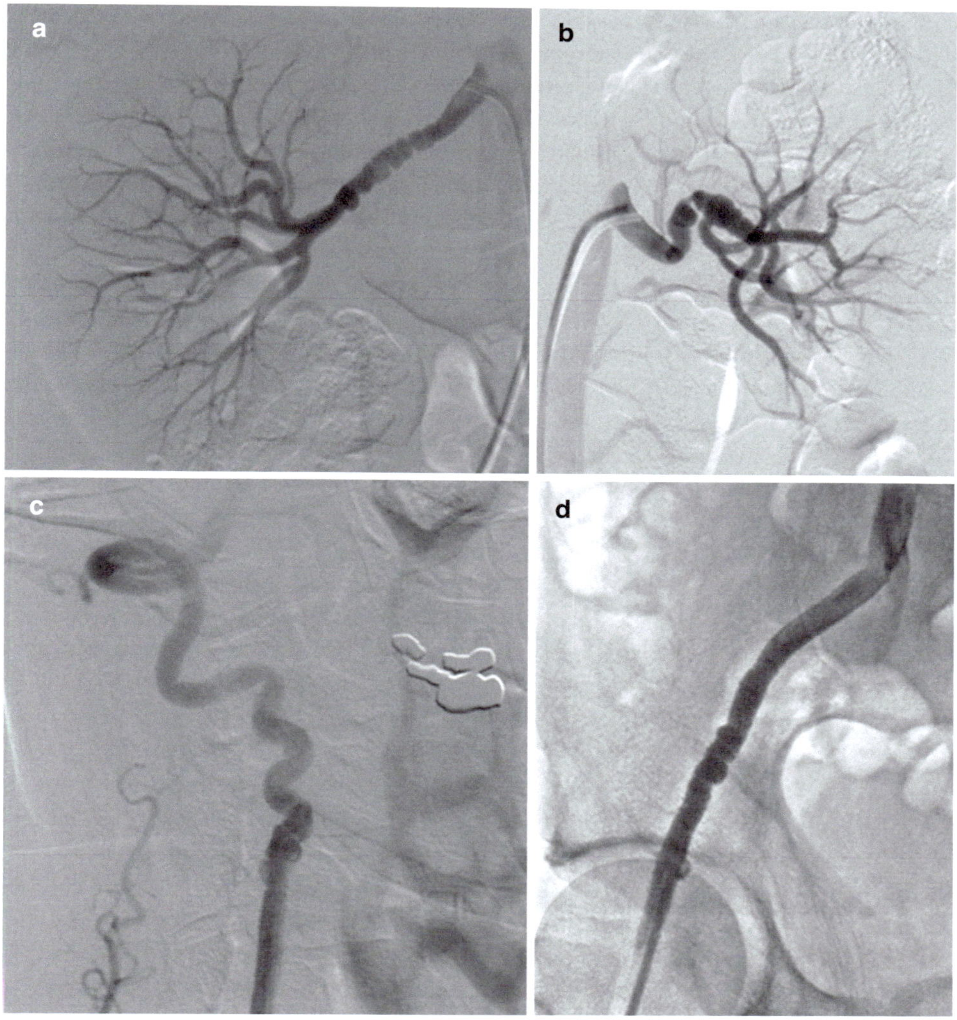

Fig. 2 Examples of extracoronary multifocal fibromuscular dysplasia (FMD): (**a**) right renal artery, (**b**) left renal artery, (**c**) right vertebral artery, and (**d**) right external iliac artery. Reused with permission from Wolters Kluwer Health [37]

string of beads pattern (Fig. 2), also known as multifocal FMD [37]. FMD can affect any arterial bed, but features are most commonly screened for in the cranial vasculature, the renal and the iliac arteries. Cohort studies have suggested a widely varying prevalence of the condition in the SCAD population, ranging from 17 to 86% depending on the imaging test used for screening [7]. There have been case reports linking the histopathological changes of FMD in coronary arteries affected by SCAD, confirming a pathophysiological link [38, 39].

Inherited vascular disorders and their associated genetic mutations can be associated with SCAD. These conditions include vascular Ehlers-Danlos syndrome, Marfan syndrome, and Loeys-Dietz syndrome among others [7]. SCAD associated with these conditions can cluster in families; however, non-syndromic SCAD does not appear to be familial [40]. In one series, a family history of SCAD was only seen in 1.2% of patients [41]. Retrospective registries have identified rates of 5–13% of patients with SCAD having underlying genetic mutations that predispose to vascular fragility and similar syndromes [42, 43]. Therefore, even though some of these genetic disorders can be diagnosed via screening, they remain relatively low yield in the absence of specific clinical characteristics [6].

In patients who have an underlying predisposition to vascular fragility and SCAD, a precipitating factor or trigger can lead to a pathological event. However, the link between these is not always clear and may not even be present in some patients for reasons which are not fully understood [7]. The most common trigger is an emotional or physical stressor, occurring in 40% and 24% of SCAD patients, respectively [24]. Emotional stressors tend to be more common in women, while men have a higher prevalence of physical stressors such as isometric exercise [44]. Any increase in thoracoabdominal pressure (Valsalva) or circulating catecholamines has been theorized to increase vascular shear stress that can trigger SCAD [6]. This hypothesis has not been specifically investigated in patients with SCAD but is mechanistically similar to other conditions such as Takotsubo syndrome [7].

4.2 Diagnosis

The overwhelming majority of patients with a SCAD event will present with symptoms and signs of ACS, with chest pain being the most common symptom presentation occurring in up to 96% of patients [45]. It should be noted however that the chest pain characteristics may not be typical for ACS, especially in women who represent the majority of SCAD presentations. Furthermore, given the patient demographics and absence of traditional cardiac risk factors, there is a higher potential for missed diagnosis which can have longer term consequences. The initial evaluation of patients should reflect standard care for any suspected ACS, including early ECG, cardiac biomarkers, and cardiac telemetry.

Invasive coronary angiography is the gold standard for diagnosis and should be used promptly when SCAD is suspected, particularly in clinically unstable patients who represent up to a third of presentations [45]. Furthermore, angiography allows further classification of the SCAD lesion into one of the three distinct angiographic subtypes, a framework which is now widely used [25, 46]. Type 1 is the pathognomonic appearance of SCAD with contrast dye staining of the arterial wall and multiple radiolucent lumens. Type 2 refers to diffuse narrowing of the affected vessel, which can be further divided into two subtypes. Type 2A SCAD is a diffuse narrowing with normal segments of vessel proximally and distally to the intramural hematoma. Type 2B is a diffuse narrowing that has normal vessel proximally but extends to the distal tip of the artery. This subtype can be misinterpreted as normal tapering of the vessel. Type 3 refers to a focal or tubular stenosis that mimics atherosclerosis and is the most difficult to accurately diagnose. It may be particularly helpful to use intracoronary imaging when this type is suspected to more accurately differentiate between plaque and intramural hematoma. Type 2 is the most commonly reported angiographic manifestation of SCAD, occurring in 67.5% of patients in one series [24]. Type 1 was reported in 29.1%, whereas type 3 was seen in 3.4%. It should also be noted that coronary angiography is not without risk in the SCAD population. The presence of an underlying vascular fragility puts these patients at an increased risk of iatrogenic catheter-induced dissection, with a reported prevalence of 3.4% [47].

Intracoronary imaging through the use of IVUS and OCT is useful, especially when the diagnosis is uncertain. OCT is particularly beneficial for diagnosing SCAD due to its higher spatial resolution than IVUS, allowing for more accurate identification of intimal tear, false lumen, and intramural hematoma. For this reason, it is the preferred imaging modality when diagnosis is uncertain and when it is technically feasible to use [7]. This is tempered by the need to use contrast injection for image acquisition, which has a theoretical risk of worsening SCAD through hydraulic dissection. IVUS is not limited by this factor and remains a good alternative to OCT when required.

CCTA has been suggested as a potential alternative to invasive angiography for diagnosing SCAD, but its use is limited by lower spatial and temporal resolution that poses difficulties in identifying features of SCAD such as intimal tears and formation of a false lumen [48]. However, it may be a useful tool for noninvasive follow-up of prior SCAD [49]. The use of CT for this indication would be limited to SCAD affecting proximal and larger caliber vessel, as the diagnostic utility reduces significantly for distal segments, side branches, and small-caliber vessels.

4.3 Management

In the majority of SCAD patients who are hemodynamically stable without evidence of ongoing ischemia, a conservative approach is the preferred management strategy [7, 11]. This recommendation is guided by observational data, particularly the finding of angiographic healing of the dissected artery that can occur in the first few days to 1 month post-event [24, 50]. Patients should be monitored in hospital for 3–5 days following the event, with hospital stay guided by the presence of left ventricular dysfunction, ventricular arrhythmia, or evidence of ongoing ischemia. There is a potential early risk of dissection extension or recurrent SCAD in this period, occurring in 5–10% of cases.

Pharmacotherapy strategies differ from traditional ACS due to differing underlying pathophysiology and a lack of clear evidence for use. Antiplatelet therapy with aspirin is generally recommended for lifetime use, although some practitioners may shorten this duration. Clopidogrel is recommended for at least 1–3 months post-event. Beta-blocker is the only pharmacotherapy that was shown to be associated with lower SCAD recurrence, demonstrating a 64% reduction in one study at a median follow-up of 3 years [22].

Therefore, it is recommended that all SCAD patients should be on maximally tolerated beta-blocker.

A conservative strategy may not be possible in patients with hemodynamic instability, ventricular arrhythmia, or involvement of proximal vessel subtending a large area of myocardium. In these situations, coronary revascularization should be considered. Percutaneous coronary intervention (PCI) in SCAD is associated with significant technical challenges and potential complications [24, 26, 50]. There is an inherent risk of propagating dissection through the use of guide catheters, guide wires, or deployment of coronary stents. Some strategies that may improve outcomes include the use of long stents extending beyond the intramural hematoma, cutting balloon fenestration to allow decompression of the false lumen, and sealing both ends of the intramural hematoma prior to stenting the middle to reduce the risk of propagation [51, 52]. Femoral access should be preferred, given that radial access may require greater manipulation to achieve coaxiality of guide catheters which can increase dissection risk. CABG has been shown to be safe when indicated and may be required following complication of PCI or involvement of the left main [26]. There is a high rate of graft failure during long-term follow-up, most likely related to healing of the native artery with competitive flow leading to graft occlusion.

Following SCAD, a number of non-pharmacological strategies can be utilized to reduce the risk of recurrence. These include limiting lifting heavy weights (avoiding >20 pounds for women and >50 pounds for men) to reduce arterial shear stress, use of psychological support to reduce the risk of depression and anxiety, and encouraging all patients to join a cardiac rehabilitation program [7]. Ideally, this would entail the use of a SCAD-specific rehabilitation program, tailored to the unique exercise and psychosocial demands of these patients. This includes baseline cardiopulmonary exercise testing, a graded aerobic exercise program, resistance training limited to weights under 20 pounds, and multidisciplinary care including support groups, psychotherapy, and educational sessions. The use of a SCAD-specific program has been shown to improve exercise capacity, reduce severity of depressive symptoms, and reduce MACE [53]. General access to a specialized SCAD rehabilitation program is limited; however, standard cardiac rehabilitation has been shown to be safe and effective in SCAD patients [54, 55].

5 Coronary Vasospasm

Coronary vasospasm is an intense, transient vasoconstriction of an epicardial coronary artery resulting in subtotal or total occlusion of myocardial blood flow that can result in angina or ACS. It can occur in vessels with and without coronary atherosclerosis, and although it is usually considered a chest pain syndrome, it can precipitate severe MI, arrhythmia, and sudden cardiac death [56, 57]. Vasospastic angina was first described by Prinzmetal in 1959, which he termed "variant angina" as the characteristics of the syndrome differed from classical exertional angina [58]. Variant angina was described as occurring in young patients without known cardiovascular risk factors and was associated with transient ECG changes. It is now known that coronary vasospasm can affect both the epicardial vessels and the microvasculature [59].

5.1 Epidemiology

The overall prevalence of coronary vasospasm is unclear due to variations in population characteristics and lack of routine coronary provocation testing in cases where a non-atherosclerotic cause for presentation is suspected [60]. It is more common in East Asian than Caucasian populations, but the underlying mechanism is unclear [61]. In one study of routine coronary provocation testing following a diagnosis of MINOCA, there were higher rates of vasospasm in Japanese and Korean patients than their white counterparts [5, 62]. Spasm is more common in males than females and is mainly diagnosed in patients aged between 40 and 70 [63]. Rates of coronary spasm may be higher than currently reported, and it remains underdiagnosed due to the lack of aforementioned routine testing. In the ACOVA study of patients with stable angina and nonobstructive coronary disease, the rate of coronary vasospasm induced by routine acetylcholine provocation was 62%, with an almost even split of epicardial or microvascular spasm [64]. When patients with MINOCA are considered, rates of spasm are similarly high with acetylcholine provocation at 79% [65].

5.2 Pathophysiology

The pathophysiology of coronary vasospasm is not fully understood but is likely multifactorial with vascular smooth muscle hyperreactivity playing a key role. Under normal physiological circumstances, the constriction and dilatation of the coronary vasculature play an important role in the regulation of myocardial blood flow and perfusion pressure. Therefore, the pathophysiological state of coronary vasospasm that leads to myocardial ischemia appears to be part of a spectrum that is underpinned by shared mechanism, albeit a malfunctioning one [59, 66].

Vascular smooth muscle hyperreactivity has been implicated as a key factor in the pathogenesis of coronary vasospasm. MLC kinase and phosphatase regulate the contraction and relaxation of vascular smooth muscle. The molecule rho kinase is implicated in the inhibition of MLC phosphatase and has been found to be upregulated in areas of spasm leading to hypercontraction of the vascular smooth muscle [60, 67]. This is mediated through enhanced sensitivity to calcium influx in response to vasoconstrictor stimuli [68].

The autonomic nervous system has been suggested to play a role due to observational data showing increased frequency of vasospastic angina after midnight into the early hours of the morning, times when vagal tone is the greatest [69, 70]. Furthermore, the use of sympathomimetic agents such as acetylcholine to precipitate spasm implies that an imbalance in parasympathetic and sympathetic may be at play. The use of surgical autonomic denervation of the heart has been shown to ameliorate refractory spasm in some case reports [71].

The normal endothelium has an important role in maintaining vascular tone through the release of vasoactive substances such as prostaglandins and nitric oxide among others [60]. Endothelial dysfunction was therefore hypothesized to contribute to the development of coronary spasm, but clear evidence is lacking. Furthermore, endothelial dysfunction is relatively common in the population while coronary vasospasm is not. Nevertheless, dysfunctional endothelium may still predispose to the formation of spasm when combined with underlying vascular smooth muscle hyperreactivity.

Chronic inflammation has been found in the coronary vascular adventitia and adipose tissue of patients with vasospastic angina and could be a marker for disease activity [72]. This finding suggests that inflammatory mediators may contribute to spasm, a hypothesis that is further strengthened by evidence demonstrating that the inflammatory mediator interleukin-B can trigger coronary vasospasm in a porcine model [73]. Other serum inflammatory markers are significantly elevated in patients with vasospasm when compared with controls, but levels are still lower than in patients with atherosclerotic ACS [74].

Reactive oxygen species and oxygen free radicals are known to damage the vascular endothelium, leading to endothelial dysfunction and reduction in nitric oxide production [60]. Thioredoxin, a biomarker of oxidative stress, is increased in patients with known vasospasm [75]. Furthermore, antioxidants such as vitamin E have been shown to be consumed at a greater rate in patients with vasospasm when compared with controls and those with atherosclerotic stable angina. This suggests a greater level of oxidative stress in the vasospastic patient [76].

5.3 Risk and Precipitating Factors

A number of factors can put individuals at increased risk of developing coronary vasospasm. As previously mentioned, people of East Asian backgrounds have a higher risk of developing coronary spasm. Cigarette smoking is strongly associated with the development of vasospasm, particularly in younger males [77, 78]. It may also develop as part of a systemic vasospastic disorder as spasm is associated with Raynaud's phenomenon and migraine [79]. Importantly, traditional atherosclerotic risk factors such as hypertension and dyslipidemia do not predict the development of vasospastic angina [78].

Although coronary vasospasm can occur spontaneously, and does so in most cases, there are also potential precipitants or triggers for discrete episodes. In particular, there are a number of substances that can induce a vasospastic episode. These include medications such as general anesthesia, bromocriptine, triptans, dobutamine, and capecitabine, as well as illicit substances such as cocaine and amphetamines [60]. Physical triggers include hyperventilation, cold exposure, early morning exercise, and Valsalva maneuver [63].

5.4 Diagnosis

Diagnosis of coronary vasospasm has been standardized by the Coronary Vasomotion Disorders International Study Group (COVADIS), combining three key components including the classical clinical manifestations, transient ECG changes, and documentation of coronary spasm either spontaneously or through provocation testing [80].

Clinically, patients present with chronic, recurrent episodes of chest pain that may be similar to classical angina. However, episodes are predominantly at rest and occur in the early hours of the morning. The pain is usually nitrate and CCB responsive but may not be relieved by beta-blocker. Patient with coronary vasospasm may also have episodes of silent ischemia, which is significant due to the risk of presentation with malignant arrhythmia or sudden cardiac death [81].

Transient ECG changes can occur with the onset of chest discomfort, and both ST elevation and depression are included as part of the diagnostic criteria. These changes rapidly return to baseline with resolution of symptoms, unlike in atherosclerotic ACS. The ECG is frequently normal between episodes of discomfort, making diagnosis more challenging. Therefore, the use of ambulatory ECG monitoring should be considered when the diagnosis is suspected. Given that the frequency of episodes can be low, longer term monitoring with an event monitor or implantable loop recorder or similar device can be useful to detect ischemic changes over extended periods. Ambulatory monitoring is also effective in monitoring treatment efficacy, given the frequency of asymptomatic episodes. Asymptomatic episodes with ECG evidence of ischemia occurred in almost 80% of patients undertaking ambulatory ECG monitoring in one cohort [82].

Provocative testing during coronary angiography is the gold standard for documenting the presence of coronary spasm when the index of suspicion is high. This is achieved through intracoronary administration of a provocative stimulus usually acetylcholine, ergonovine, or methylergonovine [60]. It should be noted that hyperventilation can be used as a provocative stimulus and has a high specificity when used with ECG monitoring, but is rarely used in the catheterization laboratory [83]. Baseline coronary angiography without provocation is also useful to exclude atherosclerotic disease as a cause for the presenting symptoms. A positive provocation test must include the reproduction of usual chest pain, ischemic ECG changes, and a greater than 90% vasoconstrictive response as imaged on angiography [60, 84]. The test is considered equivocal if all three components are not present. Intracoronary nitrate should be rapidly administered to reverse the spasm and restore coronary blood flow. Care should be taken while performing provocative testing, as serious complications can occur, although rare [85]. Registry data has shown that provocation is safe in the contemporary era, but rates of significant brady- or tachyarrhythmia occurred in 6.8% of patients [5, 86]. Even so, it should not be performed in pregnant women and those with severe hypertension, significant left main stenosis, advanced heart failure, and severe aortic stenosis [63].

Intracoronary imaging with IVUS or OCT can be useful in specific situations. Both modalities can be used to identify the presence of concomitant atherosclerotic plaque, which may not be visible on angiography. The increased spatial resolution of OCT allows interrogation of the coronary structure during spasm, including conformational changes in the intima and media [87]. However, use of intracoronary devices can also induce spasm, which may confound results.

5.5 Management

The management of coronary vasospasm aims to reduce the frequency of symptoms and also reduce the risk of serious complications. Lifestyle factors can be key in reducing potential triggers, and this includes smoking cessation and avoiding illicit drugs such as cocaine or amphetamines.

Sublingual short-acting nitrates remain the mainstay for relief of acute attacks [84]. They are effective in reducing the duration of each episode, which also limits myocardial ischemia. Calcium channel blockers are the first-line therapy for vasospastic angina, and their use has been shown to improve infarct-free survival [88]. Either dihydropyridine or non-dihydropyridine CCBs can be used to good effect, depending on the side effect profile and individual patient factors. Long-acting nitrates can be used in conjunction with CCBs, when patients have refractory symptoms that are not ameliorated by CCBs alone. They are not used as a first-line therapy, due to concerns over nitrate intolerance. Furthermore, observational data has suggested that longer term use of long-acting nitrates may not have any significant benefit over CCBs alone, but more data is required before firm recommendations can be made [89].

Rho kinase inhibitors have been developed to act directly on the vasospastic mechanisms within the coronary artery. Fasudil is a rho kinase inhibitor that has been shown to inhibit acetylcholine-induced spasm [90]. However, although useful in confirming the role of rho kinase in the pathogenesis of coronary spasm, its use is limited due to the need for intravenous administration.

Statins have a beneficial effect in the prevention of spasm, likely through beneficial effects on the vascular endothelium to improve nitric oxide release and induce relaxation of smooth muscle. A randomized trial of fluvastatin versus placebo in conjunction with CCBs showed a significant reduction in spasm on invasive provocative testing [91]. Furthermore, statin use reduced MACE at 5 years in patients on statin therapy after diagnosis of coronary vasospasm with acetylcholine provocation [92].

In patients who are refractory to medical therapy, PCI can be considered as a therapeutic option. It is indicated in patients who have significant coronary atherosclerosis which may be a trigger for focal spasm, or in patients who have clearly identifiable vasospastic segment that is refractory to medical therapy even in the absence of atherosclerosis [93]. However, many patients have diffuse or multivessel spasm and the role of a mechanical intervention in these settings is unclear.

Patients who have had a serious ventricular arrhythmia can be considered for insertion of an ICD for secondary prevention. A high rate of ventricular events with delivery of therapy was seen in one study of patients who received ICDs as secondary prevention; however, the use of ICDs did not significantly improve survival in another cohort despite a trend towards a reduction in cardiac death [94, 95]. There is currently no consensus on the use of device therapy in this population, and its use should be considered on a case-by-case basis.

6 Coronary Embolism

CE is an important etiology of NACAD but is likely underdiagnosed in clinical studies. It can be divided into three distinct types: direct, paradoxical, and iatrogenic [96]. The coronary arteries are relatively protected from embolic events compared to the systemic circulation, owing to the acute takeoff from the aortic sinuses [96]. Obstruction of myocardial blood flow leads to ischemia and ACS.

6.1 Prevalence

Early estimates of the prevalence of CE come from autopsy studies, where the rate of CE was 13% of AMI. Diagnosis was made on the basis of the presence of thrombotic material in the coronary arteries without a clear sign of plaque rupture, although this could be difficult to determine if the plaque burden was small [97]. A more contemporary study examining all comers with a first AMI showed a 3% prevalence of CE, using proposed diagnostic criteria for CE [98]. Atrial fibrillation was the most common underlying cause, followed by cardiomyopathy and valvular heart disease. There was no significant difference in the distribution of CE between the epicardial coronary arteries. Multivessel CE was present in 15%, while 23% had systemic embolization. A third of patients were found to have an intracardiac source.

6.2 Classification of Coronary Embolism

Direct CE results from thrombus originating from within a cardiac chamber, most commonly the left atrium and the left ventricle. However, there is evidence of direct embolism from the pulmonary veins, vegetations of infective and noninfective endocarditis, and cardiac tumors such as atrial myxoma [59]. The most common risk factor for direct embolism is the presence of AF without anticoagulation, which can lead to the formation of intracardiac thrombus and subsequent embolization. Prosthetic valves, particularly mechanical heart valves in the mitral position, are another important source of thrombus. This is an especially high-risk setting when there is a coexisting prothrombotic state, such as pregnancy. Infective endocarditis leads to clinically significant coronary embolism in 1.5% of cases; however, the rates of embolism at autopsy are much greater [96, 99]. The risk of a mycotic embolus increases with vegetation size >10 mm, mitral valve endocarditis, and staphylococcal or fungal infection [100].

Paradoxical CE occurs when emboli originate from the venous circulation and enter the systemic circulation through a left-to-right shunt, most commonly a PFO. The prevalence of paradoxical embolism is unknown but has been described in case reports [59].

Iatrogenic CE is the embolization of material into the coronary arteries during an interventional procedure and can comprise clot, air, or foreign material. It is most common during cardiothoracic surgery and interventional coronary procedures [96].

6.3 Diagnosis

The clinical presentation of CE is indistinguishable from atherosclerotic ACS, and therefore management should proceed as per a standard ACS pathway. In the majority of cases, patients will undergo coronary angiography which may reveal the offending thrombus and coronary occlusion. Multivessel thrombus is suggestive of an embolic source as opposed to a pathology such as plaque rupture [96]. If thrombus burden is heavy, aspiration can be considered to restore flow in the occluded coronary artery. This also allows for the assessment of any underlying atherosclerotic plaque that could have been the nidus for thrombus formation following a plaque rupture. Aspirated material should be sent for pathological evaluation in select cases where a non-thrombotic pathology is suspected, namely infected vegetation, malignancy, or foreign material [96].

Patients should be screened for the etiology of the embolism and for signs of systemic embolism. Inpatient telemetry or ambulatory ECG monitoring may be required to diagnose occult AF as a cause of intracardiac thrombus. Transthoracic echocardiography allows for the assessment of left ventricular thrombus, valvular vegetations, and presence of PFO. These pathologies can be further evaluated by transesophageal echocardiography, with the added benefit of left atrial appendage (LAA) assessment. Bubble studies with and without Valsalva maneuver using agitated saline may be used in both modalities to confirm the presence of PFO.

Routine thrombophilia testing is not useful in the setting of CE, unless there are features on clinical history and examination to suggest an underlying inherited thrombophilia.

6.4 Management

The management of CE can be divided into the acute management of the embolic event and the longer term strategy to prevent a recurrence of embolism. In the acute setting, the interventionalist can consider balloon angioplasty of the embolized material to restore flow to the affected coronary. However, this is associated with the risk of distal embolization to the microcirculation and the no-reflow phenomenon. If thrombus burden is large, aspiration can be considered as previously mentioned. This can be performed through the use of specialized catheter with manual aspiration, or with more advanced thrombectomy systems. The use of aspiration thrombectomy is controversial as randomized trials have not shown benefit in routine use in the context of STEMI, and its use is also associated with an increased risk of stroke [101, 102]. It may have a beneficial role in patients with large thrombus burden, with a reduction in cardiovascular mortality [103]. However, the small stroke risk still remains.

If aspiration is unsuccessful or partially successful, with ongoing evidence of ischemia, then other strategies should be considered. This includes the use of intracoronary agents to clear thrombotic material. The use of glycoprotein IIb/IIIa inhibitors is well studied in ACS and can be administered intracoronary and intravenously. Intracoronary thrombolysis has been used in case reports, with good outcomes [104].

Anticoagulation is an important component of therapy in the setting of thrombotic CE. Patients with AF or a persistent risk factor for thromboembolic disease should be maintained on long-term oral anticoagulation [96]. This can be achieved through the use of warfarin or DOACs. The duration of therapy when there is a transient or reversible risk factor is less clear. Expert consensus suggests oral anticoagulation for 3 months following the embolic event.

In the setting of paradoxical embolism, closure of PFO should be considered. There is observational data to suggest a long-term reduction in embolic events following closure in one observational study [105]. Recent randomized data in PFO closure for cerebral thromboembolic events has shown reduction in recurrent events out to 5 years, demonstrating the potential benefits in this setting [106].

7 Myocardial Bridging

MB is a congenital anomaly that occurs when a segment of epicardial coronary artery follows a tunneled course through the myocardium with an overlying muscular bridge. This causes compression of the bridged segment during ventricular systole, which can affect myocardial blood flow and lead to ischemic symptoms. MB is commonly found incidentally on coronary angiography and CCTA and has a benign clinical course in the majority of cases.

7.1 Epidemiology

MB was first recognized as a distinct entity on autopsy studies in 1737 and further characterized in a coronary angiography series in 1960 [107]. The prevalence of MB varies widely based on the mode of evaluation, whether in vivo or on autopsy. This discrepancy is likely due to the presence of thin bridges or myocardial loops that can be detected on autopsy, but does not cause significant systolic compression when imaging is performed in vivo. Rates on autopsy studies vary from 5 to 86%, with a mean of 25% across all studies [107]. The wide range of prevalence rates reflects the difficulty in carefully dissecting the affected vessel to appreciate the presence of a bridged segment [108]. Specific populations have a higher prevalence of MB, including patients with hypertrophic cardiomyopathy and prior heart transplantation, which reflects changes in the density of myocardial tissue.

The rate of MB is much lower when diagnosed via coronary angiography, as it is dependent on compression of the lumen during systole and the so-called milking effect of contrast. Furthermore, there are a number of factors that affect the angiographic appearance of the bridged segment. These include the length and thickness of MB, presence of connective or adipose tissue, coronary vascular tone, presence of fixed stenosis, and myocardial contractility [109]. The LAD is the most commonly affected artery, so it is also likely that MB is underdiagnosed when the circumflex or right coronary arteries are involved [110]. As a result, rates of MB on angiography range from 0.5 to 12% [111]. Diagnosis of MB can increase when provocative testing is used, up to 40% prevalence in some series [107].

The advent of CCTA has allowed for more accurate diagnosis of MB, as it reproduces the anatomical state of the artery in an in vivo setting. Contemporary studies of MB on CCTA have shown similar prevalence rates to autopsy studies, but the functional significance of these lesions cannot be ascertained by CT alone [112, 113].

7.2 Pathophysiology

There is a potential paradox in the presence of ischemia with MB, as coronary blood flow and myocardial perfusion occur predominantly in diastole when theoretically there should be no constriction of the lumen by the overlying myocardium. It is estimated that only 15% of coronary blood flow occurs in the systolic phase of the cardiac cycle [109]. However, in the presence of tachycardia, there is a potential unmasking of MB by decreasing diastolic time and coronary flow reserve [109, 114].

Angiographic and IVUS studies of patients with MB have shown that vessel compression in systole can persist into the diastolic phase, with delayed increase in luminal diameter affecting coronary blood flow [115]. This finding was especially significant during episodes of tachycardia. When atrial pacing was used as a mechanism to induce a tachycardic state in patients with MB causing greater than 70% luminal compression, an average decrease of 41% in the diastolic diameter of the vessel was seen [116]. These findings suggest that persistent diastolic luminal narrowing could explain the presence of ischemia in symptomatic patients.

Furthermore, a number of studies have shown the formation of accelerated atherosclerosis in the area just proximal to the bridged segment, with rates up to 90% when IVUS is used [110, 117]. This may be explained by increased local wall tension and changes in arterial shear stress with subsequent endothelial injury that can lead to atherosclerotic plaque formation [115, 118]. This has been shown on histological studies in a rabbit model, with evidence of endothelial structural changes suggestive of low shear stress [119]. However, it is unlikely that these lesions contribute significantly to the development of symptomatic ischemia [110]. In contrast, there is atherosclerotic sparing of the bridged segment which is most likely related to flow dynamics and its positive impact on the endothelium. The intima of the tunneled segment is thinner and contains a higher proportion of contractile smooth muscle, factors that appear to be protective against atherosclerosis [120]. There is also reduced expression of vasoactive agents such as nitric oxide synthase and endothelin-1 in the wall of the bridged segment, which have been associated with proliferation of smooth muscle and increased atherosclerotic plaque size [110, 121].

7.3 Diagnosis

The diagnosis of MB may require a multimodality approach, especially in symptomatic patients with no other clear cause for their presentation. However, it should be noted that there are no established diagnostic criteria for MB. In the majority of cases, MB is a benign incidental finding, but they can present with a wide range of symptoms ranging from stable angina to ACS, malignant arrhythmia, and sudden cardiac death [122]. Asymptomatic patients with MB can develop symptoms in the context of a separate pathology such as diastolic dysfunction, left ventricular hypertrophy, or microvascular dysfunction.

CCTA is the only reliable noninvasive method for diagnosing MB and has become a useful tool. As previously described, CCTA is the only method that is able to detect MB at similar rates to autopsy series. However, it is only able to give anatomical rather than functional information at this stage.

Coronary angiography is the most common modality for diagnosing MB [110]. It has the benefit of providing anatomical information as well as enabling the use of other modalities such as intracoronary imaging and Doppler. As previously mentioned, key features on angiography are the presence of systolic compression (sometimes referred to as "step down" and "step up" phenomena) as well as "milking" of the bridged segment. There is commonly an area of atherosclerosis proximal to the MB, and on occasion, the MB is not appreciated until PCI is performed to the proximal lesion with subsequent improvement in distal flow [123].

Intracoronary imaging with IVUS is useful for confirming MB. In one series, IVUS was able to detect MB of the LAD in 23% of patients compared with only 3% via angiography alone [124]. A characteristic "half-moon" appearance in the bridged segment can be used to identify MB. IVUS has been shown to correlate with vessel compression and impaired CFR in MB [110, 125], potentially identifying patients who may benefit from intervention.

Functional assessment of the affected artery may be utilized to assess the physiologic impact of MB. FFR can be used; however, systolic pressure can be overestimated and therefore affect the mean FFR over a single cardiac cycle [126]. Therefore, diastolic FFR is the preferred method as it more accurately reflects the hemodynamic state of the MB. Dobutamine should be used as a provocative mechanism in place of adenosine, as it is able to produce a hemodynamic state that is more likely to induce functionally important ischemia [127]. The use of iFR has been well validated against FFR in atherosclerotic cohorts and may be more useful in the setting of MB as it is a purely diastolic index. It has been shown to correlate more closely with patient symptoms when compared to FFR in one study, but further data is needed [128].

The use of intracoronary Doppler in MB can show a characteristic pattern that reflects abrupt early diastolic flow acceleration, mid-to-late diastolic plateau, and retrograde flow in systole [110, 115]. This has been termed a "spike and dome" or "fingertip" pattern [110]. CFR measurements have been shown to be abnormal distal to the bridged segment, despite being normal or slightly reduced in the proximal coronary segment [115, 129].

7.4 Management

The first-line therapy for symptomatic MB is the use of beta-blockers and non-dihydropyridine CCBs [116, 130, 131]. Evidence for their use is derived from observational data but is based on the principle of reducing heart rate and myocardial contractility to reduce symptoms in MB. Beta-blocker has been shown to reduce symptoms in small series, but the hard endpoints of morbidity and mortality have not been evaluated [110]. The use of nitrates is contraindicated in MB due to differential vasodilatation of the proximal segment, which accentuates systolic compression of the bridged segment [132].

In patients with refractory symptoms, PCI or surgery can be considered. PCI has been shown to improve hemodynamic abnormalities as well as symptoms; however, these benefits are offset by high rates of TLR especially when the stent extends into the bridged segment [110, 133]. In one study of LAD MB, patients had a TLR rate of 24% when stenting into the MB, compared with 3% when the stent only covered the area proximal to the bridge. There have been multiple case reports of coronary perforation and stent fracture when attempting PCI into these lesions [110]. Therefore, PCI should be reserved for patients with truly disabling symptoms. Surgery is indicated for patients with refractory symptoms but also deemed at high risk for a significant outcome such as AMI, ventricular arrhythmia, or sudden cardiac death. The surgical options include surgical myotomy or CABG. Surgical myotomy is the resection of the myocardium overlying the tunneled segment, essentially "deroofing" the artery. It has been shown to improve symptoms and coronary blood flow [134, 135]. CABG is most useful in MBs that are >25 mm long or >5 mm deep [122]. It typically involves anastomosis of the left internal mammary artery (LIMA) to the LAD and has an efficacy comparable to myotomy in published series [136].

8 Summary

In conclusion, NACAD is an important cause of stable angina and acute coronary syndrome. These pathologies include SCAD, coronary embolism, MB, and coronary vasospasm, which may occur in different demographic groups with different risk factors from atherosclerotic coronary artery disease. We summarized the key differences, which would aid diagnosis and management of these conditions.

References

1. Scanlon PJ, Faxon DP, Audet AM, Carabello B, Dehmer GJ, Eagle KA, et al. ACC/AHA guidelines for coronary angiography. A report of the American College of Cardiology/American Heart Association Task Force on practice guidelines (Committee on Coronary Angiography). Developed in collaboration with the Society for Cardiac Angiography and Interventions. J Am Coll Cardiol. 1999;33(6):1756–824. https://doi.org/10.1016/s0735-1097(99)00126-6.
2. Nallamothu BK, Spertus JA, Lansky AJ, Cohen DJ, Jones PG, Kureshi F, et al. Comparison of clinical interpretation with visual assessment and quantitative coronary angiography in patients undergoing percutaneous coronary intervention in contemporary practice: the Assessing Angiography (A2) project. Circulation. 2013;127(17):1793–800. https://doi.org/10.1161/CIRCULATIONAHA.113.001952.
3. De Bruyne B, Pijls NH, Kalesan B, Barbato E, Tonino PA, Piroth Z, et al. Fractional flow reserve-guided PCI versus medical therapy in stable coronary disease. N Engl J Med. 2012;367(11):991–1001. https://doi.org/10.1056/NEJMoa1205361.
4. Gotberg M, Christiansen EH, Gudmundsdottir IJ, Sandhall L, Danielewicz M, Jakobsen L, et al. Instantaneous wave-free ratio versus fractional flow reserve to guide PCI. N Engl J Med. 2017;376(19):1813–23. https://doi.org/10.1056/NEJMoa1616540.
5. Tamis-Holland JE, Jneid H, Reynolds HR, Agewall S, Brilakis ES, Brown TM, et al. Contemporary diagnosis and management of patients with myocardial infarction in the absence of obstructive coronary artery disease: a scientific statement from the American Heart Association. Circulation. 2019;139(18):e891–908. https://doi.org/10.1161/CIR.0000000000000670.
6. Saw J, Mancini GBJ, Humphries KH. Contemporary review on spontaneous coronary artery dissection. J Am Coll Cardiol. 2016;68(3):297–312. https://doi.org/10.1016/j.jacc.2016.05.034.
7. Hayes SN, Kim ESH, Saw J, Adlam D, Arslanian-Engoren C, Economy KE, et al. Spontaneous coronary artery dissection: current state of the science: a scientific statement from the American Heart Association. Circulation. 2018;137(19):e523–e57. https://doi.org/10.1161/CIR.0000000000000564.
8. Mortensen KH, Thuesen L, Kristensen IB, Christiansen EH. Spontaneous coronary artery dissection: a Western Denmark Heart Registry study. Catheter Cardiovasc Interv. 2009;74(5):710–7. https://doi.org/10.1002/ccd.22115.
9. Vanzetto G, Berger-Coz E, Barone-Rochette G, Chavanon O, Bouvaist H, Hacini R, et al. Prevalence, therapeutic management and medium-term prognosis of spontaneous coronary artery dissection: results from a database of 11,605 patients. Eur J Cardiothorac Surg. 2009;35(2):250–4. https://doi.org/10.1016/j.ejcts.2008.10.023.
10. Nishiguchi T, Tanaka A, Ozaki Y, Taruya A, Fukuda S, Taguchi H, et al. Prevalence of spontaneous coronary artery dissection in patients with acute coronary syndrome. Eur Heart J Acute Cardiovasc Care. 2016;5(3):263–70. https://doi.org/10.1177/2048872613504310.

11. Hayes SN, Tweet MS, Adlam D, Kim ESH, Gulati R, Price JE, et al. Spontaneous coronary artery dissection: JACC state-of-the-art review. J Am Coll Cardiol. 2020;76(8):961–84. https://doi.org/10.1016/j.jacc.2020.05.084.
12. McAlister C, Alfadhel M, Samuel R, Starovoytov A, Parolis JA, Grewal T, et al. Differences in baseline demographics and clinical outcomes between men and women with spontaneous coronary artery dissection. J Am Coll Cardiol. 2021;77(18_Supplement_1):38. https://doi.org/10.1016/S0735-1097(21)01397-8.
13. Buccheri D, Zambelli G, Alfonso F, Cortese B. Pulse on spontaneous coronary artery dissections: experience-based survey. JACC Cardiovasc Interv. 2017;10(14):1469–71. https://doi.org/10.1016/j.jcin.2017.05.039.
14. Saw J, Aymong E, Mancini GB, Sedlak T, Starovoytov A, Ricci D. Nonatherosclerotic coronary artery disease in young women. Can J Cardiol. 2014;30(7):814–9. https://doi.org/10.1016/j.cjca.2014.01.011.
15. Nakashima T, Noguchi T, Haruta S, Yamamoto Y, Oshima S, Nakao K, et al. Prognostic impact of spontaneous coronary artery dissection in young female patients with acute myocardial infarction: a report from the Angina Pectoris-Myocardial Infarction Multicenter Investigators in Japan. Int J Cardiol. 2016;207:341–8. https://doi.org/10.1016/j.ijcard.2016.01.188.
16. Samuel R, Alfadhel M, McAlister C, Nestelberger T, Saw J. Coronary events in the pregnant patient: who is at risk and how best to manage? Can J Cardiol. 2021. https://doi.org/10.1016/j.cjca.2021.09.009.
17. Elkayam U, Jalnapurkar S, Barakkat MN, Khatri N, Kealey AJ, Mehra A, et al. Pregnancy-associated acute myocardial infarction: a review of contemporary experience in 150 cases between 2006 and 2011. Circulation. 2014;129(16):1695–702. https://doi.org/10.1161/CIRCULATIONAHA.113.002054.
18. Smilowitz NR, Gupta N, Guo Y, Zhong J, Weinberg CR, Reynolds HR, et al. Acute myocardial infarction during pregnancy and the puerperium in the United States. Mayo Clin Proc. 2018;93(10):1404–14. https://doi.org/10.1016/j.mayocp.2018.04.019.
19. Vijayaraghavan R, Verma S, Gupta N, Saw J. Pregnancy-related spontaneous coronary artery dissection. Circulation. 2014;130(21):1915–20. https://doi.org/10.1161/CIRCULATIONAHA.114.011422.
20. Tweet MS, Hayes SN, Codsi E, Gulati R, Rose CH, Best PJM. Spontaneous coronary artery dissection associated with pregnancy. J Am Coll Cardiol. 2017;70(4):426–35. https://doi.org/10.1016/j.jacc.2017.05.055.
21. Samuel R, McAlister C, Alfadhel M, Nestelberger T, Saw J. TCT-155 de novo left main spontaneous coronary artery dissection: a case series. J Am Coll Cardiol. 2021;78(19_Supplement_S):B64-B. https://doi.org/10.1016/j.jacc.2021.09.1008.
22. Saw J, Humphries K, Aymong E, Sedlak T, Prakash R, Starovoytov A, et al. Spontaneous coronary artery dissection: clinical outcomes and risk of recurrence. J Am Coll Cardiol. 2017;70(9):1148–58. https://doi.org/10.1016/j.jacc.2017.06.053.
23. Saw J. Spontaneous coronary artery dissection. Can J Cardiol. 2013;29(9):1027–33. https://doi.org/10.1016/j.cjca.2012.12.018.
24. Saw J, Aymong E, Sedlak T, Buller CE, Starovoytov A, Ricci D, et al. Spontaneous coronary artery dissection: association with predisposing arteriopathies and precipitating stressors and cardiovascular outcomes. Circ Cardiovasc Interv. 2014;7(5):645–55. https://doi.org/10.1161/CIRCINTERVENTIONS.114.001760.
25. Saw J, Mancini GB, Humphries K, Fung A, Boone R, Starovoytov A, et al. Angiographic appearance of spontaneous coronary artery dissection with intramural hematoma proven on intracoronary imaging. Catheter Cardiovasc Interv. 2016;87(2):E54–61. https://doi.org/10.1002/ccd.26022.

26. Tweet MS, Eleid MF, Best PJ, Lennon RJ, Lerman A, Rihal CS, et al. Spontaneous coronary artery dissection: revascularization versus conservative therapy. Circ Cardiovasc Interv. 2014;7(6):777–86. https://doi.org/10.1161/CIRCINTERVENTIONS.114.001659.
27. Basso C, Morgagni GL, Thiene G. Spontaneous coronary artery dissection: a neglected cause of acute myocardial ischaemia and sudden death. Heart. 1996;75(5):451–4. https://doi.org/10.1136/hrt.75.5.451.
28. Tweet MS, Miller VM, Hayes SN. The evidence on estrogen, progesterone, and spontaneous coronary artery dissection. JAMA Cardiol. 2019;4(5):403–4. https://doi.org/10.1001/jamacardio.2019.0774.
29. Sheikh AS, O'Sullivan M. Pregnancy-related spontaneous coronary artery dissection: two case reports and a comprehensive review of literature. Heart Views. 2012;13(2):53–65. https://doi.org/10.4103/1995-705X.99229.
30. Wingrove CS, Garr E, Godsland IF, Stevenson JC. 17beta-oestradiol enhances release of matrix metalloproteinase-2 from human vascular smooth muscle cells. Biochim Biophys Acta. 1998;1406(2):169–74. https://doi.org/10.1016/s0925-4439(97)00097-5.
31. Manalo-Estrella P, Barker AE. Histopathologic findings in human aortic media associated with pregnancy. Arch Pathol. 1967;83(4):336–41.
32. Pate GE, Lowe R, Buller CE. Fibromuscular dysplasia of the coronary and renal arteries? Catheter Cardiovasc Interv. 2005;64(2):138–45. https://doi.org/10.1002/ccd.20246.
33. Saw J, Poulter R, Fung A, Wood D, Hamburger J, Buller CE. Spontaneous coronary artery dissection in patients with fibromuscular dysplasia: a case series. Circ Cardiovasc Interv. 2012;5(1):134–7. https://doi.org/10.1161/CIRCINTERVENTIONS.111.966630.
34. Saw J, Ricci D, Starovoytov A, Fox R, Buller CE. Spontaneous coronary artery dissection: prevalence of predisposing conditions including fibromuscular dysplasia in a tertiary center cohort. JACC Cardiovasc Interv. 2013;6(1):44–52. https://doi.org/10.1016/j.jcin.2012.08.017.
35. Prasad M, Tweet MS, Hayes SN, Leng S, Liang JJ, Eleid MF, et al. Prevalence of extracoronary vascular abnormalities and fibromuscular dysplasia in patients with spontaneous coronary artery dissection. Am J Cardiol. 2015;115(12):1672–7. https://doi.org/10.1016/j.amjcard.2015.03.011.
36. Olin JW, Gornik HL, Bacharach JM, Biller J, Fine LJ, Gray BH, et al. Fibromuscular dysplasia: state of the science and critical unanswered questions: a scientific statement from the American Heart Association. Circulation. 2014;129(9):1048–78. https://doi.org/10.1161/01.cir.0000442577.96802.8c.
37. Saw J, Bezerra H, Gornik HL, Machan L, Mancini GB. Angiographic and intracoronary manifestations of coronary fibromuscular dysplasia. Circulation. 2016;133(16):1548–59. https://doi.org/10.1161/CIRCULATIONAHA.115.020282.
38. Lie JT, Berg KK. Isolated fibromuscular dysplasia of the coronary arteries with spontaneous dissection and myocardial infarction. Hum Pathol. 1987;18(6):654–6. https://doi.org/10.1016/s0046-8177(87)80368-4.
39. Brodsky SV, Ramaswamy G, Chander P, Braun A. Ruptured cerebral aneurysm and acute coronary artery dissection in the setting of multivascular fibromuscular dysplasia: a case report. Angiology. 2007;58(6):764–7. https://doi.org/10.1177/0003319707303645.
40. Grond-Ginsbach C, Engelter ST. Genetics of spontaneous coronary artery dissection gains new momentum. Circ Genom Precis Med. 2018;11(4):e002148. https://doi.org/10.1161/CIRCGEN.118.002148.
41. Goel K, Tweet M, Olson TM, Maleszewski JJ, Gulati R, Hayes SN. Familial spontaneous coronary artery dissection: evidence for genetic susceptibility. JAMA Intern Med. 2015;175(5):821–6. https://doi.org/10.1001/jamainternmed.2014.8307.

42. Henkin S, Negrotto SM, Tweet MS, Kirmani S, Deyle DR, Gulati R, et al. Spontaneous coronary artery dissection and its association with heritable connective tissue disorders. Heart. 2016;102(11):876–81. https://doi.org/10.1136/heartjnl-2015-308645.
43. Kaadan MI, MacDonald C, Ponzini F, Duran J, Newell K, Pitler L, et al. Prospective cardiovascular genetics evaluation in spontaneous coronary artery dissection. Circ Genom Precis Med. 2018;11(4):e001933. https://doi.org/10.1161/CIRCGENETICS.117.001933.
44. Fahmy P, Prakash R, Starovoytov A, Boone R, Saw J. Pre-disposing and precipitating factors in men with spontaneous coronary artery dissection. JACC Cardiovasc Interv. 2016;9(8):866–8. https://doi.org/10.1016/j.jcin.2016.02.024.
45. Luong C, Starovoytov A, Heydari M, Sedlak T, Aymong E, Saw J. Clinical presentation of patients with spontaneous coronary artery dissection. Catheter Cardiovasc Interv. 2017;89(7):1149–54. https://doi.org/10.1002/ccd.26977.
46. Saw J. Coronary angiogram classification of spontaneous coronary artery dissection. Catheter Cardiovasc Interv. 2014;84(7):1115–22. https://doi.org/10.1002/ccd.25293.
47. Prakash R, Starovoytov A, Heydari M, Mancini GB, Saw J. Catheter-induced iatrogenic coronary artery dissection in patients with spontaneous coronary artery dissection. JACC Cardiovasc Interv. 2016;9(17):1851–3. https://doi.org/10.1016/j.jcin.2016.06.026.
48. Eleid MF, Tweet MS, Young PM, Williamson E, Hayes SN, Gulati R. Spontaneous coronary artery dissection: challenges of coronary computed tomography angiography. Eur Heart J Acute Cardiovasc Care. 2018;7(7):609–13. https://doi.org/10.1177/2048872616687098.
49. Roura G, Ariza-Sole A, Rodriguez-Caballero IF, Gomez-Lara J, Ferreiro JL, Romaguera R, et al. Noninvasive follow-up of patients with spontaneous coronary artery dissection with CT angiography. JACC Cardiovasc Imaging. 2016;9(7):896–7. https://doi.org/10.1016/j.jcmg.2015.06.011.
50. Tweet MS, Hayes SN, Pitta SR, Simari RD, Lerman A, Lennon RJ, et al. Clinical features, management, and prognosis of spontaneous coronary artery dissection. Circulation. 2012;126(5):579–88. https://doi.org/10.1161/CIRCULATIONAHA.112.105718.
51. Alkhouli M, Cole M, Ling FS. Coronary artery fenestration prior to stenting in spontaneous coronary artery dissection. Catheter Cardiovasc Interv. 2016;88(1):E23–7. https://doi.org/10.1002/ccd.26161.
52. Walsh SJ, Jokhi PP, Saw J. Successful percutaneous management of coronary dissection and extensive intramural haematoma associated with ST elevation MI. Acute Card Care. 2008;10(4):231–3. https://doi.org/10.1080/17482940701802348.
53. Chou AY, Prakash R, Rajala J, Birnie T, Isserow S, Taylor CM, et al. The first dedicated cardiac rehabilitation program for patients with spontaneous coronary artery dissection: description and initial results. Can J Cardiol. 2016;32(4):554–60. https://doi.org/10.1016/j.cjca.2016.01.009.
54. Silber TC, Tweet MS, Bowman MJ, Hayes SN, Squires RW. Cardiac rehabilitation after spontaneous coronary artery dissection. J Cardiopulm Rehabil Prev. 2015;35(5):328–33. https://doi.org/10.1097/HCR.0000000000000111.
55. Krittanawong C, Tweet MS, Hayes SE, Bowman MJ, Gulati R, Squires RW, et al. Usefulness of cardiac rehabilitation after spontaneous coronary artery dissection. Am J Cardiol. 2016;117(10):1604–9. https://doi.org/10.1016/j.amjcard.2016.02.034.
56. Oliva PB, Potts DE, Pluss RG. Coronary arterial spasm in Prinzmetal angina. Documentation by coronary arteriography. N Engl J Med. 1973;288(15):745–51. https://doi.org/10.1056/NEJM197304122881501.
57. Nakamura M, Takeshita A, Nose Y. Clinical characteristics associated with myocardial infarction, arrhythmias, and sudden death in patients with vasospastic angina. Circulation. 1987;75(6):1110–6. https://doi.org/10.1161/01.cir.75.6.1110.

58. Prinzmetal M, Kennamer R, Merliss R, Wada T, Bor N, Angina pectoris. I. A variant form of angina pectoris; preliminary report. Am J Med. 1959;27:375–88. https://doi.org/10.1016/0002-9343(59)90003-8.
59. Waterbury TM, Tarantini G, Vogel B, Mehran R, Gersh BJ, Gulati R. Non-atherosclerotic causes of acute coronary syndromes. Nat Rev Cardiol. 2020;17(4):229–41. https://doi.org/10.1038/s41569-019-0273-3.
60. Picard F, Sayah N, Spagnoli V, Adjedj J, Varenne O. Vasospastic angina: a literature review of current evidence. Arch Cardiovasc Dis. 2019;112(1):44–55. https://doi.org/10.1016/j.acvd.2018.08.002.
61. Beltrame JF, Sasayama S, Maseri A. Racial heterogeneity in coronary artery vasomotor reactivity: differences between Japanese and Caucasian patients. J Am Coll Cardiol. 1999;33(6):1442–52. https://doi.org/10.1016/s0735-1097(99)00073-x.
62. Pasupathy S, Air T, Dreyer RP, Tavella R, Beltrame JF. Systematic review of patients presenting with suspected myocardial infarction and nonobstructive coronary arteries. Circulation. 2015;131(10):861–70. https://doi.org/10.1161/CIRCULATIONAHA.114.011201.
63. Matta A, Bouisset F, Lhermusier T, Campelo-Parada F, Elbaz M, Carrie D, et al. Coronary artery spasm: new insights. J Interv Cardiol. 2020;2020:5894586. https://doi.org/10.1155/2020/5894586.
64. Ong P, Athanasiadis A, Borgulya G, Mahrholdt H, Kaski JC, Sechtem U. High prevalence of a pathological response to acetylcholine testing in patients with stable angina pectoris and unobstructed coronary arteries. The ACOVA Study (Abnormal COronary VAsomotion in patients with stable angina and unobstructed coronary arteries). J Am Coll Cardiol. 2012;59(7):655–62. https://doi.org/10.1016/j.jacc.2011.11.015.
65. Nakayama N, Kaikita K, Fukunaga T, Matsuzawa Y, Sato K, Horio E, et al. Clinical features and prognosis of patients with coronary spasm-induced non-ST-segment elevation acute coronary syndrome. J Am Heart Assoc. 2014;3(3):e000795. https://doi.org/10.1161/JAHA.114.000795.
66. Yasue H, Nakagawa H, Itoh T, Harada E, Mizuno Y. Coronary artery spasm—clinical features, diagnosis, pathogenesis, and treatment. J Cardiol. 2008;51(1):2–17. https://doi.org/10.1016/j.jjcc.2008.01.001.
67. Kandabashi T, Shimokawa H, Miyata K, Kunihiro I, Kawano Y, Fukata Y, et al. Inhibition of myosin phosphatase by upregulated rho-kinase plays a key role for coronary artery spasm in a porcine model with interleukin-1beta. Circulation. 2000;101(11):1319–23. https://doi.org/10.1161/01.cir.101.11.1319.
68. Shimokawa H, Sunamura S, Satoh K. RhoA/Rho-Kinase in the cardiovascular system. Circ Res. 2016;118(2):352–66. https://doi.org/10.1161/CIRCRESAHA.115.306532.
69. Yasue H, Touyama M, Shimamoto M, Kato H, Tanaka S. Role of autonomic nervous system in the pathogenesis of Prinzmetal's variant form of angina. Circulation. 1974;50(3):534–9. https://doi.org/10.1161/01.cir.50.3.534.
70. Saitoh T, Kishida H, Hanashi A, Tsukada Y, Fukuma Y, Sano J, et al. Coronary hyperreactivity to adrenergic stimulation and increased nocturnal vagal tone trigger coronary vasospasm. Jpn Circ J. 1998;62(10):721–6. https://doi.org/10.1253/jcj.62.721.
71. Bertrand ME, Lablanche JM, Tilmant PY, Ducloux G, Warembourg H Jr, Soots G. Complete denervation of the heart (autotransplantation) for treatment of severe, refractory coronary spasm. Am J Cardiol. 1981;47(6):1375–8. https://doi.org/10.1016/0002-9149(81)90271-x.
72. Ohyama K, Matsumoto Y, Takanami K, Ota H, Nishimiya K, Sugisawa J, et al. Coronary adventitial and perivascular adipose tissue inflammation in patients with vasospastic angina. J Am Coll Cardiol. 2018;71(4):414–25. https://doi.org/10.1016/j.jacc.2017.11.046.
73. Shimokawa H. Cellular and molecular mechanisms of coronary artery spasm: lessons from animal models. Jpn Circ J. 2000;64(1):1–12. https://doi.org/10.1253/jcj.64.1.

74. Hung MJ, Cherng WJ, Cheng CW, Li LF. Comparison of serum levels of inflammatory markers in patients with coronary vasospasm without significant fixed coronary artery disease versus patients with stable angina pectoris and acute coronary syndromes with significant fixed coronary artery disease. Am J Cardiol. 2006;97(10):1429–34. https://doi.org/10.1016/j.amjcard.2005.12.035.
75. Miyamoto S, Kawano H, Sakamoto T, Soejima H, Kajiwara I, Hokamaki J, et al. Increased plasma levels of thioredoxin in patients with coronary spastic angina. Antioxid Redox Signal. 2004;6(1):75–80. https://doi.org/10.1089/152308604771978363.
76. Miwa K, Igawa A, Nakagawa K, Hirai T, Inoue H. Consumption of vitamin E in coronary circulation in patients with variant angina. Cardiovasc Res. 1999;41(1):291–8. https://doi.org/10.1016/s0008-6363(98)00207-7.
77. Takaoka K, Yoshimura M, Ogawa H, Kugiyama K, Nakayama M, Shimasaki Y, et al. Comparison of the risk factors for coronary artery spasm with those for organic stenosis in a Japanese population: role of cigarette smoking. Int J Cardiol. 2000;72(2):121–6. https://doi.org/10.1016/s0167-5273(99)00172-2.
78. Nobuyoshi M, Abe M, Nosaka H, Kimura T, Yokoi H, Hamasaki N, et al. Statistical analysis of clinical risk factors for coronary artery spasm: identification of the most important determinant. Am Heart J. 1992;124(1):32–8. https://doi.org/10.1016/0002-8703(92)90917-k.
79. Miller D, Waters DD, Warnica W, Szlachcic J, Kreeft J, Theroux P. Is variant angina the coronary manifestation of a generalized vasospastic disorder? N Engl J Med. 1981;304(13):763–6. https://doi.org/10.1056/NEJM198103263041306.
80. Beltrame JF, Crea F, Kaski JC, Ogawa H, Ong P, Sechtem U, et al. International standardization of diagnostic criteria for vasospastic angina. Eur Heart J. 2017;38(33):2565–8. https://doi.org/10.1093/eurheartj/ehv351.
81. Kishida H, Tada Y, Fukuma N, Saitoh T, Kusama Y, Sano J. Significant characteristics of variant angina patients with associated syncope. Jpn Heart J. 1996;37(3):317–26. https://doi.org/10.1536/ihj.37.317.
82. Araki H, Koiwaya Y, Nakagaki O, Nakamura M. Diurnal distribution of ST-segment elevation and related arrhythmias in patients with variant angina: a study by ambulatory ECG monitoring. Circulation. 1983;67(5):995–1000. https://doi.org/10.1161/01.cir.67.5.995.
83. Previtali M, Ardissino D, Barberis P, Panciroli C, Chimienti M, Salerno JA. Hyperventilation and ergonovine tests in Prinzmetal's variant angina pectoris in men. Am J Cardiol. 1989;63(1):17–20. https://doi.org/10.1016/0002-9149(89)91068-0.
84. Group JCSJW. Guidelines for diagnosis and treatment of patients with vasospastic angina (Coronary Spastic Angina) (JCS 2013). Circ J. 2014;78(11):2779–801. https://doi.org/10.1253/circj.cj-66-0098.
85. Sueda S, Saeki H, Otani T, Mineoi K, Kondou T, Yano K, et al. Major complications during spasm provocation tests with an intracoronary injection of acetylcholine. Am J Cardiol. 2000;85(3):391–4., A10. https://doi.org/10.1016/s0002-9149(99)00754-7.
86. Takagi Y, Yasuda S, Takahashi J, Tsunoda R, Ogata Y, Seki A, et al. Clinical implications of provocation tests for coronary artery spasm: safety, arrhythmic complications, and prognostic impact: multicentre registry study of the Japanese Coronary Spasm Association. Eur Heart J. 2013;34(4):258–67. https://doi.org/10.1093/eurheartj/ehs199.
87. Tanaka A, Shimada K, Tearney GJ, Kitabata H, Taguchi H, Fukuda S, et al. Conformational change in coronary artery structure assessed by optical coherence tomography in patients with vasospastic angina. J Am Coll Cardiol. 2011;58(15):1608–13. https://doi.org/10.1016/j.jacc.2011.06.046.
88. Yasue H, Takizawa A, Nagao M, Nishida S, Horie M, Kubota J, et al. Long-term prognosis for patients with variant angina and influential factors. Circulation. 1988;78(1):1–9. https://doi.org/10.1161/01.cir.78.1.1.

89. Takahashi J, Nihei T, Takagi Y, Miyata S, Odaka Y, Tsunoda R, et al. Prognostic impact of chronic nitrate therapy in patients with vasospastic angina: multicentre registry study of the Japanese coronary spasm association. Eur Heart J. 2015;36(4):228–37. https://doi.org/10.1093/eurheartj/ehu313.
90. Masumoto A, Mohri M, Shimokawa H, Urakami L, Usui M, Takeshita A. Suppression of coronary artery spasm by the Rho-kinase inhibitor fasudil in patients with vasospastic angina. Circulation. 2002;105(13):1545–7. https://doi.org/10.1161/hc1002.105938.
91. Yasue H, Mizuno Y, Harada E, Itoh T, Nakagawa H, Nakayama M, et al. Effects of a 3-hydroxy-3-methylglutaryl coenzyme A reductase inhibitor, fluvastatin, on coronary spasm after withdrawal of calcium-channel blockers. J Am Coll Cardiol. 2008;51(18):1742–8. https://doi.org/10.1016/j.jacc.2007.12.049.
92. Ishii M, Kaikita K, Sato K, Yamanaga K, Miyazaki T, Akasaka T, et al. Impact of statin therapy on clinical outcome in patients with coronary spasm. J Am Heart Assoc. 2016;5(5). https://doi.org/10.1161/JAHA.116.003426.
93. Gaspardone A, Tomai F, Versaci F, Ghini AS, Polisca P, Crea F, et al. Coronary artery stent placement in patients with variant angina refractory to medical treatment. Am J Cardiol. 1999;84(1):96–8., A8. https://doi.org/10.1016/s0002-9149(99)00201-5.
94. Ahn JM, Lee KH, Yoo SY, Cho YR, Suh J, Shin ES, et al. Prognosis of variant angina manifesting as aborted sudden cardiac death. J Am Coll Cardiol. 2016;68(2):137–45. https://doi.org/10.1016/j.jacc.2016.04.050.
95. Meisel SR, Mazur A, Chetboun I, Epshtein M, Canetti M, Gallimidi J, et al. Usefulness of implantable cardioverter-defibrillators in refractory variant angina pectoris complicated by ventricular fibrillation in patients with angiographically normal coronary arteries. Am J Cardiol. 2002;89(9):1114–6. https://doi.org/10.1016/s0002-9149(02)02283-x.
96. Raphael CE, Heit JA, Reeder GS, Bois MC, Maleszewski JJ, Tilbury RT, et al. Coronary embolus: an underappreciated cause of acute coronary syndromes. JACC Cardiovasc Interv. 2018;11(2):172–80. https://doi.org/10.1016/j.jcin.2017.08.057.
97. Prizel KR, Hutchins GM, Bulkley BH. Coronary artery embolism and myocardial infarction. Ann Intern Med. 1978;88(2):155–61. https://doi.org/10.7326/0003-4819-88-2-155.
98. Shibata T, Kawakami S, Noguchi T, Tanaka T, Asaumi Y, Kanaya T, et al. Prevalence, clinical features, and prognosis of acute myocardial infarction attributable to coronary artery embolism. Circulation. 2015;132(4):241–50. https://doi.org/10.1161/CIRCULATIONAHA.114.015134.
99. Brunson JG. Coronary embolism in bacterial endocarditis. Am J Pathol. 1953;29(4):689–701.
100. Fabri J Jr, Issa VS, Pomerantzeff PM, Grinberg M, Barretto AC, Mansur AJ. Time-related distribution, risk factors and prognostic influence of embolism in patients with left-sided infective endocarditis. Int J Cardiol. 2006;110(3):334–9. https://doi.org/10.1016/j.ijcard.2005.07.016.
101. Jolly SS, Cairns JA, Yusuf S, Rokoss MJ, Gao P, Meeks B, et al. Outcomes after thrombus aspiration for ST elevation myocardial infarction: 1-year follow-up of the prospective randomised TOTAL trial. Lancet. 2016;387(10014):127–35. https://doi.org/10.1016/S0140-6736(15)00448-1.
102. Frobert O, Lagerqvist B, Olivecrona GK, Omerovic E, Gudnason T, Maeng M, et al. Thrombus aspiration during ST-segment elevation myocardial infarction. N Engl J Med. 2013;369(17):1587–97. https://doi.org/10.1056/NEJMoa1308789.
103. Jolly SS, James S, Dzavik V, Cairns JA, Mahmoud KD, Zijlstra F, et al. Thrombus aspiration in ST-segment-elevation myocardial infarction: an individual patient meta-analysis: thrombectomy trialists collaboration. Circulation. 2017;135(2):143–52. https://doi.org/10.1161/CIRCULATIONAHA.116.025371.
104. Mentzelopoulos SD, Kokotsakis JN, Romana CN, Karamichali EA. Intracoronary thrombolysis and intraaortic balloon counterpulsation for the emergency treatment of probable coronary

embolism after repair of an acute ascending aortic dissection. Anesth Analg. 2001;93(1):56–9. https://doi.org/10.1097/00000539-200107000-00013.
105. Wahl A, Juni P, Mono ML, Kalesan B, Praz F, Geister L, et al. Long-term propensity score-matched comparison of percutaneous closure of patent foramen ovale with medical treatment after paradoxical embolism. Circulation. 2012;125(6):803–12. https://doi.org/10.1161/CIRCULATIONAHA.111.030494.
106. Kasner SE, Rhodes JF, Andersen G, Iversen HK, Nielsen-Kudsk JE, Settergren M, et al. Five-year outcomes of PFO closure or antiplatelet therapy for cryptogenic stroke. N Engl J Med. 2021;384(10):970–1. https://doi.org/10.1056/NEJMc2033779.
107. Mohlenkamp S, Hort W, Ge J, Erbel R. Update on myocardial bridging. Circulation. 2002;106(20):2616–22. https://doi.org/10.1161/01.cir.0000038420.14867.7a.
108. Murtaza G, Mukherjee D, Gharacholou SM, Nanjundappa A, Lavie CJ, Khan AA, et al. An updated review on myocardial bridging. Cardiovasc Revasc Med. 2020;21(9):1169–79. https://doi.org/10.1016/j.carrev.2020.02.014.
109. Alegria JR, Herrmann J, Holmes DR Jr, Lerman A, Rihal CS. Myocardial bridging. Eur Heart J. 2005;26(12):1159–68. https://doi.org/10.1093/eurheartj/ehi203.
110. Lee MS, Chen CH. Myocardial bridging: an up-to-date review. J Invasive Cardiol. 2015;27(11):521–8.
111. Soran O, Pamir G, Erol C, Kocakavak C, Sabah I. The incidence and significance of myocardial bridge in a prospectively defined population of patients undergoing coronary angiography for chest pain. Tokai J Exp Clin Med. 2000;25(2):57–60.
112. Konen E, Goitein O, Sternik L, Eshet Y, Shemesh J, Di Segni E. The prevalence and anatomical patterns of intramuscular coronary arteries: a coronary computed tomography angiographic study. J Am Coll Cardiol. 2007;49(5):587–93. https://doi.org/10.1016/j.jacc.2006.09.039.
113. La Grutta L, Runza G, Lo Re G, Galia M, Alaimo V, Grassedonio E, et al. Prevalence of myocardial bridging and correlation with coronary atherosclerosis studied with 64-slice CT coronary angiography. Radiol Med. 2009;114(7):1024–36. https://doi.org/10.1007/s11547-009-0446-y.
114. Rossi L, Dander B, Nidasio GP, Arbustini E, Paris B, Vassanelli C, et al. Myocardial bridges and ischemic heart disease. Eur Heart J. 1980;1(4):239–45. https://doi.org/10.1093/oxfordjournals.eurheartj.a061125.
115. Klues HG, Schwarz ER, vom Dahl J, Reffelmann T, Reul H, Potthast K, et al. Disturbed intracoronary hemodynamics in myocardial bridging: early normalization by intracoronary stent placement. Circulation. 1997;96(9):2905–13. https://doi.org/10.1161/01.cir.96.9.2905.
116. Schwarz ER, Klues HG, vom Dahl J, Klein I, Krebs W, Hanrath P. Functional, angiographic and intracoronary Doppler flow characteristics in symptomatic patients with myocardial bridging: effect of short-term intravenous beta-blocker medication. J Am Coll Cardiol. 1996;27(7):1637–45. https://doi.org/10.1016/0735-1097(96)00062-9.
117. Ge J, Jeremias A, Rupp A, Abels M, Baumgart D, Liu F, et al. New signs characteristic of myocardial bridging demonstrated by intracoronary ultrasound and Doppler. Eur Heart J. 1999;20(23):1707–16. https://doi.org/10.1053/euhj.1999.1661.
118. Ge J, Erbel R, Gorge G, Haude M, Meyer J. High wall shear stress proximal to myocardial bridging and atherosclerosis: intracoronary ultrasound and pressure measurements. Br Heart J. 1995;73(5):462–5. https://doi.org/10.1136/hrt.73.5.462.
119. Ishikawa Y, Ishii T, Asuwa N, Masuda S. Absence of atherosclerosis evolution in the coronary arterial segment covered by myocardial tissue in cholesterol-fed rabbits. Virchows Arch. 1997;430(2):163–71. https://doi.org/10.1007/BF01008038.
120. Risse M, Weiler G. [Coronary muscle bridge and its relations to local coronary sclerosis, regional myocardial ischemia and coronary spasm. A morphometric study]. Z Kardiol 1985;74(12):700–5.

121. Masuda T, Ishikawa Y, Akasaka Y, Itoh K, Kiguchi H, Ishii T. The effect of myocardial bridging of the coronary artery on vasoactive agents and atherosclerosis localization. J Pathol. 2001;193(3):408–14. https://doi.org/10.1002/1096-9896(2000)9999:9999<::AID-PATH792>3.0.CO;2-R.
122. Corban MT, Hung OY, Eshtehardi P, Rasoul-Arzrumly E, McDaniel M, Mekonnen G, et al. Myocardial bridging: contemporary understanding of pathophysiology with implications for diagnostic and therapeutic strategies. J Am Coll Cardiol. 2014;63(22):2346–55. https://doi.org/10.1016/j.jacc.2014.01.049.
123. Tobias SL, Videlefsky SW, Misra VK. Physiological significance of a proximal coronary artery stenosis on a distal intramyocardial bridge: coronary flow velocity patterns pre- and post-angioplasty. Catheter Cardiovasc Diagn. 1995;35(2):127–30. https://doi.org/10.1002/ccd.1810350209.
124. Tsujita K, Maehara A, Mintz GS, Doi H, Kubo T, Castellanos C, et al. Comparison of angiographic and intravascular ultrasonic detection of myocardial bridging of the left anterior descending coronary artery. Am J Cardiol. 2008;102(12):1608–13. https://doi.org/10.1016/j.amjcard.2008.07.054.
125. Ge J, Erbel R, Rupprecht HJ, Koch L, Kearney P, Gorge G, et al. Comparison of intravascular ultrasound and angiography in the assessment of myocardial bridging. Circulation. 1994;89(4):1725–32. https://doi.org/10.1161/01.cir.89.4.1725.
126. Escaned J, Cortes J, Flores A, Goicolea J, Alfonso F, Hernandez R, et al. Importance of diastolic fractional flow reserve and dobutamine challenge in physiologic assessment of myocardial bridging. J Am Coll Cardiol. 2003;42(2):226–33. https://doi.org/10.1016/s0735-1097(03)00588-6.
127. Hakeem A, Cilingiroglu M, Leesar MA. Hemodynamic and intravascular ultrasound assessment of myocardial bridging: fractional flow reserve paradox with dobutamine versus adenosine. Catheter Cardiovasc Interv. 2010;75(2):229–36. https://doi.org/10.1002/ccd.22237.
128. Tarantini G, Barioli A, Nai Fovino L, Fraccaro C, Masiero G, Iliceto S, et al. Unmasking myocardial bridge-related ischemia by intracoronary functional evaluation. Circ Cardiovasc Interv. 2018;11(6):e006247. https://doi.org/10.1161/CIRCINTERVENTIONS.117.006247.
129. Schwarz ER, Klues HG, vom Dahl J, Klein I, Krebs W, Hanrath P. Functional characteristics of myocardial bridging. A combined angiographic and intracoronary Doppler flow study. Eur Heart J. 1997;18(3):434–42. https://doi.org/10.1093/oxfordjournals.eurheartj.a015263.
130. Nair CK, Dang B, Heintz MH, Sketch MH. Myocardial bridges: effect of propranolol on systolic compression. Can J Cardiol. 1986;2(4):218–21.
131. Alessandri N, Dei Giudici A, De Angelis S, Urciuoli F, Garante MC, Di Matteo A. Efficacy of calcium channel blockers in the treatment of the myocardial bridging: a pilot study. Eur Rev Med Pharmacol Sci. 2012;16(6):829–34.
132. Hongo Y, Tada H, Ito K, Yasumura Y, Miyatake K, Yamagishi M. Augmentation of vessel squeezing at coronary-myocardial bridge by nitroglycerin: study by quantitative coronary angiography and intravascular ultrasound. Am Heart J. 1999;138(2 Pt 1):345–50. https://doi.org/10.1016/s0002-8703(99)70123-7.
133. Tsujita K, Maehara A, Mintz GS, Doi H, Kubo T, Castellanos C, et al. Impact of myocardial bridge on clinical outcome after coronary stent placement. Am J Cardiol. 2009;103(10):1344–8. https://doi.org/10.1016/j.amjcard.2009.01.340.
134. Katznelson Y, Petchenko P, Knobel B, Cohen AJ, Kishon Y, Schachner A. Myocardial bridging: surgical technique and operative results. Mil Med. 1996;161(4):248–50.
135. Hill RC, Chitwood WR Jr, Bashore TM, Sink JD, Cox JL, Wechsler AS. Coronary flow and regional function before and after supraarterial myotomy for myocardial bridging. Ann Thorac Surg. 1981;31(2):176–81. https://doi.org/10.1016/s0003-4975(10)61539-1.
136. Wu QY, Xu ZH. Surgical treatment of myocardial bridging: report of 31 cases. Chin Med J. 2007;120(19):1689–93.

Evaluation of Anginal Syndromes Using Standard Clinical Procedures

Antonio Lio, Giulio Cacioli, Francesca Nicolò,
and Francesco Musumeci

1 Preface

The leading symptom of coronary artery disease (CAD) is angina pectoris, which is represented by an acute chest discomfort described as pain, pressure, tightness, and burning; typical angina is characterized by a retrosternal chest discomfort radiating to the left arm, both arms, the right arm, the neck, or the jaw. The symptom is usually associated with exertion or psychological stress, but a precipitating factor is not always present. "Atypical" chest pain description reduces the probability of a myocardial ischemic damage; the American College of Cardiology and American Heart Association (ACC/AHA) guidelines describe these conditions as atypical chest pain [1]:

- Pleural pain (acute pain related to respiratory movements)
- Abdominal localization
- Chest discomfort exacerbated by chest palpation
- Protracted pain that persists for hours
- Irradiation to lower limbs

Conversely, some patients with myocardial ischaemia may present chest pain-equivalent symptoms that include dyspnoea, epigastric pain, and isolated pain in the left arm.

A. Lio (✉) · G. Cacioli · F. Nicolò · F. Musumeci
Cardiac Surgery and Heart Transplantation Department, Azienda Ospedaliera San Camillo Forlanini, Rome, Italy
e-mail: a.lio@scamilloforlanini.rm.it; f.nicolo@scamilloforlanini.rm.it; f.musumeci@scamilloforlanini.rm.it

G. Concistrè (ed.), *Ischemic Heart Disease*,
https://doi.org/10.1007/978-3-031-25879-4_8

In this chapter, we focus our attention on the standard clinical procedures used for the evaluation of anginal syndromes. Typically, anginal syndromes could be divided into two different classes:

- Acute coronary syndromes
- Chronic coronary syndromes (formerly known as "stable angina")

2 Acute Coronary Syndromes

2.1 Introduction

Acute coronary syndromes (ACS) comprise a number of clinical scenarios, which have angina pectoris as the leading symptom. Based on the electrocardiogram (ECG), two different conditions exist:

- Acute chest pain and persistent (>20 min) ST-segment elevation: This condition is termed ST-segment elevation ACS and generally leads to a ST-segment elevation myocardial infarction (STEMI).
- Acute chest discomfort but no persistent ST-segment elevation (non-ST-segment elevation ACS—NSTE-ACS): This condition exhibits ECG changes that may include transient ST-segment elevation, persistent or transient ST-segment depression, T-wave inversion, flat T waves, or pseudo-normalization of T waves, or the ECG may be normal. The pathological correlate at the myocardial level is cardiomyocyte necrosis (non-ST-segment elevation myocardial infarction—NSTEMI) or, less frequently, myocardial ischaemia without cell damage (unstable angina).

2.2 STEMI

Acute myocardial infarction (AMI) defines cardiomyocyte necrosis in a clinical setting consistent with acute myocardial ischaemia [2, 3]. A combination of criteria is required to meet the diagnosis of AMI, namely the detection of an increase and/or decrease of a cardiac biomarker, preferably high-sensitivity cardiac troponin (hs-cTn) T or I, with at least one value above the 99th percentile of the upper reference limit and at least one of the following:

1. Symptoms of myocardial ischaemia
2. New ischaemic ECG changes
3. Development of pathological Q-waves on ECG
4. Imaging evidence of loss of viable myocardium or new regional wall motion abnormality in a pattern consistent with an ischaemic aetiology
5. Intracoronary thrombus detected on angiography or autopsy

The main objective in case of STEMI is an earlier reperfusion strategy (within 120 min).

2.2.1 Physical Examination

The typical symptom of STEMI is acute chest pain with radiation to the neck, lower jaw, or left arm. Some patients present with less typical symptoms such as shortness of breath, nausea/vomiting, fatigue, palpitations, or syncope [4]. At admission, heart rate may vary from a marked bradycardia to a rhythmic or arrhythmic tachycardia. Chest auscultation generally reveals the presence of a marked IV tone, appreciable between left sternal border and apex. The presence of the third tone is usually associated with left ventricular dysfunction, and it is generally associated with a systolic murmur due to mitral regurgitation. Mechanical complications of STEMI are life-threatening conditions; they generally occur in the first days following MI. Therefore, the occurrence of sudden hypotension, recurrence of chest pain, new cardiac murmurs suggestive of mitral regurgitation or ventricular septal defect, pulmonary congestion, or jugular vein distension should raise immediate suspicion to guide the subsequent diagnosis and treatment.

2.2.2 Electrocardiography

In case of high suspicion, 12-lead ECG recording and interpretation are indicated as soon as possible with a maximum delay of 10 min (Class I Level of Evidence B) [2, 5–7]. Main criteria for ECG diagnosis of STEMI include at least two contiguous leads with ST-segment elevation >2.5 mm in men <40 years, >2 mm in men >40 years, or >1.5 mm in women in leads V2–V3 and/or >1 mm in the other leads (in the absence of left ventricular hypertrophy or left bundle branch block) [8]. The use of additional posterior chest wall leads (V7–V9) in patients with high suspicion of posterior MI (circumflex occlusion) should be considered (Class IIa Level of Evidence B) [8–12]. In patients with inferior MI, it is recommended to record right precordial leads (V3R and V4R) to identify concomitant right ventricular (RV) infarction [8, 13].

The ECG diagnosis may be more difficult in some cases, such as bundle branch block or ventricular pacing, which nevertheless deserve prompt management and triage. Moreover, the presence of ST depression >1 mm in six or more surface leads (inferolateral ST depression), coupled with ST-segment elevation in aVR and/or V1, suggests multivessel ischaemia or left main coronary artery obstruction, particularly if the patient presents with haemodynamic compromise [14]. Patients with atypical ECG presentations and ongoing symptoms consistent with myocardial ischaemia should undergo a primary PCI strategy. Many deaths occur very early after STEMI onset due to ventricular fibrillation (VF). A primary PCI strategy is recommended in patients with resuscitated cardiac arrest and an ECG consistent with STEMI (Class I Level of Evidence B); urgent angiography (and PCI if indicated) should be considered in patients with resuscitated cardiac arrest without diagnostic ST-segment elevation but with a high suspicion of ongoing myocardial ischaemia (Class IIa Level of Evidence C) [15–18].

2.2.3 Blood Tests

After ECG recording, blood sampling for serum markers must be routinely carried out in the acute phase. This is indicated but should not delay the reperfusion strategy/treatment.

2.2.4 Echocardiography

Emergency echocardiography at presentation is indicated in patients with cardiac arrest, cardiogenic shock, haemodynamic instability, or suspected mechanical complications, and if the diagnosis of STEMI is uncertain [19].

2.2.5 Other Imaging Techniques

In the STEMI emergency setting, there is no role for routine computed tomography (CT). Use of CT should be confined to selected cases where acute aortic dissection or pulmonary embolism is suspected, but CT is not recommended if STEMI diagnosis is likely.

2.3 NSTEMI/Unstable Angina (NSTE-ACS)

In patients presenting with non-ST-segment elevation acute coronary syndrome (NSTE-ACS), typical angina symptoms are present and may have one of the following presentations:

- Prolonged (>20 min) chest discomfort at rest
- New-onset (de novo) (<3 months) angina (class II or III of the Canadian Cardiovascular Society classification) [20]
- Recent destabilization of previously stable angina with at least Canadian Cardiovascular Society Class III angina characteristics (crescendo angina)
- Post-myocardial infarction (MI) angina

Additional symptoms such as sweating, nausea, epigastric pain, dyspnoea, and syncope may be present. Less often, patients may present atypical symptoms that include isolated epigastric pain, indigestion-like symptoms, and isolated dyspnoea or fatigue. The exacerbation of symptoms by physical exertion, and their relief at rest, increases the probability of myocardial ischaemia. The relief of symptoms after nitrate administration increases the likelihood of NSTE-ACS, but this is not diagnostic [21].

Accurate initial clinical evaluation is important to identify factors associated with an increased risk of NSTE-ACS: old age, male sex, family history of CAD, diabetes, hyperlipidaemia, smoking, hypertension, renal dysfunction, previous manifestation of CAD, and peripheral or carotid artery [22, 23]. Moreover, it is important to evaluate some coexisting conditions that may exacerbate or precipitate NSTE-ACS, such as anaemia, infection, inflammation, fever, hypertensive peak, anger, emotional stress, and metabolic or endocrine (particularly thyroid) disorders.

2.3.1 Physical Examination

Physical examination is generally not useful in patients with suspected NSTE-ACS, but it could reveal signs of non-coronary causes of chest pain (e.g. pulmonary embolism, acute aortic syndromes, myopericarditis, aortic stenosis), extracardiac pathologies that could mimic angina (e.g. pneumothorax, pneumonia, musculoskeletal diseases), or precipitating conditions such as anaemia and thyrotoxicosis. Presence at cardiac auscultation of a systolic murmur is related to the presence of an ischaemic mitral regurgitation, which is associated with poor prognosis [24], or, rarely, it may indicate a mechanical complication (i.e. papillary muscle rupture or ventricular septal defect) of a sub-acute and possibly undetected MI. Signs of heart failure or haemodynamic or electrical instability mandate a quick diagnosis and treatment.

2.3.2 Electrocardiography

The resting 12-lead ECG is the first-line diagnostic tool in the assessment of patients with suspected ACS. It is recommended to perform it within 10 min of the patient's arrival in the emergency room or, ideally, at first contact with the emergency medical services in the pre-hospital setting and to have it immediately interpreted by a qualified physician. Typical ECG abnormalities include ST-segment depression, transient ST-segment elevation, and T-wave changes [25–27]. However, the ECG in the setting of NSTE-ACS may be normal in more than 30% of patients. If the standard leads are inconclusive and the patient has signs or symptoms suggestive of ongoing myocardial ischaemia, additional leads should be recorded; left circumflex artery occlusion may be detected only in V7–V9 or right ventricular MI only in V3R and V4R [3].

2.3.3 Blood Tests

Measurement of a biomarker of cardiomyocyte injury is mandatory in all patients with suspected NSTE-ACS [2, 8, 28, 29]; cardiac troponins are more sensitive and specific markers of cardiomyocyte injury than creatine kinase (CK), its myocardial band isoenzyme (CK-MB), and myoglobin [2, 8, 28–30].

Particularly, an elevation of cardiac troponin above the 99th percentile of healthy individuals indicates MI. Measurement of high-sensitivity cardiac troponin (hs-cTn) has shown in large studies an increased diagnostic accuracy for MI compared with conventional assays, especially in patients presenting early after chest pain onset [2, 8, 22, 23, 28–30].

However, it is important to consider that many other cardiac pathologies may result in cardiac troponin elevations due to cardiomyocyte injury, such as tachyarrhythmias, heart failure, hypertensive emergencies, myocarditis, Takotsubo syndrome, aortic dissection, pulmonary embolism, and valvular heart disease, which should be considered in the differential diagnosis. Moreover, in patients presenting with suspected NSTE-ACS, three important clinical variables could affect hs-cTn levels: age, renal dysfunction, and sex [22, 23, 31].

Due to the higher sensitivity and diagnostic accuracy for the detection of MI at presentation, the time interval to the second cardiac troponin assessment can be shortened with the use of hs-cTn assays. The European Society of Cardiology (ESC) Guidelines recommend the use of the 0-h/1-h algorithm (best option, blood draw at 0 h and 1 h) or the 0-h/2-h algorithm (second best option, blood draw at 0 h and 2 h): these algorithms have very high sensitivity (99%) also in patients with early chest pain onset (e.g. <2 h) [2, 23]. However, due to the time dependency of troponin release, in patients presenting <1 h after chest pain, an additional assessment of cardiac troponin concentration at 3 h should be considered [2].

2.3.4 Echocardiography

Transthoracic echocardiography should be routinely performed in all patients with NSTE-ACS to identify abnormalities suggestive of myocardial ischaemia or necrosis (i.e. segmental hypokinesia or akinesia). Moreover, echocardiography is useful for differential diagnosis with other conditions associated with chest pain such as acute aortic dissection, pericardial effusion, aortic valve stenosis, hypertrophic cardiomyopathy, mitral valve prolapse, or acute pulmonary embolism [32].

2.3.5 Other Imaging Techniques

Chest X-ray is recommended in all patients in whom NSTE-ACS is considered unlikely in order to detect pneumonia, pneumothorax, rib fractures, or other thoracic disorders. Conditions that should always be considered in the differential diagnosis of NSTE-ACS, because they are potentially life-threatening, include aortic dissection and pulmonary embolism; therefore, in case of high suspicion, CT scan is recommended. Coronary computed tomography angiography (CCTA) allows visualization of the coronary arteries: CCTA has a high negative predictive value to exclude ACS, and a normal scan excludes CAD [33].

3 Chronic Coronary Syndromes

3.1 Introduction

Chronic coronary syndromes (CCS) represent a large and heterogeneous group of clinical conditions associated with myocardial ischaemia, which are thought to be stable, in contrast with acute (or unstable) disease. Acute and chronic coronary syndromes could be considered as two different points on the same line. Ischaemic heart disease is in fact characterized by a slow and progressive course, with a balance that can be broken at any time by an acute event, generally a complication of a coronary atherosclerotic plaque. Multiple pathophysiologic mechanisms may cause CCS. The most common is atherosclerotic epicardial coronary artery obstruction. However, as many as one-third of patients may have no significant epicardial disease and often have microvascular disease as the underlying pathophysiology. Angina pectoris is the classical clinical presentation of CCS. Most patients can be given the diagnosis of CCS based on a history of angina in the presence of either risk factors for or known atherosclerotic cardiovascular disease [34]. However, given the variable nature of the disease, the current ESC Guidelines recognize some of the most frequently encountered clinical scenarios in patients with suspected or established CCS [35]; patients with suspected CAD and "stable" anginal symptoms and/or dyspnoea; patients with new onset of heart failure (or left ventricular dysfunction) and suspected CAD; asymptomatic and symptomatic patients with stabilized symptoms either less or more than 1 year after an acute coronary syndrome and/or previous revascularization; patients with angina and suspected vasospastic or microvascular disease; and asymptomatic subjects in whom CAD is detected at screening.

A comprehensive clinical evaluation is the key to diagnosing CCS. Detailed medical history, physical examination, and analysis and interpretation of laboratory and instrumental tests are essential tools for an effective differential diagnosis, as well as to exclude an acute coronary syndrome, with which a significant overlap exists.

3.2 Medical History

Angina pectoris refers to chest discomfort that occurs when myocardial oxygen demand exceeds oxygen supply. It is the cornerstone of myocardial ischaemia and must be sought in every suspect of coronary artery disease. Several studies have reported that the majority of patients suspected of having CAD present with atypical or non-anginal chest pain, with as few as 10–15% presenting with typical angina. The prevalence of anginal symptoms varies and is thought to be lower among community-dwelling patients than trial participants. Furthermore, among older individuals, which represent a growing proportion of patients with CCS, recognition of disease can be more challenging due to a higher prevalence of atypical symptoms, including exertional dyspnoea or silent myocardial ischaemia [36–39]. Talking to the patient, asking the right questions, is paramount for the detection of angina. Essential elements for the characterization of anginal pain include site and irradiation, relationship with effort or alternative triggers, duration, and character.

- *Site and irradiation:* Usually located in the chest, across the sternum, but may be felt anywhere from the epigastrium to the lower jaw or teeth, between the shoulder blades, or in either arm to the wrist and fingers.
- *Relationship with effort: "Stable"* angina occurs predictably and reproducibly at a certain level of exertion and is relieved with rest or nitroglycerine. Angina classically appears or becomes more severe with increased levels of exertion such as walking up an incline or against a breeze or in cold weather and rapidly disappears within a few minutes when these causal factors abate. Exacerbations of symptoms after a heavy meal or after waking up in the morning are classic features of angina. Angina may paradoxically be reduced with further exercise (walk-through angina) or on second exertion (warm-up angina) [20]. The angina threshold, and hence symptoms, may vary considerably from day to day and even during the same day.
- *Duration:* The duration of the discomfort is brief <10 min in the majority of cases, and more commonly just a few minutes or less so that chest pain lasting for seconds is

unlikely to be due to CAD. No less important is the time necessary for its regression with rest or administration of nitrates, typically less than 5 min.
- *Character:* Angina is often described as pressure, tightness, or heaviness, sometimes strangling, constricting, and less frequently as burning.

In summary, angina could be defined typical when it meets three characteristics: constricting discomfort in the front of the chest or in the neck, jaw, shoulder, or arm; is precipitated by physical exertion; and is relieved by rest or nitrates within 5 min. Angina is considered atypical when it meets only two of these three main characteristics. It is non-anginal pain when it meets only one or none of the characteristics listed above. This classification, reported in the Guidelines [35], is practical and of proven value in determining the likelihood of obstructive CAD [40].

The Canadian Cardiovascular Society classification is used to quantify the threshold of effort at which symptoms occur [20]:

- **Grade I**: Ordinary physical activity does not cause angina, such as walking and climbing stairs. Angina with strenuous or rapid or prolonged exertion at work or recreation
- **Grade II:** Slight limitation of ordinary activity. Walking or climbing stairs rapidly, walking uphill, walking or stair climbing after meals, or in cold, or in wind, or under emotional stress, or only during the few hours after awakening. Walking more than two blocks on the level and climbing more than one flight of ordinary stairs at a normal pace and in normal conditions
- **Grade III**: Marked limitation of ordinary physical activity. Walking one or two blocks on the level and climbing one flight of stairs in normal conditions and at normal pace
- **Grade IV**: Inability to carry on any physical activity without discomfort, anginal syndrome may be present at rest

Symptoms are unrelated to breathing, position, or palpation. These represent distinctive elements for the differential diagnosis with:

- *Pericardial pain:* exacerbated by deep inhalation and eased by bending the torso on the abdomen
- *Pleural pain:* frequently stinging, with preferential sub-mammary and/or suprascapular localization

Sublingual nitrates could rapidly relieve angina. However, this feature does not always lead to a certain diagnosis. In fact, even motor disorders of the oesophagus can be related to pain, which is attenuated by or regressed with the administration of nitrates. In such cases, other information will need to be considered for the differential diagnosis.

3.3 Stable vs. Unstable Angina

The patient with stable angina reports the onset of discomfort after a certain reproducible level of exertion or activity. It is advisable to research the trend of the symptoms and identify the exercise threshold at which angina (hence myocardial ischaemia) appears. This allows the patient's risk of events to be stratified and guides the diagnostic and therapeutic path. On the contrary, diagnosis of unstable angina should be considered in the case of either resting angina, with typical characteristics and longer duration (>20 min); new-onset angina; or recent (2 months) onset of moderate-to-severe angina (Canadian Cardiovascular Society grade II or III). Additional features suggestive of instability include increased intensity, duration, number, and/or frequency of anginal episodes. Whenever a patient reports these characteristics, then he or she should be classified as having acute disease, and therefore be managed according to the appropriate guidelines [41].

3.4 Alternative Presentations

The patient may report shortness of breath, difficult to distinguish from shortness of breath of other origin. Otherwise, the patient may present symptoms suggestive of heart failure including those related to reduced cardiac output such as fatigue, with difficulty in making efforts such as climbing stairs or walking uphill, or those related to pulmonary (orthopnoea and paroxysmal nocturnal dyspnoea, bendopnoea) or systemic congestion (reduced appetite and weight reduction, vice versa weight gain linked to fluid accumulation). A possible but infrequent clinical presentation of CCS is represented by arrhythmias and syncope. Ventricular arrhythmias are a frequent complication of both the early and late phases of acute coronary syndromes. However, any finding of ventricular arrhythmias (resting ECG, exercise test, or ambulatory ECG monitoring) reinforces the suspicion of ischaemic heart disease and classifies the patient as at high risk of events. Less specific symptoms such as nausea, burning, restlessness, or a sense of impending doom may also be present.

Moreover, the role of history in diagnosing ischaemic heart disease goes beyond the search for angina and its equivalents. It is advisable to research and characterize the patient's cardiovascular risk factors, i.e. arterial hypertension, dyslipidaemia, diabetes mellitus, smoking, and consumption of illicit drugs and therefore familial history of cardiovascular disease and/or of sudden cardiac death, and to search for alternative comorbidities such as endocrinopathies (thyroid disorders) and haematological and inflammatory diseases.

3.5 Physical Examination

Physical examination of a patient with suspected CAD is important to assess the presence of signs of heart failure as well as of comorbidities such as anaemia, hypertension, valvular heart disease, hypertrophic cardiomyopathy (see below), or arrhythmias. It is also recommended to obtain the body mass index (BMI) and search for signs of comorbid conditions such as thyroid disease, renal disease, or diabetes. This should be used in the context of other clinical information, such as the presence of cough or stinging pain, making CAD more unlikely. One should also try to reproduce the symptoms by palpation and test the effect of sublingual nitroglycerine in order to classify the symptoms.

3.6 Differential Diagnoses

3.6.1 Angina Without Obstructive Coronary Artery Disease

Angina means myocardial ischaemia; thus, its finding is not synonymous with obstructive coronary artery disease. Ischaemia can occur as a consequence of many different pathological processes, which can involve both the epicardial coronaries and the coronary microcirculation, even in the context of myocardial diseases.

- *Microvascular and vasospastic angina:* A distinction between symptoms caused by an epicardial stenosis and symptoms caused by microvascular or vasospastic disease cannot be made with reasonable certainty. Reliance on ischaemia testing or depiction of the coronary anatomy is often unavoidable to exclude obstructive CAD, which can be absent in symptomatic patients. Patients with microvascular angina typically have exercise-related angina, evidence of ischaemia in non-invasive tests, and either no stenoses or mild-to-moderate stenoses (40/60%), revealed by invasive coronary angiography or computed tomography angiography, that are deemed functionally non-relevant [42]. Some patients may also have a mixed pattern of angina, with occasional episodes at rest, particularly associated with exposure to cold. Vasospastic angina should be suspected in patients with anginal symptoms occurring predominantly at rest, with maintained effort tolerance. Attacks may follow a circadian pattern, with more episodes at night and in the early morning hours [35]. Patients are frequently younger and have fewer cardiovascular risk factors than patients with effort angina. The diagnosis of vasospastic angina relies on detecting transient ischaemic ST-segment changes during an angina attack (usually at rest). Prinzmetal angina represents a special subset with resting symptoms accompanied by transient ST-segment elevation.

  Aortic stenosis and hypertrophic cardiomyopathy, through (concentric) myocardial hypertrophy, could determine secondary microvascular angina:
- *Aortic stenosis:* Angina, dyspnoea, and syncope are clinical and prognostic defining elements in patients with aortic valve stenosis. Angina has typical characteristics; therefore, the suspicion of aortic valve disease will have to be guided by other clinical signs: the classic systolic ejective murmur, harsh, radiated to the carotids; possible absence of the second heart sound; and the well-known "parvus and tardus" pulse.
- *Hypertrophic cardiomyopathy:* Patients with hypertrophic cardiomyopathy (HCM) are susceptible to myocardial ischaemia attributable to a mismatch between myocardial oxygen supply and demand. Anatomical remodelling of the intra-myocardial coronary

arterioles has been observed, associated with severely decreased luminal area. Along with microvascular remodelling, reduced capillary density, myocyte disarray, interstitial fibrosis, and increased oxygen demand of the hypertrophied cardiomyocytes constitute the anatomical basis for microvascular dysfunction and represent the substrate for ischaemia in HCM [43]. Most HCM patients complain of atypical chest pain or tightness occurring at rest or during exercise. Clinical pearls for the differential diagnosis include a family history of cardiomyopathy or sudden death, a history of transient loss of consciousness especially after intense exertion, and the presence of symptoms and signs of heart failure (with eventual appearance and worsening after meals, typical of obstructive forms). Physical examination could reveal a systolic murmur, prominent apical point of maximal impulse shifted laterally and either bifid or trifid, carotid double pulsation known as *"pulsus bisferiens"*, and an S4 from a noncompliant left ventricle. Systolic anterior motion of the mitral valve leads to left ventricular outflow tract obstruction (LVOTO) and resultant harsh crescendo-decrescendo systolic murmur best heard over the lower left sternal border. Physical findings of LVOTO should be sought both at rest and with provocative manoeuvres (Valsalva manoeuvre, standing from the squatting position). Those without LVOTO may have a normal physical examination [44]. Clinical evaluation, together with instrumental examinations such as ECG and echocardiography, usually allows the differential diagnosis with obstructive coronary disease. Nonetheless, typical angina, even if rarely reported by HCM patients, should be carefully evaluated. Coronary arteriography should be considered, in order to exclude causes of ischaemia involving the epicardial coronary circulation, such as atherosclerotic disease in the adults, intra-myocardial bridges, or anomalous origin of coronary arteries in the young.

3.6.2 Obstructive Coronary Artery Disease Without Angina

Conversely, the absence of angina does not rule out the diagnosis of CAD but, as reported above, makes it more difficult. This group includes patients whose coronary artery disease is diagnosed as part of screening tests, as well as patients who, due to a previous silent myocardial infarction or the presence of extensive coronary artery disease, develop symptoms of heart failure.

- *Diabetes mellitus:* It often compromises anginal symptoms. In the diabetic patient, angina is muffled due to neuropathic complications, even in the presence of obstructive coronary artery disease (either in the acute or the chronic context).
- *Coronary allograft vasculopathy (CAV):* Coronary artery disease is a major determinant of the long-term prognosis of heart-transplant recipients. Angiographically significant CAV is associated with shorter graft survival and high mortality rate [45]. Innate and adaptive immune responses are involved in the pathogenesis of CAV. Vascular lesions are the result of cumulative endothelial injuries induced both by alloimmune responses and by non-specific insults (including ischemia-reperfusion injury, viral infections, and metabolic disorders) in the context of impaired repair mechanisms [46].

Early detection of CAV is challenging because symptoms of myocardial ischemia secondary to CAV are typically absent or atypical due to afferent and efferent allograft denervation [47] (regardless of the variable degree of re-innervation by a few years after transplantation). As a result, angina pectoris is rarely referred by patients with CAV. Premonitory symptoms associated with exertion such as chest pain, dyspnoea, diaphoresis, gastrointestinal distress, pre-syncope, or syncope are often missing or atypical, so symptoms do not provide a reliable warning of disease [48]. As a consequence, symptoms and signs of progressive heart failure due to allograft dysfunction, silent myocardial infarction detected on testing, or sudden death are common initial clinical presentations of CAV. CAV may also present with asymptomatic changes in allograft function detected on routine imaging studies or right-heart catheterization. Thus, CAV must be detected by screening studies rather than by waiting for the onset of symptoms.

3.7 Electrocardiography

The electrocardiographic diagnosis of myocardial ischaemia is based on repolarization abnormalities (classically, ST-segment depression). The latter can be found in a resting ECG, or be absent at rest and appear in the course of a provocative test (such as exercise stress test rather than stress echocardiography), or be found in the context of ambulatory ECG monitoring. In the electrocardiogram of a patient with chronic coronary syndrome, we can otherwise find alterations suggestive of a previous acute myocardial infarction (Q waves) or find ventricular arrhythmias that, properly contextualized, may suggest the presence of current myocardial ischemia. Indirect signs of CAD could be conduction abnormalities (mainly left bundle branch block and impairment of atrio-ventricular conduction). Since they could be non-specific, when found, such alterations must be integrated with clinical information so that the correct meaning can be given. The finding of dynamic changes in ventricular repolarization can be diagnostic of myocardial ischaemia (for example the classic ST-segment transient elevation that characterizes Prinzmetal angina). Atrial fibrillation is a frequent finding in patients with chest pain (usually atypical). ST-segment depression during supraventricular tachyarrhythmias is not predictive of obstructive CAD.

3.8 Blood Tests

Blood tests are useful in identifying any triggers of myocardial ischaemia, comorbidities, and risk factors for ischaemic heart disease. Blood tests that every patient with suspected CAD should undergo (as part of an initial screening or as part of periodic follow-up), include full blood count, electrolytes and renal function indices, lipid profile, and diabetes mellitus indices (fasting blood glucose, HbA1c, oral glucose tolerance test). To these, we can add the assessment of thyroid function.

3.9 Echocardiography

In chronic coronary syndromes, echocardiography may give important information about cardiac structure and function. It may show regional wall motion abnormalities suggesting the presence of CAD (current, or as a result of a previous acute coronary event). It also allows highlighting valvular heart disease and a set of structural abnormalities that can sustain or exclude alternative causes of angina (for example, cardiomyopathies). Furthermore, echocardiography is recommended for the evaluation of diastolic function and the measurement of left ventricular ejection fraction, a mean of prognostic stratification [35]. However, biochemical testing, ECG, and echocardiography of a patient with CCS could be completely normal.

4 Conclusions

In summary, history and physical examination are essential to establish the clinical likelihood of ischaemic heart disease. Clinical findings, together with laboratory and instrumental examinations, help in stratifying the patient's risk and defining the subsequent diagnostic and therapeutic path. When the clinical likelihood of CAD is high (once an acute coronary syndrome has been ruled out), current guidelines suggest a functional non-invasive imaging test, with the purpose of evaluating myocardial perfusion and detecting myocardial ischaemia through ECG changes or wall motion abnormalities [35]. Conversely, when the clinical probability is low, we can opt for an anatomical non-invasive imaging test (cardiac computed tomography angiography), which describes the coronary anatomy but does not provide information on any perfusion defects. When the clinical probability and the risk of events are very high, in selected cases, it is reasonable to use invasive coronary angiography. History and physical examination are valuable tools both at the time of diagnosis and at each subsequent follow-up visit. Any change in physical activity and in the frequency, severity, or pattern of angina; modification of risk factors; and development of new or worsened comorbid illnesses should be investigated.

References

1. Braunwald E, Antman EM, Beasley JW, et al. ACC/AHA guidelines for the management of patients with unstable angina and non-ST-segment elevation myocardial infarction. J Am Coll Cardiol. 2000;36(3):970–1062.
2. Roffi M, Patrono C, Collet JP, Mueller C, Valgimigli M, Andreotti F, et al. 2015 ESC Guidelines for the management of acute coronary syndromes in patients presenting without persistent ST-segment elevation: Task Force for the Management of Acute Coronary Syndromes in Patients Presenting without Persistent ST-Segment Elevation of the European Society of Cardiology (ESC). Eur Heart J. 2016;37:267–315.

3. Thygesen K, Alpert JS, Jaffe AS, Chaitman BR, Bax JJ, Morrow DA, et al. Fourth universal definition of myocardial infarction (2018). Eur Heart J. 2019;40:237–69.
4. De Torbal A, Boersma E, Kors JA, van Herpen G, Deckers JW, van der Kuip DA, et al. Incidence of recognized and unrecognized myocardial infarction in men and women aged 55 and older: the Rotterdam Study. Eur Heart J. 2006;27(6):729–36.
5. Diercks DB, Peacock WF, Hiestand BC, Chen AY, Pollack CV Jr, Kirk JD, et al. Frequency and consequences of recording an electrocardiogram >10 minutes after arrival in an emergency room in non-ST-segment elevation acute coronary syndromes (from the CRUSADE Initiative). Am J Cardiol. 2006;97(4):437–42.
6. Ibanez B, James S, Agewall S, Antunes MJ, Bucciarelli-Ducci C, Bueno H, et al. 2017 ESC Guidelines for the management of acute myocardial infarction in patients presenting with ST-segment elevation: the Task Force for the management of acute myocardial infarction in patients presenting with ST-segment elevation of the European Society of Cardiology (ESC). Eur Heart J. 2018;39(2):119–77.
7. Rokos IC, French WJ, Koenig WJ, Stratton SJ, Nighswonger B, Strunk B, et al. Integration of pre-hospital electrocardiograms and ST-elevation myocardial infarction receiving center (SRC) networks: impact on door-to-balloon times across 10 independent regions. JACC Cardiovasc Interv. 2009;2(4):339–46.
8. Thygesen K, Alpert JS, Jaffe AS, Simoons ML, Chaitman BR, White HD, Writing Group on the Joint ESC/ACCF/AHA/WHF Task Force for the Universal Definition of Myocardial Infarction, Thygesen K, Alpert JS, White HD, Jaffe AS, Katus HA, Apple FS, Lindahl B, Morrow DA, Chaitman BA, Clemmensen PM, Johanson P, Hod H, Underwood R, Bax JJ, Bonow RO, Pinto F, Gibbons RJ, Fox KA, Atar D, Newby LK, Galvani M, Hamm CW, Uretsky BF, Steg PG, Wijns W, Bassand JP, Menasché P, Ravkilde J, Ohman EM, Antman EM, Wallentin LC, Armstrong PW, Simoons ML, Januzzi JL, Nieminen MS, Gheorghiade M, Filippatos G, Luepker RV, Fortmann SP, Rosamond WD, Levy D, Wood D, Smith SC, Hu D, Lopez-Sendon JL, Robertson RM, Weaver D, Tendera M, Bove AA, Parkhomenko AN, Vasilieva EJ, Mendis S, ESC Committee for Practice Guidelines (CPG). Third universal definition of myocardial infarction. Eur Heart J. 2012;33(20):2551–67.
9. Dixon WC 4th, Wang TY, Dai D, Shunk KA, Peterson ED, Roe MT. Anatomic distribution of the culprit lesion in patients with non-ST-segment elevation myocardial infarction undergoing percutaneous coronary intervention: findings from the National Cardiovascular Data Registry. J Am Coll Cardiol. 2008;52(16):1347–8.
10. Rokos IC, Farkouh ME, Reiffel J, Dressler O, Mehran R, Stone GW. Correlation between index electrocardiographic patterns and pre-intervention angiographic findings: insights from the HORIZONS-AMI trial. Catheter Cardiovasc Interv. 2012;79(7):1092–8.
11. Stribling WK, Kontos MC, Abbate A, Cooke R, Vetrovec GW, Dai D, et al. Left circumflex occlusion in acute myocardial infarction (from the National Cardiovascular Data Registry). Am J Cardiol. 2011;108(7):959–63.
12. Wang TY, Zhang M, Fu Y, Armstrong PW, Newby LK, Gibson CM, et al. Incidence, distribution, and prognostic impact of occluded culprit arteries among patients with non-ST elevation acute coronary syndromes undergoing diagnostic angiography. Am Heart J. 2009;157(4):716–23.
13. Lopez-Sendon J, Coma-Canella I, Alcasena S, Seoane J, Gamallo C. Electrocardiographic findings in acute right ventricular infarction: sensitivity and specificity of electrocardiographic alterations in right precordial leads V4R, V3R,V1, V2, and V3. J Am Coll Cardiol. 1985;6(6):1273–9.
14. Yan AT, Yan RT, Kennelly BM, Anderson FA Jr, Budaj A, Lopez-Sendon J, et al. Relationship of ST elevation in lead aVR with angiographic findings and outcome in non-ST elevation acute coronary syndromes. Am Heart J. 2007;154(1):71–8.

15. Garot P, Lefevre T, Eltchaninoff H, Morice MC, Tamion F, Abry B, et al. Six-month outcome of emergency percutaneous coronary intervention in resuscitated patients after cardiac arrest complicating ST-elevation myocardial infarction. Circulation. 2007;115(11):1354–62.
16. Kern KB, Rahman O. Emergent percutaneous coronary intervention for resuscitated victims of out-of-hospital cardiac arrest. Catheter Cardiovasc Interv. 2010;75(4):616–24.
17. Larsen JM, Ravkilde J. Acute coronary angiography in patients resuscitated from out-of-hospital cardiac arrest: a systematic review and meta-analysis. Resuscitation. 2012;83(12):1427–33.
18. Spaulding CM, Joly LM, Rosenberg A, Monchi M, Weber SN, Dhainaut JF, et al. Immediate coronary angiography in survivors of out-of-hospital cardiac arrest. N Engl J Med. 1997;336(23):1629–33.
19. Neskovic AN, Hagendorff A, Lancellotti P, Guarracino F, Varga A, Cosyns B, et al. Emergency echocardiography: the European Association of Cardiovascular Imaging recommendations. Eur Heart J Cardiovasc Imaging. 2013;14(1):1–11.
20. Campeau L. Letter: grading of angina pectoris. Circulation. 1976;54:522–3.
21. Rubini Gimenez M, Reiter M, Twerenbold R, Reichlin T, Wildi K, Haaf P, et al. Sex specific chest pain characteristics in the early diagnosis of acute myocardial infarction. JAMA Intern Med. 2014;174:241.
22. Boeddinghaus J, Nestelberger T, Twerenbold R, Neumann JT, Lindahl B, Giannitsis E, et al. Impact of age on the performance of the ESC 0/1h-algorithms for early diagnosis of myocardial infarction. Eur Heart J. 2018;39:3780–94.
23. Twerenbold R, Badertscher P, Boeddinghaus J, Nestelberger T, Wildi K, Puelacher C, et al. 0/1-hour triage algorithm for myocardial infarction in patients with renal dysfunction. Circulation. 2018;137:436–51.
24. Persson A, Hartford M, Herlitz J, Karlsson T, Omland T, Caidahl K. Long-term prognostic value of mitral regurgitation in acute coronary syndromes. Heart. 2010;96:1803–8.
25. Chapman AR, Shah ASV, Lee KK, Anand A, Francis O, Adamson P, et al. Long-term outcomes in patients with type 2 myocardial infarction and myocardial injury. Circulation. 2018;137:1236–45.
26. Mandelzweig L, Battler A, Boyko V, Bueno H, Danchin N, Filippatos G, et al. The second Euro Heart Survey on acute coronary syndromes: characteristics, treatment, and outcome of patients with ACS in Europe and the Mediterranean Basin in 2004. Eur Heart J. 2006;27:2285–93.
27. Neumann JT, Sorensen NA, Rubsamen N, Ojeda F, Renne T, Qaderi V, et al. Discrimination of patients with type 2 myocardial infarction. Eur Heart J. 2017;38:3514–20.
28. Reichlin T, Twerenbold R, Maushart C, Reiter M, Moehring B, Schaub N, et al. Risk stratification in patients with unstable angina using absolute serial changes of 3 high-sensitive troponin assays. Am Heart J. 2013;165:371–8.e3.
29. Reichlin T, Twerenbold R, Reiter M, Steuer S, Bassetti S, Balmelli C, et al. Introduction of high-sensitivity troponin assays: impact on myocardial infarction incidence and prognosis. Am J Med. 2012;125:1205–13.e1.
30. Mueller C, Giannitsis E, Mockel M, Huber K, Mair J, Plebani M, et al. Rapid rule out of acute myocardial infarction: novel biomarker-based strategies. Eur Heart J Acute Cardiovasc Care. 2017;6:218–22.
31. Sorensen NA, Neumann JT, Ojeda F, Schafer S, Magnussen C, Keller T, et al. Relations of sex to diagnosis and outcomes in acute coronary syndrome. J Am Heart Assoc. 2018;7:e007297.
32. Lancellotti P, Price S, Edvardsen T, Cosyns B, Neskovic AN, Dulgheru R, et al. The use of echocardiography in acute cardiovascular care: recommendations of the European Association of Cardiovascular Imaging and the Acute Cardiovascular Care Association. Eur Heart J Acute Cardiovasc Care. 2015;4:3.

33. Samad Z, Hakeem A, Mahmood SS, Pieper K, Patel MR, Simel DL, et al. A meta-analysis and systematic review of computed tomography angiography as a diagnostic triage tool for patients with chest pain presenting to the emergency department. J Nucl Cardiol. 2012;19:364–76.
34. Ford TJ, Corcoran D, Berry C. Stable coronary syndromes: pathophysiology, diagnostic advances and therapeutic need. Heart. 2018;104:284.
35. Knuuti J, Wijns W, Saraste A, Capodanno D, Barbato E, Funck-Brentano C, et al. 2019 ESC Guidelines for the diagnosis and management of chronic coronary syndromes. Eur Heart J. 2020;41(3):407–77. https://doi.org/10.1093/eurheartj/ehz425. Erratum in: Eur Heart J. 2020 Nov 21;41(44):4242.
36. Cheng VY, Berman DS, Rozanski A, Dunning AM, Achenbach S, Al-Mallah M, et al. Performance of the traditional age, sex, and angina typicality-based approach for estimating pretest probability of angiographically significant coronary artery disease in patients undergoing coronary computed tomographic angiography: results from the multinational coronary CT angiography evaluation for clinical outcomes: an international multicenter registry (CONFIRM). Circulation. 2011;124(2423–32):2421–8.
37. Ferraro R, Latina JM, Alfaddagh A, et al. Evaluation and management of patients with stable angina: beyond the ischemia paradigm: JACC state-of-the-art review. J Am Coll Cardiol. 2020;76:2252.
38. Reeh J, Therming CB, Heitmann M, Hojberg S, Sorum C, Bech J, et al. Prediction of obstructive coronary artery disease and prognosis in patients with suspected stable angina. Eur Heart J. 2018;40:1426–35.
39. SCOT-HEART Investigators. CT coronary angiography in patients with suspected angina due to coronary heart disease (SCOT-HEART): an open-label, parallel-group, multicentre trial. Lancet. 2015;385:2383–91.
40. Genders TS, Steyerberg EW, Hunink MG, Nieman K, Galema TW, Mollet NR, et al. Prediction model to estimate presence of coronary artery disease: retrospective pooled analysis of existing cohorts. BMJ. 2012;344:e3485.
41. Collet JP, Thiele H, Barbato E, Barthélémy O, Bauersachs J, Bhatt DL, et al. 2020 ESC Guidelines for the management of acute coronary syndromes in patients presenting without persistent ST-segment elevation. Eur Heart J. 2021;42(14):1289–367. https://doi.org/10.1093/eurheartj/ehaa575. Erratum in: Eur Heart J. 2021 May 14;42(19):1908. Erratum in: Eur Heart J. 2021 May 14;42(19):1925. Erratum in: Eur Heart J. 2021 May 13.
42. Ong P, Camici PG, Beltrame JF, Crea F, Shimokawa H, Sechtem U, et al. Coronary Vasomotion Disorders International Study Group (COVADIS). International standardization of diagnostic criteria for microvascular angina. Int J Cardiol. 2018;250:16–20.
43. Ommen SR, Mital S, Burke MA, Day SM, Deswal A, Elliott P, et al. 2020 AHA/ACC guideline for the diagnosis and treatment of patients with hypertrophic cardiomyopathy: a report of the American College of Cardiology/American Heart Association Joint Committee on Clinical Practice Guidelines. J Am Coll Cardiol. 2020;76(25):e159–240.
44. Cecchi F, Sgalambro A, Baldi M, Sotgia B, Antoniucci D, Camici PG, et al. Microvascular dysfunction, myocardial ischemia, and progression to heart failure in patients with hypertrophic cardiomyopathy. J Cardiovasc Transl Res. 2009;2(4):452–61.
45. Khush KK, Cherikh WS, Chambers DC, et al. The International Thoracic Organ Transplant Registry of the International Society for Heart and Lung Transplantation: thirty-sixth adult heart transplantation report—2019; Focus theme: donor and recipient size match. J Heart Lung Transplant. 2019;38:1056.
46. Schmauss D, Weis M. Cardiac allograft vasculopathy: recent developments. Circulation. 2008;117(16):2131–41.

47. Ades PA, Keteyian SJ, Balady GJ, et al. Cardiac rehabilitation exercise and self-care for chronic heart failure. JACC Heart Fail. 2013;1:540.
48. Gao SZ, Schroeder JS, Hunt SA, et al. Acute myocardial infarction in cardiac transplant recipients. Am J Cardiol. 1989;64:1093.

Cardiovascular Biomarkers in Acute Myocardial Infarction

Cristina Vassalle, Laura Sabatino, and Alessia Pepe

Abbreviations

AACC	American Association for Clinical Chemistry
ACC	American College of Cardiology
AHA	American Heart Association
AMI	Acute myocardial infarction
ANP	Atrial natriuretic peptide
AST	Aspartate aminotransferase
AST	Aspartate transaminase
BNP	B-type (or brain) natriuretic peptide
CAD	Coronary artery disease
CK	Creatine kinase
CNP	C-type natriuretic peptide
CRP	C-reactive protein
c-Tn	Cardiac troponins
CVD	Cardiovascular disease

C. Vassalle (✉)
Fondazione CNR-Regione Toscana, G. Monasterio, Pisa, Italy
e-mail: cristina.vassalle@ftgm.it

L. Sabatino
Institute of Clinical Physiology, National Research Council, Pisa, Italy
e-mail: laura.sabatino@ifc.cnr.it

A. Pepe
Department of Medicine, Institute of Radiology, University of Padua, Padua, Italy
e-mail: alessia.pepe@unipd.it

G. Concistrè (ed.), *Ischemic Heart Disease*,
https://doi.org/10.1007/978-3-031-25879-4_9

ESC	European Society of Cardiology
HBT	Heterophilic blocking tubes
HF	Heart failure
IL	Interleukin
LDH	Lactate dehydrogenase
MB	Myoglobin
miRNAs	MicroRNAs
MPV	Mean platelet volume
ncRNA	Noncoding RNA
NLR	Neutrophil-to-lymphocyte ratio
NP	Natriuretic peptides
NT-proBNP	N-terminal fragment of precursor BNP
PDW	Platelet distribution width
PLR	Platelet-to-lymphocyte ratio
POCT	Point-of-care testing
RDW	Red cell distribution width
WBC	White blood cells
WHO	World Health Organization

1 Introduction

According to the World Health Organization (WHO), cardiovascular disease (CVD), as the leading cause of death in the world, is responsible for 32% of all deaths, corresponding to 17.9 million deaths per year [1]. Thus, CVD has been the object of intense research to improve diagnosis, risk stratification, and patient management, especially for acute myocardial infarction (AMI) that together with heart failure (HF) is the most common and studied CV condition [2, 3]. Circulating biomarkers associated with these diseases (e.g., cardiac troponins (cTns) and natriuretic peptides (NPs)) represent important references in the routine clinical practice [4]. Really, biomarkers such as myoglobin (MB), lactate dehydrogenase (LDH), aspartate aminotransferase (AST), and creatine kinase (CK) were firstly used for AMI diagnosis, then abandoned for their low specificity and sensibility, and replaced by cardiac troponins (cTnI and T). In fact, cTns have radically changed AMI diagnosis and are nowadays considered the most reliable available biomarkers of myocardial ischemia/necrosis, especially with the development of high-sensibility assays (hs-cTn, able to detect lower and lower levels of troponins) [5]. However, whereas the use of hs-cTn has greatly improved diagnostic sensitivity, it has in parallel entailed a decrease in diagnostic specificity, since cTn increase results elevated in a number of other diseases (e.g., acute or chronic heart failure, aortic dissection, myocarditis, takotsubo cardiomyopathy, atrial fibrillation, and stroke) [6].

NP family includes three structurally similar peptides, atrial natriuretic peptide (ANP), B-type (or brain) natriuretic peptide (BNP), and C-type natriuretic peptide (CNP), whose levels increase in response to enhanced cardiac wall stretching due to volume or load stress [7]. In particular, levels of BNP and the N-terminal fragment of its precursor (NT-proBNP) contribute to AMI patient's prognosis (death, acute heart failure: according to 2020 ESC Guidelines for the management of acute coronary syndromes in patients presenting without persistent ST-segment elevation) and are commonly used for HF diagnosis, risk stratification, and management of HF patients [8].

Although the importance of cTn and BNP/NT-proBNP is widely recognized, it is also clear that the involvement of these markers is not sufficient to include the complexity of CV pathophysiology. Thus, the efforts in the identification and validation of new reliable biomarkers are extremely active in various pathophysiological contexts (e.g., myocardial stress or necrosis, neurohormonal activation, inflammation/oxidative stress, fibrosis, plaque instability), which use, also in a multimarker approach, may ultimately improve patient well-being.

Accordingly, the aim of this chapter is to explore the literature on cardiac biomarkers, mainly focusing on the role and applications of cTn and NP in the diagnosis, risk stratification, and management of patients with AMI, discussing some additional available routine biomarkers and newer biomarkers with relevant potential clinical value in the future.

2 Brief Notes on Historical Cardiac Biomarkers

The first biomarkers (AST, LDH, CK, creatine kinase MB isoenzyme-CK-MB, or MB) of cardiac damage were considered with low specificity since, in addition to the heart, they were also localized in skeletal muscle. In fact, the continuous turnover of the skeletal muscle cells generates a baseline level of these biomarkers into the circulation, rendering the diagnosis of AMI difficult, especially in case of small infarction, which often does not cause a detectable change over the baseline value.

2.1 Aspartate Transaminase (AST)

AST is an enzyme that catalyzes the conversion of aspartate and alpha-ketoglutarate to oxaloacetate and glutamate, and it was the first circulating biomarker used for AMI diagnosis and introduced in the clinical practice since the half of the past century [9]. Kinetics of AST implies an increase in blood within 3–4 h after AMI, peaking in 15–28 h and returning towards normal values within 5 days [10]. Although AST retains high sensitivity for AMI, it is not so specific for myocardial tissue, since it can also increase in several other diseases [11].

2.2 Lactate Dehydrogenase (LDH)

LDH belongs to the class of oxidoreductases, catalyzing the synthesis of lactate and pyruvate in a reversible reaction [12]. The LDH trend during IMA showed an increase in blood 5–10 h after AMI, achievement of the maximum value in blood in 60–144 h, and returning to normal values in 12 days [10]. LDH is widely expressed in different organs and is not heart specific. Therefore, LDH assays assume a higher clinical significance when its five isoenzymes are evaluated. In particular, LDH1 is present in cardiac myocytes and erythrocytes, and retains more organ specificity than total LDH activity. For this reason, LDH1 activity was also initially used for AMI diagnosis; however, it is no longer used [13]. Generally, levels of LDH1 are lower than isoenzyme LDH2 (highest content in white blood cells), but after AMI, LDH1 exceeds the LDH2 values. Thus, a reversal of the LDH1:LDH2 ratio was considered suggestive of myocardial necrosis. Nonetheless, since also hemolysis produces this characteristic inversion pattern, and since LDH is present in erythrocytes, it is important to verify the lack of sample hemolysis before the analysis [14].

2.3 Creatine Kinase (CK) Total Enzyme Activity and Isoforms

CK is an enzyme expressed by various tissues, catalyzing the conversion of creatinine by using ATP to give phosphocreatine and adenosine diphosphate, in a reversible reaction, which can also generate ATP [15]. Trend of CK in AMI involves its appearance in blood 3–9 h after the event, maximum value in 10–20 h, and return to normal values in about 72 h [10]. CK shows a good sensitivity, although not specific for the heart, with its activity considerably increased in many diseases and tissues other than myocardium (e.g., liver, kidneys, and skeletal muscle) [16]. Another limitation is represented by the difficulty to detect minor myocardial damage, due to its high molecular weight (diffuse at a slower rate).

Measurement of CK isoforms (BB, MM, and MB), named according to the various combinations of the M-muscle and B-brain isoforms, is also possible [17]. In particular, the CK-MB isoenzyme, normally undetectable or present at very low concentration in the blood, is found mostly in the myocardium and may be useful in heart disease as an AMI early specific biomarker [18]. However, it can increase in skeletal muscle disorders, and its assay is affected by many pre-analytical/analytical interferences (e.g., prolonged storage or inadequate sample preservation, interference from other enzymes or drugs, pH and ionic concentration used in the analyses, and assay temperature), as well as cross-reactivity can occur with other different compounds (e.g., rheumatoid factor) [19, 20]. CK-MB has different isoforms (CK-MB1 in myocardium, CK-MB2 in blood) [21]. The determination of CK-MB mass appears a more stable and reliable value than the measurement of enzyme activity, as it increases more rapidly than CK or CK-MB activity [10, 22]. CK-MB clinical relevance is attributable to its more rapid decline after AMI with respect to cTn, which gives to CK-MB an added value for a correct determination of myocardial injury onset and early detection of reinfarction [8].

2.4 Myoglobin

Myoglobin is a protein found exclusively in the heart tissue and in the skeletal muscle cells, acting as a local oxygen reserve and providing oxygen under intense muscular activity [23]. It can be found in the blood of AMI patients 1–3 h after the cardiac event, reaching its maximum within 4–7 h, and returning to basal values after 1–1.5 days [10]. Its rapid rise facilitates early AMI diagnosis or exclusion of any cardiac damage [24]. Myoglobin is characterized by a rapid clearance from blood; therefore, if on one side it is no more detectable in late-presenting patients, its rapid kinetics may help to diagnose reinfarction in patients [24]. However, it is not highly cardiac specific [24].

3 Troponins

Troponins are proteins characteristic of skeletal and heart muscle, where they are involved in muscular contraction [25]. History of troponins began in the 1960s with identification, purification, and characterization of a new sarcomeric protein complex, including the TnC, TnI, and TnT, named in view of their specific characteristics: Ca^{2+}-binding capacity of TnC, inhibition of ATPase activity by TnI, and tropomyosin binding by TnT [25, 26]. When their structure was defined, and skeletal and cardiac isoforms were identified (cTnT and cTnI for heart), the significance of cTnT and cTnI as cardiac biomarkers began to grow [27]. First assays were developed some years later utilizing RIA methodology and evidenced the trend of cTn during AMI—increased within 4–6 h, a peak at 18 h, and returned to normal value in up to 8 days [10, 28]. Then, cTn immunoassays were developed and considerably optimized during the time, so for example the actual cTnT fifth-generation assays reached an analytical sensitivity almost 100-fold higher than the first commercial assay [10, 28]. Actual hs-cTn assays measure lower concentration ranges making evaluation of changes more reliable, with a low analytical imprecision (<10% CV) at the 99th percentile concentration of the reference population, which is the recommended upper reference limit (URL), thus with a very high degree of analytical sensitivity. Circulating troponin levels are very low in healthy subjects; thus, its elevation in blood accounts for even the smallest cardiac injury [29]. It has been estimated that hs-cTnT and hs-cTnI are able to evidence myocardial damage (cTns in blood over the 99th percentile) provoked by the necrosis of about 0.015% of heart tissue, at amounts significantly lower than the limit of the spatial resolution of the most sensitive noninvasive cardiac imaging techniques (e.g., magnetic resonance imaging or positron-emission tomography) [30, 31].

Troponin is essentially located in the contractile apparatus and, in a more limited amount, in the cytosol. During AMI, it is released in the blood initially from the cytosolic pool and later from the contractile apparatus [32].

Due to the number of cTnI assay methods available, results obtained for the same patient through different methods may not be in agreement [33]. This fact makes cTnI standardization a critical issue [34, 35]. In 2000, the consensus document of the Joint

European Society of Cardiology/American College of Cardiology Committee for the redefinition of myocardial infarction unequivocally recommended cTnI and T as the best options for the differential diagnosis [36]. The clinical cutoff value for the diagnosis was defined as a value exceeding the 99th percentile in a cTn distribution of a reference control population (99th percentile URL), with an acceptable imprecision at this value corresponding to 10 CV% [37]. In the 2018 Fourth Universal Definition of Myocardial Infarction, myocardial injury was confirmed when at least one cTn value was above the 99th percentile URL [37]. Laboratory experts, in May 2018, evidenced two critical points to be considered: (a) the %CV at the 99th percentile URL should be <10% (e.g., using the Elecsys-Roche analyzer, at the 99th percentile value corresponding to 13.5 ng/L, the CV resulted 9%) [38] and (b) measurable cTn concentrations should be reachable at a value equal or above the assay's LoD for 50% of healthy individuals belonging to both genders [39]. Nonetheless, the most recent hs assays have been able to detect troponin up to 95% of healthy subjects in the reference population, with imprecision (coefficient of variation for repeated analyses of the sample) values of 2–5% [40]. Guidelines by the American Heart Association (AHA), the American College of Cardiology (ACC), and the European Society of Cardiology (ESC) also advised on the use of hs-cTn and defined AMI in the presence of myocardial injury by an elevation of cardiac troponin values with at least one value above the 99th percentile upper reference limit [3]. The establishment of the 99th percentile value must be taken according to gender, and troponin values should be measured in at least 300 female and 300 male subjects. Ideally, this value should be established by each laboratory, considering not only the method and instrumentation used but also the specific characteristics of the population in which the test is performed. Clearly, this procedure is very complex and implies elevated costs; thus, generally parameters provided by the manufacturers are accepted. Notably, the improved sensitivity of the new-generation immunoassays corresponds to a decreased specificity for AMI. Nonetheless, the use of hs-cTn assays does not aim to identify more AMI patients but, rather, to shorten the time required for AMI diagnosis and quickly identify AMI patients and discharge those without AMI on the basis of hs-cTn levels (rule-in/rule-out) [8]. Preferably, AMI diagnosis in the clinical practice considers standard clinical rule-out/rule-in algorithms (as 0/1-h and 0/2-h algorithms, recommended by the 2020 European Society of Cardiology-ESC-Guidelines-class I recommendation) based on the difference between two (or more) hs-cTn samples, collected during fixed time periods after admission in patients who present more than 2–3 h after symptom onset (thus not recommended in "very early presenters," with onset of symptoms <3 h, due to a potential time shift in cTn release) [8]. Further serial testing, in parallel to careful clinical and instrumental evaluation, is currently adopted in the clinical practice to stratify patients with elevated cTn, but without satisfying rule-in/rule-out AMI criteria (e.g., values over the upper range limit at admission, but with remission of chest pain, or without typical changes of electrocardiogram-ECG) [8]. A value lower than the limit of detection (LoD, by using method-specific cutoff) at admission, always evaluated together with ECG and clinical symptoms, has a high negative predictive value and allows safe and sure AMI rule-out in patients [8]. Another important issue is that hs-cTn must be intended as a quantitative biomarker related to the extension of cardiac damage, and not as a categorical parameter (positive/negative), according to the assertion that the higher the value, the higher the risk for AMI and the worse the prognosis [41]. Typically, high hs-cTn, which usually occurs within 3–12 h, especially in the presence of ECG changes, is suggestive of AMI, and the patient should be treated as soon as possible [37]. Moreover, serial sampling may not increase positive predictive values in patients with very high cTn elevation at admission (e.g., values greater than 80 ng/L) [42].

Beyond diagnostic utility, cTn retains short- and long-term prognostic values, as two meta-analyses suggested, evidencing as this biomarker may assist in the early identification of higher risk patients [43, 44]. Specifically, a meta-analysis conducted in non-ST-segment elevation myocardial infarction (NSTEMI) patients evidenced that the short-term odds of death are increased up to eightfold for patients with an abnormal troponin test, as well as another meta-analysis suggested that hs-Tn elevation predicted a higher risk of death in suspected acute coronary syndrome patients [43, 44].

Since hs-cTn is very sensitive to evidence an extremely limited myocardial tissue injury, underlying pathology may be of different nature (ischemic as well as nonischemic), and thus, this biomarker is *not disease specific* at all [45, 46]. However, as acute cardiac events presented a pattern of changes (rising or falling levels), chronic cardiac disorders (e.g., heart failure, valvular heart disease, or renal insufficiency) showed stable elevations, generally lower than in AMI (around two- or threefold upper normality limits) [45, 46]. Excluding patients with frank elevation of cTn, the others need serial sampling to distinguish acute from chronic elevation characteristic of other conditions. The hs-cTn retest could permit better stratification of an acute cardiac event from a chronic cardiac disease characterized by stable hs-cTn trend. hs-cTn assays allow the detection of circulating troponins in the majority of patients with stable coronary artery disease (CAD), whereas higher cTn values seem to suggest a worse prognosis in this population [47–49]. Similarly, an elevated cTn is frequent in HF patients, where it represents an independent predictor of adverse outcomes when compared with HF patients who showed low hsTnT or decreased levels on follow-up [50–52]. Moreover, elevated hsTn can be commonly found in patients with renal failure, likely reflecting reduced renal elimination and/or increased cardiac, where it confers adverse prognosis, even in asymptomatic patients [53–55]. Elevated hsTn is also common in patients with cardiac amyloid, where higher concentration is associated with adverse outcomes [56]. Patients under chemotherapy may also present increased hsTn, and in this setting, the opportunity of pharmacological intervention, as enalapril, can be beneficial to prevent left ventricular dysfunction, at least in selected patients [57, 58]. Intense acute exercise may increase cTn, although this transient and often moderate elevation may rather suggest a physiological response to acute exercise, than a real damage of cardiomyocytes [59]. Nonetheless, even in asymptomatic healthy subjects, an increase of cTn may have a prognostic role [60, 61]. Moreover, there is a gradient of risk across the reference range even for those who are within the normal interval limit [62]. Many underlying mechanisms

Table 1 Troponin take-home messages

Detectable release of cTnI or cTnT indicates some degree of cardiac injury, but not its underlying condition (cardiac injury specificity, but not disease specificity)
Adoption of 99th percentile of a reference population (higher sensitivity) and measurement uncertainty $\leq 10\%$ at this concentration represent the desirable goal
Finding of a rising pattern of values over time is critical to detect patients with acute diseases
hs-cTnT/I assays (vs. conventional ones) increase the diagnostic AMI accuracy, which means that it is now possible to measure smaller concentrations of cardiac troponin
Improved (analytical) sensitivity of hs-cTn assays means that it is possible to measure smaller concentrations of cTn (thus different from "clinical sensitivity")
hs-cTnT/I should always be interpreted as a quantitative variable; the higher the concentration, the higher the AMI probability
hs-cTn can remain elevated up to 10–14 days after an acute event
Higher hs-cTnT/I sensitivity with respect to all available cardiac imaging techniques (including cardiac magnetic resonance), thus unexpected hs-cTnT/I elevations are more likely true positive, than "*false elevations*" due to analytical problems
Values obtained with one method cannot be directly extrapolated to other methods
hs-cTn levels are higher in men and increase with age
hs-cTnT/I concentrations should always be interpreted within the context of the clinical presentation with all the other available medical information
In majority of patients, a definitive diagnosis can be made within 2 h (the ESC 0/1-h algorithm, published in the NSTE-ACS guidelines in 2015, being the preferred algorithm, validated for all clinically available hs-cTnT/I assays)

for this increase in the general population have been proposed, including apoptosis, cardiomyocyte turnover, strain, increased cardiac mass, and subclinical plaque rupture [63] (Table 1 summarized main important points to consider in cTn interpretation).

3.1 Troponin Test in Laboratory Medicine

Elevated concentrations of cTnT and I indicate cardiomyocyte injury, but do not necessarily indicate an acute coronary event, because many other conditions may induce an elevation of cTn. However, beyond the challenge of the nonspecific etiology, there are other aspects that must be considered in cTn interpretation, surely including the extent of false-positive results, pre-analytical and analytical confounders, biological variability, and lack of standardization of methods. If troponin values are discrepant with the clinical and instrumental findings, the possibility of an analytical error must be considered. Moreover, whether hs-cTnI and T are concordant and both elevated is likely the case of "true elevations," whereas if they are discordant, a suspicion of "false elevations" is reasonable. Moreover, due to between-method differences, values for troponins should be preferably performed in the same laboratory, to avoid misinterpretation [64]. This fact may create problems in case a patient needs to be transferred from a hospital to another where different methods of Tn determination are used, because the results may not agree.

3.2 Pre-analytical and Analytical Interferences, and Method Standardization

In the interpretation of cTn values, it is important to remember that the definition of 99th percentile marks a value at which 1 sample/100 may give a false-positive result, a fact caused by many factors, including pre-analytical and analytical interferences. One of the most common pre-analytical interferences is sample hemolysis, which can cause both false-negative and false-positive results [65–68]. Other interferences can be due to fibrin clots, also in this case causing both false-positive and false-negative cTn findings [69]. Moreover, heparin can interfere with cTnI and cTnT determination when a heparinized tube is used (a fact that can be overcome by dosing another sample with a different anticoagulant) or in patients on heparin therapy (an effect avoidable only by discontinuing the heparinization), as heparin may bind cTnI and impair its association with the antibodies in the immunoassays [70, 71]. Macrotroponin I, macro-complex produced by the binding of cTnI molecule to circulating immunoglobulins, characterized by a delayed clearance, may provoke unreal increased circulating troponin levels [72].

Blood TnI and T are full-sized forms (high MW) and proteolytic fragments of different lengths (low MW) (e.g., in view of proteolytic cleavage, posttranslational modifications) [73]. Thus, producers aimed to develop assays using antibodies directed against parts of the molecule that are not subject to proteolytic degradation, since coexistent circulating degradation products may cause interference and differences between assays. For example, it seems that the elevation of cTn which characterized intense exercise in healthy subjects is essentially due to fragments, whereas intact cTnI and T predominate in patients with AMI, likely reflecting different forms of injury [74, 75]. Consequently, the future development of assays capable of discriminating specific forms may allow better distinguishing of different pathophysiological conditions, increasing the specificity of AMI diagnosis, as well as the time course of cTn degradation, which may give information on the different temporal phases of the acute ischemic event [76, 77].

One of the most common analytical interferences causing false-positive results is the presence of heterophilic antibodies. In high titers, they can bind other species of antibodies, such as those used as reagents in immunoassays, giving positivity regardless of the concentration of the true analyte, even in the absence of the antigen to be detected (particularly regarding hs-cTnI assays) [78]. This interference can be excluded by pretreatment of samples with heterophilic blocking tubes (HBT), or PEG precipitation, although an alternative measurement with another hs-cTn method may represent a simple possibility to confirm/exclude the interference, which generally is method dependent [6].

The lack of standardization, particularly critical for hs-cTnI assays for which many methods are currently available, is related to several factors, including (1) the availability of assays with different stabilities, (2) the use of different antibodies recognizing different epitopes, and (3) the different coefficients of variability between methods [79]. There are several immunoassays for measuring cTnI, implemented on a number of instruments ranging from small point-of-care testing (POCT) instruments to large and automated analytical platforms, essentially belonging to two categories: "high-sensitivity" and "contemporary" (conventional) methods. The difference is due to the total imprecision at which a cTn method can measure the 99th reference percentile and the proportion of healthy subjects showing cTn values over the LoD [39]. While hs-cTn assays can measure low values and small increases above the 99th percentile URL, many contemporary and POCT cTn assays may not be able to detect small increasing values within the reference interval or slightly above the 99th percentile URL, causing significant differences in the frequency of events if the judgment is based exclusively on the cTn result. Nonetheless, their utilization is consented, although the clinical use of an assay with an imprecision $\geqslant$20% is not acceptable [31]. However, continuous encouraging improvement for cTn POCT may greatly benefit quicker decision-making strategies inside as well as outside the emergency department in the near future [80, 81].

To note, the American Association for Clinical Chemistry (AACC) Troponin I Standardization and the Subcommittee IFCC Working Group on Standardization of Cardiac Troponin I are working to propose a commutable reference material for cTnI to standardize cTnI measurements and reduce inter-assay bias [82].

3.3 Biological Variability

The intraindividual variation of cTnI in healthy adults, evaluated with a high-sensitivity method, is on average about 8–10%, lower than the intersubject variation, which may account for 50% of variation [83]. In view of the low intraindividual variation, the measurement of hs-cTn in a single subject/patient acquires importance, especially when compared to a clinical cutoff estimated in a large reference population (e.g., the 99th percentile URL), with a higher interindividual variation. Thus, the use of temporal changes in hs-cTn is recommended for early AMI diagnosis, as chronic myocardial injury is a status that implies the stability of Tn values, whereas an even slight change from baseline could be clinically relevant.

hs-cTnI and T showed a circadian rhythm, characterized by higher values in the morning, gradually decreasing until evening [84, 85]. Exact pathophysiological mechanisms for this rhythm are not completely clear, although sympathoadrenal, renin-angiotensin-aldosterone, and hypothalamic-pituitary-thyroid systems may have a role [31]. Nonetheless, this trend does not seem to significantly affect the diagnostic accuracy for AMI, although it could reduce the difference between cTn in non-AMI versus AMI conditions, as well as affect the changes from the first to the second blood draw [85, 86]. For hs-TnI, some studies reported that levels of this biomarker do not significantly differ with time of presentation [85].

Aging causes a progressive increase of hs-cTn levels, as elevated cTn values are found more frequently observed in older individuals, especially after 65 years [87,

88]. In fact, it is possible that some subjects with asymptomatic cardiac dysfunction (e.g., increased left ventricular mass or decreased left ventricular ejection fraction) are anyway present in the reference healthy population. Moreover, in elderly, there is a higher prevalence of cardiovascular risk factors, or reduced kidney functionality, although the relationship between age and cTn increase seems even independent from these risk factors [89].

Moreover, it is known that men have higher cTn concentration than women, as men present higher myocardial mass [90]. On this basis, the use of specific gender-related cutoff is recommended (e.g., by the Global Task Force for the Diagnosis of MI and the International Federation of Clinical Chemistry and Laboratory Medicine (IFCC) Task Force on Cardiac Biomarkers), but still not endorsed by all scientific societies (e.g., European Society of Cardiology Guideline (ESC) for management of non-ST-segment elevation ACS (NSTE-ACS)) [8, 39]. Interestingly, there may be significant discordant classifications between the hs-cTnT and hs-cTnI methods (e.g., in one study including 3588 patients, 21% were classified as having myocardial injury by hs-cTnT, but not by hs-cTnI) that the use of sex-specific thresholds is capable to reduce [91, 92]. Clearly, the use of specific gender-related cutoffs leads to a reclassification of AMI patients, increasing the number of diagnoses in women, despite increasing the risk of overdiagnosis in the elderly, who may have higher cTn values. As an example, using biological sex-specific hs-cTnI cutoffs, the AMI diagnoses changed from 16.6 to 22.6% in women, and from 23.1 to 21.1% in men, in a population of 1282 chest pain patients [93]. Interestingly, the predictive role of hs-cTn-specific gender cutoff improves the identification of women (but not men) at risk for 1-year adverse outcomes and all-cause mortality [94, 95].

Although at present there is still too controversial data to definitively adopt the use of gender-specific cutoffs, cutoffs including not only gender but also age, symptoms, and renal function have been proposed, towards a more personalized diagnosis. For this purpose, development of algorithms, which consider relative or absolute concentration changes and determine the optimal individual cutoff, is needed, but it is still impractical for clinical use.

4 Natriuretic Peptides

Natriuretic peptides belong to a family of hormones, which includes the brain natriuretic peptide (BNP), a quantitative biomarker of hemodynamic cardiac stress and ventricular dysfunction [96]. BNP is synthesized by cardiomyocytes as prohormone (proBNP) and then cleaved into the active BNP hormone and an inactive NT-proBNP fragment [96]. NT-proBNP represents the entire N-terminal fragment of proBNP (amino acids 1–76), and this molecule may be detected in both myocardium and blood. NT-proBNP has a longer half-life than BNP (60–120 versus 20–40 min, respectively), and its concentration is about 20 times greater than that of BNP, characteristics which make its use and result interpretation appreciable [96]. Commercially available assays to measure either BNP or NT-proBNP are immunometric double-antibody sandwich assays [97]. Pre-analytical phase is important for natriuretic peptide assessment. Samples for NT-proBNP can be collected in ethylenediaminetetraacetic acid on ice and are stable for days if refrigerated or stored at −80 °C, with NT-proBNP samples more stable than BNP in the longer period [97].

Considering the biological aspect, natriuretic peptides and cardiac troponins may be differently affected by mechanisms related to cardiac dysfunction and/or damage, respectively [95]. An increase of both biomarkers may suggest alterations on cardiac function (i.e., increased BNP/NT-proBNP levels), together with cellular structural damage (i.e., increased hs-cTn levels) [98]. Accordingly, patients with elevation of both biomarker species showed worse prognosis than those with only one altered biomarker [99].

NT-proBNP levels increase with age and are higher in women and in patients with kidney dysfunction [100–102]. Reasons for this gender-related differences have been attributed, almost partially, to sexual hormones, as testosterone could lower cardiac natriuretic peptide levels, whereas estrogen may increase cardiac natriuretic peptide gene expression and NP release [103, 104]. This effect might be mediated by neprilysin activity (a transmembrane zinc metallopeptidase that degrades a wide range of peptide substrates), affected by the action of sexual hormones [105]. Moreover, some evidence suggested that free testosterone may directly decrease natriuretic peptide synthesis [106]. As it is known that obese subjects may present lower NP levels, emerging data from a general population study showed that the relationship between NT-proBNP and obesity had a significant sex-related behavior [100, 107]. In fact, the inverse association between NT-proBNP and obesity was stronger among females than males, especially in women (but not in men) with abdominal obesity [100, 107].

BNP and NT-proBNP are elevated in patients with AMI, correlating with acute and chronic myocardial infarct size [108–111]. Nonetheless, for their low specificity (e.g., high levels in heart failure, renal dysfunction, and pulmonary embolism), their values for AMI diagnosis are low. Moreover, from a laboratory medicine point of view, natriuretic peptides have a shorter blood half-life and a reduced sample stability (especially BNP) than cTn, and circadian variations and trends during the time of natriuretic peptides vary more with respect to hs-cTn [86, 112–115]. For these reasons, hs-cTn remains the elective biomarker for AMI diagnosis. Instead, the value of NP in predicting post-AMI adverse events is demonstrated by many findings [116–119]. Accordingly, in the 2020 ESC Guidelines for the management of acute coronary syndromes in patients presenting without persistent ST-segment elevation, both BNP and NT-proBNP are indicated as biomarkers significantly contributing to patient's prognosis (death, acute heart failure), and as such their assessment may be helpful for this clinical purpose [8].

5 Additive Biomarkers

5.1 C-Reactive Protein

CRP is an acute-phase reactant protein produced by the liver in response to inflammation and stimulation by inflammatory cytokines, primarily interleukin-6 (IL-6). This molecule is one of the most widely used inflammatory biomarkers in routine clinical practice. However, many factors are known to modulate CRP levels, including lifestyle behaviors (e.g., gender, smoking, exercise, alcohol), whereas elevation is associated with increased body mass index and obesity [120–125]. Moreover, serum concentration of CRP (actually measured by hsCRP assays) can be found increased in AMI patients and closely associated with the severity of coronary artery lesions [126]. However, the significance of these associations is far less to that of the cardiac-specific biomarkers (NT-proBNP and especially cTn); thus, CRP, not considered with sufficient specificity and sensitivity for this clinical setting, is not absolutely recommended as a reliable marker for AMI diagnostic purposes [8]. Rather, CRP may represent an independent prognostic marker of poor outcome (e.g., nonfatal MI, heart failure, or cardiac death) in this setting [127–129]. As the prognostic value of CRP is independent from other biomarkers, such as cTn, and for its pathophysiological significance and advantages (e.g., low costs, availability), simultaneous evaluation of C-reactive protein with other biomarkers might allow a better prognostic assessment [130]. Thus, hsCRP has been often tested in combined multimarker panels (also including not only laboratory biomarkers) to evaluate whether this approach may better identify patients at high risk for adverse prognosis, provide prognostic information beyond that of established clinical risk scores, or improve clinical decision-making [131–133]. For example, the combination of hsCRP with hsTnT and NT-proBNP may improve risk stratification accuracy of the Global Registry of Acute Coronary Events (GRACE) score in patients with acute coronary syndrome [134]. Nonetheless, other studies suggested that the assessment of CRP as that of other recently proposed biomarkers did not significantly improve AMI patient management, with a value in risk assessment which seems marginal [8]. For these reasons, the routinary use of CRP for prognostic assessment is not recommended by the current AMI guidelines [8].

5.2 Hemochrome-Related Biomarkers

The complete blood cell count is one of the most common laboratory tests, because it is simple to perform and cheap, and it is a part of the overall general patient evaluation and thus practically always available. Many parameters can be easily obtained or calculated by hemochrome, which, although difficult to use for AMI diagnosis, has shown good predictive power for adverse events such as white blood cells (WBC), neutrophil-to-lymphocyte ratio (NLR), red cell distribution width (RDW), and platelet-derived parameters, such as platelet-to-lymphocyte ratio (PLR), mean platelet volume (MPV), and platelet distribution width (PDW) [135].

One of the most studied factors is MPV (which means the average size of platelets), a biomarker that may increase during platelet activation, which correlates with an increased incidence of long-term adverse events, including all-cause mortality in NSTEMI patients [136]. From a laboratory point of view, the assessment of the MPV parameter is widely discussed, in view of the number of physiological determinants for platelet size and the poor standardization of MPV methods. In particular, as MPV may vary depending on the instrument and technology used, it is important to state that all hemochromes were performed by using the same automated counter. The use of different anticoagulants has been found to affect MPV, as other hematological parameters (e.g., PDW) [137]. Moreover, some drugs (e.g., statins) or other diseases (e.g., chronic renal failure, anemia, thrombocytopenia, thyroid dysfunction, dyslipidemia, diabetes, and hypertension) may affect levels of these hemochrome-related biomarkers [138]. Interestingly, the variability affecting MPV may be reduced in a ratio with other hematological biomarkers. Accordingly, the MPV-to-platelet count ratio (MPV/PLT ratio) retains a better prognostic capacity in the prediction of adverse prognosis compared to MPV alone in predicting adverse outcomes in patients with NSTEMI, similar to the GRACE score, but with the advantage of being easier to be calculated [136, 139]. In addition, hematological biomarkers may have an additional prognostic value for AMI patients if they are considered with other inflammatory markers (e.g., CRP and fibrinogen) or with GRACE, SYNTAX, and TIMI risk scores [135, 139].

6 Emerging Biomarkers

6.1 Other Biomarkers

A number of other biomarkers have been proposed and are actually under study for a possible use in AMI diagnosis and prediction of CV outcome after AMI. These biomarkers evidenced different aspects and underlying pathways involved in the complexity of the AMI, some of the important ones being given in Table 2 [8, 24, 32, 98, 140–157]. Whether for cTnI or T the value in diagnosis, prognosis, and risk stratification is recognized, for all the other biomarkers evidence is unclear. The 2020 ESC Guidelines for the management of acute coronary syndromes in NSTEMI patients evidence the incremental prognostic value of BNP/NT-proBNP, which may therefore help in risk stratification [8]. However, the measurement of additional biomarkers, such as hs-C-reactive protein, mid-regional pro-adrenomedullin, GDF-15, copeptin, and hFABP is not recommended, because it remains to establish their incremental role and effective utility in the clinical practice, in addition to validated risk predictors [8]. It is noteworthy that most of these new proposed biomarkers are not specific for myocardium tissue and their circulating levels may be

Table 2 Conventional and new proposed biomarkers related to different AMI pathophysiological underlying mechanisms

Abbreviation	Biomarker	Pathway	Ref.
cTnT-I	Cardiac troponin I and T	Myocardial necrosis	[8]
BNP/ NT-proBNP	Brain natriuretic peptide/N-terminal proBNP	Myocardial stress	[8]
cMyC	Cardiac myosin-binding protein C	Myocardial necrosis	[140]
H-FABP	Heart-type fatty acid-binding protein	Myocardial necrosis	[141]
IMA	Ischemia-modified albumin	Myocardial necrosis	[141]
sST2	ST2 soluble	Myocardial stress, fibrosis	[142]
S100A	S100 calcium-binding protein A	Myocardial damage	[143]
IR	Irisin	Myocardial repair	[144]
CT-proAVP	Copeptin	Neurohormonal activation	[32]
MR-proADM	Mid-regional-pro-adrenomedullin	Neurohormonal activation	[145]
CRP	C-reactive protein	Inflammation	[32]
IL-6	Interleukin-6	Inflammation	[24]
FIB	Fibrinogen	Inflammation	[32]
TNF-α	Tumor necrosis factor-α	Inflammation	[24]
UA	Uric acid	Inflammation	[146]
GDF-15	Growth differentiation factor 15	Inflammation, apoptosis	[32]
Lp-PLA2	Lipoprotein-associated phospholipase-A2	Platelet activation	[32]
GAL-3	Galectin-3	Inflammation, fibrosis	[32]
GDF-15	Growth differentiation factor-15	Inflammation, modulation of growth, and cell differentiation	[147]
WBC	White blood cell count	Inflammation	[148]
SYND	Syndecan-1-4	Inflammation, fibrosis, cardiac remodeling	[149]
PIGF	Placental growth factor	Growth factors, inflammation	[150]
PLT	Platelet count	Platelet biomarkers	[148]
MPV	Mean platelet volume	Platelet biomarkers	[148]
LPLT	Large platelets	Platelet biomarkers	[148]
sPLA2	Secretory phospholipase A2	Platelet activation	[145]
sCD40L	Soluble CD40 ligand	Platelet activation	[142]
PAPP-A	Pregnancy-associated plasma protein-A	Plaque instability	[145]
MMPs	Matrix metalloproteinases	Plaque instability	[145]
MPO	Myeloperoxidase	Plaque instability	[143]
CER	Ceramides	Cellular death, apoptosis	[151]
Cytc	Cytochrome c	Mitochondrial biomarkers	[152]
mtDNA	Mitochondrial DNA	Mitochondrial biomarkers	[152]
Hcy	Homocysteine	Oxidative stress	[32]

(continued)

Table 2 (continued)

Abbreviation	Biomarker	Pathway	Ref.
VCAM-1 and ICAM-1	Vascular cell adhesion molecule 1 and intercellular adhesion molecule 1	Vascular cell adhesion molecules	[153, 154]
ADM	Adrenomedullin	Natriuresis and vasodilation	[98]
P-sel	P-selectin	Cell adhesion molecule	[98]
GPBB	Glycogen phosphorylase isoenzyme	Myocardial damage	[24]
NGAL	Neutrophil gelatinase-associated lipocalin	Renal function	[155]
FGF-23	Fibroblast growth factor 23	Phosphate and vitamin D metabolism	[156]
PCT	Procalcitonin	Calcium homeostasis, inflammation	[141]
ET1/CT-proET1	Endothelin 1/C-terminal pro-endothelin-1	Vasoconstriction	[140]
Cys-c	Cystatin-C	Renal damage	[142]
PACAP	Pituitary adenylate cyclase-activating polypeptide	Neuropeptide	[157]
miRNAs	MicroRNA	Other	[174, 175]

affected by different determinants (e.g., age, gender, or renal dysfunction). Nonetheless, a multimarker panel, including some of these biomarkers, may theoretically increase the diagnostic accuracy and improve risk stratification, especially if applied in particular subgroups where traditional scores may not optimally work (e.g., women, elderly population). In particular, this approach may be more effective if selected biomarkers have a low degree of correlation and it is even better if each biomarker belongs to totally unrelated contributing pathophysiological pathways, providing different levels of information [158, 159]. This multimarker approach has been tested by adding to cTn values other biomarkers related to different pathophysiological pathways involved in AMI (e.g., markers of inflammation like CPR and leukocyte activation, myeloperoxidase, or earlier cardiac biomarkers such as CK-MB, myoglobin, hFABP, or copeptin). However, the diagnostic and prognostic additive value of the other biomarkers with respect to cTn, when measured with hs-assays, is not significant [160]. For example, the incremental gain suggested for hFABP addition to cTn, also in view of the higher sensitivity of hFABP with respect to cTn, was never definitively proven, and consequently its use in the patient with chest pain for AMI diagnosis and rule-out [161–164]. In fact, two meta-analyses, comparing the diagnostic performance of hFABP both alone and together with hsTn in the early AMI diagnosis and exclusion, do not prove a significant gain over hs-cTn diagnostic accuracy [165, 166]. Instead, copeptin use within a dual-marker approach together with conventional cTn, increases in particular the negative predictive value of cTn alone for AMI, but not the incremental value, also in this case not justifying its measurement in great number of patients [167]. However, current AMI guidelines advocate the use of copeptin as an alternative biomarker for the early rule-out of AMI when hs-cTn assays are not available [8]. Other multimarker combinations (e.g., IL-10/MPO/PGF/cTnT or ST2/GDF-15/hFABP/hs-TnT) have also been tested, although they need further validation to assess their effective prognostic advantage [168, 169].

Another intriguing aspect is to determine which of these biomarkers may act as pharmacological targets. Increasing data suggested this possibility, as in the case of successful inhibition of MPO activity by the orally administered drug PF-1355 in parallel to structural and functional heart improvement in a mice experimental model [170]. Moreover, administration of CP-471,474, a matrix metalloproteinase inhibitor, reduced left ventricular remodeling and dilation in an AMI rabbit model [171]. Similarly, fluvastatin may improve left ventricle structural remodeling and contractile function, reducing AMI-related increase of matrix metalloproteinase-2 and -13 activity in a mice model [172]. Other evidences suggested that anti-inflammatory therapy (canakinumab at a dose of 150 mg every 3 months) targeting the interleukin-1β innate immunity pathway (an IL-6 inductor) reduced the rate of recurrent AMI in patients with previous myocardial infarction and ongoing inflammation (hsCRP higher than 2 mg/L) [173].

6.2 Noncoding RNAs

About 99% of the human genome is not encoding but transcriptionally active and gives rise to noncoding RNA (ncRNA) with regulatory and structural functions. A very interesting aspect is that the same ncRNAs may not have the same functions in different species; thus, in many cases, their pathogenic relevance in humans cannot be investigated in animal models. It is therefore fundamental to conduct screening studies for ncRNAs clinically interesting in humans. On this basis, genome-wide association studies and transcriptome mapping are two of the most useful technologies to identify ncRNAs involved in cardiovascular disease pathogenesis. ncRNAs include different classes of small regulatory RNAs, the best studied of which is composed of microRNAs (miRNAs), short (20–25 nucleotides) single stranded, which modulate gene expression and have fundamental roles in many key biological processes, including those related to CV pathophysiology (e.g., oxidative stress, inflammation, lipid metabolism, glucose homeostasis, vascular and endothelial cell function) [174]. Advantages are that different cardiac miRNAs can be easily found in blood samples, stable at room temperature as well as after sample frozen and thawed cycles [175]. In particular, miR-15 appears involved in the regulation of cardiac cell death and regeneration after myocardial ischemia; in fact, its inhibition has been proven to reduce infarct size and cardiac remodeling and enhances cardiac function in response to AMI [176].

Furthermore, members of miR-17–92 cluster (formed by miR-17, miR-18a, miR-19a, miR-20a, miR-19b-1, and miR-92a) are involved in cardiomyocyte cell death and neovascularization after ischemia. Particularly, miR-92a is active in response to ischemic injury and its pharmacological inhibition increases capillary density and improves heart function in a mouse model [177].

Analogously, miR-26a is upregulated after AMI in mice and inhibits angiogenesis; however, the administration of a specific anti-miRNA stimulates angiogenesis and reduces the infarct size, improving cardiac function [178]. A large spectrum of miRNAs are also involved in mitochondrial function regulation, as miR-140 impairs mitochondrial fission and, consequently, cardiomyocyte survival [179]. Moreover, miR-1, miR-133a, miR-208a/b, and miR-499 are among the most studied miRNAs associated with cardiac function. They are involved in differentiation of myocytes and fibroblasts and maintain activity and survival of cardiac muscle cells [180].

Since circulating miR-1 levels are particularly high in AMI patients, it has been adopted as a selective biomarker for early AMI diagnosis and used to distinguish the cardiac event from other cardiovascular diseases [181]. Furthermore, circulating miR-1 levels strongly correlate with cTnT in AMI patients and downregulation of miR-1 would be beneficial for heart ischemia and post-MI complications. Also circulating levels of miR-133 are upregulated in AMI patients, making it a valuable diagnostic marker for AMI; however, it is not as much efficient with TnT, and thus, miR-133a has a weaker prognostic power than miR-1 [182]. Recently, it has been found that miRNA-499 and miR-22 are highly expressed in the heart of AMI patients. miR-499 overexpression is associated with cardiac myosin heavy-chain gene upregulation, together with many inflammatory cytokines, whereas miR-22 is believed to protect cardiomyocytes by promoting autophagy and inhibiting apoptosis. Furthermore, in AMI patients, both miRNAs' sensitivity and specificity for diagnosis result to be extremely high [183].

Emerging data also suggest that the variation of miRNA during the acute ischemic event may be helpful to evaluate the risk for subsequent adverse events in the follow-up [184]. Important in this setting will be the serial assessments to evaluate longitudinal changes in circulating miRNAs. At present, in addition to the many technical and bioinformatics aspects that need to be improved, as well as the assessment of the clinical gain of these biomarkers over current diagnostic tools/scores, available miRNA detection techniques require time, which may not fit with the need for the fast diagnosis required in patients with AMI. Nonetheless, some miRNAs may have a prognostic role in the prediction of left ventricular remodeling, CV events, and death (e.g., miR-133a, miR-208b) [185]. Another interesting issue to be exploited is that miRNAs may act not only as disease biomarkers, but also as pharmacological targets. Some efforts in this direction are in progress and tested on experimental models. Accordingly, injection of human microRNA-590 and human microRNA-199a improves cardiomyocyte proliferation and cardiac tissue repair, with a recovery of cardiac functional parameters in both neonatal and adult infarcted mice, likely through effects on target genes (Homer1, homeodomain-only protein X, and chloride intracellular channel 5) [186, 187]. Another example is the delivery of anti-miR-34a to neonatal and adult infarcted mouse hearts, which significantly improves post-AMI remodeling by facing miR-34 upregulation and modulating miR-34a targets (such as Bcl2, cyclin D1, and Sirt1) [188].

Other ncRNAs (e.g., long noncoding RNAs-lncRNAs and circular RNAs-circRNAs) appear correlated to cardiac pathophysiology, in particular participating in events related to ischemic heart disease, and cardiac fibrosis, although the research in these fields is at an even earlier levels of development with respect to miRNAs [189, 190].

7 Conclusion

Biochemical markers represent the core to the diagnosis of early risk stratification and guidance of therapy for AMI, with cTn as the reference standard biomarker. In fact, through cTn assessment, the majority of patients can be ruled out quickly in 1–2-h algorithms. Whether cTn is cardiac specific, accurately reflecting myocardial injury, it is otherwise well known that cTn may increase in several other clinical situations without overt cardiac disease involvement, and even following particular exercise sessions (thus sensitivity is not completely satisfactory). Moreover, it is clear that the early diagnosis of AMI is critical to maximally shorten the time of AMI treatment and save as much myocardium tissue at risk as possible. However, troponin blood levels are detectable in blood samples about 2–4 h after AMI onset, leaving a "troponin gap," where the use of other biomarkers, which could further benefit diagnosis, risk stratification, and prognosis, may be desired. Accordingly, the efforts to identify additive biomarkers improving AMI diagnosis and risk assessment are intense at present. Really, a number of emerging biomarkers have been proposed and are under evaluation to be translated into clinical practice, including biochemical biomarkers belonging to different underlying pathways and molecular biomarkers, some promising with diagnostic and/or prognostic utility, also in a multimarker approach view. Moreover, several challenges must be overcome before entering into a clinical workflow algorithm. Surely, the added value of each biomarker over conventional utilized tools must be carefully evaluated (none at present superior to cTn), as well as the development of standardized methods and quality control schemes, and an appropriate estimation of cost and test run time. Nonetheless, the efforts towards the identification of additive biomarkers have the potential to improve diagnosis and risk stratification and may be informative on underlying biological pathways contributing to improving knowledge of the onset and development of acute cardiac events as well as the management of patients in the clinical practice.

References

1. https://www.who.int/health-topics/cardiovascular-diseases#tab=tab_1.
2. Seferović PM, Vardas P, Jankowska EA, Maggioni AP, Timmis A, Milinković I, Polovina M, Gale CP, Lund LH, Lopatin Y, Lainscak M, Savarese G, Huculeci R, Kazakiewicz D, Coats AJS, National Heart Failure Societies of the ESC member countries (see Appendix). The Heart Failure Association Atlas: Heart Failure Epidemiology and Management Statistics 2019. Eur J Heart Fail. 2021;23:906–14.

3. Ibanez B, James S, Agewall S, Antunes MJ, Bucciarelli-Ducci C, Bueno H, ALP C, Crea F, Goudevenos JA, Halvorsen S, Hindricks G, Kastrati A, Lenzen MJ, Prescott E, Roffi M, Valgimigli M, Varenhorst C, Vranckx P, Widimský P, ESC Scientific Document Group. ESC Guidelines for the management of acute myocardial infarction in patients presenting with ST-segment elevation: the Task Force for the management of acute myocardial infarction in patients presenting with ST-segment elevation of the European Society of Cardiology (ESC). Eur Heart J. 2017;2018(39):119–77.
4. Khan S, Rasool ST. Current use of cardiac biomarkers in various heart conditions. Endocr Metab Immune Disord Drug Targets. 2021;21:980–93.
5. Danese E, Montagnana M. An historical approach to the diagnostic biomarkers of acute coronary syndrome. Ann Transl Med. 2016;4:194.
6. Clerico A, Zaninotto M, Passino C, Padoan A, Migliardi M, Plebani M. High-sensitivity methods for cardiac troponins: the mission is not over yet. Adv Clin Chem. 2021;103:215–52.
7. Clerico A, Passino C, Franzini M, Emdin M. Natriuretic peptides as biomarkers of cardiac endocrine function in heart failure: new challenges and perspectives. Futur Cardiol. 2016;12:573–84.
8. Collet JP, Thiele H, Barbato E, Barthélémy O, Bauersachs J, Bhatt DL, Dendale P, Dorobantu M, Edvardsen T, Folliguet T, Gale CP, Gilard M, Jobs A, Jüni P, Lambrinou E, Lewis BS, Mehilli J, Meliga E, Merkely B, Mueller C, Roffi M, Rutten FH, Sibbing D, Siontis GCM, ESC Scientific Document Group. 2020 ESC Guidelines for the management of acute coronary syndromes in patients presenting without persistent ST-segment elevation. Eur Heart J. 2021;42(14):1289–367. https://doi.org/10.1093/eurheartj/ehaa575. Erratum in: Eur Heart J. 2021 May 14;42(19):1908. Erratum in: Eur Heart J. 2021;42:1925.
9. Ladue JS, Wrŏblewski F, Karmen A. Serum glutamic oxaloacetic transaminase activity in human acute transmural myocardial infarction. Science. 1954;120:497–9.
10. Penttilä I, Penttilä K, Rantanen T. Laboratory diagnosis of patients with acute chest pain. Clin Chem Lab Med. 2000;38:187–97.
11. Ndrepepa G. Aspartate aminotransferase and cardiovascular disease—a narrative review. J Lab Precis Med. 2021;6:6.
12. Schumann G, Bonora R, Ceriotti F, Clerc-Renaud P, Ferrero CA, Férard G, Franck PF, Gella FJ, Hoelzel W, Jørgensen PJ, Kanno T, Kessner A, Klauke R, Kristiansen N, Lessinger JM, Linsinger TP, Misaki H, Panteghini M, Pauwels J, Schimmel HG, Vialle A, Weidemann G, Siekmann L. IFCC primary reference procedures for the measurement of catalytic activity concentrations of enzymes at 37 degrees C. Part 3. Reference procedure for the measurement of catalytic concentration of lactate dehydrogenase. Clin Chem Lab Med. 2002;40:643–8.
13. Wróblewski F, Ruegsegger P, LaDue JS. Serum lactic dehydrogenase activity in acute transmural myocardial infarction. Science. 1956;123:1122–3.
14. Galbraith LV, Leung FY, Jablonsky G, Henderson R. Time-related changes in the diagnostic utility of total lactate dehydrogenase, lactate dehydrogenase isoenzyme-1, and two lactate dehydrogenase isoenzyme-1 ratios in serum after myocardial infarction. Clin Chem. 1990;36:1317–2132.
15. McLeish MJ, Kenyon GL. Relating structure to mechanism in creatine kinase. Crit Rev Biochem Mol Biol. 2005;40:1–20.
16. Apple FS. The specificity of biochemical markers of cardiac damage: a problem solved. Clin Chem Lab Med. 1999;37:1085–9.
17. Cabaniss CD. Creatine Kinase. In: Walker HK, Hall WD, Hurst JW, editors. Clinical methods: the history, physical, and laboratory examinations. 3rd ed. Boston: Butterworths; 1990. Chapter 32.
18. Lin JC, Apple FS, Murakami MM, Luepker RV. Rates of positive cardiac troponin I and creatine kinase MB mass among patients hospitalized for suspected acute coronary syndromes. Clin Chem. 2004;50:333–8.

19. Rittoo D, Jones A, Lecky B, Neithercut D. Elevation of cardiac troponin T, but not cardiac troponin I, in patients with neuromuscular diseases: implications for the diagnosis of myocardial infarction. J Am Coll Cardiol. 2014;63:2411–20.
20. Perović A, Dolčić M. Influence of hemolysis on clinical chemistry parameters determined with Beckman Coulter tests—detection of clinically significant interference. Scand J Clin Lab Invest. 2019;79:154–9.
21. Achar SA, Kundu S, Norcross WA. Diagnosis of acute coronary syndrome. Am Fam Physician. 2005;72:119–26.
22. Marwah SA, Shah H, Chauhan K, Trivedi A, Haridas N. Comparison of mass versus activity of creatine kinase MB and its utility in the early diagnosis of re-infarction. Indian J Clin Biochem. 2014;29:161–6.
23. Zafar Gondal A, Foris LA, Richards JR. Serum myoglobin. In: StatPearls. Treasure Island, FL: StatPearls Publishing; 2021.
24. Aydin S, Ugur K, Aydin S, Sahin İ, Yardim M. Biomarkers in acute myocardial infarction: current perspectives. Vasc Health Risk Manag. 2019;15:1–10.
25. Ebashi S. Calcium binding and relaxation in the actomyosin system. J Biochem. 1960;48:150–1.
26. Greaser ML, Gergely J. Reconstitution of troponin activity from three protein components. J Biol Chem. 1971;246:4226–33.
27. Cummins B, Auckland ML, Cummins P. Cardiac-specific troponin-I radioimmunoassay in the diagnosis of acute myocardial infarction. Am Heart J. 1987;113:1333–44.
28. Giannitsis E, Kurz K, Hallermayer K, Jarausch J, Jaffe AS, Katus HA. Analytical validation of a high-sensitivity cardiac troponin T assay. Clin Chem. 2010;56:254–61.
29. Clerico A, Zaninotto M, Ripoli A, Masotti S, Prontera C, Passino C, Plebani M, on the behalf of the Study Group on Cardiovascular Risk Biomarkers of the Italian Society of Clinical Biochemistry (SIBioC). The 99th percentile of reference population for cTnI and cTnT assay: methodology, pathophysiology and clinical implications. Clin Chem Lab Med. 2017;55:1634–51.
30. Marjot J, Kaier TE, Martin ED, Reji SS, Copeland O, Iqbal M, Goodson B, Hamren S, Harding SE, Marber MS. Quantifying the release of biomarkers of myocardial necrosis from cardiac myocytes and intact myocardium. Clin Chem. 2017;63:990–6.
31. Chaulin A. Cardiac troponins: contemporary biological data and new methods of determination. Vasc Health Risk Manag. 2021;17:299–316.
32. Zoltani CK. Chapter 11—Cardiovascular toxicity biomarkers. In: Gupta RC, editor. Biomarkers in toxicology. Academic Press; 2014. p. 199–215.
33. Clerico A, Ripoli A, Masotti S, Musetti V, Aloe R, Dipalo M, Rizzardi S, Dittadi R, Carrozza C, Storti S, Belloni L, Perrone M, Fasano T, Canovi S, Correale M, Prontera C, Guiotto C, Cosseddu D, Migliardi M, Bernardini S. Evaluation of 99th percentile and reference change values of a high-sensitivity cTnI method: a multicenter study. Clin Chim Acta. 2019;493:156–61.
34. Ko DH, Hyun J, Kim HS, Park MJ, Shin DH. Harmonization of Cardiac Troponin I: significance of sample types. Clin Lab. 2019;65.
35. Clerico A, Ripoli A, Masotti S, Prontera C, Storti S, Fortunato A, Buzzi P, Casagranda I, Franzini M, Ndreu R, Zucchelli GC, Zaninotto M, Plebani M. Pilot study on harmonization of cardiac troponin I immunoassays using patients and quality control plasma samples. On behalf of the Italian Section of the European Ligand Assay Society (ELAS) and of the Study Group on Cardiovascular Biomarkers of the Società Italiana di Biochimica Clinica (SIBioC). Clin Chim Acta. 2016;456:42–8.
36. Alpert JS, Thygesen K, Antman E, Bassand JP. Myocardial infarction redefined—a consensus document of The Joint European Society of Cardiology/American College of Cardiology Committee for the redefinition of myocardial infarction. J Am Coll Cardiol. 2000;36:959–69.

37. Thygesen K, Alpert JS, Jaffe AS, Chaitman BR, Bax JJ, Morrow DA, White HD, Executive Group on behalf of the Joint European Society of Cardiology (ESC)/American College of Cardiology (ACC)/American Heart Association (AHA)/World Heart Federation (WHF) Task Force for the Universal Definition of Myocardial Infarction. Fourth Universal Definition of Myocardial Infarction (2018). Circulation. 2018;138:e618–51.
38. Apple FS, Collinson PO, IFCC Task Force on Clinical Applications of Cardiac Biomarkers. Analytical characteristics of high-sensitivity cardiac troponin assays. Clin Chem. 2012;58:54–61.
39. Wu AHB, Christenson RH, Greene DN, Jaffe AS, Kavsak PA, Ordonez-Llanos J, Apple FS. Clinical Laboratory Practice Recommendations for the Use of Cardiac Troponin in Acute Coronary Syndrome: expert opinion from the Academy of the American Association for Clinical Chemistry and the Task Force on Clinical Applications of Cardiac Bio-Markers of the International Federation of Clinical Chemistry and Laboratory Medicine. Clin Chem. 2018;64:645–55.
40. Apple FS, Ler R, Murakami MM. Determination of 19 cardiac troponin I and T assay 99th percentile values from a common presumably healthy population. Clin Chem. 2012;58:1574–81.
41. Muzyk P, Twerenbold R, Morawiec B, Ayala PL, Boeddinghaus J, Nestelberger T, Mueller C, Kawecki D. Use of cardiac troponin in the early diagnosis of acute myocardial infarction. Kardiol Pol. 2020;78:1099–106.
42. Mueller-Hennessen M, Mueller C, Giannitsis E, Biener M, Vafaie M, deFilippi CR, Christ M, Ordóñez-Llanos J, Panteghini M, Plebani M, Verschuren F, Melki D, French JK, Christenson RH, Body R, McCord J, Dinkel C, Katus HA, Lindahl B, TRAPID-AMI Investigators. Serial sampling of high-sensitivity cardiac troponin T may not be required for prediction of acute myocardial infarction diagnosis in chest pain patients with highly abnormal concentrations at presentation. Clin Chem. 2016;63:542–51.
43. Heidenreich PA, Alloggiamento T, Melsop K, McDonald KM, Go AS, Hlatky MA. The prognostic value of troponin in patients with non-ST elevation acute coronary syndromes: a meta-analysis. J Am Coll Cardiol. 2001;38:478–85.
44. Chatterjee S, Kim J, Dahhan A, Choudhary G, Sharma S, Wu WC. Use of high-sensitivity troponin assays predicts mortality in patients with normal conventional troponin assays on admission-insights from a meta-analysis. Clin Cardiol. 2013;36:649–53.
45. Kontos MC, Turlington JS. High-sensitivity troponins in cardiovascular disease. Curr Cardiol Rep. 2020;22:30.
46. Park KC, Gaze DC, Collinson PO, Marber MS. Cardiac troponins: from myocardial infarction to chronic disease. Cardiovasc Res. 2017;113:1708–18.
47. Brown AJ, Shah ASV, West NEJ, Costopoulos C, Orzalkiewicz M, Newby DE, Bennett MR, Mills NL, Calvert PA. High-sensitivity troponin I is associated with high-risk plaque and MACE in stable coronary artery disease. JACC Cardiovasc Imaging. 2017;10:1200–3.
48. Beatty AL, Ku IA, Christenson RH, DeFilippi CR, Schiller NB, Whooley MA. High-sensitivity cardiac troponin t levels and secondary events in outpatients with coronary heart disease from the heart and soul study. JAMA Intern Med. 2013;173:763–9.
49. White HD, Tonkin A, Simes J, Stewart R, Mann K, Thompson P, Colquhoun D, West M, Nestel P, Sullivan D, Keech AC, Hunt D, Blankenberg S, LIPID Study Investigators. Association of contemporary sensitive troponin I levels at baseline and change at 1 year with long-term coronary events following myocardial infarction or unstable angina: results from the LIPID study (Long-Term Intervention with Pravastatin in Ischaemic Disease). J Am Coll Cardiol. 2014;63:345–54.
50. Kociol RD, Pang PS, Gheorghiade M, Fonarow GC, O'Connor CM, Felker GM. Troponin elevation in heart failure prevalence, mechanisms, and clinical implications. J Am Coll Cardiol. 2010;28:1071–8.

51. Evans JDW, Dobbin SJH, Pettit SJ, Di Angelantonio E, Willeit P. High-sensitivity cardiac troponin and new-onset heart failure: a systematic review and meta-analysis of 67,063 patients with 4, 165 incident heart failure events. JACC Heart Fail. 2018;6:187–97.
52. Masson S, Anand I, Favero C, Barlera S, Vago T, Bertocchi F, Maggioni AP, Tavazzi L, Tognoni G, Cohn JN, Latini R, Valsartan Heart Failure Trial (Val-HeFT) and Gruppo Italiano per lo Studio della Sopravvivenza nell'Insufficienza Cardiaca–Heart Failure (GISSI-HF) Investigators. Serial measurement of cardiac troponin T using a highly sensitive assay in patients with chronic heart failure: data from 2 large randomized clinical trials. Circulation. 2012;125:280–8.
53. Apple FS, Murakami MM, Pearce LA, Herzog CA. Predictive value of cardiac troponin I and T for subsequent death in end-stage renal disease. Circulation. 2002;106:2941–5.
54. Devereaux PJ, Szczeklik W. Myocardial injury after non-cardiac surgery: diagnosis and management. Eur Heart J. 2020;41:3083–91.
55. de Filippi CR, Herzog CA. Interpreting cardiac biomarkers in the setting of chronic kidney disease. Clin Chem. 2017;63:59–65.
56. Dispenzieri A, Gertz MA, Kumar SK, Lacy MQ, Kyle RA, Saenger AK, Grogan M, Zeldenrust SR, Hayman SR, Buadi F, Greipp PR, Leung N, Russell SR, Dingli D, Lust JA, Rajkumar SV, Jaffe AS. High sensitivity cardiac troponin T in patients with immunoglobulin light chain amyloidosis. Heart. 2014;100:383–8.
57. Sawaya H, Sebag IA, Plana JC, Januzzi JL, Ky B, Tan TC, Cohen V, Banchs J, Carver JR, Wiegers SE, Martin RP, Picard MH, Gerszten RE, Halpern EF, Passeri J, Kuter I, Scherrer-Crosbie M. Assessment of echocardiography and biomarkers for the extended prediction of cardiotoxicity in patients treated with anthracyclines, taxanes, and trastuzumab. Circ Cardiovasc Imaging. 2012;5:596–603.
58. Cardinale D, Ciceri F, Latini R, Franzosi MG, Sandri MT, Civelli M, Cucchi G, Menatti E, Mangiavacchi M, Cavina R, Barbieri E, Gori S, Colombo A, Curigliano G, Salvatici M, Rizzo A, Ghisoni F, Bianchi A, Falci C, Aquilina M, Rocca A, Monopoli A, Milandri C, Rossetti G, Bregni M, Sicuro M, Malossi A, Nassiacos D, Verusio C, Giordano M, Staszewsky L, Barlera S, Nicolis EB, Magnoli M, Masson S, Cipolla CM. ICOS-ONE Study Investigators. Anthracycline-induced cardiotoxicity: a multicenter randomised trial comparing two strategies for guiding prevention with enalapril: the International CardioOncology Society-one trial. Eur J Cancer. 2018;94:126–37.
59. Vassalle C, Masotti S, Lubrano V, Basta G, Prontera C, Di Cecco P, Del Turco S, Sabatino L, Pingitore A. Traditional and new candidate cardiac biomarkers assessed before, early, and late after half marathon in trained subjects. Eur J Appl Physiol. 2018;118:411–7.
60. McEvoy JW, Chen Y, Nambi V, Ballantyne CM, Sharrett AR, Appel LJ, Post WS, Blumenthal RS, Matsushita K, Selvin E. High-sensitivity cardiac troponin t and risk of hypertension. Circulation. 2015;132:825–33.
61. McEvoy JW, Chen Y, Ndumele CE, Solomon SD, Nambi V, Ballantyne CM, Blumenthal RS, Coresh J, Selvin E. Six-year change in high-sensitivity cardiac troponin t and risk of subsequent coronary heart disease, heart failure, and death. JAMA Cardiol. 2016;1:519–28.
62. Collinson PO. The role of cardiovascular biomarkers in cardiovascular disease risk assessment. Curr Opin Cardiol. 2014;29:366–71.
63. Mair J, Lindahl B, Hammarsten O, Müller C, Giannitsis E, Huber K, Möckel M, Plebani M, Thygesen K, Jaffe AS. How is cardiac troponin released from injured myocardium? Eur Heart J Acute Cardiovasc Care. 2018;7:553–60.
64. Clerico A, Ripoli A, Zaninotto M, Masotti S, Musetti V, Ciaccio M, Aloe R, Rizzardi S, Dittadi R, Carrozza C, Fasano T, Perrone M, de Santis A, Prontera C, Riggio D, Guiotto C, Migliardi M, Bernardini S, Plebani M. Head-to-head comparison of plasma cTnI concentration values measured with three high-sensitivity methods in a large Italian population of healthy volunteers

and patients admitted to emergency department with acute coronary syndrome: a multi-center study. Clin Chim Acta. 2019;496:25–34.
65. Harley K, Bissonnette S, Inzitari R, Schulz K, Apple FS, Kavsak PA, Gunsolus IL. Independent and combined effects of biotin and hemolysis on high-sensitivity cardiac troponin assays. Clin Chem Lab Med. 2021;59:1431–43.
66. Sodi R, Darn SM, Davison AS, Stott A, Shenkin A. Mechanism of interference by haemolysis in the cardiac troponin T immunoassay. Ann Clin Biochem. 2006;43:49–56.
67. Masimasi N, Means RT Jr. Elevated troponin levels associated with hemolysis. Am J Med Sci. 2005;330:201–3.
68. Saenger AK, Jaffe AS, Body R, Collinson PO, Kavsak PA, Lam CSP, Lefèvre G, Omland T, Ordóñez-Llanos J, Pulkki K, Apple FS. Cardiac troponin and natriuretic peptide analytical interferences from hemolysis and biotin: educational aids from the IFCC Committee on Cardiac Biomarkers (IFCC C-CB). Clin Chem Lab Med. 2019;57:633–40.
69. Vafaie M, Biener M, Mueller M, Schnabel PA, André F, Steen H, Zorn M, Schueler M, Blankenberg S, Katus HA, Giannitsis E. Analytically false or true positive elevations of high sensitivity cardiac troponin: a systematic approach. Heart. 2014;100:508–14.
70. Krintus M, Kozinski M, Boudry P, Capell NE, Köller U, Lackner K, Lefèvre G, Lennartz L, Lotz J, Herranz AM, Nybo M, Plebani M, Sandberg MB, Schratzberger W, Shih J, Skadberg Ø, Chargui AT, Zaninotto M, Sypniewska G. European multicenter analytical evaluation of the Abbott ARCHITECT STAT high sensitive troponin I immunoassay. Clin Chem Lab Med. 2014;52:1657–65.
71. Gerhardt W, Nordin G, Herbert AK, Burzell BL, Isaksson A, Gustavsson E, Haglund S, Müller-Bardorff M, Katus HA. Troponin T and I assays show decreased concentrations in heparin plasma compared with serum: lower recoveries in early than in late phases of myocardial injury. Clin Chem. 2000;46:817–21.
72. Warner JV, Marshall GA. High incidence of macrotroponin I with a high-sensitivity troponin I assay. Clin Chem Lab Med. 2016;54:1821–9.
73. Katrukha IA, Katrukha AG. Myocardial injury and the release of troponins I and T in the blood of patients. Clin Chem. 2021;67:124–30.
74. Damen SAJ, Vroemen WHM, Brouwer MA, Mezger STP, Suryapranata H, van Royen N, Bekers O, Meex SJR, Wodzig WKWH, Verheugt FWA, de Boer D, Cramer GE, Mingels AMA. Multi-site coronary vein sampling study on cardiac troponin T degradation in non-ST-segment-elevation myocardial infarction: toward a more specific cardiac troponin T assay. J Am Heart Assoc. 2019;8:e012602.
75. Vroemen WHM, Mezger STP, Masotti S, Clerico A, Bekers O, de Boer D, Mingels A. Cardiac troponin T: only small molecules in recreational runners after marathon completion. J Appl Lab Med. 2019;3:909–11.
76. Madsen LH, Christensen G, Lund T, Serebruany VL, Granger CB, Hoen I, Grieg Z, Alexander JH, Jaffe AS, Van Eyk JE, Atar D. Time course of degradation of cardiac troponin I in patients with acute ST-elevation myocardial infarction: the ASSENT-2 troponin substudy. Circ Res. 2006;99:1141–7.
77. Cardinaels EP, Mingels AM, van Rooij T, Collinson PO, Prinzen FW, van Dieijen-Visser MP. Time-dependent degradation pattern of cardiac troponin T following myocardial infarction. Clin Chem. 2013;59:1083–90.
78. Bolstad N, Warren DJ, Nustad K. Heterophilic antibody interference in immunometric assays. Best Pract Res Clin Endocrinol Metab. 2013;27:647–61.
79. Bhoi S, Verma P, Vankar S, Galwankar S. High sensitivity troponins and conventional troponins at the bedside. Int J Crit Illn Inj Sci. 2014;4:253–6.
80. Clerico A, Zaninotto M, Plebani M. High-sensitivity assay for cardiac troponins with POCT methods. The future is soon. Clin Chem Lab Med. 2021;59:1477–8.

81. Collinson P. Cardiac biomarker measurement by point of care testing—development, rationale, current state and future developments. Clin Chim Acta. 2020;508:234–9.
82. Tate JR, Bunk DM, Christenson RH, Barth JH, Katrukha A, Noble JE, Schimmel H, Wang L, Panteghini M, IFCC Working Group on Standardization of Cardiac Troponin I. Evaluation of standardization capability of current cardiac troponin I assays by a correlation study: results of an IFCC pilot project. Clin Chem Lab Med. 2015;53:677–90.
83. van der Linden N, Hilderink JM, Cornelis T, Kimenai DM, Klinkenberg LJJ, van Doorn WP, Litjens EJR, van Suijlen JDE, van Loon LJC, Bekers O, Kooman JP, Meex SJR. Twenty-four-hour biological variation profiles of cardiac troponin I in individuals with or without chronic kidney disease. Clin Chem. 2017;63:1655–6.
84. Klinkenberg LJ, Wildi K, van der Linden N, Kouw IW, Niens M, Twerenbold R, Rubini Gimenez M, Puelacher C, Daniel Neuhaus J, Hillinger P, Nestelberger T, Boeddinghaus J, Grimm K, Sabti Z, Bons JA, van Suijlen JD, Tan FE, Ten Kate J, Bekers O, van Loon LJ, van Dieijen-Visser MP, Mueller C, Meex SJ. Diurnal rhythm of cardiac troponin: consequences for the diagnosis of acute myocardial infarction. Clin Chem. 2016;62:1602–11.
85. Wildi K, Singeisen H, Twerenbold R, Badertscher P, Wussler D, Klinkenberg LJJ, Meex SJR, Nestelberger T, Boeddinghaus J, Miró Ò, Martin-Sanchez FJ, Morawiec B, Muzyk P, Parenica J, Keller DI, Geigy N, Potlukova E, Sabti Z, Kozhuharov N, Puelacher C, du Fay de Lavallaz J, Rubini Gimenez M, Shrestha S, Marzano G, Rentsch K, Osswald S, Reichlin T, Mueller C, APACE Investigators. Circadian rhythm of cardiac troponin I and its clinical impact on the diagnostic accuracy for acute myocardial infarction. Int J Cardiol. 2018;270:14–20.
86. Zaninotto M, Padoan A, Mion MM, Marinova M, Plebani M. Short-term biological variation and diurnal rhythm of cardiac troponin I (Access hs-TnI) in healthy subjects. Clin Chim Acta. 2020;504:163–7.
87. Eggers KM, Lind L, Ahlström H, Bjerner T, Ebeling Barbier C, Larsson A, Venge P, Lindahl B. Prevalence and pathophysiological mechanisms of elevated cardiac troponin I levels in a population-based sample of elderly subjects. Eur Heart J. 2008;29:2252–8.
88. de Lemos JA, Drazner MH, Omland T, Ayers CR, Khera A, Rohatgi A, Hashim I, Berry JD, Das SR, Morrow DA, McGuire DK. Association of troponin T detected with a highly sensitive assay and cardiac structure and mortality risk in the general population. J Am Med Assoc. 2010;304:2503–12.
89. Wallace TW, Abdullah SM, Drazner MH, Das SR, Khera A, McGuire DK, Wians F, Sabatine MS, Morrow DA, de Lemos JA. Prevalence and determinants of troponin T elevation in the general population. Circulation. 2006;113:1958–65.
90. de Simone G, Devereux RB, Daniels SR, Meyer RA. Gender differences in left ventricular growth. Hypertension. 1995;26:979–83.
91. Mueller T, Egger M, Peer E, Dieplinger B. 5th generation cardiac troponin I and T assays in clinical routine—a head-to-head comparison with data from the Linz troponin (LITROP) study. Clin Chim Acta. 2018;485:195–204.
92. Mueller T, Egger M, Peer E, Jani E, Dieplinger B. Evaluation of sex-specific cut-off values of high-sensitivity cardiac troponin I and T assays in an emergency department setting—results from the Linz Troponin (LITROP) study. Clin Chim Acta. 2018;487:66–74.
93. Mueller-Hennessen M, Lindahl B, Giannitsis E, Biener M, Vafaie M, deFilippi CR, Christ M, Santalo-Bel M, Panteghini M, Plebani M, Verschuren F, Jernberg T, French JK, Christenson RH, Body R, McCord J, Dilba P, Katus HA, Mueller C, TRAPID-AMI Investigators. Diagnostic and prognostic implications using age- and gender-specific cut-offs for high-sensitivity cardiac troponin T—sub-analysis from the TRAPID-AMI study. Int J Cardiol. 2016;209:26–33.
94. Shah AS, Griffiths M, Lee KK, McAllister DA, Hunter AL, Ferry AV, Cruikshank A, Reid A, Stoddart M, Strachan F, Walker S, Collinson PO, Apple FS, Gray AJ, Fox KA, Newby DE,

Mills NL. High sensitivity cardiac troponin and the under-diagnosis of myocardial infarction in women: prospective cohort study. Br Med J. 2015;350:g7873.
95. Cullen L, Greenslade JH, Carlton EW, Than M, Pickering JW, Ho A, Greaves K, Berndt SL, Body R, Ryan K, Parsonage WA. Sex-specific versus overall cut points for a high sensitivity troponin I assay in predicting 1-year outcomes in emergency patients presenting with chest pain. Heart. 2016;102:120–6.
96. Clerico A, Vittorini S, Passino C. Circulating forms of the b-type natriuretic peptide prohormone: pathophysiologic and clinical considerations. Adv Clin Chem. 2012;58:31–44.
97. Vasile VC, Jaffe AS. Natriuretic Peptides and Analytical Barriers. Clin Chem. 2017;63:50–8.
98. Lyngbakken MN, Myhre PL, Røsjø H, Omland T. Novel biomarkers of cardiovascular disease: applications in clinical practice. Crit Rev Clin Lab Sci. 2019;56:33–60.
99. Tello-Montoliu A, Marín F, Roldán V, Mainar L, López MT, Sogorb F, Vicente V, Lip GY. A multimarker risk stratification approach to non-ST elevation acute coronary syndrome: implications of troponin T, CRP, NT pro-BNP and fibrin D-dimer levels. J Intern Med. 2007;262:651–8.
100. Choi HI, Lee MY, Oh BK, Lee SJ, Kang JG, Lee SH, Lee JY, Kim BJ, Kim BS, Kang JH, Sung KC. Effects of age, sex, and obesity on N-terminal pro B-type natriuretic peptide concentrations in the general population. Circ J. 2021;85:647–54.
101. Hogenhuis J, Voors AA, Jaarsma T, Hillege HL, Boomsma F, van Veldhuisen DJ. Influence of age on natriuretic peptides in patients with chronic heart failure: a comparison between ANP/NT-ANP and BNP/NT-proBNP. Eur J Heart Fail. 2005;7:81–6.
102. Luchner A, Hengstenberg C, Löwel H, Riegger GA, Schunkert H, Holmer S. Effect of compensated renal dysfunction on approved heart failure markers: direct comparison of brain natriuretic peptide (BNP) and N-terminal pro-BNP. Hypertension. 2005;46:118–23.
103. Bachmann KN, Huang S, Lee H, Dichtel LE, Gupta DK, Burnett JC Jr, Miller KK, Wang TJ, Finkelstein JS. Effect of testosterone on natriuretic peptide levels. J Am Coll Cardiol. 2019;73:1288–96.
104. Firmes LB, Belo NO, Reis AM. Conjugated equine estrogens and estradiol benzoate differentially modulate the natriuretic peptide system in spontaneously hypertensive rats. Menopause. 2013;20:554–60.
105. Yao M, Nguyen TV, Rosario ER, Ramsden M, Pike CJ. Androgens regulate neprilysin expression: role in reducing beta-amyloid levels. J Neurochem. 2008;105:2477–88. https://doi.org/10.1111/j.1471-4159.2008.05341.x.
106. Chang AY, Abdullah SM, Jain T, Stanek HG, Das SR, McGuire DK, Auchus RJ, de Lemos JA. Associations among androgens, estrogens, and natriuretic peptides in young women: observations from the Dallas Heart Study. J Am Coll Cardiol. 2007;49:109–16.
107. Suthahar N, Meijers WC, Ho JE, Gansevoort RT, Voors AA, van der Meer P, Bakker SJL, Heymans S, van Empel V, Schroen B, van der Harst P, van Veldhuisen DJ, de Boer RA. Sex-specific associations of obesity and N-terminal pro-B-type natriuretic peptide levels in the general population. Eur J Heart Fail. 2018;20:1205–14.
108. Luchner A, Hengstenberg C, Löwel H, Trawinski J, Baumann M, Riegger GA, Schunkert H, Holmer S. N-terminal pro-brain natriuretic peptide after myocardial infarction: a marker of cardio-renal function. Hypertension. 2002;39:99–104.
109. Mayr A, Mair J, Schocke M, Klug G, Pedarnig K, Haubner BJ, Nowosielski M, Grubinger T, Pachinger O, Metzler B. Predictive value of NT-pro BNP after acute myocardial infarction: relation with acute and chronic infarct size and myocardial function. Int J Cardiol. 2011;147:118–23.
110. Steen H, Futterer S, Merten C, Jünger C, Katus HA, Giannitsis E. Relative role of NT-pro BNP and cardiac troponin T at 96 hours for estimation of infarct size and left ventricular function after acute myocardial infarction. J Cardiovasc Magn Reson. 2007;9:749–58.

111. Arakawa N, Nakamura M, Aoki H, Hiramori K. Relationship between plasma level of brain natriuretic peptide and myocardial infarct size. Cardiology. 1994;85:334–40.
112. Mueller T, Gegenhuber A, Dieplinger B, Poelz W, Haltmayer M. Long-term stability of endogenous B-type natriuretic peptide (BNP) and amino terminal proBNP (NT-proBNP) in frozen plasma samples. Clin Chem Lab Med. 2004;42:942–4.
113. Wu AH, Shea E, Lu QT, Minyard J, Bui K, Hsu JC, Agee SJ, Todd J. Short- and long-term cardiac troponin I analyte stability in plasma and serum from healthy volunteers by use of an ultrasensitive, single-molecule counting assay. Clin Chem. 2009;55:2057–9.
114. Melzi d'Eril G, Tagnochetti T, Nauti A, Klersy C, Papalia A, Vadacca G, Moratti R, Merlini G. Biological variation of N-terminal pro-brain natriuretic peptide in healthy individuals. Clin Chem. 2003;49:1554–5.
115. Nordenskjöld AM, Ahlström H, Eggers KM, Fröbert O, Venge P, Lindahl B. Short- and long-term individual variation in NT-proBNP levels in patients with stable coronary artery disease. Clin Chim Acta. 2013;422:15–20.
116. Radosavljevic-Radovanovic M, Radovanovic N, Vasiljevic Z, Marinkovic J, Mitrovic P, Mrdovic I, Stankovic S, Kružliak P, Beleslin B, Uscumlic A, Kostic J. Usefulness of NT-proBNP in the follow-up of patients after myocardial infarction. J Med Biochem. 2016;35:158–65.
117. Clerico A, Passino C. Predictive value of NT-proBNP in patients with acute myocardial infarction. Clin Chem. 2017;63:1045–6.
118. Gong X, Zhang T, Feng S, Song D, Chen Y, Yao T, Han P, Liu Y, Li C, Song Z, Gao J, Cui Z, Ma J, Liu Y. Association between N-terminal pro-BNP and 12 months major adverse cardiac events among patients admitted with NSTEMI. Ann Palliat Med. 2021;10:5231–43.
119. Wolsk E, Claggett B, Pfeffer MA, Diaz R, Dickstein K, Gerstein HC, Lawson FC, Lewis EF, Maggioni AP, McMurray JJV, Probstfield JL, Riddle MC, Solomon SD, Tardif JC, Køber L. Role of B-type natriuretic peptide and N-terminal prohormone BNP as predictors of cardiovascular morbidity and mortality in patients with a recent coronary event and type 2 diabetes mellitus. J Am Heart Assoc. 2017;6:e004743.
120. Chen M, Li Y, Zhang D, Wu Y. Gender difference in the association between smoking and lung function: exploring the role of C-reactive protein as a mediating factor. Public Health. 2020;183:88–93.
121. Mangnus L, van Steenbergen HW, Nieuwenhuis WP, Reijnierse M, van der Helm-van Mil AHM. Moderate use of alcohol is associated with lower levels of C reactive protein but not with less severe joint inflammation: a cross-sectional study in early RA and healthy volunteers. RMD Open. 2018;4:e000577.
122. Hammonds TL, Gathright EC, Goldstein CM, Penn MS, Hughes JW. Effects of exercise on c-reactive protein in healthy patients and in patients with heart disease: a meta-analysis. Heart Lung. 2016;45:273–82.
123. McConnell JP, Branum EL, Ballman KV, Lagerstedt SA, Katzmann JA, Jaffe AS. Gender differences in C-reactive protein concentrations confirmation with two sensitive methods. Clin Chem Lab Med. 2002;40:56–9.
124. Khera A, McGuire DK, Murphy SA, Stanek HG, Das SR, Vongpatanasin W, Wians FH Jr, Grundy SM, de Lemos JA. Race and gender differences in C-reactive protein levels. J Am Coll Cardiol. 2005;46:464–9.
125. Vigna L, Vassalle C, Tirelli AS, Gori F, Tomaino L, Sabatino L, Bamonti F. Gender-related association between uric acid, homocysteine, γ-glutamyltransferase, inflammatory biomarkers and metabolic syndrome in subjects affected by obesity. Biomark Med. 2017. https://doi.org/10.2217/bmm-2017-0072. Epub ahead of print.
126. Ma QQ, Yang XJ, Yang NQ, Liu L, Li XD, Zhu K, Fu Q, Wei P. Study on the levels of uric acid and high-sensitivity C-reactive protein in ACS patients and their relationships with the extent of the coronary artery lesion. Eur Rev Med Pharmacol Sci. 2016;20:4294–8.

127. Lindahl B, Toss H, Siegbahn A, Venge P, Wallentin L. Markers of myocardial damage and inflammation in relation to long-term mortality in unstable coronary artery disease. FRISC Study Group. Fragmin during Instability in Coronary Artery Disease. N Engl J Med. 2000;343:1139–47.
128. Zhang X, Wang S, Fang S, Yu B. Prognostic role of high sensitivity C-reactive protein in patients with acute myocardial infarction. Front Cardiovasc Med. 2021;8:659446.
129. Mani P, Puri R, Schwartz GG, Nissen SE, Shao M, Kastelein JJP, Menon V, Lincoff AM, Nicholls SJ. Association of initial and serial C-reactive protein levels with adverse cardiovascular events and death after acute coronary syndrome: a secondary analysis of the VISTA-16 trial. JAMA Cardiol. 2019;4:314–20.
130. Morrow DA, Rifai N, Antman EM, Weiner DL, McCabe CH, Cannon CP, Braunwald E. C-reactive protein is a potent predictor of mortality independently of and in combination with troponin T in acute coronary syndromes: a TIMI 11A Substudy. J Am Coll Cardiol. 1998;31:1460–5.
131. Jia L, Yuan JQ, Zhu L, Zhang Y. High high-sensitivity C-reactive protein/BMI ratio predicts future adverse outcomes in patients with acute coronary syndrome. Coron Artery Dis. 2019;30:448–54.
132. O'Donoghue ML, Morrow DA, Cannon CP, Jarolim P, Desai NR, Sherwood MW, Murphy SA, Gerszten RE, Sabatine MS. Multimarker risk stratification in patients with acute myocardial infarction. J Am Heart Assoc. 2016;5:e002586.
133. Sabatine MS, Morrow DA, de Lemos JA, Gibson CM, Murphy SA, Rifai N, McCabe C, Antman EM, Cannon CP, Braunwald E. Multimarker approach to risk stratification in non-ST elevation acute coronary syndromes: simultaneous assessment of troponin I, C-reactive protein, and B-type natriuretic peptide. Circulation. 2002;105:1760–3.
134. Klingenberg R, Aghlmandi S, Räber L, Gencer B, Nanchen D, Heg D, Carballo S, Rodondi N, Mach F, Windecker S, Jüni P, von Eckardstein A, Matter CM, Lüscher TF. Improved risk stratification of patients with acute coronary syndromes using a combination of hsTnT, NT-proBNP and hsCRP with the GRACE score. Eur Heart J Acute Cardiovasc Care. 2018;7:129–38.
135. Budzianowski J, Pieszko K, Burchardt P, Rzeźniczak J, Hiczkiewicz J. The role of hematological indices in patients with acute coronary syndrome. Dis Markers. 2017;2017:3041565.
136. Azab B, Torbey E, Singh J, Akerman M, Khoueiry G, McGinn JT, Widmann WD, Lafferty J. Mean platelet volume/platelet count ratio as a predictor of long-term mortality after non-ST-elevation myocardial infarction. Platelets. 2011;22:557–66.
137. Pizzulli L, Yang A, Martin JF, Lüderitz B. Changes in platelet size and count in unstable angina compared to stable angina or non-cardiac chest pain. Eur Heart J. 1998;19:80–4.
138. Sivri N, Tekin G, Yalta K, Aksoy Y, Senen K, Yetkin E. Statins decrease mean platelet volume irrespective of cholesterol lowering effect. Kardiol Pol. 2013;71:1042–7.
139. Wan ZF, Zhou D, Xue JH, Wu Y, Wang H, Zhao Y, Zhu L, Yuan ZY. Combination of mean platelet volume and the GRACE risk score better predicts future cardiovascular events in patients with acute coronary syndrome. Platelets. 2014;25:447–51.
140. Chan D, Ng LL. Biomarkers in acute myocardial infarction. BMC Med. 2010;8:34.
141. Chen Y, Tao Y, Zhang L, Xu W, Zhou X. Diagnostic and prognostic value of biomarkers in acute myocardial infarction. Postgrad Med J. 2019;95:210–6.
142. Wang XY, Zhang F, Zhang C, Zheng LR, Yang J. The biomarkers for acute myocardial infarction and heart failure. Biomed Res Int. 2020;2020:2018035.
143. Gong XJ, Song XY, Wei H, Wang J, Niu M. Serum S100A4 levels as a novel biomarker for detection of acute myocardial infarction. Eur Rev Med Pharmacol Sci. 2015;19:2221–5.
144. Ho MY, Wang CY. Role of irisin in myocardial infarction, heart failure, and cardiac hypertrophy. Cell. 2021;10:2103.

145. Wang J, Tan GJ, Han LN, Bai YY, He M, Liu HB. Novel biomarkers for cardiovascular risk prediction. J Geriatr Cardiol. 2017;14:135–50.
146. Yan L, Liu Z, Zhang C. Uric acid as a predictor of in-hospital mortality in acute myocardial infarction: a meta-analysis. Cell Biochem Biophys. 2014;70:1597–601.
147. Wang Y, Zhen C, Wang R, Wang G. Growth-differentiation factor-15 predicts adverse cardiac events in patients with acute coronary syndrome: a meta-analysis. Am J Emerg Med. 2019;37:1346–52.
148. Kamińska J, Koper OM, Siedlecka-Czykier E, Matowicka-Karna J, Bychowski J, Kemona H. The utility of inflammation and platelet biomarkers in patients with acute coronary syndromes. Saudi J Biol Sci. 2018;25:1263–71.
149. Wernly B, Fuernau G, Masyuk M, Muessig JM, Pfeiler S, Bruno RR, Desch S, Muench P, Lichtenauer M, Kelm M, Adams V, Thiele H, Eitel I, Jung C. Syndecan-1 predicts outcome in patients with ST-segment elevation infarction independent from infarct-related myocardial injury. Sci Rep. 2019;9:18367.
150. Armstrong EJ, Morrow DA, Sabatine MS. Inflammatory biomarkers in acute coronary syndromes: part III: biomarkers of oxidative stress and angiogenic growth factors. Circulation. 2006;113:e289–92.
151. Gaggini M, Sabatino L, Vassalle C. Conventional and innovative methods to assess oxidative stress biomarkers in the clinical cardiovascular setting. BioTechniques. 2020;68:223–31.
152. Cosentino N, Campodonico J, Moltrasio M, Lucci C, Milazzo V, Rubino M, De Metrio M, Marana I, Grazi M, Bonomi A, Veglia F, Lauri G, Bartorelli AL, Marenzi G. Mitochondrial biomarkers in patients with ST-elevation myocardial infarction and their potential prognostic implications: a prospective observational study. J Clin Med. 2021;10:275.
153. Hayek A, Paccalet A, Mechtouff L, Da Silva CC, Ivanes F, Falque H, Leboube S, Varillon Y, Amaz C, de Bourguignon C, Prieur C, Tomasevic D, Genot N, Derimay F, Bonnefoy-Cudraz E, Bidaux G, Mewton N, Ovize M, Bochaton T. Kinetics and prognostic value of soluble VCAM-1 in ST-segment elevation myocardial infarction patients. Immun Inflamm Dis. 2021;9:493–501.
154. Freitas IA, Lima NA, Silva GBD Jr, Castro RL Jr, Patel P, Lima CCV, Lino DODC. Novel biomarkers in the prognosis of patients with atherosclerotic coronary artery disease. Rev Port Cardiol (Engl Ed). 2020;39:667–72.
155. Šabanović-Bajramović N, Hodžić E, Iglica A, Begić E, Resić N, Aganović K, Halilčević M, Bajramović S. Neutrophil gelatinase-associated lipocalin is a predictor of complications in the early phase of ST-elevation myocardial infarction. Med Glas (Zenica). 2020;17:328–34.
156. Stöhr R, Schuh A, Heine GH, Brandenburg V. FGF23 in cardiovascular disease: innocent bystander or active mediator? Front Endocrinol (Lausanne). 2018;9:351. https://doi.org/10.3389/fendo.2018.00351. Erratum in: Front Endocrinol (Lausanne). 2018;9:422.
157. Szabo D, Sarszegi Z, Polgar B, Saghy E, Nemeth A, Reglodi D, Makkos A, Gorbe A, Helyes Z, Ferdinandy P, Herczeg R, Gyenesei A, Cziraki A, Tamas A. PACAP-38 in acute ST-segment elevation myocardial infarction in humans and pigs: a translational study. Int J Mol Sci. 2021;22:2883.
158. Vassalle C. New biomarkers and traditional cardiovascular risk scores: any crystal ball for current effective advice and future exact prediction? Clin Chem Lab Med. 2018;56:1803–5.
159. Vassalle C. Oxidative stress and cardiovascular risk prediction: the long way towards a "radical" perspective. Int J Cardiol. 2018;273:252–3.
160. Aldous SJ. Cardiac biomarkers in acute myocardial infarction. Int J Cardiol. 2013;164:282–94.
161. Young JM, Pickering JW, George PM, Aldous SJ, Wallace J, Frampton CM, Troughton RW, Richards MA, Greenslade JH, Cullen L, Than MP. Heart fatty acid binding protein and cardiac troponin: development of an optimal rule-out strategy for acute myocardial infarction. BMC Emerg Med. 2016;16.

162. Reiter M, Twerenbold R, Reichlin T, Mueller M, Hoeller R, Moehring B, Haaf P, Wildi K, Merk S, Bernhard D, Mueller CZ, Freese M, Freidank H, Campodarve Botet I, Mueller C. Heart-type fatty acid-binding protein in the early diagnosis of acute myocardial infarction. Heart. 2013;99:708–14.
163. Carroll C, Al Khalaf M, Stevens JW, Leaviss J, Goodacre S, Collinson PO, Wang J. Heart-type fatty acid binding protein as an early marker for myocardial infarction: systematic review and meta-analysis. Emerg Med J. 2013;30:280–6.
164. Colli A, Josa M, Pomar JL, Mestres CA, Gherli T. Heart fatty acid binding protein in the diagnosis of myocardial infarction: where do we stand today? Cardiology. 2007;108:4–10.
165. Xu LQ, Yang YM, Tong H, Xu CF. Early diagnostic performance of heart-type fatty acid binding protein in suspected acute myocardial infarction: evidence from a meta-analysis of contemporary studies. Heart Lung Circ. 2018;27(4):503–12.
166. Liou K, Ho S, Ooi SY. Heart-type fatty acid binding protein in early diagnosis of myocardial infarction in the era of high-sensitivity troponin: a systematic review and meta-analysis. Ann Clin Biochem. 2015;52:370–81.
167. Mueller C, Möckel M, Giannitsis E, Huber K, Mair J, Plebani M, Thygesen K, Jaffe AS, Lindahl B. ESC Study Group on Biomarkers in Cardiology of the Acute Cardiovascular Care AssociationUse of copeptin for rapid rule-out of acute myocardial infarction. Eur Heart J Acute Cardiovasc Care. 2018;7:570–6.
168. Oemrawsingh RM, Lenderink T, Akkerhuis KM, Heeschen C, Baldus S, Fichtlscherer S, Hamm CW, Simoons ML, Boersma E, CAPTURE Investigators. Multimarker risk model containing troponin-T, interleukin 10, myeloperoxidase and placental growth factor predicts long-term cardiovascular risk after non-ST-segment elevation acute coronary syndrome. Heart. 2011;97:1061–6.
169. Schernthaner C, Lichtenauer M, Wernly B, Paar V, Pistulli R, Rohm I, Jung C, Figulla HR, Yilmaz A, Cadamuro J, Haschke-Becher E, Pernow J, Schulze PC, Hoppe UC, Kretzschmar D. Multibiomarker analysis in patients with acute myocardial infarction. Eur J Clin Investig. 2017;47:638–48.
170. Ali M, Pulli B, Courties G, Tricot B, Sebas M, Iwamoto Y, Hilgendorf I, Schob S, Dong A, Zheng W, Skoura A, Kalgukar A, Cortes C, Ruggeri R, Swirski FK, Nahrendorf M, Buckbinder L, Chen JW. Myeloperoxidase inhibition improves ventricular function and remodeling after experimental myocardial infarction. JACC Basic Transl Sci. 2016;1:633–43.
171. Lindsey ML, Gannon J, Aikawa M, Schoen FJ, Rabkin E, Lopresti-Morrow L, Crawford J, Black S, Libby P, Mitchell PG, Lee RT. Selective matrix metalloproteinase inhibition reduces left ventricular remodeling but does not inhibit angiogenesis after myocardial infarction. Circulation. 2002;105:753–8.
172. Hayashidani S, Tsutsui H, Shiomi T, Suematsu N, Kinugawa S, Ide T, Wen J, Takeshita A. Fluvastatin, a 3-hydroxy-3-methylglutaryl coenzyme a reductase inhibitor, attenuates left ventricular remodeling and failure after experimental myocardial infarction. Circulation. 2002;105:868–73.
173. Ridker PM, Everett BM, Thuren T, JG MF, Chang WH, Ballantyne C, Fonseca F, Nicolau J, Koenig W, Anker SD, JJP K, Cornel JH, Pais P, Pella D, Genest J, Cifkova R, Lorenzatti A, Forster T, Kobalava Z, Vida-Simiti L, Flather M, Shimokawa H, Ogawa H, Dellborg M, Rossi PRF, Troquay RPT, Libby P, Glynn RJ, CANTOS Trial Group. Antiinflammatory therapy with canakinumab for atherosclerotic disease. N Engl J Med. 2017;377:1119–31.
174. Fung EC, Butt AN, Eastwood J, Swaminathan R, Sodi R. Circulating microRNA in cardiovascular disease. Adv Clin Chem. 2019;91:99–122.
175. Feinberg MW, Moore KJ. MicroRNA regulation of atherosclerosis. Circ Res. 2016;118:703–20.

176. Hullinger TG, Montgomery RL, Seto AG, Dickinson BA, Semus HM, Lynch JM, Dalby CM, Robinson K, Stack C, Latimer PA, Hare JM, Olson EN, van Rooij E. Inhibition of miR-15 protects against cardiac ischemic injury. Circ Res. 2012;110:71–81.
177. Bonauer A, Carmona G, Iwasaki M, Mione M, Koyanagi M, Fischer A, Burchfield J, Fox H, Doebele C, Ohtani K, Chavakis E, Potente M, Tjwa M, Urbich C, Zeiher AM, Dimmeler S. MicroRNA-92a controls angiogenesis and functional recovery of ischemic tissues in mice. Science. 2009;324:1710–3.
178. Icli B, Wara AK, Moslehi J, Sun X, Plovie E, Cahill M, Marchini JF, Schissler A, Padera RF, Shi J, Cheng HW, Raghuram S, Arany Z, Liao R, Croce K, MacRae C, Feinberg MW. MicroRNA-26a regulates pathological and physiological angiogenesis by targeting BMP/SMAD1 signaling. Circ Res. 2013;113:1231–41.
179. Li J, Li Y, Jiao J, Wang J, Li Y, Qin D, Li P. Mitofusin 1 is negatively regulated by microRNA 140 in cardiomyocyte apoptosis. Mol Cell Biol. 2014;34:1788–99.
180. Piubelli C, Meraviglia V, Pompilio G, D'Alessandra Y, Colombo GI, Rossini A. microRNAs and cardiac cell fate. Cell. 2014;3:802–23.
181. Wang GK, Zhu JQ, Zhang JT, Li Q, Li Y, He J, Qin YW, Jing Q. Circulating microRNA: a novel potential biomarker for early diagnosis of acute myocardial infarction in humans. Eur Heart J. 2010;31:659–66.
182. Devaux Y, Mueller M, Haaf P, Goretti E, Twerenbold R, Zangrando J, Vausort M, Reichlin T, Wildi K, Moehring B, Wagner DR, Mueller C. Diagnostic and prognostic value of circulating microRNAs in patients with acute chest pain. J Intern Med. 2015;277:260–71.
183. Wang X, Tian L, Sun Q. Diagnostic and prognostic value of circulating miRNA-499 and miRNA-22 in acute myocardial infarction. J Clin Lab Anal. 2020;34:2410–7.
184. Badacz R, Kleczyński P, Legutko J, Żmudka K, Gacoń J, Przewłocki T, Kabłak-Ziembicka A. Expression of miR-1-3p, miR-16-5p and miR-122-5p as possible risk factors of secondary cardiovascular events. Biomedicine. 2021;9:1055.
185. Tanase DM, Gosav EM, Ouatu A, Badescu MC, Dima N, Ganceanu-Rusu AR, Popescu D, Floria M, Rezus E, Rezus C. Current knowledge of microRNAs (miRNAs) in Acute Coronary Syndrome (ACS): ST-Elevation Myocardial Infarction (STEMI). Life (Basel). 2021;11:1057.
186. Hodgkinson CP, Kang MH, Dal-Pra S, Mirotsou M, Dzau VJ. MicroRNAs and cardiac regeneration. Circ Res. 2015;116:1700–11.
187. Eulalio A, Mano M, Dal Ferro M, Zentilin L, Sinagra G, Zacchigna S, Giacca M. Functional screening identifies miRNAs inducing cardiac regeneration. Nature. 2012;492:376–81.
188 Yang Y, Cheng HW, Qiu Y, Dupee D, Noonan M, Lin YD, Fisch S, Unno K, Sereti KI, Liao R. MicroRNA-34a plays a key role in cardiac repair and regeneration following myocardial infarction. Circ Res. 2015;117:450–9.
189. Yin L, Tang Y, Jiang M. Research on the circular RNA bioinformatics in patients with acute myocardial infarction. J Clin Lab Anal. 2021;35:e23621.
190. Wang S, Wang E, Chen Q, Yang Y, Xu L, Zhang X, Wu R, Hu X, Wu Z. Uncovering potential lncRNAs and mRNAs in the progression from acute myocardial infarction to myocardial fibrosis to heart failure. Front Cardiovasc Med. 2021;8:664044.

Electrocardiogram in Ischemic Heart Disease

Andrea Rossi

1 Introduction

The feasibility of recording the cardiac electrical activity via the limbs and directly from the chest in intact animals and humans was demonstrated by Augustus Desiré Waller in 1887. Inspired by this discovery, Willem Einthoven, using a modified version of the galvanometer, obtained a device able to record an ECG from a human and published his findings between 1902 and 1903 labelling the P, Q, R, S, and T waves of the ECG. The work by Einthoven and Sir Thomas Lewis, one of the first to use a commercially available string galvanometer from the Cambridge Scientific Instrument Company, led to the electrocardiographic description of sinus arrhythmia, heart block, atrial fibrillation, and hypertrophy. Einthoven also studied the spread of action potentials introducing the three standard limb leads and the concept of "Einthoven's triangle," father of vectorcardiography. In 1938, the American Heart Association recommended six positions for placement of electrodes named V1–V6, which were then adopted for routine use. Finally, in 1942, Goldberger using unipolar limb leads (first described by Wilson in 1931) produced augmented unipolar limb leads. These derivations were added to the standard limb leads and the unipolar chest leads to give the so-called standard 12-leads ECG.

2 ECG Findings During Acute Myocardial Ischemia

The electrocardiogram (ECG) remains a fundamental tool in the diagnosis of acute and chronic coronary artery syndromes. Typical findings depend on (1) the *duration* of the ischemic process (acute vs. chronic), (2) the *extent* of ischemia, (3) the *topography*, and (4) the *presence of underlying arrhythmic conditions* (masking or altering the classic ECG patterns).

A. Rossi (✉)
Electrophysiology Division, Fondazione Toscana Gabriele Monasterio, Pisa, Italy
e-mail: andrea.rossi@ftgm.it

G. Concistrè (ed.), *Ischemic Heart Disease*,
https://doi.org/10.1007/978-3-031-25879-4_10

2.1 Repolarization Abnormalities (ST-T Wave)

Ischemia is defined as inadequate blood flow, which reduces oxygen delivery to tissue leading to hypoxia state and decrease in intracellular adenosine triphosphate (ATP) level [1]. This condition induces a K^+ outflow and increases extracellular K^+ levels, consequently leading to a depolarized state of the cell. Furthermore, intracellular ATP reduction decreases the activity of the Na/K-ATPase pump, leading to extracellular accumulation of K^+ and a loss of the electrogenic contribution of the pump to the membrane potential. This condition may contribute to depolarization.

During acute ischemia, myocardial ischemic cells present resting membrane potential reduction, shortening of action potential duration in the ischemic area, and upslope phase 0 potential slowing and depression [2]. As for the depolarized state, Na channels responsible for the "phase 0" of action potentials become inactivated inducing reduction of the phase 0 slope. In this condition, inward current derives from slow L-type Ca channels that become responsible for phase 0. Finally, ischemic depolarization also shortens the action potential duration, which may be related to the opening of K-ATP channels, leading to earlier phase 3 repolarization [1, 3, 4].

Ischemia can alter the ECG in several different ways. Changes in depolarization and repolarization lead to ST deviation and T wave alterations, changes in rate and rhythm, and conduction disturbances depending on the location of the ischemic region. Conduction blocks in the left or right branches lead to alteration of ventricular activation or prolongation of activation times and QRS duration. Localized altered conduction may also lead to the development of reentry circuits and tachyarrhythmias [5]. The earliest and typical ECG sign during acute cardiac ischemia is the deviation of the ST segment. This is the result of "*current of injury*" mechanism. Normally, healthy myocardial cells have the same potential at the early repolarization phase and ST segment is nearly isoelectric in the normal ECG. Cellular alterations induced by hypoxia and acidosis causing modification of the action potential determine a voltage gradient between normal and ischemic zones leading to a current flow. This current is represented by the ST-segment deviation on the surface ECG. When acute ischemia is transmural, the resultant ST vector is usually shifted in the direction of the epicardial layers and ST elevation is associated sometimes with tall positive (hyperacute) T waves in the ischemic zones. As previously described by Harold E.B. Pardee in his original paper in 1920, upsloping convex ST elevation during acute phase of myocardial infarction is considered a typical electrocardiographic finding of the acute transmural ischemic process (*Pardee's sign*) [6]. Reciprocal ST depression can appear in leads reflecting the contralateral surface of the heart (reciprocal ST depression can be often more apparent than primary ST elevation) [7, 8].

The amplitude of ST depression or elevation gives information about the severity of myocardial ischemia. Profound ST deviation in multiple leads indicates very severe ischemia. Conversely, prompt resolution of ST elevation following reperfusion strategy (thrombolytic therapy or primary angioplasty) is a specific marker of successful reperfusion [9, 10].

Ventricular ischemia can alter repolarization and produce *T wave inversion*. In the normal heart, the sequence of ventricular repolarization differs from depolarization leading to the explanation for why the T wave presents a different appearance with respect to QRS. T wave is normally upright in the left-sided leads (I, II, V3–V6) and has a longer duration than the QRS. The reason is that the last cells to depolarize are the first cells to repolarize. The last cells to depolarize are located in the subepicardial region of the upper left ventricular free wall. The subepicardial cells repolarize first because they have shorter action potential duration than subendocardial cells. Therefore, although an overlying electrode would record a positive QRS, the wave of repolarization normally travels away from the recording electrode leading to a positive deflection [11]. Finally, T wave is longer in duration than the QRS because the repolarization is longer than the depolarization phase. In effect, depolarization involves the high-speed Purkinje system to rapidly conduct action potentials throughout the ventricles, whereas the propagation of repolarization uses slower cell-to-cell conduction outside of Purkinje system.

During ischemic process, the action potential of the cell is shortened leading to early repolarization phase than normal. As the subendocardial layers are more susceptible to ischemia [12], these cells may repolarize before those in subepicardial regions. In this condition, the propagation of repolarization travels from the subendocardial to subepicardial surface of the ventricle causing a negative deflection in the T wave recording by electrode overlying that region (Fig. 5). T wave inversion does not necessarily indicate myocardial ischemia but is often observed clinically during ischemic events.

2.2 Depolarization Abnormalities (QRS Changes)

Changes in depolarization propagation accompany ST-T abnormality during myocardial infarction. Necrosis of sufficient amount of myocardial tissue can reduce R wave or generate abnormal Q wave as result of the loss of relevant component of electromotive forces in infarcted area. Local conduction delays caused by acute ischemia could contribute sometimes to Q wave pathogenesis. The historical definition of "Q wave" or "non-Q wave" myocardial infarction (also deemed useful to estimate the severity and the extension of infarcted area) as differentiation between transmural and subendocardial ischemia has been overcome by the evidence that Q wave finding is not always related with transmural ischemia as reported in ECG-pathological correlative studies [13, 14]. Q waves are often found in normal ECGs. Abnormal Q waves suggesting a myocardial infarction, however, usually have a greater negative deflection and a longer duration (Fig. 1). The presence of any Q waves in leads V1 through V3 that are at least 30 ms in duration or Q waves in at least 2 contiguous leads in leads I, II, aVL, aVF, or V4 through V6 that are at least 1 mm in depth is considered to be worrisome for a myocardial infarction. Pathologic Q waves typically appear within the first 9 h of infarction, with a range of only a few minutes to 24 h [15].

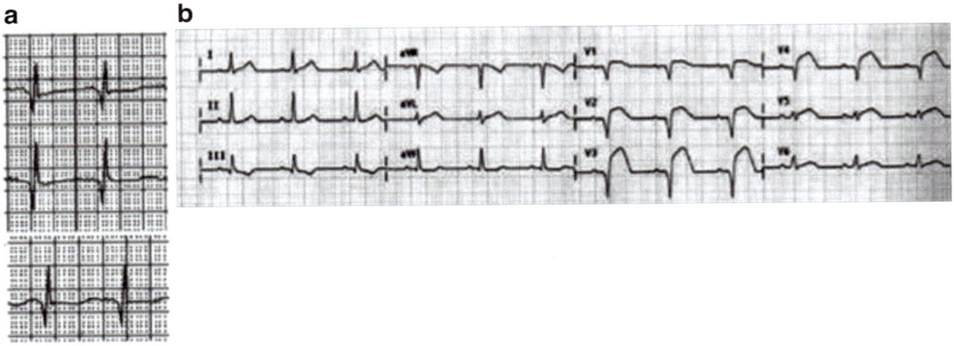

Fig. 1 (**a**) Pathologic Q waves indicative of past myocardial infarction. (**b**) Anterolateral ST-elevation myocardial infarction with Q waves in leads V1–V4. From: Nable JV, Brady W. The Evolution of electrocardiographic changes in ST-segment elevation myocardial infarction. American Journal of Emergency Medicine 2009;27:734–46

In case of posterior or lateral infarction, typically with concomitant Q waves, loss of depolarization forces in ischemic region may be associated with reciprocal R wave amplitude increase in right precordial leads (V1–V3) [16]. Tall R waves in right precordial leads require differential diagnosis with particular conditions with prominent anterior electromotive forces (i.e., right ventricular hypertrophy, hypertrophic cardiomyopathy, Wolff-Parkinson-White preexcitation, Duchenne's progressive muscular dystrophy).

2.3 Evolution of ECG Changes

During acute ischemia, findings of hyperacute T waves associated with ST elevation are followed by changes within a period ranging from hours to days evolving T wave inversion and sometimes Q waves in the same leads. Evolutionary T wave changes after acute myocardial infarction are attributed to abnormal prolongation of ventricular action potential in the region adjacent to the necrotic area, so that the degree of prolonged repolarization may influence T wave voltage and polarity [17]. The T wave inversion can resolve after days or week or persist indefinitely. As previously reported, persistent negative T waves in leads with Q waves in advanced stages of myocardial infarction indicate the presence of a transmural infarction with a thin fibrotic layer whereas positive T waves can be found in non-transmural infarct containing viable myocardium within the layer [18] (Fig. 2).

In the days to weeks or longer following infarction, the QRS changes can persist or begin to resolve. Complete normalization of ECG after Q wave infarction is uncommon but can occur, especially in case of smaller infarcts and when the left ventricular ejection fraction and regional wall motion improve. This happens with good collateral circulation, spontaneous recanalization, or prompt revascularization and is a good prognostic sign

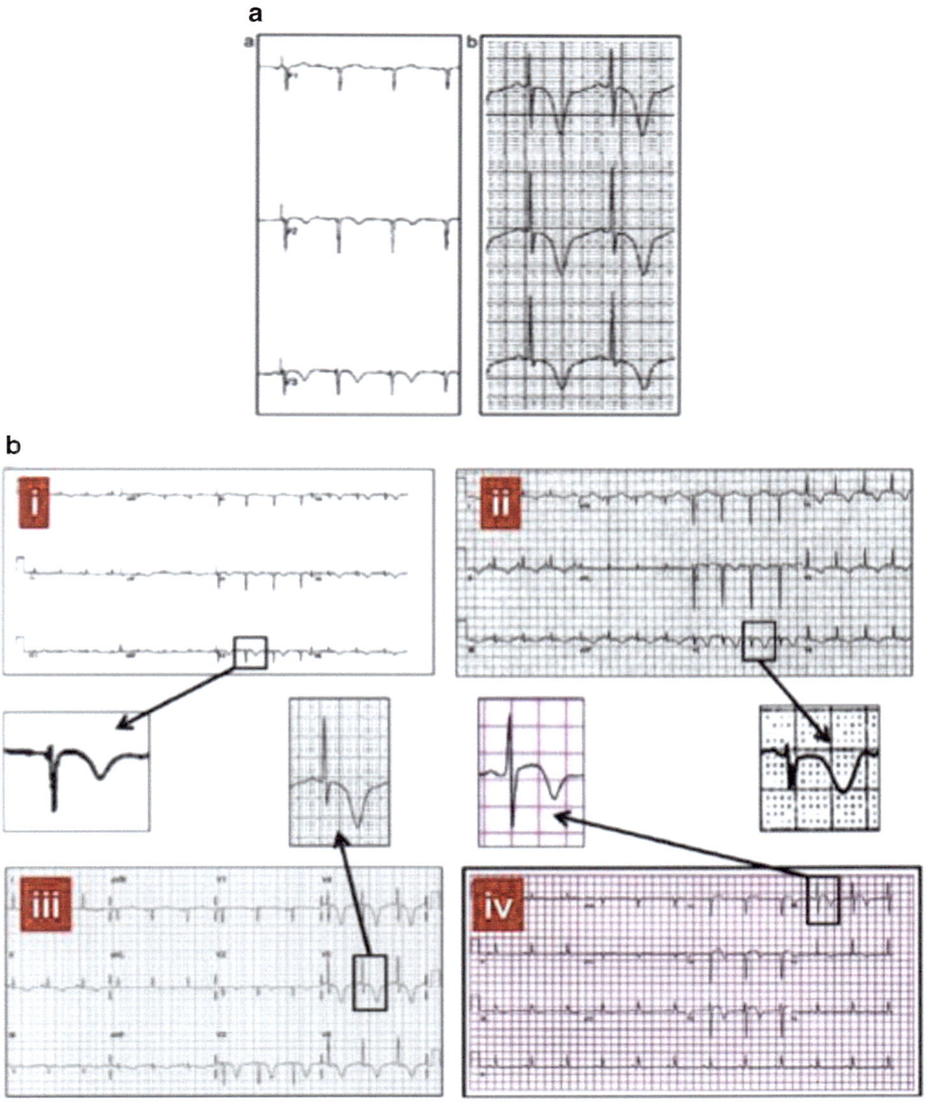

Fig. 2 (**a**) Infarct-related T wave inversion. Inverted T waves resulting from ischemia or infarction are symmetric in morphology with similar down- and upsloping limbs; a, minimally inverted T waves; b, deeply inverted T waves. (**b**) Infarct-related T wave inversion; "i" anterior T wave inversion; "ii" anterolateral T wave inversion; "iii" anterolateral T wave deeply inverted; "iv" anterior biphasic T waves. From: Maeda S, Imai T, Kuboki K, et al. Pathologic Implications of Restored Positive T Waves and Persistent Negative T Waves after Q wave Myocardial Infarction. J Am Coll Cardiol;28:1514–8, 1996

[19]. In case of persistence of Q waves and ST elevation several weeks after myocardial infarction, the yield of severe underlying wall motion disorder (akinetic or dyskinetic zones) is very high. The presence of an rSR' or similar complex in the mid-left chest leads or in lead I is a specific marker of left ventricular aneurysm (*"El-Sherif" sign*) [20].

2.4 Other Ischemic Patterns

Reversible transmural ischemia caused by coronary vasospasm may induce transient ST elevation pattern (*Prinzmetal variant angina*) [21]. Depending on the duration and the severity of the underlying condition, the ST elevation can resolve completely within minutes or could be followed by T wave inversion that persists for hours or days with or without elevation of cardiac enzyme markers.

The baseline ECG is usually normal or can depict nonspecific ST changes, or flat or negative T wave in the leads showing ST elevation during attacks. The most frequent and typical ECG changes are related to repolarization as a consequence of progressive ischemia provoked by abrupt coronary spasm. In more than 50% of the cases, the first ECG change is a tall, symmetrical, and usually peaked T wave, which is accompanied by a mild increase in the QT interval (Fig. 3). These findings are followed by ST elevation typically

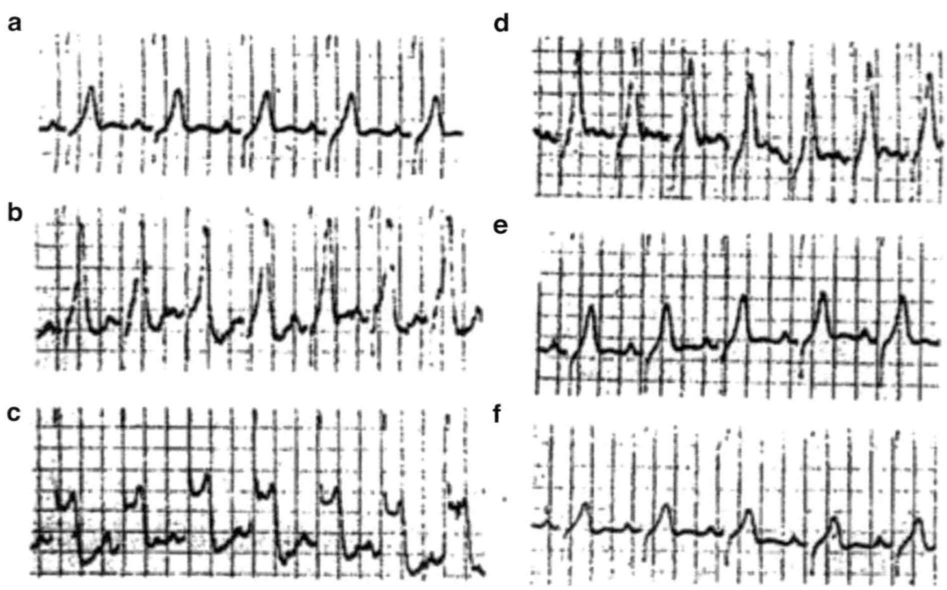

Fig. 3 Crisis of coronary spasm (Prinzmetal angina). (**a**) Control. (**b**) Initial pattern of a very tall T wave (subendocardial ischemia). (**c**) Huge pattern of ST elevation. (**d–f**) Resolution toward normal values. Total duration of the crisis was 2 min. From: Bayes de Luna A, Cygankiewicz I, Baranchuk A, et al. Prinzmetal Angina: ECG Changes and Clinical Considerations: a Consensus Paper. Ann Noninvasive Electrocardiol;19(5):442–443, 2014

associated with angina periods. Due to the transient nature of the phenomenon, ECG findings can be better appreciated with ECG Holter monitoring [22].

In case of the presence of T wave inversion in the baseline, normalization of the T waves can be found during episodes of acute myocardial ischemia (*T wave pseudonormalization*) [23].

QT lengthening and increased QT dispersion may be present in Prinzmetal angina. QT dispersion was reported in patients who experienced cardiac arrest due to triggered ventricular arrhythmias [24].

Transient intraventricular conduction disorders, especially right bundle branch block in case of proximal left anterior descending coronary artery spasm and hemiblocks, may exist but they are very rare. Pathologic Q waves appear occasionally, especially in case of preexisting occlusive coronary artery disease with acute coronary syndromes. However, in most cases, the Q waves are transient and do not represent permanent necrosis because of the brief period of myocardial ischemia.

2.5 Localization of Ischemia or Infarction

The ECG leads are helpful in localizing regions of transmural than subendocardial ischemia. 12-Leads ECG and modified leads can offer a topographic tool in recognizing the ischemic zones and the specific coronary vessels involved in the ischemic process (Fig. 4).

While ECG is limited by its inadequate representation of the posterior, lateral, and apical walls of the left ventricle, culprit vessel occlusion recognition may be possible according to ST elevation in specific ECG leads (Table 1).

ST elevation or hyperacute T waves are seen in one or more of the precordial leads (V1 through V6); lead I with acute transmural anterior or anterolateral wall ischemia; leads V1–V3 with anteroseptal ischemia; leads II, III, and aVF with inferior wall ischemia; right-sided precordial leads with right ventricular ischemia; and V7 through V9 (posterior leads) with posterior wall infarction (Fig. 11). Localization of ischemic area in non-ST-elevation acute coronary syndrome/non-ST-elevation myocardial infarction (NSTE-ACS/NSTEMI) is more difficult because leads with ST depression do not point exactly to the ischemic area. Therefore, it is commonly stated that ST depression (as well as T wave inversion) cannot be used to localize the ischemic area. In exception to this rule, "*Wellens syndrome*" is caused by proximal occlusion in the LAD and thus causes anterior wall ischemia [25] (Figs. 5 and 6).

In patients with inferior wall myocardial infarction, the presence of ST-segment elevation in lead III exceeding lead II associated with ST elevation in V1 may be a useful predictor of an occlusion in the proximal right coronary artery. Right-sided ST elevation is indicative of acute right ventricular injury and usually correlates with occlusion of the proximal right coronary artery (Fig. 7). Not uncommonly, ECG can show characteristic findings of acute myocardial ischemia in leads pointing different regions. Inferior lead ST elevation associated with acute anterior wall infarction suggests occlusion of a left anterior descending coronary artery that extends onto the inferior wall of the left ventricle ("wraparound" vessel).

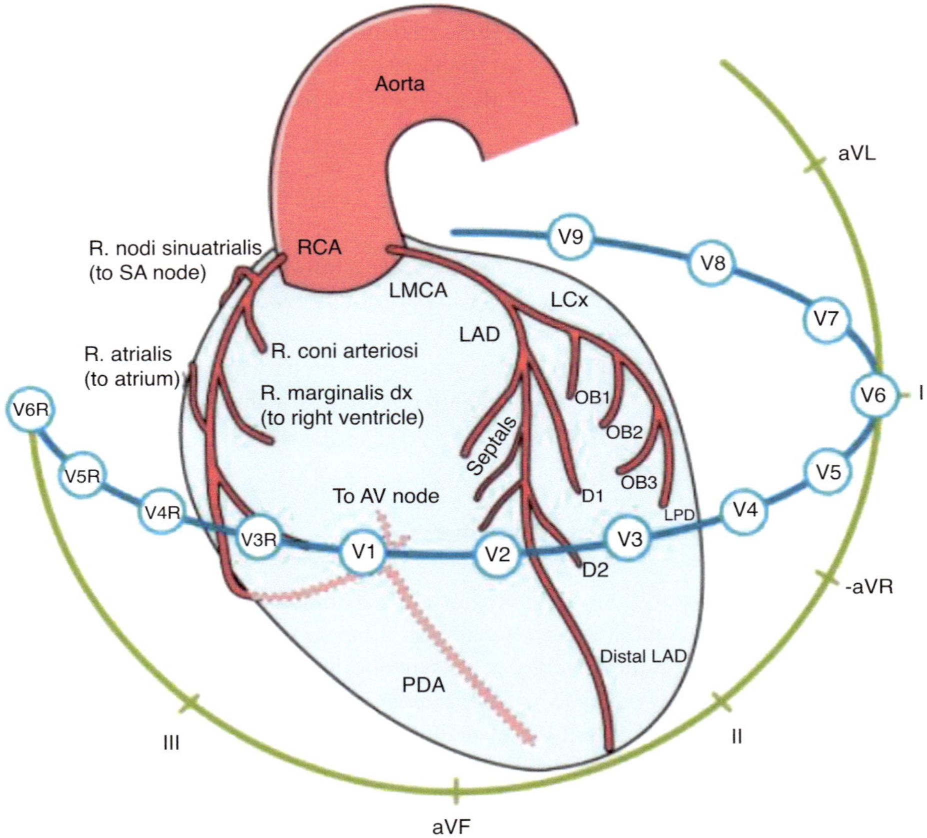

Fig. 4 Topographic representation of the heart and coronary vessel distribution according to ECG leads. RCA (right coronary artery), PDA (posterior descending artery), LMCA (left main coronary artery), LAD (left anterior descending artery), D (diagonal branches (D1, D2)), Septals (septal branches), LCx (left circumflex artery), OB (obtuse marginals (OB1, OB2, OB3)), LPD (left posterior descending artery), V3R through V6R (right-sided leads), V7 through V9 (posterior leads)

Table 1 Localization of ischemic area in ST-segment elevation myocardial infarction. LAD (left anterior descending coronary artery), LCx (left circumflex coronary artery), RCA (right coronary artery)

Leads with ST-segment elevation	Affected myocardial area	Occluded coronary artery (culprit)
V1–V2	Septal	Proximal LAD
V3–V4	Anterior	LAD
V5–V6	Apical	Distal LAD
I, aVL	Lateral	LCx
II, aVL, III	Lateral	90% RCA, 10% LCx
V7, V8, V9 (reciprocal ST depression is frequently evident in V1–V3)	Posterolateral (also referred to as inferobasal or posterior)	RCA or LCx

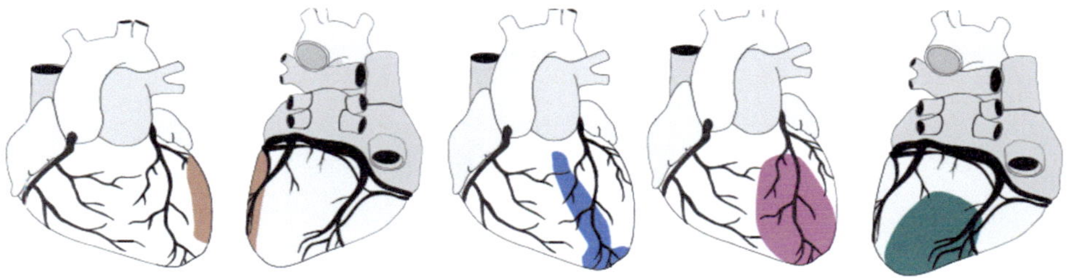

Fig. 5 Localization of infarct area according to the topographic distribution of coronary vessels. From the left: lateral infarction (brown area), septal infarction (blue area), anterior-apical infarction (purple area), inferior infarction (green area)

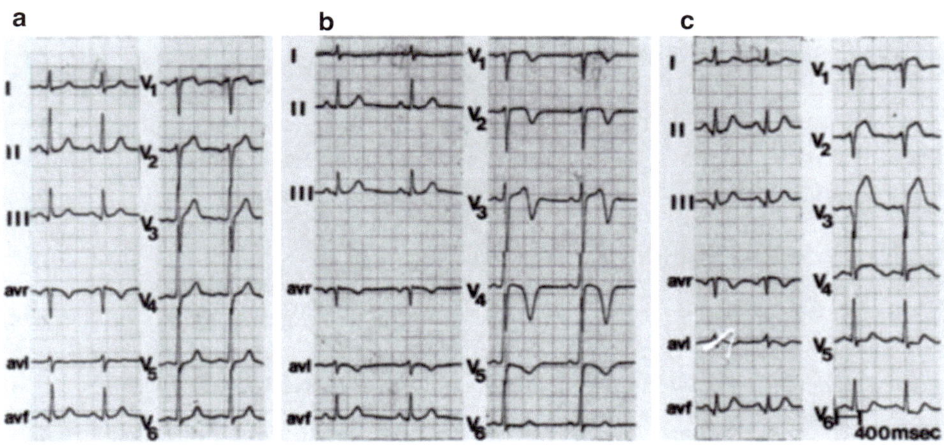

Fig. 6 "Wellens syndrome." Tracing recorded on the same patient. (**a**) ECG recorded on admission. (**b**) ECG recorded 23 h later. The patient was without chest pain in the interval between tracings **a** and **b**. During tracing **b**, the patient experienced transient chest pain. **c**: Tracing captured hours after. The patient died from a massive anterior myocardial infarction. Note huge T wave inversion in precordial leads V1 through V4 in tracing B followed by hyperacute T waves in V2–V3 (**c**), typical sign of pre-infarction stage. From: De Zwaan C, Bar FHM, Wellens HJJ. Characteristic electrocardiographic pattern indicating a critical stenosis high in left anterior descending coronary artery in patients admitted because of impeding myocardial infarction. Am Heart J;103:730. 1982

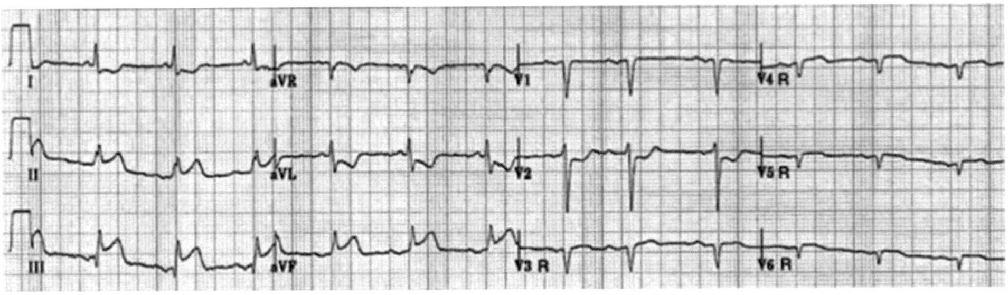

Fig. 7 Right ventricular myocardial infarction. ST elevation of >1 mm in lead V4R with upright T wave in that lead typically found in the acute stage of right ventricular infarction. From: Rafla S, Kamal A. Localization of the occluded vessel in acute myocardial infarction. J Cardiol Cardiovasc Med. 2020; 5: 029–033

2.6 Conduction System Disease in the Setting of Myocardial Infarction

Disturbances of cardiac rhythm and conduction are a frequent component of the usual course of myocardial infarction, making knowledge of the cardiac conduction system and its blood supply essential [26] (Fig. 8).

2.6.1 Anteroseptal Myocardial Infarction

Neither the sinus node nor the AV (atrioventricular) node (and His bundle) is normally supplied by the anterior descending artery, and atrial arrhythmias or AV block is virtually never the consequence of occlusion in this vessel alone. If an atrial arrhythmia or AV block occurs during anteroseptal infarction, there is always associated disease in either the left circumflex or the right coronary artery. During anteroseptal infarction, typical pathological ECG signs are often accompanied by right bundle branch block (RBBB). RBBB mainly affects the terminal portion of the QRS complex, resulting in a second R-wave (R') in V1–V3 and a broad and deep S wave in V5–V6. RBBB also causes secondary ST-T changes in leads V1–V3, but these forces are not strong enough to mask ischemic ST-T changes arising from the left ventricle. The classical ECG changes (and ECG criteria) used for acute myocardial infarction diagnosis can be applied also in the presence of RBBB. It is interesting to note that RBBB is often accompanied by a fascicular block indicating concomitant anterior fascicle damage. The typical association between RBBB and left anterior hemiblock happens because the left posterior fascicle receives dual blood supply but both right bundle and left anterior fascicle receive same blood supply.

2.6.2 Lateral Infarcts

Lateral infarct is nearly always due to occlusion of the circumflex artery (LCx), but significant anatomic variations of this vessel are frequent. In 10% of the human hearts, left circumflex artery crosses the crux and supplies all the diaphragmatic surface of the left ventricle (in 90% of the cases, right coronary artery crosses the crux cordis and supplies the diaphragmatic wall of the left ventricle).

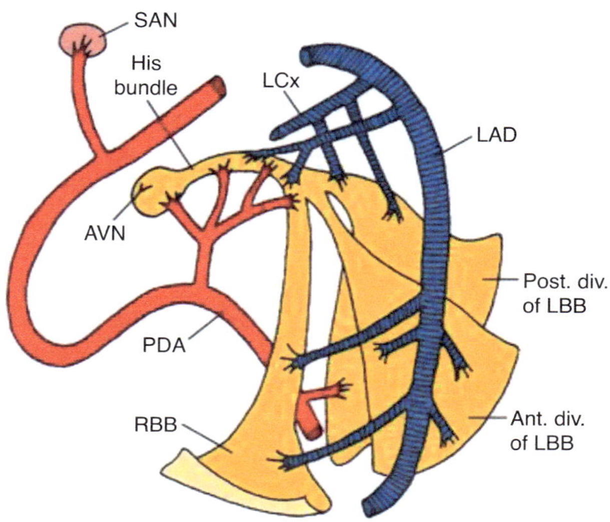

Fig. 8 Diagrammatic representation of the conduction system and its blood supply. Abbreviation: *Ant. div.* anterior division; *AVN* atrioventricular node; *LAD* left anterior descending artery; *LBB* left bundle branch; *LCx* left circumflex artery; *PDA* posterior descending artery; *Post. div.* posterior division; *RBB* right bundle branch; *SAN* sinoatrial node

LCx often supplies the AV node and the His bundle. The occurrence of AV block during lateral infarction indicates a long LCx or a concomitant involvement of the right coronary artery disease. In about 45% of the cases, LCx supplies the sinoatrial node. The occurrence of atrial arrhythmia during acute lateral infarction suggests that the occlusion of the LCx is very near the origin of the vessel (the branch to sinoatrial node originates proximally from the LCx).

2.6.3 Posterior Infarcts

Right coronary artery (RCA) occlusion happens in 90% of the cases. These infarcts are inevitably associated with ischemia of the AV node and His bundle, including the cholinergic nerves and ganglia present there [26]. Furthermore, in 55% of human hearts, proximal RCA supplies sinoatrial node. Both neuroreflexes and arrhythmias and conduction disturbances are frequently associated with acute inferior infarcts inducing sudden arrhythmic death especially in the acute stage.

2.7 ECG Diagnosis of Myocardial Infarction in the Presence of Bundle Branch Blocks

The presence of bundle branch blocks (BBBs) makes diagnosis of acute myocardial ischemia more difficult. Moreover, the presence of BBB pattern develops as a complication of the infarct. A new BBB in a patient with chest discomfort is strongly suggestive of ongoing ischemia.

The right bundle branch block (RBBB) mainly affects the terminal portion of the QRS complex, resulting in a second R-wave (namely R') in V1–V3 and a broad and deep S wave in V5–V6. Given that the RBBB only affects the depolarization of the right ventricle, the left ventricle will be depolarized and consequently typical criteria for the diagnosis of infarct (pathological Q waves) will be applied in the presence of RBBB. The RBBB also causes secondary ST-T changes in leads V1 through V3, but these forces are not strong enough to mask ischemic ST-T changes arising from left ventricle. In conclusion, the classical diagnostic ECG changes and ECG criteria can be used in the presence of RBBB.

The diagnosis of ischemia/infarction in the presence of left bundle branch block (LBBB) is more complicated and confusing because LBBB alters the early and the late depolarization phase of the left ventricle. Secondary ST-T changes provoked by LBBB may imitate and/or mask ischemia. In uncomplicated LBBB, the ventricles are activated sequentially (right ventricle depolarizes before the left ventricle). The normal direction of septal depolarization is reversed (from right to left) and forces spread first to the right ventricle through the right bundle branch and then to the left ventricle via slow activation of the septum. This activation extends the duration of QRS (≥120 ms) and eliminates the normal initial septal Q waves in the lateral leads. The overall direction of depolarization produces monophasic wide R waves in the lateral leads (I, V5–V6) and concomitant rS or QS waves from V1 through V3. In normal uncomplicated LBBB, the ST-segment and T wave vectors are opposite to the greater deflection of the QRS: positive from V1 to V3 and negative in lateral leads.

In normal LBBB setting, overall vector forces are directed posteriorly and to the left within the range from −90° to −40°. On the horizontal plane, maximal vector of the QRS is located in the left posterior quadrant (−40° and −80°) with increased magnitude (2 mV); main portions of QRS loop have a clockwise rotation. On a vectorcardiographic analysis, T wave loop is directed rightward and anteriorly with counterclockwise rotation (this is why T wave is typically positive in right precordial leads and diphasic in V4 through V6). On the frontal plane, overall vector is directed usually between +30° and −30°; T wave loops are opposite to the QRS with counterclockwise rotation.

Given the normal features in uncomplicated LBBB, some ECG signs can be used to diagnose myocardial ischemia. ST elevations in lateral leads or ST depressions or deep T wave inversions in leads V1 to V3 strongly suggest underlying ischemia. More pronounced ST elevation (≥0.5 mV) in leads with QS or rS waves may also be due to acute ischemia. As described by Sgarbossa et al. [27], the presence of specific ECG features (*Sgarbossa criteria*) is strictly associated with the diagnosis of myocardial infarction in LBBB pattern:

1. **Concordant ST elevation > 1 mm in leads with a positive QRS complex**
2. **Concordant ST depression > 1 mm in V1–V3**
3. **Excessively discordant ST elevation > 5 mm in leads with a negative QRS complex**

2.8 ECG Differential Diagnosis of Ischemia and Infarction

2.8.1 ST-Segment Elevation

The diagnosis of acute myocardial infarction with ST elevation (STEMI) should be made by a 12-leads ECG. The presence of ST-segment elevation (STE) in a patient with acute chest pain should be considered as STEMI. If uncertainty about diagnosis exists, repetitive

Table 2 Differential diagnosis of ST-segment elevation

Myocardial Ischemia/Infarction
Non-infarction transmural ischemia (Prinzmetal angina)
Acute myocardial infarction
Ventricular aneurysm pattern
Acute Pericarditis
Normal variant ("early repolarization pattern")
Left ventricular hypertrophy/LBBB pattern (in V1–V2 or V3 only)
Other rare pathological conditions
Myocardial trauma
Acute myocarditis
Cardiac tumors invading the left ventricle
Hypothermia
Post-electrical cardioversion pattern
Intracranial hemorrhage
Hyperkalemia (usually V1–V2)
Channelopathies (Brugada's pattern)
Hypercalcemia

ECG recordings and echocardiographic and additional laboratory information can be included in order not to add delay in reperfusion strategy. The differential diagnosis of ST elevation includes some pathological situations listed in Table 2.

During acute diffuse inflammatory process affecting pericardial sac or myocardial muscle (acute pericarditis/myocarditis), the current of injury sign may be recognized without correspondence to a specific coronary territory. STE will be present in most leads (not in aVR and V1 where ST-segment depression can be seen due to its distant and opposite position of the normal heart axis). STE in acute pericarditis/myocarditis has mainly a concave morphology and unaltered R wave amplitude. Often, PR segment depression can be typically seen as the inflammatory process involves the atria [28].

2.8.2 T Wave Inversion

When caused by physiological variants, T wave inversion is sometimes mistaken for ischemia. T wave inversion in V1 through V2 may be inverted normally at any age, and it is sometimes normally negative. T waves can be negative in leads aVR, V1, and III in subjects without cardiac diseases. Diagnostic approach should be tailored according to the clinical presentation and medical and family history [29]. Differential diagnosis of prominent T wave inversion is listed in Table 3.

When the presence of T wave inversion represents a pathological finding, we define *primary T wave inversion* when abnormalities are due to alteration in myocardial cellular electrophysiology (ischemia or injury). Primary T wave changes are caused by alteration in duration and morphology of ventricular action potentials without changes in cardiac conduction sequence. Ischemia, drug effect, and metabolic disorders can be included. Primary T wave inversion is described sometimes in acute cerebrovascular accidents, particularly in case of stroke or subarachnoid hemorrhage ("cerebral T waves"); it is known that acute cerebrovascular accidents can drive alterations in the autonomic nervous system

Table 3 Differential diagnosis of prominent T wave inversion

Normal variants
Juvenile T wave pattern
Early repolarization
Myocardial ischemia/infarction
Cerebrovascular accident (especially intracranial bleeds)
Left or right overload ECG patterns
"Strain" pattern
Cardiomyopathies
Post-tachycardia T wave pattern
Secondary T wave alterations: bundle branch blocks, Wolff-Parkinson-White patterns
"Memory" T waves
Intermittent left bundle branch block
Preexcitation
Ventricular pacing
Electroconvulsive therapy

involving changes in cardiac cellular action potentials inducing often conduction disturbances and mechanical ventricular dysfunction [30].

Secondary T wave inversion refers to a presence of alterations depending on the sequence of ventricular activation without changes of action potential characteristics. Examples include bundle branch block, preexcitation syndromes, and paced rhythms. The term "memory T wave changes" has been used to describe repolarization changes induced by depolarization changes caused by intermittent preexcitation, left bundle branch block, and paced beats.

3 Cardiac Arrhythmias in the Setting of Ischemic Heart Disease

Coronary artery disease (CAD) represents the leading cause of death in the industrialized world. Many of these deaths are attributed to the development of ventricular tachyarrhythmias during periods of myocardial ischemia or infarction. Myocardial ischemia is characterized by ionic and biochemical alterations, creating an unstable electrical substrate capable of initiating and sustaining arrhythmias. The infarct process creates areas of electrical inactivity and blocks conduction, which also promotes arrhythmogenesis [31]. During acute myocardial ischemia, several biochemical and metabolic changes alter inward and outward transmembrane ionic current fluxes, causing profound alterations of the resting membrane and action potential characteristics of the myocyte. These changes induce slow conduction, decreased excitability, shortening of action potential duration, refractoriness dishomogeneity, dispersion of repolarization, and abnormal automaticity. These factors represent electrophysiological triggers and anatomic substrate necessary to induce arrhythmias (Fig. 9).

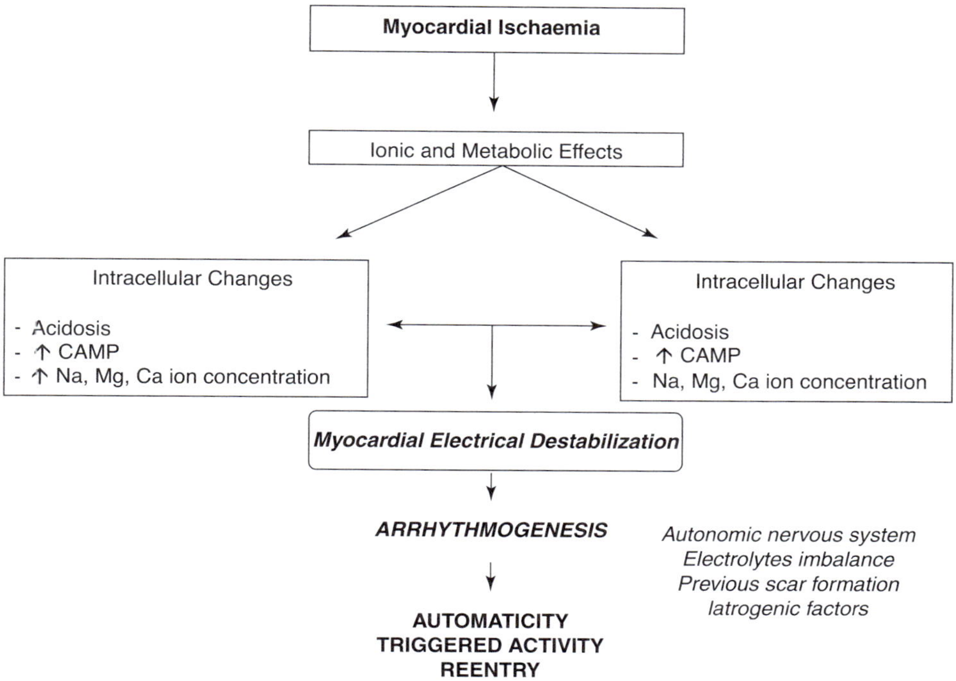

Fig. 9 Mechanisms of ischemia-induced arrhythmogenesis. *CAMP* cyclic adenosine monophosphate

3.1 Supraventricular Arrhythmias

3.1.1 Sinus Bradycardia

Sinus bradycardia (<60 beats/min) is common, occurring in 25–40% of patients with the first hour of a myocardial infarction. It is more common with inferior wall myocardial infarction and is often due to hypervagotonia induced by stimulation of vagal afferent receptors (more commonly represented in the infero-posterior than the anterior and lateral portions of the left ventricle) with resulting efferent cholinergic stimulation of the heart. This is a manifestation of the *Bezold-Jarisch reflex* [32] that is mediated by the vagus nerves and occurs during reperfusion, particularly of the right coronary artery [33].

3.1.2 Sinus Tachycardia

This arrhythmia is typically associated with augmented sympathetic activity and may provoke transient hypertension or hypotension. Contributing factors are anxiety, persistent thoracic pain, fever, pericarditis, hypovolemia, pulmonary embolism, and drugs. Sinus tachycardia is frequently associated with large anterior infarction especially with left ventricular dysfunction. It is an unfavorable rhythm in patients with acute myocardial infarction because of augmented oxygen consumption induction and reduction in the time available for coronary perfusion, intensifying myocardial ischemic process.

3.1.3 Atrial Tachyarrhythmias

The incidence of atrial tachyarrhythmias during the peri-infarction period is estimated at 10–20%, with atrial fibrillation as the commonest occurring in 10–15% of cases. Atrial flutter occurs in less than 5% of cases [34]. These arrhythmias usually occur within 72 h of the index infarction with less than 3% arising in the very early phase (<3 h) [35]. Atrial fibrillation has been shown to be independently associated with in-hospital and long-term mortality, reinfarction rates, ventricular arrhythmias, conduction disturbances, asystole, cardiogenic shock, and ischemic strokes [36, 37]. Contributing factors to peri-infarction atrial fibrillation development are atrial infarction/ischemia, sinus node dysfunction, older age, metabolic abnormalities, pericarditis, pericardial effusion, right ventricular infarction, congestive heart failure, increased heart rate, diabetes, history of hypertension, and iatrogenic factors.

3.2 Ventricular Arrhythmias

The knowledge of the mechanisms of ventricular arrhythmias (VAs) in acute myocardial ischemia and infarction derives from animal studies. The acute phase includes a very early period (2–10 min from artery occlusion) in which the pathophysiology is most likely to be related to alterations in cellular electrophysiology and reentrant mechanisms. In the period between 10 and 30 min from the beginning of ischemic process, principal mechanisms seem to be related to local accumulation of catecholamines and increased automaticity [38]. The late phase of VAs occurs up to 72 h after coronary artery occlusion and may be caused by abnormal automaticity within surviving Purkinje fibers, triggered activity from surviving cells, or ischemic myocardium. Chronic-phase VAs develop after 72 h and usually depend on reentry mechanisms.

3.2.1 Premature Ventricular Complexes (PVCs)

PVCs commonly develop during ischemic period. Some studies report an incidence of 10–93% of PVCs in the acute phase of infarction [39]. Their presence in late postinfarction phase (usually >10 per hour) represents a strong predictor of all-cause and arrhythmic mortality [40].

3.2.2 Accelerated Idioventricular Rhythm

This is a ventricular rhythm with a rate of 60–125 beats/min and is frequently called "slow ventricular tachycardia" (Fig. 10) presenting in 20% of patients with acute myocardial infarction, probably caused by enhanced automaticity of Purkinje fibers. Accelerated idioventricular rhythm is commonly seen early after reperfusion therapy.

3.2.3 Ventricular Tachycardia (VT)

VT is conventionally described according to its temporal and morphological presentation. Nonsustained ventricular tachycardia (NSVT) is usually defined as three or more consecutive ventricular beats at a rate > 100 beats/min and lasting for <30 s. Sustained ventricular

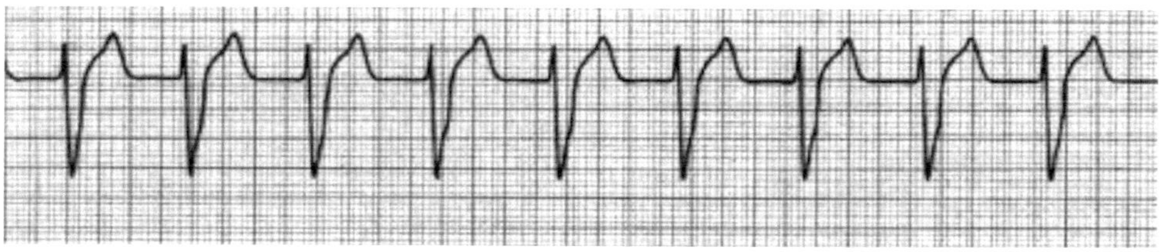

Fig. 10 Accelerated idioventricular rhythm

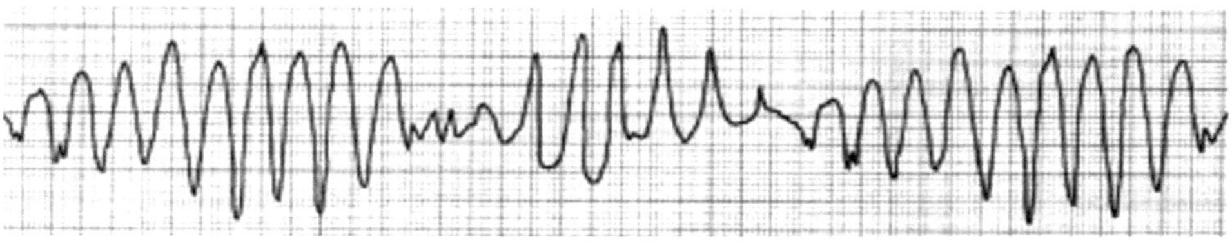

Fig. 11 Polymorphic VT. Note the frequent changes in QRS complex morphology

tachycardia (SVT) refers to ventricular rhythm at a rate > 100 beats/min lasting for more than 30 s or causing hemodynamic compromise that requires intervention. VT is described as "monomorphic" if the QRS complexes have one morphology, "multiple monomorphic" if there are two or more runs of different QRS morphologies, and "polymorphic" if the QRS morphology is variable during one episode [41] (Fig. 11).

Peri-infarction VT has an incidence of 0.3–2%. It is associated with a higher in-hospital mortality but is not considered to be a prognostic factor among hospital survivors [42]. The occurrence of SVT in peri-infarction period is uncommon and usually an indicator of extensive myocardial damage or recurrent ischemia [43].

3.2.4 Ventricular Fibrillation (VF)

VF is characterized by rapid, disorganized, multiple reentrant wavelets in the ventricle resulting in no uniform ventricular contraction and no cardiac output. Untreated, this arrhythmia is lethal and it is the main mechanism of sudden cardiac death. It has been reported to occur in 3% of acute myocardial infarction with 60% of episodes occurring within 4 h and 80% within 12 h [44].

References

1. Carmeliet E. Cardiac ionic currents and acute ischemia: from channels to arrhythmias. Physiol Rev. 1999;79:917–1017.
2. Kablunde RE. Cardiac electrophysiology: normal and ischemic ionic current and the ECG. Adv Physiol Educ. 2017;41:29–37.
3. Akar JG, Akar FG. Regulation of ion channels and arrhythmias in the ischemic heart. J Electrocardiol. 2007;40(Suppl):S37–41.
4. Shaw RM, Rudy Y. Electrophysiologic effects of acute myocardial ischemia: a theoretical study of altered cell excitability and action potential duration. Cardiovasc Res. 1997;35:256–72.

5. Fischer DB, Lilly LS. The electrocardiogram. In: Lilly LS, editor. Pathophysiology of heart disease. 6th ed. Philadelphia, PA: Wolters Kluwer; 2016. p. 74–111.
6. Pardee HEB. An electrocardiographic sign of coronary artery obstruction. Arch Intern Med. 1920;26:244e257.
7. Goldberger AL, Erickson R. A subtle ECG sign in myocardial infarction: Prominent reciprocal ST depression with minimal ST elevation. Pacing Clin Elctrophysiol. 1981;4:709–12.
8. Kracoff OH, Adelman AG, Oettinger M, et al. Reciprocal changes as the presenting electrocardiographic manifestation of acute myocardial ischaemia. Am J Cardiol. 1993;71:1359–62.
9. Hohnloser SH, Zabel M, Kasper W, et al. Assessment of coronary artery patency after thrombolytic therapy: Accurate prediction utilizing the combined analysis of three noninvasive markers. J Am Coll Cardiol. 1991;18:44–9.
10. Krucoff MW, Croll MA, Pope JE, et al. Continuous 12-lead ST-segment recovery analysis in the TAMI 7 study: Performance of noninvasive method for real-time detection of failed myocardial reperfusion. Circulation. 1993;88:437–46.
11. Nerbonne JM, Kass RS. Molecular physiology of cardiac repolarization. Physiol Rev. 2005;85:1205–53.
12. Kjekshus JK. Mechanism for flow distribution in normal and ischemic myocardium during increased ventricular preload in the dog. Circ Res. 1973;33:489–99.
13. Mirvis DM, Ingram LA, Ramanathan KB, Wilson JL, et al. R and S wave changes produced by experimental nontransmural and transmural myocardial infarction. J Am Coil Cardiol. 1986;8:675–8.
14. Phibbs B, Marcus F, Marriott HJ, et al. Q-wave versus non-Q-wave myocardial infarction: A meaningless distinction. J Am Coll Cardiol. 1999;33:576–82.
15. Nable JV, Brady W. The Evolution of electrocardiographic changes in ST-segment elevation myocardial infarction. Am J Emerg Med. 2009;27:734–46.
16. Zema M. Electrocardiographic Tall R Waves in the Right Precordial Leads. J Electrocardiol. 1990;23
17. Bosimini E, Giannuzzi P, Temporelli PL, et al. Electrocardiographic evolutionary changes and left ventricular remodeling after acute myocardial infarction. J Am Coll Cardiol. 2000;35:127–35.
18. Maeda S, Imai T, Kuboki K, et al. Pathologic implications of restored positive T waves and persistent negative T waves after Q wave myocardial infarction. J Am Coll Cardiol. 1996;28:1514–8.
19. Nagase K, Tamura A, Mikuriya Y, et al. Significance of Q-wave regression after anterior wall acute myocardial infarction. Eur Heart J. 1998;19:742–6.
20. El-Sherif N. The rsR' pattern in left surface leads in ventricular aneurysm. Br Heart J. 1970;32:440–8.
21. Prinzmetal M, Kennamer R, Merliss R, et al. Angina pectoris. I. A variant form of angina pectoris. Preliminary report. Am J Med. 1959;27:375–88.
22. Crea P, Kaski JC, Maseri A, et al. Key references on coronary artery spasm. Circulation. 1994;89:2442–6.
23. Goldberger AL. Myocardial infarction: electrocardiographic differential diagnosis. 4th ed. St Louis: Mosby; 1991.
24. Suzuki M, Nishizaki M, Arita M, et al. Increased QT dispersion in patients with vasospastic angina. Circulation. 1988;98:435–40.
25. De Zwaan C, Bar FHM, Wellens HJJ. Characteristic electrocardiographic pattern indicating a critical stenosis high in left anterior descending coronary artery in patients admitted because of impeding myocardial infarction. Am Heart. 1982;J;103:730.
26. James T. The coronary circulation and conduction system in acute myocardial infarction. Prog Cardiovasc Dis. 1968;10(5):410.

27. Sgarbossa EB, Pinski SL, Barbagelata A, et al. Electrocardiographic diagnosis of evolving acute myocardial infarction in the presence of left bundle branch block. GUSTO-1. N Engl J Med. 1996;334:481–7.
28. de Bliek EC. ST elevation: Differential Diagnosis and caveats. A comprehensive review to help distinguish ST myocardial infarction from non-ischaemic etiologies of ST elevation. Turkish J Emerg Med. (18) 2018.
29. Said SAM, Bloo R, Slootweg A. Cardiac and non-cardiac causes of T-wave inversion in the precordial leads in adult subjects: A Dutch case series and review of the literature. World J Cardial. 2015;7(2):86–100.
30. Stone J, Mor-Avi V, Ardelt A, et al. Frequency of inverted electrocardiographic T-waves (Cerebral T waves) in patients with acute stroke and their relation to left ventricular wall motion abnormalities. Am J Cardiol. 2017;121(1):120–4.
31. Ghuran AV, Camm AJ. Ischaemic heart disease presenting as arrhythmias. Br Med Bull. 2001;59:193–210.
32. Mark AL. The Bezold-Jarisch reflex revisited: Clinical implication of inhibitory reflexes originating in the heart. J Am Coll Cardiol. 1983;1:90.
33. Chiladakis JA, Patsouras N, Manolis AS. The Bezold-Jarisch reflex in acute inferior myocardial infarction. Clinical and sympathovagal spectral correlates. Clini Cardiol. 2003;26:323–8.
34. Liberthson RR, Salisbury KW, Hutter AM Jr, DeSanctis RW. Atrial tachyarrhythmias in acute myocardial infarction. Am J Med. 1976;60:956–60.
35. Hod H, Lew AS, Keltai M, et al. Early atrial fibrillation during evolving myocardial infarction: a consequence of impaired left atrial perfusion. Circulation. 1987;75:146–50.
36. Crenshaw BS, Ward SR, Granger CB, Stebbins AL, Topol EJ, Califf RM. Atrial fibrillation in the setting of acute myocardial infarction: the GUSTO-I experience. Global Utilization of Streptokinase and TPA for Occluded Coronary Arteries. J Am Coll Cardiol. 1997;30:406–13.
37. Sakata K, Kurihara H, Iwamori K, et al. Clinical and prognostic significance of atrial fibrillation in acute myocardial infarction. Am J Cardiol. 1997;80:1522–7.
38. Janse MJ, Wit AL. Electrophysiological mechanisms of ventricular arrhythmias resulting from myocardial ischemia and infarction. Physiol Rev. 1989;69:1049–169.
39. Bigger JT Jr, Dresdale FJ, Heissenbuttel RH, Weld FM, Wit AL. Ventricular arrhythmias in ischemic heart disease: mechanism, prevalence, significance, and management. Prog Cardiovasc Dis. 1977;19:255–300.
40. Maggioni AP, Zuanetti G, Franzosi MG, et al. Prevalence and prognostic significance of ventricular arrhythmias after acute myocardial infarction in the fibrinolytic era. GISSI-2 results. Circulation. 1993;87:312–22.
41. Wolfe CL, Nibley C, Bhandari A, et al. Polymorphous ventricular tachycardia associated with acute myocardial infarction. Circulation. 1991;84:1543–51.
42. Eldar M, Sievner Z, Goldbourt U, Reicher-Reiss H, Kaplinsky E, Behar S. Primary ventricular tachycardia in acute myocardial infarction: clinical characteristics and mortality. The SPRINT Study Group. Ann Intern Med. 1992;117:31–6.
43. Mont L, Cinca J, Blanch P, et al. Predisposing factors and prognostic value of sustained monomorphic ventricular tachycardia in the early phase of acute myocardial infarction. J Am Coll Cardiol. 1996;28:1670–6.
44. Campbell RW, Murray A, Julian DG. Ventricular arrhythmias in first 12 hours of acute myocardial infarction. Natural history study. Br Heart J. 1981;46:351–7.

Exercise Testing and Its Role in Ischemic Heart Disease

Giuseppe Vergaro, Valentina Spini, and Iacopo Fabiani

Abbreviations

CFR	Coronary flow reserve
CO	Cardiac output
CPET	Cardiopulmonary exercise testing
HR	Heart rate
LV	Left ventricular
LVEF	LV ejection fraction
METS	Metabolic equivalents
RWM	Regional wall motion
SE	Stress echocardiography
SV	Stroke volume
WMSI	Wall motion score index

G. Vergaro (✉)
Division of Cardiology and Cardiovascular Medicine, Fondazione Toscana Gabriele Monasterio, Pisa, Italy

Health Science Interdisciplinary Center, Scuola Superiore Sant'Anna, Pisa, Italy
e-mail: vergaro@ftgm.it

V. Spini · I. Fabiani
Division of Cardiology and Cardiovascular Medicine, Fondazione Toscana Gabriele Monasterio, Pisa, Italy
e-mail: vspini@ftgm.it; ifabiani@ftgm.it

G. Concistrè (ed.), *Ischemic Heart Disease*,
https://doi.org/10.1007/978-3-031-25879-4_11

1 Principles of Exercise Testing

Exercise testing has been used as a provocative test in patients with known or suspected cardiovascular disease since decades. Although recent recommendations have reappraised the utility of exercise testing in ischemic heart disease, it is still used for diagnostic purposes in patients with chest pain syndromes or potential anginal equivalents, to predict cardiovascular events and all-cause death, to evaluate exercise-related symptoms, and to assess response to interventions.

Aerobic exercise up to maximal individual tolerance is the most commonly used stress to unmask cardiovascular abnormalities that can be absent at rest. The increased metabolic demand following exercise initiation elicits cardiovascular responses characterized by a rise in cardiac output following augmentation in stroke volume and, especially at moderate to high intensity, in heart rate. As the exercise intensity progresses toward a maximum level, sympathetic discharge becomes maximal and parasympathetic stimulation is inhibited, resulting in vasoconstriction in most circulatory body systems, except in exercising muscle and in the cerebral and coronary circulations, and skeletal muscle blood flow and oxygen extraction increase. Maximal oxygen uptake (Vo2max) corresponds to the product of maximum cardiac output and maximum arteriovenous oxygen difference. While systolic blood pressure increases with exercise, diastolic pressure remains unchanged or slightly decreases in healthy subjects.

Myocardial metabolic demand, mainly determined by intramyocardial wall stress, contractility, and heart rate, is also increased by exercise, which can elicit up to a fivefold increase in coronary blood flow above resting values. In patients with obstructive coronary artery disease (CAD), an adequate coronary blood flow may not be provided to the affected myocardial tissue, leading to myocardial ischemia.

2 Clinical Indications to Exercise Testing

Latest European guidelines on chronic coronary syndromes suggest a stepwise approach to the assessment of patients with suspected CAD [1]. The first steps are the evaluation of signs and symptoms, investigation on comorbidities and possible alternative causes of symptoms, basic testing with biochemistry, resting electrocardiogram (ECG), echocardiography, assessment of pretest probability, and clinical likelihood of CAD based on age, sex, and nature of symptoms. In patients in whom CAD cannot be excluded by clinical assessment alone, noninvasive diagnostic tests, either functional imaging of ischemia or anatomical imaging, are recommended to establish the diagnosis and assess the event risk. ECG changes can be detected during a conventional exercise testing or, as discussed later

Table 1 Summary of characteristics of the most commonly used exercise test for the detection of coronary artery disease. *ECG* electrocardiogram. See text for references

Test	Sensitivity (%)	Specificity (%)	Advantages	Limitations
Exercise stress testing	68	77	Wide availability, limited costs	Limited diagnostic accuracy, especially in patients with abnormal resting ECG and previous coronary revascularization
Stress echocardiography	79	87	Assessment or regional wall motion abnormalities, as well as of valves. Does not require radiations	Dependent on quality of images and on operator
Exercise single photon emission computed tomography	85	85	Evaluation of regional perfusion, prognostic assessment	Cannot assess valves, affected by heart rhythm, requires radiations

in this chapter, can be combined with echocardiography or nuclear imaging (e.g., with single photon emission computed tomography - SPECT) to detect wall motion abnormalities or perfusion defects.

Exercise ECG has limited diagnostic performance and is less powerful for the ruling-in and ruling-out of CAD, compared to imaging tests [2]. As some randomized clinical trials have demonstrated that imaging tests (either functional or anatomical) have superior diagnostic yield [3, 4], allow the targeting of therapeutic intervention (such as coronary revascularization), and potentially reduce the risk of myocardial infarction, they should be preferred as the initial test in patients with suspected CAD [1]. Table 1 summarizes the characteristics of the most commonly used exercise tests for the detection of CAD. Nonetheless, exercise ECG may be considered when imaging tests are not available, or when information about exercise tolerance, arrhythmias, and blood pressure response is sought.

Importantly, some characteristics of resting ECG further limit the diagnostic value of exercise ECG for the detection of CAD, such as the presence of left bundle branch block, paced rhythm, or repolarization abnormalities [5–7]. Alternative tests should therefore be preferred in these settings. Moreover, some patient characteristics and clinical conditions, especially recent acute cardiovascular events, may represent absolute and relative contraindication to exercise testing, as summarized in Table 2 [5, 6].

Table 2 Absolute and relative contraindication to exercise testing

Absolute	Relative
Acute myocardial infarction (within 2 days)	Known obstructive left main coronary artery stenosis
Ongoing unstable angina	Moderate-to-severe aortic stenosis
Uncontrolled arrhythmia with hemodynamic compromise	Tachyarrhythmias with uncontrolled ventricular rates
Active endocarditis	Acquired advanced or complete heart block
Symptomatic severe aortic stenosis	Hypertrophic obstructive cardiomyopathy with severe resting gradient
Decompensated heart failure	Recent stroke or transient ischemic attack
Acute pulmonary embolism, pulmonary infarction, or deep vein thrombosis	Mental impairment with impaired ability to cooperate
Acute myocarditis or pericarditis	Resting hypertension (systolic/diastolic blood pressure > 200/110 mmHg)
Acute aortic dissection	Uncorrected significant medical conditions (e.g., anemia, electrolyte imbalance, hyperthyroidism)

3 Setup and Performance of Exercise Testing

Whether it is associated with ECG monitoring only or it is complemented by an imaging technique, the setting up and performance of exercise testing are similar. Preparation to the exam should follow the following steps [5, 8]:

- Indications to the test should be clarified.
- Patient should be fasting for at least 3 h before the test and should dress comfortably.
- Although no formal recommendation exists on the management of background medications, when ischemia is searched, especially in patients without a known history of ischemic heart disease, some drug classes (in particular beta-blockers) may be suspended, as they can reduce blood pressure and heart rate response and further limit the diagnostic accuracy of the test.
- A brief history and physical examination should be routinely taken, in order to exclude absolute or relative contraindications to the test.
- A resting supine ECG should be recorded before exercise to be initiated.
- Informed consent should be systematically obtained before the test.

Although some differences exist in relation to the dynamics of exercise consumption and in muscular groups involved, both treadmill and cycle ergometers are universally accepted as exercise equipment and are the most commonly used dynamic exercise testing devices [5, 6].

Exercise protocols generally include an initial warm-up at low workload, followed by an increasing graded exercise at higher workload up to the individual maximal functional

Table 3 Absolute and relative indication to exercise termination

Absolute	Relative
Central nervous system symptoms (e.g., ataxia, dizziness, near syncope)	Other arrhythmias (such as frequent/repetitive premature ventricular beats, supraventricular tachycardia, bradyarrhythmias) potentially evolving into more relevant rhythm disorders
Decrease in systolic blood pressure > 10 mmHg with other signs of ischemia	Bundle branch block that cannot immediately be distinguished from ventricular tachycardia
Sustained ventricular tachycardia or other brady/tachyarrhythmia potentially affecting cardiac output	Decrease in systolic blood pressure > 10 mmHg without other signs of ischemia
ST-segment elevation (>1.0 mm) in leads without preexisting Q waves (other than aVR, aVL, and V1)	Marked hypertensive response (systolic blood pressure > 250 mm Hg and/or diastolic blood pressure > 115 mm Hg)
Signs of peripheral hypoperfusion	Marked ST-segment displacement (horizontal or downsloping >2 mm, measured 60–80 ms after the J point)
Technical difficulties in ECG monitoring	
Increasing/severe angina	
Willingness of the patient	

capacity, and a low/no workload recovery period [5]. The Bruce protocol, consisting of 3 steps at increasing speed and slope, is the most commonly used with treadmill. Conversely, steps with increasing workload of 25 W every 1–3 min are frequently used with cycle ergometry. The test should be performed under the supervision of an experienced physician and should be symptom limited (usually conducted up to maximum exercise tolerance). The test may be interrupted earlier when absolute or relative indications to exercise termination appear (listed in Table 3) [5, 8].

4 Interpretation of Exercise Testing in Patients with Suspected Ischemic Heart Disease

ST-segment depression is the traditional manifestation of exercise-induced myocardial ischemia [9, 10]. The standard criteria for test positivity include horizontal or downsloping ST depression ≥1 mm (0.1 mV) assessed at 60–80 ms after the J point (Fig. 1). Still, a marked upsloping ST depression may also be associated with underlying coronary artery disease in high-risk subsets and in patients with angina [11]. Characteristics of ST displacement associated with the probability and severity of disease are the extent, workload, and number of leads where ST displacement appears and should therefore be all considered. Occasionally, ST-segment elevation may occur during exercise in leads where postinfarction Q waves are present, possibly accounting for perinecrotic ischemia. When ST elevation occurs in patients without signs of myocardial infarction, it should be

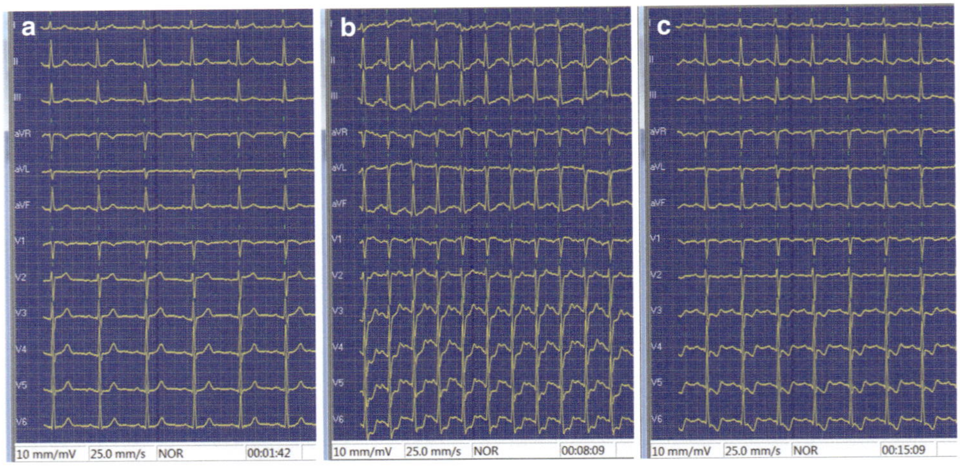

Fig. 1 Exercise electrocardiogram. ECG recording at baseline (panel **a**), at peak exercise (150 W, panel **b**), and during recovery (5′, panel **c**) in a patient with angina and angiographic documentation of stenosis >75% of right coronary artery. Panel **b** shows marked ST-segment depression in D2–D3–aVF and V3–V6 leads at peak exercise; marked ventricular repolarization abnormalities in precordial leads

regarded as an index of severe (both subendocardial and subepicardial) ischemia [12] or as a sign of coronary artery spasm [13]. Moreover, normalization of repolarization abnormalities present at rest, such as T wave inversion or ST depression, may also indicate the presence of myocardial ischemia.

Tachyarrhythmia, in particular either isolated or repetitive premature ventricular beats [14], and less frequently bradyarrhythmias, such as advanced atrioventricular block, can be suggestive of underlying myocardial ischemia, irrespective of ST-segment displacement.

Each of the aforementioned abnormalities should be regarded with more attention when it is associated with exercise-induced angina, especially when symptoms occur at low workload.

Further to diagnostic information, exercise testing is also of clinical utility for risk stratification purposes [7]. Exercise capacity itself holds prognostic relevance, as it can predict all-cause death [15, 16]. With regard to ischemic heart disease, the lower the workload and rate–pressure product at which ST depression occurs, the worse the prognosis [17]. Further, ventricular ectopy in the recovery period can also be an independent predictive marker for death [14, 18]. In the early 1990s, the Duke treadmill score was developed, based on a weighted combination of exercise duration, ST-segment depression, and presence and nature of angina during testing, as a tool for death prediction [19].

5 Exercise Echocardiography and Nuclear Medicine

SE provides a dynamic evaluation of myocardial structure and function by the combination of 2D echocardiography with a physical, pharmacological, or electrical stress [20]. The diagnostic endpoint for the detection of myocardial ischemia is the appearance of a transient change in regional function during stress. The underlying pathophysiological mechanism is the reduction of CFR due to an imbalance between oxygen demand and supply that usually results in the typical ischemic "cascade", which is a chain of events hierarchically ranked in a well-defined time sequence [21]. Flow heterogeneity, especially between the subendocardial and subepicardial perfusion, is the forerunner of ischemia, followed by metabolic changes, by alteration in regional mechanical function, and only at a later stage by electrocardiographic changes and pain. Regardless of the stress used and the morphological substrate, ischemia propagates centrifugally with respect to the ventricular cavity: it involves primarily the subendocardial layer, whereas the subepicardial layer is affected only in a subsequent phase if the ischemia persists, as extravascular pressure is higher in the subendocardial than in the subepicardial layer with a higher metabolic demand and an increased resistance to flow. CFR can be reduced in the presence of CAD, but also in other conditions such as microvascular disease (e.g., in syndrome X) or LV hypertrophy (e.g., arterial hypertension). In this condition, angina with ST-segment depression can occur with regional perfusion changes, typically in the absence of any regional wall motion abnormalities during stress.

For assessment of regional myocardial function, either the 16- or the 17-segment model of the LV may be used [22]. In clinical practice in which RWM and thickening are assessed, the 16-segment model is commonly used. The 17-segment model, which includes the apical cap, an area beyond the LV cavity, is recommended if myocardial perfusion is evaluated or if echocardiography is compared with another imaging modality [22]. The function of each segment is graded at rest and with stress according to a 5-point scoring system. Scores are as follows: normal or hyperkinesis =1 (systolic increase in thickness > 50%), hypokinesis =2 (<40%), severe hypokinesis or akinesis =3 (<10%), dyskinesis (paradoxical systolic motion away from the center of the LV) =4, and aneurysmal (diastolic deformation) =5. The WMSI can be calculated by dividing the sum of the scores of individual segments by the number of segments visualized. However, a resting akinesia becoming dyskinesia during stress reflects purely passive phenomenon of increased intraventricular pressure developed by normally contracting walls and should not be considered a true active ischemia [20].

The most frequently used stressors for echocardiographic are exercise, dobutamine, and dipyridamole. Exercise echocardiography can be performed using either a treadmill or a bicycle protocol and provide information on exercise capacity, heart rate response, rhythm, and blood pressure trend; all these changes are analyzed together with wall motion analysis and become part of the final interpretation [23]. ESC Guidelines on stable CAD have posed a new emphasis on the clinical utility of SE [24]; in a meta-analysis of 55 studies with 3714 patients, exercise, dobutamine, dipyridamole, and adenosine echocardiography showed a sensitivity of 83, 81, 72, and 79%, respectively, and a specificity of 84, 84, 95, and 91%, respectively [25]. When compared to standard exercise electrocardiography, stress echocardiography has a particularly relevant advantage in terms of specificity [26]. Compared to nuclear perfusion imaging, SE at least has similar accuracy, with a moderate sensitivity gap that is more than balanced by a markedly higher specificity [25]. Current indications for stress echocardiography include [27]:

(a) CAD diagnosis
(b) Prognosis and risk stratification in patients with established diagnosis (e.g., after myocardial infarction)
(c) Preoperative risk assessment
(d) Evaluation for cardiac etiology of exertional dyspnea
(e) Evaluation after revascularization
(f) Ischemia localization in patients with multivessel disease
(g) Viability assessment

As a rule, the less informative the exercise ECG test is, the stricter the indication for stress echocardiography will be. Out of five patients, one is unable to exercise, one exercises submaximally, and one exercises maximally but the ECG is uninterpretable.

Indications in the individual patient can be optimized, after careful consideration of relative and absolute contraindications for each test. For instance, a patient with severe hypertension and/or atrial or ventricular arrhythmias can more reasonably undergo dipyridamole stress test, which, unlike dobutamine, has no arrhythmogenic or hypertensive effect. In contrast, a patient with severe conduction disturbances or advanced asthmatic disease should undergo the dobutamine stress test, since adenosine has a negative chronotropic and dromotropic effect, as well as a documented bronchoconstrictor activity. Patients either taking xanthine medication or under the effect of caffeine contained in drinks (tea, coffee, cola) should undergo the dobutamine test. Both dipyridamole and dobutamine have overall good tolerance and feasibility. The choice of one test over the other depends on patient characteristics, local drug cost, and physician's preference. Antianginal medical therapy (in particular, beta-blocking agents) significantly affects the diagnostic accuracy of all forms of stress; therefore, it is recommended, whenever possible, to withhold medical therapy at the time of testing to avoid a false-negative result [28, 29].

Although SE is routinely used for the diagnosis of CAD, an equally important role is to identify patients at risk for future cardiac events and to assess prognosis. Several studies have demonstrated that a normal stress echocardiogram (normal regional wall motion at rest and with stress) is associated with a good prognosis [29–32]. Exercise capacity and heart rate response can be used to further stratify risk in patients undergoing exercise SE [33–35]. Peak WMSI and EF have been identified on multivariate analysis as the best predictors of cardiac events [29]. The extent and severity of wall motion abnormalities by stress echocardiography are both independent and cumulative predictors of prognosis [36].

SE allows assessment of viability: a sign of myocardial viability is a stress-induced improvement of function during low levels of stress in a region that is abnormal at rest. By far, the widest experience is available with low-dose dobutamine stress echocardiography [37–39]. Sensitivity and specificity of low-dose dobutamine test are 86% and 90%, respectively, for the prediction of spontaneous functional recovery after an acute myocardial infarction (stunning) [37], and 84 and 81% for the prediction of functional recovery following revascularization in patients with chronic CAD (hibernation) [38]. However, it is also possible to assess the presence of myocardial viability using low-dose dipyridamole [40–42], low-level exercise [43], or enoximone [44, 45].

For the detection of left main or multivessel CAD, stress echocardiography had greater sensitivity compared with nuclear myocardial perfusion imaging, which compares relative differences in perfusion and may miss ischemia that is balanced or globally reduced [46]. Another meta-analysis revealed that dipyridamole and dobutamine SE had similar sensitivity and specificity for detection of CAD [47].

Most recently, the American College of Cardiology has directed appropriate use criteria not to focus on a given imaging modality, but instead to have considered the role of multimodality imaging in the case of a diagnosis or disease state [48]. From this point of view, SE and nuclear perfusion scintigraphy were rated as similarly appropriate for diagnosis or risk stratification of patients with symptoms of suspected cardiac etiology.

SPECT allows evaluation of regional myocardial perfusion and viability [49–52]. An abnormal reduction in regional myocardial perfusion, a disturbance in cell membrane transport, a lack of energy production, or an abnormality in cellular energy utilization results in diminished myocardial uptake of radionuclide tracers. Severe myocardial ischemia or infarction can damage cells so these will not take up radionuclide agents even if flow is still intact. Major clinical application of myocardial perfusion imaging using SPECT technology is the detection of CAD in patients presenting with chest pain or other symptoms considered suggestive (Fig. 2). Either exercise or pharmacologic stress is employed, and most commonly, one of the Tc-99m-labeled tracers is used. Pooled sensitivity of stress SPECT is 87% with a specificity of 73% [53]. Some areas of myocardial tracer uptake can be reduced in normal subjects, such as in inferior-basal segment and in anterior wall in women who have overlying breast tissue, that attenuates the photons coming from the heart. Interpretation of SPECT images also depends on adequate image quality, reader expertise, and well-functioning equipment with trained and accredited laboratory staff. It should be pointed out that functional data such as regional thickening abnormalities due to ischemia or scar, LVEF, and LV systolic and diastolic volumes can accurately be determined on gated SPECT images in most patients [54].

A great deal of data has accumulated over the past few decades pertaining to the prognostic value of exercise and pharmacologic stress myocardial perfusion imaging. First, it has been shown that patients with normal SPECT scans have a low risk of cardiac death or

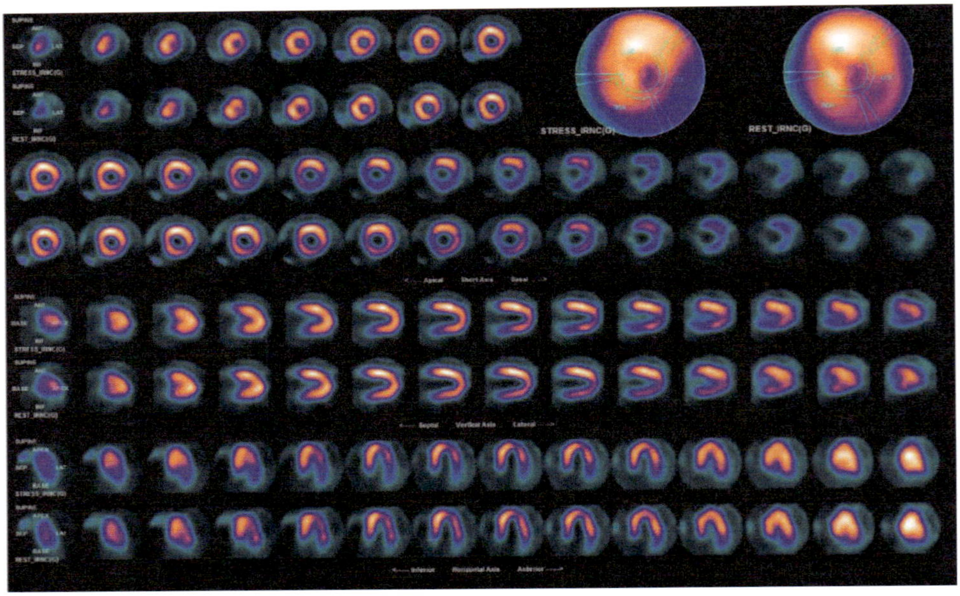

Fig. 2 Single photon emission computed tomography (SPECT). Rest and stress myocardial SPECT images demonstrating lateral ischemia accounting for 12% of left ventricular mass in a patient with angiographic documentation of stenosis >75% of circumflex coronary artery

nonfatal infarction during follow-up. A pooled analysis from 19 studies involving 39,173 patients reported a hard event rate of 0.6% per year for patients with normal scans [55]. Stress perfusion imaging is particularly effective in separating high- and low-risk subsets that have an intermediate Duke treadmill score [56]. However, the value of exercise SPECT is questionable in patients who achieve ≥10 METS of workload. One study showed that patients achieving a workload of 10 METS or more had a very low prevalence of significant ischemia [57]. The prognostic value of stress SPECT is enhanced by assessing functional variables on gated images [54]. A reduced post-stress LVEF and an increased LV end-systolic volume add supplemental prognostic information. Postischemic stunning manifested by a lower LVEF on the post-stress compared to the rest images is a high-risk finding.

Stress SPECT may assist in identifying which patients with CAD may benefit more from revascularization than medical therapy [58]. It appears that an ischemia involving at least 10% of left ventricular mass may identify the group of patients with more benefit from revascularization than from medical therapy. It must be emphasized that SPECT underestimates the extent of significant coronary artery stenoses, particularly with the Tc-99m-labeled perfusion agents, Tc-99m-sestamibi, and Tc-99m-tetrofosmin. It has been shown that only 10% of patients with three-vessel CAD had perfusion abnormalities identified in the supply regions of all three coronary arteries and only 25% had perfusion and/or regional wall motion abnormalities on gated SPECT images in three coronary territories [59]. In the same study, 12% of the patients with angiographic three-vessel disease (>50%

stenosis) had normal scans. On the other hand, exercise or pharmacologic SPECT for risk assessment can be useful for patients who have high coronary calcium scores (>400) on CT scanning, particularly if they are diabetic [60]. Some patients with intermediate stenoses (50–70%) on CT angiography may benefit from stress perfusion imaging to determine the physiologic significance of such noncritical stenoses. There is no indication for stress perfusion imaging as the first test for primary risk assessment in asymptomatic patients [61].

6 Cardiopulmonary Exercise Testing in Ischemic Heart Disease

CPET enables the assessment of gas exchange during exercise, providing a thorough description of the system responsible for O_2 transport and usage. This information is crucial for clinical decision-making in various clinical settings, since CPET provides information on functional capacity, training prescription, treatment effectiveness, and outcome prediction across a wide range of cardiopulmonary disorders [62, 63]. CPET is also a useful technique for the noninvasive assessment of CAD, since many CPET parameters give diagnostic and prognostic information with potential therapeutic implications [64].

The diagnostic utility of CPET in detecting exercise-induced cardiac dysfunction is based on variables that are surrogates for CO (i.e., oxygen consumption, VO_2) and SV (i.e., O_2 pulse) as well as on direct measure of the HR response in real time (*Fick equation*) [63]. Briefly, exertional myocardial oxygen deficiency (i.e., ischemia) induces mechanical dysfunction beyond the ischemic threshold, resulting in an SV decrease with increasing activity. As a compensatory mechanism, the autonomic nervous system increases sympathetic activity (HR increase). This increase, occurring during late exercise, is measured as the shift in the HR to work-rate slope parameter (HR–WR slope), which is calculated by comparing the HR slope during the last 2 min of exercise to the HR slope during the first 2 min of exercise [65].

In late exercise, ischemic patients experience an acceleration of their HR response (positive HR–WR slope; values more than 15% are pathological). Conversely, in patients who are unable to augment their HR response (including advanced CAD), the abrupt plateau or decrease in SV is accompanied by a reduction in CO, as measured by VO_2 relative to work-rate (flattening of the VO_2/WR slope) and minute ventilation (i.e., the oxygen uptake efficiency slope). Overall, combining standard exercise testing variables with gas exchange parameters, CPET offers a higher accuracy in diagnosing myocardial ischemia in patients presenting with chest pain [66, 67].

Peak VO_2 is the most accredited cardiorespiratory fitness indicator [68], with a strong and independent relationship with the risk of nonfatal myocardial infarction and heart failure, and considerable risk stratification potential [69]. In addition, cardiorespiratory fitness has a significant long-term prognostic role in males following myocardial infarction or coronary revascularization [70, 71]. A continuous, 1 mL O_2/kg/min increase in early peak VO_2 is associated with a 10% reduction in cardiac mortality [71], and patients with a peak VO_2 < 16 mL O_2/kg/min at the time of discharge following MI or percutaneous coronary intervention have an increased risk of events at follow-up [69]. Peak VO_2 is a therapy-responsive variable, and serial measurements may be beneficial in the careful monitoring of cardiovascular health status. Patients with peak VO_2 increase at follow-up have a reduced risk of events [68]. Several drugs have a beneficial effect on peak VO2 increase, including ranolazine and ACE inhibitors [72, 73]. Beta-blockers blunt the HR response to exercise, but an increase in peak VO_2 is observed in CAD and heart failure patients involved in a correct exercise training strategy [74].

The combination of exercise SE and CPET, a recent acquisition of stress echocardiography, provides further information for differential diagnosis and therapeutic management of patients with exertional dyspnea in various clinical settings including CAD [63]. CPET and SE allow a simultaneous, noninvasive, cost-effective, and widely available evaluation of several echocardiographic and CPET variables, providing a deeper phenotyping. In the field of CAD, recent papers allowed for the differentiation of coronary circulatory disease from deconditioning [75, 76]: in detail, many CPET parameters (in particular VE/VCO_2 slope) showed correlation with a poor stroke volume response to exercise, refining the identification and prognostic stratification of CAD.

7 Special Populations

Clinical significance and interpretation of exercise testing can be largely influenced by patient characteristics. Women often present with resting ECG abnormalities and have more atypical symptoms, thus resulting in a lower accuracy of exercise testing for the detection of coronary artery disease. A meta-analysis of studies published between 1966 and 1995 has shown that exercise ECG had a weighted mean sensitivity and specificity of 0.61 (95% confidence intervals 0.54–0.68) and 0.70 (0.64–0.75), respectively [77].

Although advanced age *per se* is not a contraindication to exercise testing, the use of pharmacological stressors is more common in the elderly population, due to functional limitations and comorbidities. Yet, the association of exercise SPECT perfusion defects with cardiac death supports the use of myocardial perfusion imaging in older patients [78, 79].

Finally, diabetic patients are at higher risk of coronary artery disease, yet they present with a higher prevalence of silent ischemia or with atypical symptoms [80]. Exercise ECG has been shown to have similar diagnostic yield in diabetic and nondiabetic patients [81], while a particularly high rate of SPECT perfusion abnormalities, approaching 50%, has been documented in patients with diabetes and mild symptoms [82].

8 Conclusions

Recent technological advances have provided clinicians with an increasing number of diagnostic tools in patients with suspected CAD. While imaging modalities have a better diagnostic yield, exercise testing still represents an option in patients with interpretable electrocardiograms who are able to exercise and enables efficient prognostic stratification. The choice of the optimal test requires a patient-centered approach accounting for local availabilities and risk-benefit and cost-effectiveness ratio.

References

1. Knuuti J, Wijns W, Saraste A, Capodanno D, Barbato E, Funck-Brentano C, et al. 2019 ESC guidelines for the diagnosis and management of chronic coronary syndromes. Eur Heart J. 2020;41:407–77.
2. Knuuti J, Ballo H, Juarez-Orozco LE, Saraste A, Kolh P, Rutjes AWS, et al. The performance of non-invasive tests to rule-in and rule-out significant coronary artery stenosis in patients with stable angina: a meta-analysis focused on post-test disease probability. Eur Heart J. 2018;39:3322–30.
3. Zacharias K, Ahmed A, Shah BN, Gurunathan S, Young G, Acosta D, et al. Relative clinical and economic impact of exercise echocardiography vs. exercise electrocardiography, as first line investigation in patients without known coronary artery disease and new stable angina: a randomized prospective study. Eur Heart J Cardiovasc Imaging. 2017;18:195–202.
4. Jørgensen ME, Andersson C, Nørgaard BL, Abdulla J, Shreibati JB, Torp-Pedersen C, et al. Functional testing or coronary computed tomography angiography in patients with stable coronary artery disease. J Am Coll Cardiol. 2017;69:1761–70.
5. Fletcher GF, Ades PA, Kligfield P, Arena R, Balady GJ, Bittner VA, et al. Exercise standards for testing and training: a scientific statement from the American Heart Association. Circulation. 2013;128:873–934.
6. Garner KK, Pomeroy W, Arnold JJ. Exercise stress testing: indications and common questions. Am Fam Physician. 2017;96:293–9.
7. Bourque JM, Beller GA. Value of exercise ECG for risk stratification in suspected or known CAD in the era of advanced imaging technologies. JACC Cardiovasc Imaging. 2015;8:1309–21.
8. Gibbons RJ, Balady GJ, Bricker JT, Chaitman BR, Fletcher GF, Froelicher VF, et al. ACC/AHA 2002 guideline update for exercise testing: summary article. A report of the American College of Cardiology/American Heart Association Task Force on Practice Guidelines (Committee to Update the 1997 Exercise Testing Guidelines). J Am Coll Cardiol. 2002;40:1531–40.
9. Okin PM, Bergman G, Kligfield P. Effect of ST segment measurement point on performance of standard and heart rate-adjusted ST segment criteria for the identification of coronary artery disease. Circulation. 1991;84:57–66.
10. Gianrossi R, Detrano R, Mulvihill D, Lehmann K, Dubach P, Colombo A, et al. Exercise-induced ST depression in the diagnosis of coronary artery disease. A meta-analysis. Circulation. 1989;80:87–98.
11. Stuart RJ, Ellestad MH. Upsloping S-T segments in exercise stress testing. Six year follow-up study of 438 patients and correlation with 248 angiograms. Am J Cardiol. 1976;37:19–22.
12. Beinart R, Matetzky S, Shechter M, Fefer P, Rozen E, Beinart T, et al. Stress-induced ST-segment elevation in patients without prior Q-wave myocardial infarction. J Electrocardiol. 2008;41:312–7.
13. Widlansky S, McHenry PL, Corya BC, Phillips JF. Coronary angiographic, echocardiographic, and electrocardiographic studies on a patient with variant angina due to coronary artery spasm. Am Heart J. 1975;90:631–5.
14. Beckerman J, Mathur A, Stahr S, Myers J, Chun S, Froelicher V. Exercise-induced ventricular arrhythmias and cardiovascular death. Ann Noninvasive Electrocardiol. 2005;10:47–52.
15. Gulati M, Black HR, Shaw LJ, Arnsdorf MF, Merz CN, Lauer MS, et al. The prognostic value of a nomogram for exercise capacity in women. N Engl J Med. 2005;353:468–75.

16. Morris CK, Morrow K, Froelicher VF, Hideg A, Hunter D, Kawaguchi T, et al. Prediction of cardiovascular death by means of clinical and exercise test variables in patients selected for cardiac catheterization. Am Heart J. 1993;125:1717–26.
17. Goldschlager N, Selzer A, Cohn K. Treadmill stress tests as indicators of presence and severity of coronary artery disease. Ann Intern Med. 1976;85:277–86.
18. Dewey FE, Kapoor JR, Williams RS, Lipinski MJ, Ashley EA, Hadley D, et al. Ventricular arrhythmias during clinical treadmill testing and prognosis. Arch Intern Med. 2008;168:225–34.
19. Mark DB, Shaw L, Harrell FE Jr, Hlatky MA, Lee KL, Bengtson JR, et al. Prognostic value of a treadmill exercise score in outpatients with suspected coronary artery disease. N Engl J Med. 1991;325:849–53.
20. Picano E. Stress echocardiography. 6th ed. Heidelberg: Springer Verlag; 2015.
21. Picano E. Dipyridamole-echocardiography test: historical background and physiologic basis. Eur Heart J. 1989;10:365–76.
22. Lang RM, Bierig M, Devereux RB, Flachskampf FA, Foster E, Pellikka PA, et al. Recommendations for chamber quantification: a report from the American Society of Echocardiography's guidelines and Standards Committee and the Chamber quantification Writing group, developed in conjunction with the European Association of echocardiography, a branch of the European Society of Cardiology. J Am Soc Echocardiogr. 2005;18:1440–63.
23. Nihoyannopoulos P, Kaski J-C, Crake T, Maseri A. Absence of myocardial dysfunction during stress in patients with syndrome X. J Am Coll Cardiol. 1991;18:1463–70.
24. Montalescot G, Sechtem U, Achenbach S, Andreotti F, Arden C, Budaj A, et al. 2013 ESC guidelines on the management of stable coronary artery disease: the Task Force on the management of stable coronary artery disease of the European Society of Cardiology. Eur Heart J. 2013;34:2949–3003.
25. Heijenbrok-Kal MH, Fleischmann KE, Hunink MG. Stress echocardiography, stress single-photon-emission computed tomography and electron beam computed tomography for the assessment of coronary artery disease: a meta-analysis of diagnostic performance. Am Heart J. 2007;154:415–23.
26. Severi S, Picano E, Michelassi C, Lattanzi F, Landi P, Distante A, et al. Diagnostic and prognostic value of dipyridamole echocardiography in patients with suspected coronary artery disease. Comparison with exercise electrocardiography. Circulation. 1994;89:1160–73.
27. Sicari R, Nihoyannopoulos P, Evangelista A, Kasprzak J, Lancellotti P, Poldermans D, et al. Stress echocardiography expert consensus statement. Eur J Echocardiogr. 2008;9:415–37.
28. Lattanzi F, Picano E, Bolognese L, Piccinino C, Sarasso G, Orlandini A, et al. Inhibition of dipyridamole-induced ischemia by antianginal therapy in humans. Correlation with exercise electrocardiography. Circulation. 1991;83:1256–62.
29. Yao SS, Qureshi E, Sherrid MV, Chaudhry FA. Practical applications in stress echocardiography: risk stratification and prognosis in patients with known or suspected ischemic heart disease. J Am Coll Cardiol. 2003;42:1084–90.
30. Marwick TH, Case C, Sawada S, Rimmerman C, Brenneman P, Kovacs R, et al. Prediction of mortality using dobutamine echocardiography. J Am Coll Cardiol. 2001;37:754–60.
31. Marwick TH, Case C, Vasey C, Allen S, Short L, Thomas JD. Prediction of mortality by exercise echocardiography: a strategy for combination with the Duke treadmill score. Circulation. 2001;103:2566–71.
32. McCully RB, Roger VL, Mahoney DW, Karon BL, Oh JK, Miller FA Jr, et al. Outcome after normal exercise echocardiography and predictors of subsequent cardiac events: follow-up of 1,325 patients. J Am Coll Cardiol. 1998;31:144–9.
33. McCully RB, Ommen SR, Klarich KW, Burger KN, Mahoney DW, Pellikka PA. Prognosis of patients with good exercise capacity and mildly abnormal exercise echocardiography results: identification of an at-risk subgroup. J Am Soc Echocardiogr. 2005;18:644–8.

34. McCully RB, Roger VL, Ommen SR, Mahoney DW, Burger KN, Freeman WK, et al. Outcomes of patients with reduced exercise capacity at time of exercise echocardiography. Mayo Clin Proc. 2004;79:750–7.
35. Elhendy A, Mahoney DW, Khandheria BK, Burger K, Pellikka PA. Prognostic significance of impairment of heart rate response to exercise: impact of left ventricular function and myocardial ischemia. J Am Coll Cardiol. 2003;42:823–30.
36. Arruda-Olson A, Juracan E, Mahoney D, McCully R, Roger V, Pellikka P. Prognostic value of exercise echocardiography in 5,798 patients: is there a gender difference? J Am Coll Cardiol. 2002;39:625–31.
37. Smart SC, Sawada S, Ryan T, Segar D, Atherton L, Berkovitz K, et al. Low-dose dobutamine echocardiography detects reversible dysfunction after thrombolytic therapy of acute myocardial infarction. Circulation. 1993;88:405–15.
38. Bax JJ, Cornel JH, Visser FC, Fioretti PM, van Lingen A, Reijs AE, et al. Prediction of recovery of myocardial dysfunction after revascularization. Comparison of fluorine-18 fluorodeoxyglucose/thallium-201 SPECT, thallium-201 stress-reinjection SPECT and dobutamine echocardiography. J Am Coll Cardiol. 1996;28:558–64.
39. Bax JJ, Wijns W, Cornel JH, Visser FC, Boersma E, Fioretti PM. Accuracy of currently available techniques for prediction of functional recovery after revascularization in patients with left ventricular dysfunction due to chronic coronary artery disease: comparison of pooled data. J Am Coll Cardiol. 1997;30:1451–60.
40. Picano E, Pingitore A, Conti U, Kozàkovà M, Boem A, Cabani E, et al. Enhanced sensitivity for detection of coronary artery disease by addition of atropine to dipyridamole echocardiography. Eur Heart J. 1993;14:1216–22.
41. Dal Porto R, Faletra F, Picano E, Pirelli S, Moreo A, Varga A. Safety, feasibility, and diagnostic accuracy of accelerated high-dose dipyridamole stress echocardiography. Am J Cardiol. 2001;87:520–4.
42. Zoghbi WA, Cheirif J, Kleiman NS, Verani MS, Trakhtenbroit A. Diagnosis ofischemic heart disease with adenosine echocardiography. J Am Coll Cardiol. 1991;18:1271–9.
43. Hoffer EP, Dewe W, Celentano C, Pierard LA. Low-level exercise echocardiography detects contractile reserve and predicts reversible dysfunction after acute myocardial infarction: comparison with low-dose dobutamine echocardiography. J Am Coll Cardiol. 1999;34:989–97.
44. Lu C, Carlino M, Fragasso G, Maisano F, Margonato A, Cappelletti A, et al. Enoximone echocardiography for predicting recovery of left ventricular dysfunction after revascularization: a novel test for detecting myocardial viability. Circulation. 2000;101:1255–60.
45. Ghio S, Constantin C, Raineri C, Fontana A, Klersy C, Campana C, et al. Enoximone echocardiography: a novel test to evaluate left ventricular contractile reserve in patients with heart failure on chronic betablocker therapy. Cardiovasc Ultrasound. 2003;1:13.
46. Mahajan N, Polavaram L, Vankayala H, Ference B, Wang Y, Ager J, et al. Diagnostic accuracy of myocardial perfusion imaging and stress echocardiography for the diagnosis of left main and triple vessel coronary artery disease: a comparative meta-analysis. Heart. 2010;96:956–66.
47. Picano E, Molinaro S, Pasanisi E. The diagnostic accuracy of pharmacological stress echocardiography for the assessment of coronary artery disease: a meta-analysis. Cardiovasc Ultrasound. 2008;6:30.
48. Pellikka PA, Arruda-Olson A, Chaudhry FA, Chen MH, Marshall JE, Porter TR, et al. Guidelines for performance, interpretation, and application of stress echocardiography in ischemic heart disease: from the American Society of Echocardiography. J Am Soc Echocardiogr. 2020;33:1–41.
49. Watson DD, Glover DK. Overview of tracer kinetics and cellular mechanisms of uptake. In: Zaret BL, Beller GA, editors. Clinical nuclear cardiology. 4th ed. Elsevier: Mosby; 2020. p. 3–13.
50. Grunwald AM, Watson DD, Holzgrefe HH Jr, Irving JF, Beller GA. Myocardial thallium-201 kinetics in normal and ischemic myocardium. Circulation. 1981;64:610–8.

51. Beller GA, Holzgrefe HH, Watson DD. Effects of dipyridamole-induced vasodilation on myocardial uptake and clearance kinetics of thallium-201. Circulation. 1983;68:1328–38.
52. Pohost GM, Zir LM, Moore RH, McKusick KA, Guiney TE, Beller GA. Differentiation of transiently ischemic myocardium from infracted myocardium by serial imaging after a single dose of thallium-201. Circulation. 1977;55:294–302.
53. Klocke FJ, Baird MG, Lorell BH, Bateman TM, Messer JV, Berman DS, et al. ACC/AHA/ASNC guidelines for the clinical use of cardiac radionuclide imaging—executive summary: a report of the American College of Cardiology/American Heart Association Task Force on Practice Guidelines (ACC/AHA/ASNC Committee to Revise the 1995 Guidelines for the Clinical Use of Cardiac Radionuclide Imaging). Circulation. 2003;108:1404–18.
54. Sharir T, Germano G, Kavanagh PB, Shenan L, Cohen I, Lewin HC, et al. Incremental prognostic value of poststress left ventricular ejection fraction and volume by gated myocardial perfusion single photon emission computed tomography. Circulation. 1999;100:1035–42.
55. Shaw LJ, Iskandrian AE. Prognostic value of gated myocardial perfusion SPECT. J Nucl Cardiol. 2004;11:171–85.
56. Hachamovitch R, Berman DS, Kiat H, Cohen I, Friedman JD, Shaw LJ. Value of stress myocardial perfusion single photon emission computed tomography in patients with normal resting electrocardiograms: an evaluation of incremental prognostic value and cost-effectiveness. Circulation. 2002;105:823–9.
57. Bourque JM, Holland BH, Watson DD, Beller GA. Achieving an exercise workload of ≥10 metabolic equivalents predicts a very low risk of inducible ischemia: does myocardial perfusion imaging have a role? J Am Coll Cardiol. 2009;54:538–45.
58. Hachamovitch R, Hayes SW, Friedman JD, Cohen I, Berman DS. Comparison of the short-term survival benefit associated with revascularization compared with medical therapy in patients with no prior coronary artery disease undergoing stress myocardial perfusion single photon emission tomography. Circulation. 2003;107:2900–7.
59. Lima RS, Watson DD, Goode AR, Siadaty MS, Ragosta M, Beller GA, et al. Incremental value of combined perfusion and function over perfusion alone by gated SPECT myocardial perfusion imaging for detection of severe three vessel coronary artery disease. J Am Coll Cardiol. 2003;42:64–70.
60. Anand DV, Lim E, Hopkins D, Corder R, Shaw LJ, Sharp P, et al. Risk stratification in uncomplicated type 2 diabetes: prospective evaluation of the combined use of coronary artery calcium imaging and selective myocardial perfusion scintigraphy. Eur Heart J. 2006;27:713–21.
61. Greenland P, Alpert JS, Beller GA, Benjamin EJ, Budoff MJ, Fayad ZA, et al. 2010 ACCF/AHA guideline for assessment of cardiovascular risk in asymptomatic adults: executive summary: a report of the American College of Cardiology Foundation/American Heart Association Task Force on Practice Guidelines. J Am Coll Cardiol. 2010;56:2182–99.
62. Guazzi M, Arena R, Halle M, Piepoli MF, Myers J, Lavie CJ. 2016 focused update: clinical recommendations for cardiopulmonary exercise testing data assessment in specific patient populations. Circulation. 2016;133:e694–711.
63. Guazzi M, Bandera F, Ozemek C, Systrom D, Arena R. Cardiopulmonary exercise testing: what is its value? J Am Coll Cardiol. 2017;70:1618–36.
64. Chaudhry S, Arena R, Bhatt DL, Verma S, Kumar N. A practical clinical approach to utilize cardiopulmonary exercise testing in the evaluation and management of coronary artery disease: a primer for cardiologists. Curr Opin Cardiol. 2018;33:168–77.
65. Chaudhry S, Kumar N, Behbahani H, Bagai A, Singh BK, Menasco N, et al. Abnormal heart-rate response during cardiopulmonary exercise testing identifies cardiac dysfunction in symptomatic patients with non-obstructive coronary artery disease. Int J Cardiol. 2017;228:114–21.

66. Belardinelli R, Lacalaprice F, Carle F, Minnucci A, Cianci G, Perna G, et al. Exercise-induced myocardial ischaemia detected by cardiopulmonary exercise testing. Eur Heart J. 2003;24:1304–13.
67. Belardinelli R, Lacalaprice F, Tiano L, Mucai A, Perna GP. Cardiopulmonary exercise testing is more accurate than ECG-stress testing in diagnosing myocardial ischemia in subjects with chest pain. Int J Cardiol. 2014;174:337–42.
68. Ross R, Blair SN, Arena R, Church TS, Despres JP, Franklin BA, et al. Importance of assessing cardiorespiratory fitness in clinical practice: a case for fitness as a clinical vital sign: a scientific statement from the American Heart Association. Circulation. 2016;134:e653–e99.
69. Khan H, Jaffar N, Rauramaa R, Kurl S, Savonen K, Laukkanen JA. Cardiorespiratory fitness and nonfatal cardiovascular events: a population-based follow-up study. Am Heart J. 2017;184:55–61.
70. Kavanagh T, Mertens DJ, Hamm LF, Beyene J, Kennedy J, Corey P, et al. Prediction of long-term prognosis in 12 169 men referred for cardiac rehabilitation. Circulation. 2002;106:666–71.
71. Kavanagh T, Mertens DJ, Hamm LF, Beyene J, Kennedy J, Corey P, et al. Peak oxygen intake and cardiac mortality in women referred for cardiac rehabilitation. J Am Coll Cardiol. 2003;42:2139–43.
72. Pauly DF, Johnson BD, Anderson RD, Handberg EM, Smith KM, Cooper-DeHoff RM, et al. In women with symptoms of cardiac ischemia, nonobstructive coronary arteries, and microvascular dysfunction, angiotensin-converting enzyme inhibition is associated with improved microvascular function: a double-blind randomized study from the National Heart, Lung and Blood Institute Women's Ischemia Syndrome Evaluation (WISE). Am Heart J. 2011;162:678–84.
73. Chaudhry S, Arena R, Wasserman K, Hansen JE, Lewis GD, Myers J, et al. The utility of cardiopulmonary exercise testing in the assessment of suspected microvascular ischemia. Int J Cardiol. 2011;148:e7–9.
74. Pavia L, Orlando G, Myers J, Maestri M, Rusconi C. The effect of beta-blockade therapy on the response to exercise training in postmyocardial infarction patients. Clin Cardiol. 1995;18:716–20.
75. Rozenbaum Z, Khoury S, Aviram G, Gura Y, Sherez J, Man A, et al. Discriminating circulatory problems from deconditioning: echocardiographic and cardiopulmonary exercise test analysis. Chest. 2017;151:431–40.
76. Contini M, Andreini D, Agostoni P. Cardiopulmonary exercise test evidence of isolated right coronary artery disease. Int J Cardiol. 2006;113:281–2.
77. Kwok Y, Kim C, Grady D, Segal M, Redberg R. Meta-analysis of exercise testing to detect coronary artery disease in women. Am J Cardiol. 1999;83:660–6.
78. Valeti US, Miller TD, Hodge DO, Gibbons RJ. Exercise single-photon emission computed tomography provides effective risk stratification of elderly men and elderly women. Circulation. 2005;111:1771–6.
79. Iskandrian AS, Heo J, Decoskey D, Askenase A, Segal BL. Use of exercise thallium-201 imaging for risk stratification of elderly patients with coronary artery disease. Am J Cardiol. 1988;61:269–72.
80. Albers AR, Krichavsky MZ, Balady GJ. Stress testing in patients with diabetes mellitus: diagnostic and prognostic value. Circulation. 2006;113:583–92.
81. Lee DP, Fearon WF, Froelicher VF. Clinical utility of the exercise ECG in patients with diabetes and chest pain. Chest. 2001;119:1576–81.
82. Wiersma JJ, Verberne HJ, Trip MD, En Holt WL, van Eck-Smit BL, Piek JJ, et al. Prevalence of myocardial ischaemia as assessed with myocardial perfusion scintigraphy in patients with diabetes mellitus type 2 and mild angina symptoms. Eur J Nucl Med Mol Imaging. 2006;33:1468–76.

Echocardiography Evaluation of Ischemic Heart Disease

Antonio Boccellino and Eustachio Agricola

Abbreviations

AMI	Acute myocardial infarction
CAD	Coronary artery disease
CE	Contrast echocardiography
CFR	Coronary flow reserve
CFVR	Coronary flow velocity reserve
ECG	Electrocardiogram
EROA	Effective regurgitant orifice area
ESL	Early systolic lengthening
GLS	Global longitudinal strain
HF	Heart failure
IHD	Ischemic heart disease
LAD	Left anterior descending coronary artery
LCx	Left circumflex
LM	Left main coronary artery

A. Boccellino
Cardiovascular Imaging Unit, Cardiothoracic Department, San Raffaele Hospital, IRCCS, Milan, Italy
e-mail: Boccellino.Antonio@hsr.it

E. Agricola (✉)
Cardiovascular Imaging Unit, Cardiothoracic Department, San Raffaele Hospital, IRCCS, Milan, Italy

Vita-Salute San Raffaele University, Milan, Italy
e-mail: agricola.eustachio@hsr.it

G. Concistrè (ed.), *Ischemic Heart Disease*,
https://doi.org/10.1007/978-3-031-25879-4_12

LV	Left ventricle
LVO	LV opacification
MCE	Myocardial contrast echocardiography
MR	Mitral regurgitation
MW	Myocardial work
PDA	Posterior descending branch
PL	Posterolateral
PMR	Papillary muscle rupture
PSS	Postsystolic shortening
RCA	Right coronary artery
RegFr	Regurgitant fractions
RV	Right ventricle
RWMA	Regional wall motion abnormality
SE	Stress echocardiography
STE	Speckle tracking echocardiography
TAPSE	Tricuspid annular plane systolic excursion
TDI	Tissue Doppler imaging
TOE	Transesophageal echocardiography
WMSI	Wall motion score index

1 Echocardiographic Assessment of Myocardial Ischemia

1.1 Coronary Artery Anatomy

The LAD coronary artery branches off the LM coronary artery and supplies the major portion of the LV. Its diagonal branches perfuse the entire anterior wall, and its septal branches supply the anterior septum. The LAD continues distally until the tip of the LV to supply the apex. Ischemia may impair the motion of basal and mid-cavity segments of anterior septum and anterior wall, apical segments of the septum and anterior wall, and apical cap. Depending on which diagonal branches supply the lateral wall, the basal and mid-cavity segments of anterolateral wall and the apical lateral segment may be involved. If the LAD artery extends around the apex, also the inferior apical segment may be affected.

The LCx artery branches off the LM coronary artery, runs in the left atrioventricular groove, and, via its obtuse marginal branches, perfuses the basal and mid-cavity segments of the anterolateral and inferolateral walls and the apical lateral segment.

The RCA originates from the aortic right coronary sinus and travels anteriorly around the right atrioventricular groove at the base of the heart. Its proximal branches, acute marginal branches, supply the RV. Once it reaches the posterior interventricular groove, the right PDA runs in the groove towards the apex and supplies the basal and mid-cavity segments of the inferior septum and inferior wall in approximately 85% of the general population (referred to as "right-dominant"). In approximately 15% of the population termed "left-dominant," the left PDA originates from the LCx. In some cases, the PDA extends around the apex to supply the apical segment of the anterior wall. The remainder of the RCA may travel further along the left atrioventricular groove as right PL branch. In most individuals, this is a minor branch, but in some patients (referred to as "super right-dominant"), the right PL branch is large and supplies the territory usually supplied by the LCx.

1.2 Pathophysiology of Myocardial Ischemia

As a consequence of the interruption in coronary blood flow, pathophysiologic changes occur in a well-defined time sequence (described as the "ischemic cascade") [1]. Resting blood flow may be preserved until a coronary artery stenosis approaches a 90% diameter narrowing. At lesser stenosis degree, the CFR may be reduced leading to an oxygen supply-demand mismatch and subsequent myocardial ischemia (during stress). This inadequate increase in blood flow leads to a sequential reduction in myocardial perfusion, reduced myocardial systolic strain, RWMA, ECG changes, and symptoms eventually [1]. This translates clinically into a gradient of sensitivity of the available clinical markers and imaging modalities for ischemia detection, with regional perfusion being the most and chest pain the least sensitive markers. Regardless of the stress used, ischemia tends to propagate centrifugally with respect to the ventricular cavity involving primarily the subendocardial layer and finally the subepicardial layer [2]. Indeed, extravascular pressure is higher in the subendocardial than in the subepicardial layer; this provokes a higher metabolic demand and an increased resistance to flow [3]. In the absence of CAD, CFR can be reduced in microvascular disease. In this condition, regional perfusion changes, angina, and ST-segment depression can occur usually in the absence of any RWMA during stress [2].

After a prolonged period of ischemia due to transient occlusion of blood flow with minimal infarction, recovery of function of the affected myocardial segments may be delayed due to myocardial stunning [4]. Repetitive episodes of ischemia may also lead to stunning. Myocardial stunning manifests as a persistent RWMA soon after restoration of blood flow, followed by the recovery of contraction over time. In some patients with ischemic LV dysfunction, there may be areas of dysfunctional but viable myocardium that result from a state of chronic reduced coronary flow. These areas of hibernating myocardium can recover the contractile function following revascularization [4]. If severe ischemia persists, myocardial necrosis develops, followed by scarring and permanent dysfunction.

1.3 Stress Echocardiography in Ischemic Heart Disease

SE is a well-established noninvasive technique for diagnosis and risk stratification of patients with IHD [5]. SE requires a high level of expertise to achieve accurate and reproducible results, and it is recognized that performing the technique requires additional training beyond proficiency in transthoracic echocardiography [6]. The advantage of SE is that it can virtually detect each one of the abnormalities that make up the ischemic "cascade": abnormal perfusion, regional wall motion abnormalities, global systolic dysfunction, ECG changes, and symptoms [7].

Physiologic exercise is the preferred method of stress testing for ambulant patients, and this can be achieved either by treadmill exercise or by bicycle ergometry [8]. For treadmill exercise, the Bruce protocol is most commonly used, and the workload achieved provides useful clinical and prognostic information [9]. Imaging under these circumstances is performed at rest and immediately after exercise, allowing a time interval of 90 s to acquire the stress images. Upright or semisupine bicycle ergometry offers the advantage of continuous monitoring of wall motion. However, the test may be limited by suboptimal patient position for image acquisition or leg fatigue, preventing the achievement of target heart rate. Indeed, higher workload is usually evoked by treadmill exercise than bicycle ergometry [8].

Pharmacologic stress testing, using inotropic or vasodilator stress agents, is a suitable alternative for those unable to exercise and provides similar diagnostic accuracy to exercise echocardiography. The stress images can be obtained at a constant and controlled heart rate at peak stress and without the challenges posed by exercise, such as hyperventilation and excessive chest wall movement. Dobutamine is the most widely used stressor agent. It increases heart rate, blood pressure, and myocardial inotropic activity by stimulating α-1, β-1, and β-2 adrenoceptors. The protocol uses a weight-adjusted intravenous continuous infusion [5]. Echocardiographic images are acquired at rest, mid-dose, peak dose, and recovery. Endpoints of the test include achievement of 85% of age-predicted target heart rate, development of cardiac symptoms or ischemia, severe arrhythmias, hypotension, severe hypertension, or intolerable side effects. If target heart rate has not been achieved at maximal dobutamine dose, intravenous atropine may be given to a maximum dose of 2 mg. Short-acting intravenous β-blockade may be needed to reverse the effects of dobutamine. Any rate-limiting medications should be withheld for at least 48 h to achieve target heart rate.

Vasodilator SE is typically performed with either dipyridamole or adenosine (that has a shorter duration of action). Both agents are contraindicated in patients with significant conduction disease and reactive airway obstruction. Under these circumstances, dobutamine may be the stress agent of choice. On the other hand, vasodilators may be safer in those with a history of atrial or ventricular tachyarrhythmias [5]. The standard dipyridamole protocol consists of intravenous infusion of 0.84 mg/kg over 10 min, while standard adenosine protocol consists of infusion of adenosine at a maximum dose of 140 mg/kg/min over 6 min [5, 7].

In patients with a permanent pacemaker, stress testing can be performed by programming the pacing rate to increase every 2–3 min until the target heart rate is achieved. This technique can be used in conjunction with dobutamine to further increase inotropic activity and myocardial oxygen consumption [10].

Four basic responses are possible in SE [11]: (1) Normal response: a segment is normokinetic at rest and normal or hyperkinetic during stress; (2) Ischemic response: the function of a segment worsens during stress from normokinesia to hypokinesia, akinesia, or dyskinesia (paradoxical systolic movement); (3) Necrotic response: an akinetic segment remains fixed during stress (a resting akinesia becoming dyskinesia during stress reflects passive phenomenon of increased intraventricular pressure and should not be considered active ischemia); and (4) Viability response: a segment with resting dysfunction may constantly improve during stress indicating myocardial stunning or may show a biphasic response (improvement during early stress with subsequent deterioration at peak), the last suggestive of viability and ischemia (myocardium fed by a coronary with a critically coronary stenosis) [11, 12].

1.4 Assessment of Regional Wall Motion Abnormalities

Analysis of regional wall function must include assessment of the wall thickening rather than just assessment of the extent of wall motion [13]. Indeed, it is recognized that myocardial movements may be caused by adjacent segment tethering or LV displacement. The LV is divided along the long-axis plane into six (anterior, anterolateral, inferolateral, inferior, inferior septum, and anterior septum) and in the orthogonal short-axis plane into thirds (basal, mid-cavity, and apical) with an additional single distal apical cap segment. The cumulative result is the 17-segment model used by most cardiac imaging modalities [13]. Optimally, both long- and short-axis images of the heart should be inspected, from base to apex, in multiple windows to evaluate all segments. The function of each segment is graded at rest and with stress according to a 5-point scoring system. Scores are as follows: normal or hyperkinesis = 1 (systolic increase in thickness >40%); hypokinesis = 2 (<40%); severe hypokinesis or akinesis = 3 (<10%); dyskinesis (paradoxical systolic motion away from the center of the LV) = 4; and aneurysmal (diastolic deformation) = 5 [14]. The WMSI should be derived by dividing the sum of the scores of individual segments by the number of segments visualized. In normal nonischemic myocardium, WMSI equals 1 (Fig. 1).

The development of RWMA during early stages of stress indicates the presence of severe coronary stenosis [15], and the persistence of abnormalities in the recovery period may represent stunning and indicates more severe ischemia [16]. A severe resting RWMA with no change with stress (including no biphasic response) is considered a fixed wall motion response and represents a transmurally infarcted region.

Assessment of RV lateral wall motion (better by dedicated RV view), primarily supplied by the marginal branches of the RCA, either by measurement of TAPSE or by peak

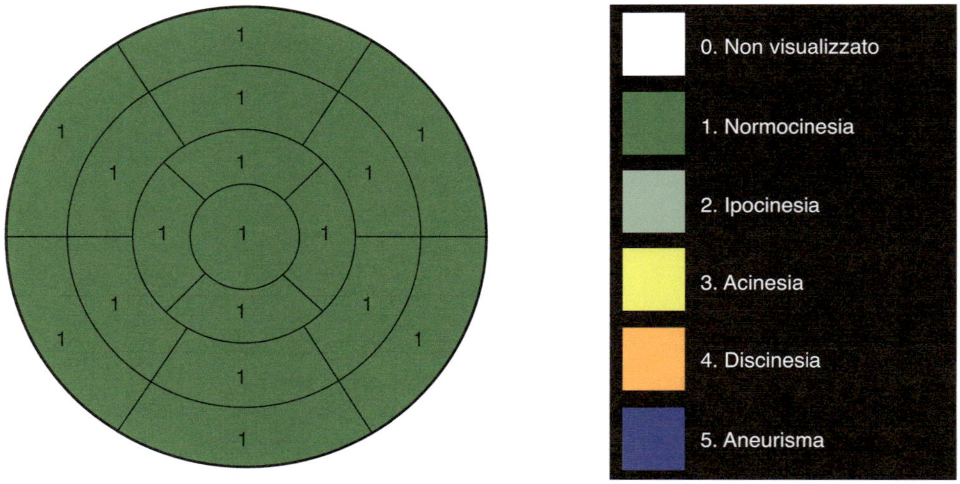

Fig. 1 Bull's-eye representation of the 17-segment model in a normal patient (WMSI = 1)

systolic velocity by TDI, can be useful for detection of right CAD [17, 18]. A decline in TAPSE of >4 mm with exercise has reasonable sensitivity for proximal RCA critical stenosis [5].

1.4.1 Assessment of Coronary Flow Velocity Reserve

CFVR represents the ratio between maximal coronary blood flow, induced by coronary vasodilators (adenosine or dipyridamole), and resting blood flow. Ideally, all three coronary arteries could be visualized by TTE, but the LAD is the more technically feasible to investigate (90% of cases in experienced hands). Blood flow velocity is measured by PW Doppler echocardiography, using a sample volume of 3–4 mm, placed on the color signal in the LAD, in a low parasternal long-axis view and/or modified apical two-, three-, or four-chamber views [19] (Fig. 2). Like the invasive fractional flow reserve, the TTE-derived CFVR reflects the coronary atherosclerotic burden and the status of the microvasculature. The functional significance of a stenosis is best evaluated by the coronary flow in the tract distal to the lesion, as proximally to the stenosis CFVR can be normal (because of the existence of side coronary branches). In contrast to wall motion analysis which is qualitative or semiquantitative and sometimes difficult to interpret, TTE-derived CFVR provides a quantitative interpretation of a Doppler signal. The CFVR value ≤2, measuring the diastolic velocity of the PW Doppler signal, is the best cutoff value for detecting a significant epicardial coronary stenosis [20] (Fig. 2). TTE-derived CFVR is a bedside test, safe and reproducible, and, compared to other tests, less time consuming, without irradiation, and can be regularly repeated without additional risk to patients.

Dual-imaging vasodilator stress echocardiography is an independent predictor of death conferring useful prognostic information in subjects with CAD (RWMA plus impaired CFR on LAD identifies a patient category with a risk >10% for annual mortality) [21]. In

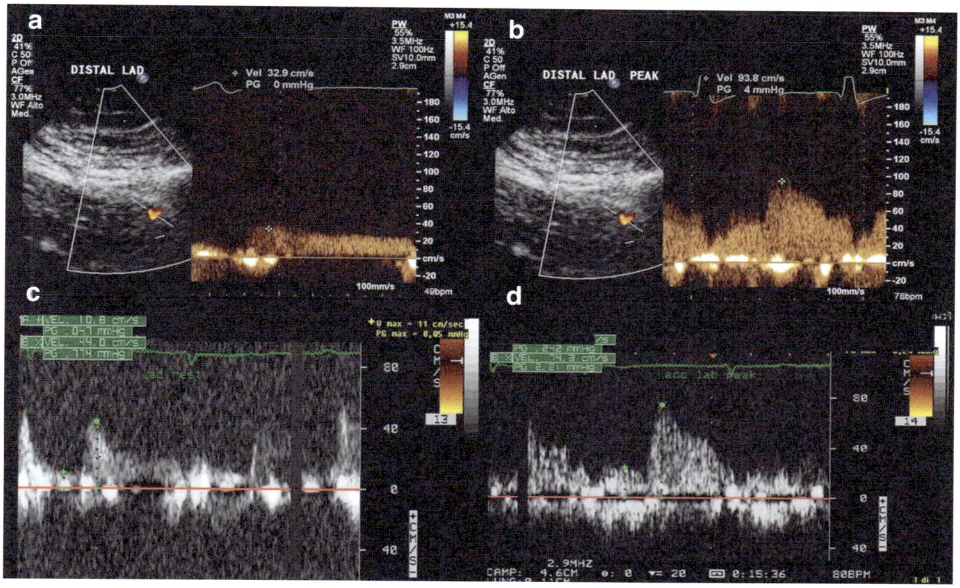

Fig. 2 Pulse-wave Doppler of the left anterior descending artery (LAD). (**a**, **b**) Coronary flow at the distal LAD with normal CFVR (CFVR = 2.8). A rest and B during stress with dipyridamole. (**c**, **d**) Coronary flow at the distal LAD in a patient pathological CFVR (CFVR = 1.7). C rest and D during stress with dipyridamole

patients with proximal LAD or LM stenosis of intermediate severity, the TEE-derived CFVR >2 was shown to be a good prognostic parameter and the deferral of revascularization was associated with low cardiac event rates [22, 23].

The addition of TTE-derived CFVR to standard WM analysis yielded higher values for the prediction of total cardiac events [24]. For these reasons, the combination of conventional WM analysis and CFVR of mid-distal LAD is now the recommended technique during vasodilator stress echocardiography [21].

1.5 Assessment of Viability

The assessment of myocardial viability is important in evaluating patients with chronic ischemic LV dysfunction. Myocardial viability refers to reversible LV systolic dysfunction, which could be secondary to myocardial stunning, myocardial hibernation, or a combination of both. Low-dose DSE is a commonly used method for assessing myocardial viability [25]. Compared to nuclear techniques, dobutamine SE has lower sensitivity, but higher specificity [26, 27], as a larger mass of viable myocytes (at least 50% viable myocytes in a given segment) is required to generate a contractility change compared to scintigraphic methods.

Assessment for viability may provide crucial information for the identification of patients who could possibly benefit from myocardial revascularization. The use of echocardiography in the myocardial viability approach is based on three parameters: wall thickness, contrast enhancement by myocytes, and contractile reserve with inotropic stimulation.

A severe decreased diastolic wall thickness (<70% of the thickness in normal segments or absolute thickness <6 mm) is suggestive of transmural infarction and scar and showed a high negative predictive value for contractile recovery after revascularization [28].

In recent years, the use of myocardial contrast echocardiography (MCE) has increased. Contrast enhancement assesses myocardial perfusion and, subsequently, cellular integrity.

Low-dose dobutamine SE, however, is the most studied and experienced method to access the contractile reserve of a dysfunctional ischemic segment at rest. Low-dose dobutamine (5–10 mcg/kg) is enough to assess the contractile reserve [11]. The possible findings include 1. sustained improvement in function at low dose, which persists at higher doses, suggestive of viable myocardium with no critical stenosis of the coronary artery supplying the region (stunned myocardium); 2. biphasic response: after an initial improvement, contractility worsens at higher doses of dobutamine (20 mcg/kg), highly suggestive of viable myocardium with flow-limiting stenosis of the coronary artery supplying the segment [29–31] (hibernated myocardium); and 3. non-phasic response: no change in function is observed, suggestive of nonviable scarred myocardium. Low-dose dobutamine SE has clinically useful sensitivity (up to 80%) and specificity (up to 85%) for identification of viable hibernated segments that will functionally recover after revascularization [32, 33]. Moreover low-dose dobutamine SE showed good sensitivity and specificity (86% and 90%) for predicting spontaneous functional recovery of a stunned segment after an AMI [34]. Finally, patients with larger area of dysfunctional but viable myocardium (six segments or more) have higher likelihood of LVEF improvement and lower cardiac event rate after revascularization compared to those with minimal or no viable myocardium [35].

1.6 Contrast Echocardiography in Ischemic Heart Disease

CE relies on the administration of acoustically active contrast agents to complement standard echocardiography in many scenarios. Contrast agents approved for clinical use are composed of gas-filled microbubbles encapsulated within a stabilizing exterior lipid shell. The microbubbles administered in humans are smaller than red blood cells, which allows their passage through the pulmonary circulation and distribution throughout the myocardial intravascular compartment after intravenous injection [36].

CE is performed for the assessment of regional and global LV function both at rest and under stress, for the assessment of myocardial perfusion and for the optimal evaluation of LV structures. For assessment of RWMA and myocardial perfusion, a low mechanical index is preferred (MI 0.1) [36]. Several studies have demonstrated the ability of ultrasound contrast agents to improve the myocardial border detection and improve study quality and reproducibility [37]. The impact of LVO is particularly relevant in segments that more commonly suffer from poor endocardial discrimination, such as the anterior wall, basal lateral, and basal inferior segments. The ability to ensure that the true LV apex is imaged and not foreshortened is also a valuable contribution of LVO [37]. Contrast 2D echocardiography should be considered when two or more contiguous LV segments are not adequately visualized on non-contrast echocardiography and management of the patient will depend on whether there are RWMA [37].

Following destruction of microbubbles from the myocardium during a brief burst of high-power imaging, contrast replenishment within the myocardium can be observed. A functionally significant stenosis is most likely present when an area of myocardium does not replenish within approximately 2 s after a high MI impulse [38]. CE improves sensitivity of SE by contemporarily improving the detection of RWMA and the identification of perfusion defects [39, 40].

Ultrasound contrast agents increase the accuracy for the detecting of resting RWMA [41]. Performing perfusion imaging when there is already a RWMA allows characterization of the flow status as either complete lack of perfusion, hypoperfusion with some antegrade or collateral flow, or stunning where perfusion has normalized but the RWMA persists [42]. The analysis of myocardial perfusion with MCE during stress has been shown to be more sensitive than RWMA assessment for the detection of moderate stenosis [43]. It has also been shown to be superior to RWMA for determining the area of ischemia and for the detection of multivessel CAD [37, 44].

1.6.1 Risk Stratification and Prognosis

A normal SE (normal wall motion at rest and with stress) is associated with a benign prognosis with a low annual rate of major cardiac events (0.9% per year) [45, 46]. Peak WMSI and LVEF have been identified as the best predictors of cardiac events. Intermediate WMSI (1.1–1.7) and high WMSI (>1.7), as well as an EF <45%, further stratified risk (from 3% per year to 6% per year, respectively, in intermediate- and high-risk patients) [45, 47]. Exercise capacity and heart rate response can be further used in risk stratification. Anti-ischemic therapy modifies the prognostic impact of pharmacological SE. Inducible myocardial ischemia in patients on medical therapy identifies patients at highest risk of fatal cardiac events [48]. Those patients with a negative test on medical therapy or a positive test off medical therapy are at intermediate risk [48]. Patients with transient ischemic dilation (reminding that increase in end-systolic size is more commonly observed with ESE rather than with DSE) had greater extent and severity of RWMA, higher percentage of coronary multivessel disease, and higher adverse event rate compared to patients with ischemia without dilation [49].

RV wall motion analysis should be routinely performed in patients referred for SE for effective risk stratification. RV wall motion analysis provides prognostic value independently of LV ischemia and LVEF and offers incremental value over rest and conventional SE variables. Patients with both abnormal RV and LV have worse outcomes [50].

1.7 Emerging Echocardiographic Approaches to the Assessment of Ischemia

The use of deformation imaging, nowadays mostly using the strain and strain rate derived from STE, allows less subjective evaluation of myocardial contraction as compared to simple visual assessment. The STE replaced techniques based on TDI overcoming its limitations (sensitivity to passive translational movements of the myocardial segments, angle dependence, decrease of myocardial velocities from base to the apex) [51].

The strain and strain rate derived from two-dimensional (2D) STE are based on computer algorithms tracking the movement of "speckles" (acoustic markers generated within the myocardium). These techniques allow evaluation of longitudinal (from apical views), radial, and circumferential (from short-axis views) strains. The technique requires higher frame rates (50–70/s) and a good image quality for accurate tracking. In the normal myocardium, strain and strain rate are nearly homogenously distributed.

In chronic ischemia, despite structural changes such as fibrosis and loss of myocytes, conventional measures of LV contractile function may be unaffected. Indeed, in the early phases, impairment in longitudinal systolic function is known to be compensated by augmentation of circumferential deformation, which can explain why the LVEF is preserved. The myocardial fibers most susceptible to ischemia are the longitudinally orientated fibers that are located in the subendocardium. Measurements of longitudinal motion and deformation are, therefore, sensitive markers of CAD [52, 53] (Fig. 3). Assessment of LV function through measurement of GLS by STE allows detection of early myocardial dysfunction before an explicit reduction in LVEF, thus revealing a subclinical LV dysfunction [54, 55].

To date, stable CAD was the major setting of investigation of STE among the IHD spectrum. Particularly, the importance of the reduction of LV longitudinal strain has been shown with rest and SE in both symptomatic and asymptomatic patients for the prediction of significant CAD (GLS) and detection and localization of ischemic myocardium according to coronary perfusion territories (segmental longitudinal strain) [53, 56, 57] (Fig. 3).

The application of STE to SE is still debated, since its feasibility could be limited by high heart rate and poor acoustic window due to patients' position; moreover, it lacks

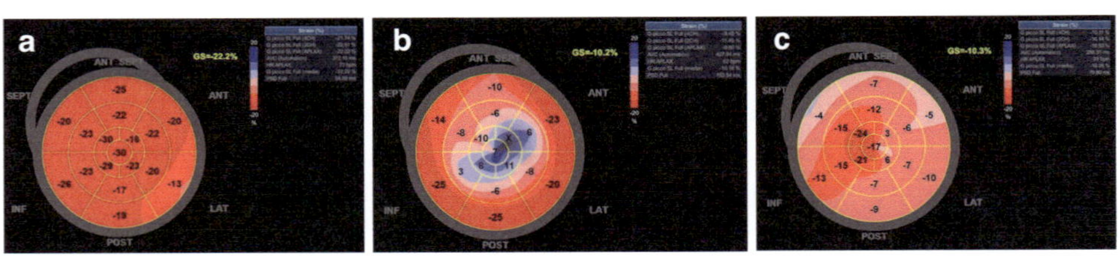

Fig. 3 Peak global longitudinal strain (GLS) in bull's-eye diagram derived by speckle tracking echocardiography. (**a**) Normal patient; (**b**) patient with an extensive apical myocardial infarction resulting from occlusion of the left anterior descending coronary artery; (**c**) patient with a multivessel coronary artery disease

standardization and reference cutoffs and strongly depends on the experience of the operator. However, to date, there are evidences supporting its use in clinical practice [58, 59]. Recovery LV GLS was the strongest predictor of obstructive CAD and was associated with nuclear imaging findings (extent, localization, and depth of myocardial ischemia) [59].

ESL is a novel STE-derived predictor of cardiovascular events defined as the time from the onset of the QRS complex to the peak positive systolic strain [60]. ESL reflects a passive lengthening of an ischemic myocardial region before the beginning of systolic shortening, due to its reduced ability to generate an adequate active force during the pressure increase in the isovolumic contraction phase. ESL may discern between viable and nonviable segments, with akinetic segments displaying significantly higher ESL values [61]. PSS is an STE-derived marker that reflects a longitudinal shortening occurring after aortic valve closure. PSS may be found in ischemic viable myocardium reflecting some degree of active contraction, whereas necrotic myocardium remains passive [62]. PSS provides information about the ischemic burden and is a predictor of major cardiac events in patients with acute MI [63] and chronic CAD [62]. PSS may not be ready to be adopted as a standalone to identify CAD, as it may be found in healthy individuals and, in scar tissue, can represent the passive recoil of adjacent viable segment.

The application of STE to the RV could help in allowing the detection of subtle RV dysfunction. RV strain is a reliable and accurate tool for the evaluation of RV systolic function when validated against RVEF assessed by MRI [64]. RV strain is obtained from the apical four-chamber view (the RV free wall has the largest body of evidence). RV strain is useful for the detection of occult RV dysfunction in patients with chronic RCA stenosis [64].

A limitation of strain imaging is load dependency, which can affect the diagnostic accuracy of myocardial function evaluation. The recently proposed MW can overcome these limitations taking into account global and regional deformation as well as afterload through interpretation of strain in relation to LV pressure. Preliminary results have showed an appealing usefulness of MW in predicting critical coronary artery stenosis in patients with CAD [65].

2D echocardiography algorithms rely on geometric assumptions about the LV shape and have limitations in asymmetric or aneurysmal left ventricles. Conversely, 3-dimensional (3D) echocardiography overcomes these limitations limiting the foreshortening of apex and analyzing all the amount of LV myocardium with increased reproducibility and accuracy [66]. Therefore, the recent guidelines for cardiac chamber quantification with echocardiography advice the 3D measurement of LV volumes and LVEF [13, 14]. Indeed, when measured by 3D echocardiography, volumes and LVEF are comparable to those assessed by cardiac MRI [67]. The 3D acquisitions during DSE could be useful by allowing more accurate assessment of LV volume and EF, especially in patients with resting WMA and aneurysm (Fig. 4). With its ability to acquire the entire LV volume in a single beat, 3D SE may become a reference standard in the evaluation of patients with suspected IHD. However, the 3D image quality is greatly dependent on the 2D image and on the ability to obtain artifact-free 3D datasets. The advantages of 3D SE in comparison to

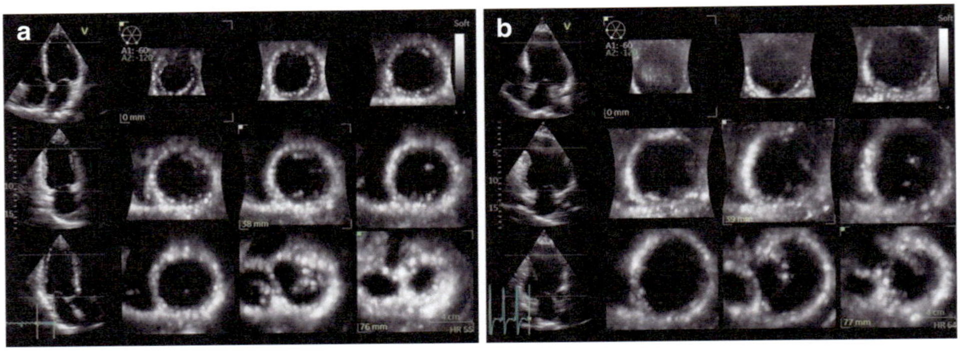

Fig. 4 Multi-slice display of the left ventricle (LV) derived by 3D full-volume datasets. (**a**) Normal patient; (**b**) patient with ischemic heart disease complicated by dilation of the LV and apical aneurysm

conventional 2D SE for detecting myocardial ischemia both during exercise and pharmacological stress have been evaluated and validated in a few studies [68]. Moreover, an integrated 2D/3D contrast-enhanced dobutamine SE is technically feasible and showed the best prognostic value for acute cardiac events in a large contemporary study [69].

Recently, a new standard of practice in stress echocardiography, the ABCDE protocol, has been proposed, merging five different parameters with different pathophysiological targets [70]. It allows the assessment of inducible myocardial ischemia (step A), pulmonary congestion (step B), contractile reserve (step C), CFVR (step D), and cardiac sympathetic reserve (step E). Step A includes assessment of RWMA as previously described. Step B of the protocol includes the assessment of B lines with lung ultrasound by scan from midaxillary to midclavicular lines on the third intercostal space, each site scored from 0 (normal horizontal A lines) to 10 (white lung with coalescent B lines) [71, 72]. Step C includes the assessment of LV contractile reserve as the stress/rest ratio of force (calculated as systolic blood pressure/end-systolic volume). Step D includes calculation of CFVR as previously described. Step E includes the assessment of heart rate reserve, calculated as the peak/rest heart rate from 12-leads ECG [71]. The ABCDE-SE protocol can detect sources of vulnerability of the patient with CAD other than RWMA [71, 73]. Each pathophysiological variable contributes independently and incrementally to the prognosis of the individual patient as the outcome progressively worsens with the increasing number of abnormal steps [71].

2 Echocardiographic Assessment of Myocardial Infarction

2.1 Diagnosis of Myocardial Infarction

Myocardial infarction is defined as an injury to the myocardium due to prolonged ischemia, usually secondary to acute thrombotic occlusion of an epicardial coronary artery. Diagnosis of an acute MI is typically based upon the history, ECG, and serum troponins

[74]. In the acute setting, echocardiography enables fast evaluation of global ventricular function and hemodynamic status of the patients, and detection of RWMA caused by ischemia [75, 76]. In addition, it is useful in excluding other possible causes of acute chest pain, such as aortic dissection, massive pulmonary embolism, aortic stenosis, hypertrophic cardiomyopathy, and pericardial effusion [76]. Evaluation of RWMA while a patient is experiencing chest pain can be useful when the ECG is nondiagnostic; evaluation of RWMA may also be useful if there is ECG or laboratory evidence of AMI in the absence of chest pain [76]. The myocardial segments affected and the echocardiographic views for the assessment of myocardial infarction are the same as described for the evaluation of myocardial ischemia. During AMI, affected segments could appear hypo- or akinetic while the unaffected walls could be hyperkinetic (raising the risk of acute dynamic left ventricular outflow tract obstruction). Moreover, echocardiography is essential to access RV dysfunction. RV MI occurs in one-third to one-half of patients presenting with inferior MI and cause RV dilation, depressed RV systolic function, and RV akinesia or dyskinesia [77]. RV akinesia or dyskinesia was found to be a surrogate marker of hemodynamically significant RV MI [78].

2.2 Mechanical Complications of MI

Acute mitral regurgitation in the setting of MI can be secondary to papillary muscle dysfunction, abnormal wall motion of the segment underlying a papillary muscle, or papillary muscle rupture (Fig. 5). The anterolateral (AL) papillary muscle receives a dual blood supply from both the LAD and LCx, while the posteromedial (PM) papillary muscle is supplied only by the PDA (from the LCx artery or the RCA, depending on dominance).

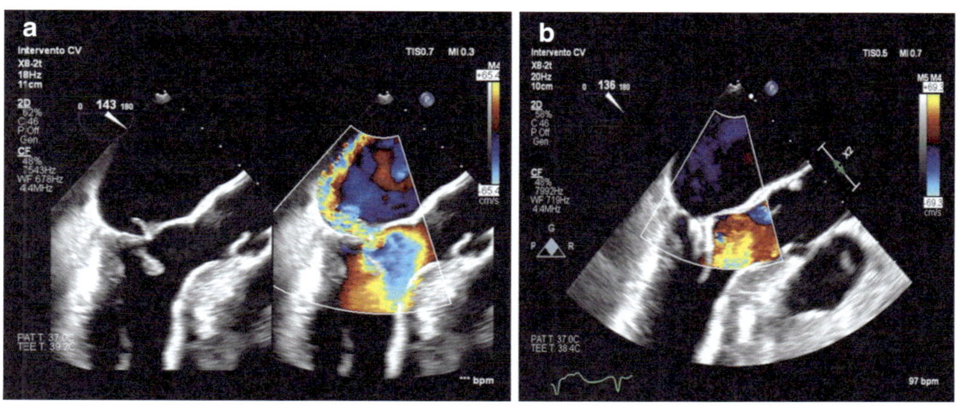

Fig. 5 Rupture of the posteromedial papillary muscle. (**a**) Transesophageal three-chamber view demonstrating the ruptured posteromedial papillary muscle and the flail of the anterior mitral leaflet with severe mitral regurgitation. (**b**) Effective percutaneous mitral valve repair with MitraClip in the same patient

Inferior MI can cause dysfunction of the PM and MR that can resolve entirely following effective revascularization. PMR is a rare (range, 0.05–0.26%) and catastrophic (hospital mortality rate ranges between 10% and 40%) complication of inferior or lateral MI [79]. PMR commonly occurs within 3–5 days after AMI and may be complete or partial, and roughly half of the patients present with progressive severe acute HF. In this setting, TOE has a high diagnostic sensitivity. Although surgical treatment remains the standard for severe MR secondary to PMR, surgical risk may be prohibitive in selected patients and percutaneous mitral valve edge-to-edge repair guided by TOE may be a therapeutic option [80].

Ventricular septal defect (VSD) after MI has an incidence of ≈0.3% and typically occurs 3–5 days after infarction [79] (Fig. 6). VSDs occurring after MI are typically detected by a color-flow jet directed from the left to right ventricle. VSDs may be simple or complex when there are multiple, irregular, and variable interventricular connections. VSDs caused by anterior MIs are typically simple and arise apically, whereas VSDs caused by inferior MIs are complex and usually involve the basal segment of the septum. The jet between the left and right ventricles can be interrogated by continuous-wave Doppler: smaller (restrictive) VSDs will have higher gradients compared to larger (nonrestrictive) VSDs. Moreover, the RV systolic pressure may be calculated by knowing the systolic

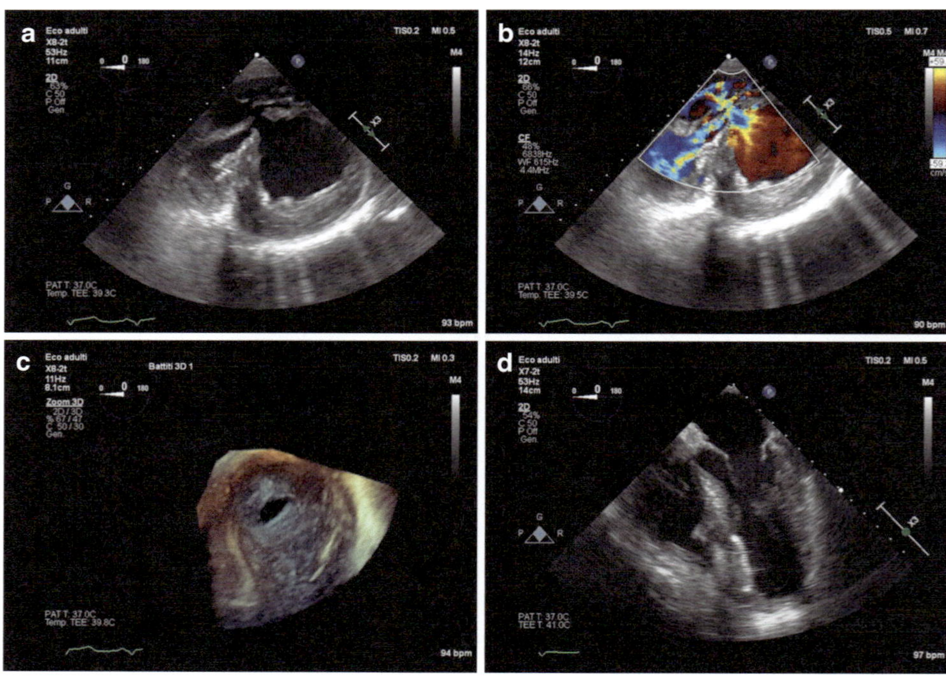

Fig. 6 Post-myocardial infarction ventricular septal defect (VSD). (**a**) Transgastric mid-short-axis view showing the VSD. (**b**) Color-flow jet is directed from the left to right ventricle; (**c**) en face view of VSD by real-time 3D imaging; (**d**) VSD repair with Amplatzer occluder device

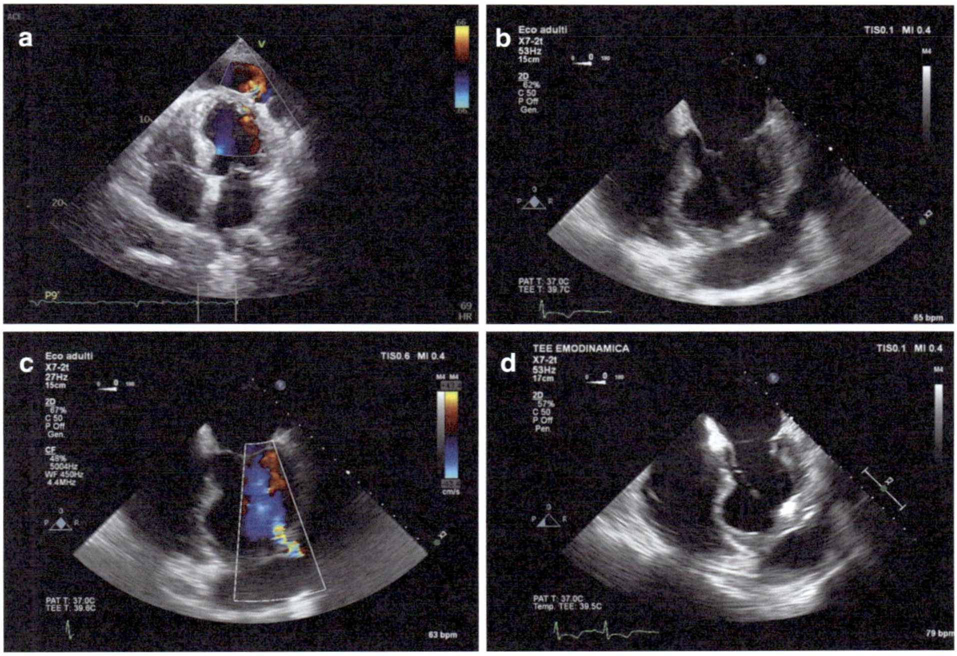

Fig. 7 Left ventricular pseudoaneurysm. (**a**) Transthoracic apical four-chamber view showing blood flow into a cavity contained by pericardium; (**b**, **c**) transesophageal four-chamber view demonstrating a narrow neck connecting the ventricle to the cavity; (**d**) pseudoaneurysm repair with Amplatzer occluder device

blood pressure. Finally, the pulsed-wave Doppler technique allows the noninvasive evaluation of Qp/Qs with a high degree of accuracy [81]. Treatment is generally surgical; in cases where the surgical risk is prohibitive, percutaneous closure with a device, using echocardiographic guidance, can be a valuable alternative [82].

Free wall rupture is a devastating complication of MI, most frequently detected within 5 days post-MI [79]. The findings include an acute pericardial effusion associated with thin and akinetic myocardium. The actual point of rupture may not be easy to demonstrate. Echocardiographic contrast injection may be useful in identifying the rupture [83].

A *pseudoaneurysm* is a discrete ventricular free wall perforation that is locally contained by pericardial adhesions [79] (Fig. 7). Most pseudoaneurysms are found after inferior MIs, and less commonly in the lateral or apical regions. On echocardiogram, they appear as echo-free chambers or spaces adjacent to the LV and can be distinguished from true aneurysms by a narrow neck (specifically less than 50% of the maximum diameter of the aneurysm itself) and the abrupt transition from normal to thinned walls. CE can be helpful in the diagnosis.

LV thrombus formation is a well-recognized complication of MI, tending to occur more commonly after large anterior infarction (up to 25% in patients with anterior MI)

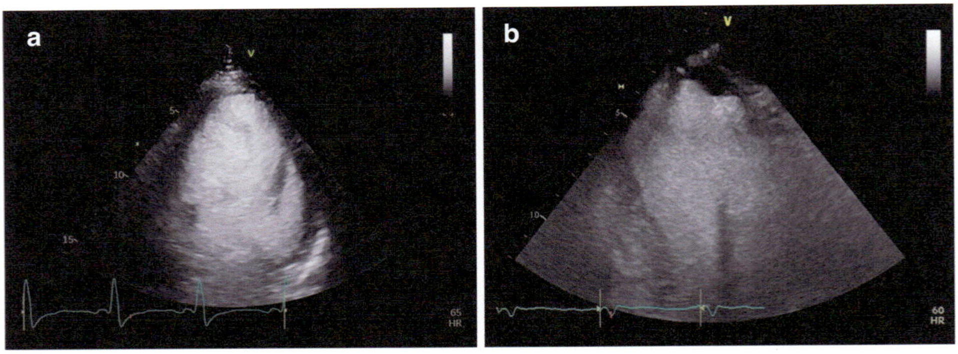

Fig. 8 Use of contrast echocardiography (CE) in the diagnosis of apical mural thrombus. (**a**) Normal control; (**b**) thrombus in the left ventricle as viewed by CE

usually within the first 1–2 weeks after the MI [84]. On echocardiography, thrombus is identified as a discrete echo dense mass with clear margins that are distinct from the endocardium. Thrombus also tends to form over dysfunctional segments. Spontaneous echo contrast can be sometimes visualized. Thrombus can be laminar and nonmobile, showing a flattened appearance, or pedunculated and mobile with a greater likelihood of embolization. On occasion, there may be uncertainty as to whether thrombus is present over the apex, due to difficult echo windows or near-field artifacts. Non-contrast echocardiography has a low sensitivity (approximately 30%) for LV thrombus diagnosis [85] when compared with delayed-enhancement cardiac MRI. In this context, the addition of intravenous contrast to TTE may improve sensitivity (up to 64%), while providing similar specificity [85] (Fig. 8). Cardiac thrombi may be indistinguishable from tumors, especially when occurring adjacent to a normally contracting myocardium. Presence of significant vascularization detected by MCE establishes a cardiac tumor diagnosis [86].

2.3 Prognostic Role of Echocardiography After Acute Myocardial Infarction

Transthoracic echocardiography plays a fundamental role in early risk stratification of patients with AMI. More recently, advanced echocardiography (mainly 2D STE, CE, and 3D echocardiography) has shown to predict long-term adverse outcomes and to provide additional information beyond conventional echocardiographic parameters [87].

LVEF has a very-well-established short-term and long-term prognostic value in this clinical setting. LVEF <40% is an important risk factor for post-discharge mortality and hospital readmission [88]. In addition to LVEF, overall LV size (as assessed by LV end-diastolic volume and diameter) and sphericity are important prognostic indicators [89].

Owing to the compensatory hyperkinesia of normal myocardial segments, LVEF may underestimate the true amount of myocardial damage after AMI. In patients with preserved LVEF, assessment of RWMA is useful as a predischarge resting WMSI >1.50 was prognostically superior to LVEF in identifying patients at risk for post-AMI cardiac events [90]. Other measurements independently predictive of HF include significant diastolic dysfunction (restrictive filling pattern or E/e' >15 predischarge), left atrial volume index >32 mL/m^2, and pulmonary artery systolic pressure >35 mmHg. RV systolic function by RV fractional area (RVFAC <32%) independently predicted hard endpoints post-AMI [91].

GLS has shown an incremental value for risk stratification after AMI. Impaired systolic GLS was independently associated with cardiac endpoints irrespective of LVEF and volumes [92, 93]. Moreover, sophisticated measures derived by STE may have a prognostic role. High value of mechanical dispersion (MD ≥75 ms) was found highly predictive of ventricular arrhythmias and sudden cardiac death in patients with moderate and severe LV systolic dysfunction [94, 95]. The assessment of RV myocardial function by RV free wall LS has shown a prognostic value after AMI [91].

SE performed early after AMI has been demonstrated to predict the recovery of global and regional systolic function [87, 96, 97]. STE applied to low-dose dobutamine SE after AMI appears to be promising for prediction of LV functional recovery, also in the presence of normal LVEF.

In the setting of acute MI, MCE could be useful in the recognition of the no-reflow phenomenon after revascularization (similar to MRI, but with the advantages of lower cost and performance at the bedside in a coronary care unit) and to predict LV remodeling and cardiac endpoints [98].

The role of 3D echocardiography in the risk stratification of patients post-AMI has not been extensively evaluated. 3D derived sphericity index may predict LV remodeling, and the 3D strain technology can help in the detection of nonviable myocardial segments and the prediction of global LV function recovery [99].

3 Echocardiographic Assessment of Ischemic Heart Failure

IHD is the main cause of HF in high-income countries (CAD is the main cause of HF in roughly 60% of the patients) [100]. After AMI, anatomical changes in the LV myocardium occur, including scar formation (replacement fibrosis), dilation of the infarcted region, reactive LV hypertrophy, and finally dilation of the remote zones [101]. Further LV remodeling and dysfunction cause distortion of the mitral valve (MV) apparatus and mitral regurgitation. The LV volume overload and increased filling pressures are transmitted to the pulmonary vasculature leading to pulmonary hypertension, finally causing pressure overload, dilation and dysfunction of the RV, and functional tricuspid regurgitation [100].

3.1 Assessment of Ventricular Remodeling and Dysfunction

Echocardiography is the leading imaging technique to evaluate LV remodeling in routine clinical practice. LV remodeling is defined by the changes in the typical anatomy and structures of the LV. Firstly, increased volumes and alterations in wall thickness are observed. With more extensive remodeling, the heart often becomes more spherical in shape (as calculated by the sphericity index) and the dilation is accompanied by a severe depression of LVEF. LVEF, end-diastolic, and end-systolic dimensions have been associated with all-cause mortality [102, 103]. LVEF assessed by 3D echocardiography is an independent predictor of clinical and arrhythmic events in comparison with conventional 2D echocardiography in patients with LV dysfunction [94, 95]. Ultrasound contrast agents (for enhanced endocardial border detection) have resulted in improved accuracy of LV volumes and EF quantification, and CE should be recommended, irrespective of image quality, when clinical management depends on accurate measurements of LVEF (such as monitoring of patients when implantation of ICD or CRT devices is considered) [36].

GLS provides the largest evidence on the diagnostic and prognostic incremental value over EF [104] in ischemic HF. LV GLS may be impaired at an earlier stage of the remodeling process, while EF is still within the normal values; therefore, GLS is considered a more sensitive marker of myocardial damage with an incremental prognostic value over EF [104, 105].

A transmural infarct will result in a myocardial scar, seen on echocardiography as an akinetic or dyskinetic segment with thinning and increased echo signal intensity. One or more infarcted segments may form an aneurysm defined as a segment with diastolic deformation, with preservation of all three heart layers (endocardium, residual myocardium, and epicardium) (Fig. 9). Because there is no acute mechanical disruption of tissue, the transition from normal myocardium to aneurysm tends to be smooth and gradual compared to pseudoaneurysm.

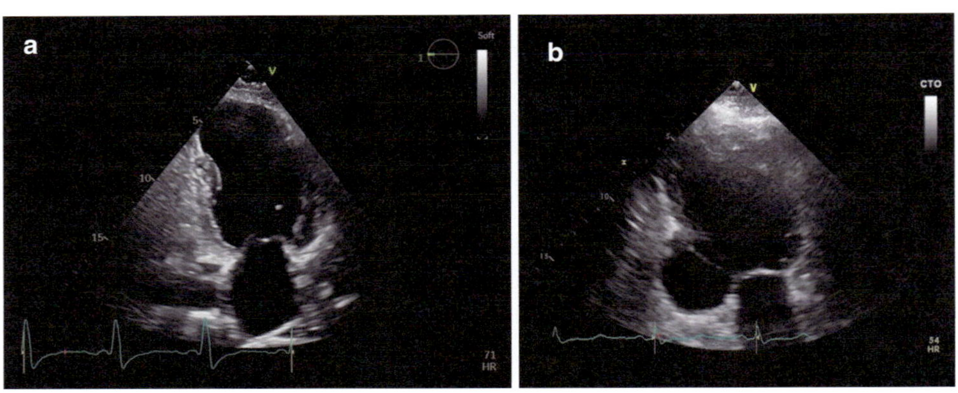

Fig. 9 Post-myocardial infarction left ventricle aneurysm. (**a**) Apical aneurysm; (**b**) basal inferior wall aneurysm

Progression of LV systolic dysfunction due to CAD may be accompanied by widening of the QRS duration, most commonly with an LBBB pattern. The prolonged interventricular and intraventricular conduction may cause dyssynchronous contraction, therapeutic target of CRT. Many echocardiographic parameters of mechanical dyssynchrony have been studied to predict the response to CRT. However, when assessed individually, these parameters do not demonstrate significant predictive value in dyssynchrony–resynchrony evaluation [106, 107]. Moreover, in LV dysfunction due to CAD, response to CRT is affected by other factors including location and extent of myocardial scar, LV lead position, RV function, extent of cavity dilation, and mitral regurgitation.

3.2 Secondary Ischemic Mitral Regurgitation

Ischemic MR is a common complication of CAD and is caused by alteration of the geometrical relationship between the LV and mitral valve apparatus. The mitral annular dilation and dysfunction, the LV dysfunction, and the LV mechanical dyssynchrony can also affect the degree of MR.

The closure of mitral leaflets is determined by the balance between the closing forces generated by the LV systolic contraction and the tethering forces, which restrain the leaflets avoiding leaflet prolapse [108].

LV dysfunction reduces the closure forces, while the LV remodeling causes displacement of the papillary muscles increasing the tethering forces. When tethering forces overcome closure forces, malcoaptation of the MV leaflets and finally MR develops. The direction and degree of tethering determine the MR severity. Local remodeling in the posterior-lateral region creates the major leaflet tension and explains why ischemic MR incidence is higher in inferior than in anterior MI [108]. Indeed, the leaflet tethering is frequently asymmetric, affecting the medial scallop of the posterior mitral leaflet (Fig. 10). Tethering of the anterior mitral leaflet by strut chordae leads to the characteristic "seagull sign." The tenting area and the coaptation depth (measured in mid-systole) quantify the degree of MV remodeling.

Ischemic MR is an independent predictor of cardiovascular death, and the increased mortality risk relates to the degree of MR. Moreover, ischemic MR is a dynamic lesion and frequently increases in severity over time, and its progression is a powerful independent predictor of adverse events in patients with ischemic heart failure [109].

Echocardiography is pivotal for diagnosis and severity assessment of MR and for accurate characterization of the geometry of the valvular apparatus. EACVI and ASE guidelines for native valve regurgitation should be followed for the preprocedural evaluation of MR severity [110, 111]. Qualitative, semiquantitative, and quantitative methods have different strengths and should be combined in a multiparametric approach for grading MR severity. Moreover, careful evaluation of LV volume, ejection fraction, and effective stroke volumes is essential. Indeed, ventricles of different volumes can have similar EROAs but different RegFr. This is at the base of the distinction of secondary MR in proportionate and

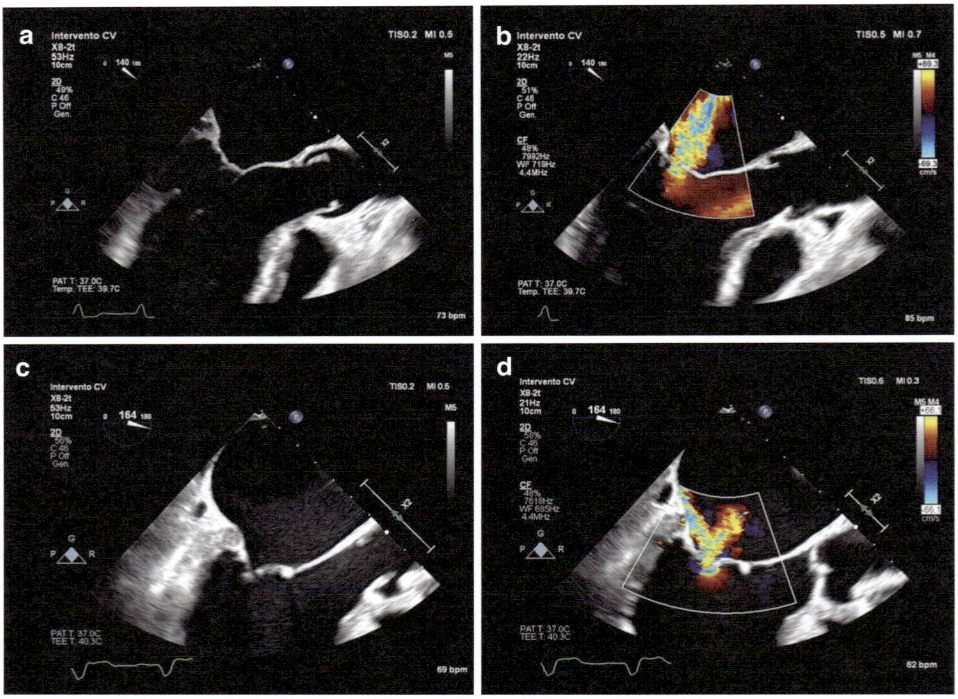

Fig. 10 Secondary mitral regurgitation (MR). (**a**, **b**) Transesophageal three-chamber view showing MR secondary to the symmetric tethering of the leaflets; (**c**, **d**) transesophageal three-chamber view showing MR secondary to the asymmetric tethering of the leaflets (mainly the posterior) with a regurgitant jet directed posteriorly

disproportionate according to the LV end-diastolic volume; this theory, proposed by Greybun, can, at least in part, explain the different outcomes of the contemporary RCTs on percutaneous correction of secondary MR [112]. An algorithm for quantitative assessment of secondary MR has been proposed [113] to further stratify the patients among those within the grey area (EROA between 20 and 30 mm^2 and a RVol between 30 and 44 mL), identifying patients with RegFr >50% as at high risk.

References

1. Stillman AE, Oudkerk M, Bluemke DA, de Boer MJ, Bremerich J, Garcia EV, et al. Imaging the myocardial ischemic cascade. Int J Cardiovasc Imaging. 2018;34(8):1249–63.
2. Sicari R, Nihoyannopoulos P, Evangelista A, Kasprzak J, Lancellotti P, Poldermans D, et al. Stress echocardiography expert consensus statement—executive summary: European Association of Echocardiography (EAE) (a registered branch of the ESC). Eur Heart J. 2009;30(3):278–89.
3. Duncker DJ, Koller A, Merkus D, Canty JM Jr. Regulation of coronary blood flow in health and ischemic heart disease. Prog Cardiovasc Dis. 2015;57(5):409–22.

4. Heusch G. Myocardial stunning and hibernation revisited. Nat Rev Cardiol. 2021;18(7):522–36.
5. Pellikka PA, Arruda-Olson A, Chaudhry FA, Chen MH, Marshall JE, Porter TR, et al. Guidelines for performance, interpretation, and application of stress echocardiography in ischemic heart disease: from the American Society of Echocardiography. J Am Soc Echocardiogr. 2020;33(1):1–41 e8.
6. Writing Committee M, Wiegers SE, Ryan T, Arrighi JA, Brown SM, Canaday B, et al. 2019 ACC/AHA/ASE Advanced Training Statement on Echocardiography (Revision of the 2003 ACC/AHA Clinical Competence Statement on Echocardiography): a report of the ACC Competency Management Committee. J Am Soc Echocardiogr. 2019;32(8):919–43.
7. Steeds RP, Wheeler R, Bhattacharyya S, Reiken J, Nihoyannopoulos P, Senior R, et al. Stress echocardiography in coronary artery disease: a practical guideline from the British Society of Echocardiography. Echo Res Pract. 2019;6(2):G17–33.
8. Peteiro J, Bouzas-Mosquera A, Estevez R, Pazos P, Pineiro M, Castro-Beiras A. Head-to-head comparison of peak supine bicycle exercise echocardiography and treadmill exercise echocardiography at peak and at post-exercise for the detection of coronary artery disease. J Am Soc Echocardiogr. 2012;25(3):319–26.
9. Fine NM, Pellikka PA, Scott CG, Gharacholou SM, McCully RB. Characteristics and outcomes of patients who achieve high workload (>/=10 metabolic equivalents) during treadmill exercise echocardiography. Mayo Clin Proc. 2013;88(12):1408–19.
10. Gligorova S, Agrusta M. Pacing stress echocardiography. Cardiovasc Ultrasound. 2005;3:36.
11. Sicari R, Cortigiani L. The clinical use of stress echocardiography in ischemic heart disease. Cardiovasc Ultrasound. 2017;15(1):7.
12. Senior R, Lahiri A. Enhanced detection of myocardial ischemia by stress dobutamine echocardiography utilizing the "biphasic" response of wall thickening during low and high dose dobutamine infusion. J Am Coll Cardiol. 1995;26(1):26–32.
13. Lang RM, Badano LP, Mor-Avi V, Afilalo J, Armstrong A, Ernande L, et al. Recommendations for cardiac chamber quantification by echocardiography in adults: an update from the American Society of Echocardiography and the European Association of Cardiovascular Imaging. Eur Heart J Cardiovasc Imaging. 2015;16(3):233–70.
14. Pellikka PA, Nagueh SF, Elhendy AA, Kuehl CA, Sawada SG, American Society of E. American Society of Echocardiography recommendations for performance, interpretation, and application of stress echocardiography. J Am Soc Echocardiogr. 2007;20(9):1021–41.
15. Sawada SG, Safadi A, Gaitonde RS, Tung N, Mahenthiran J, Gill W, et al. Stress-induced wall motion abnormalities with low-dose dobutamine infusion indicate the presence of severe disease and vulnerable myocardium. Echocardiography. 2007;24(7):739–44.
16. Tsoukas A, Ikonomidis I, Cokkinos P, Nihoyannopoulos P. Significance of persistent left ventricular dysfunction during recovery after dobutamine stress echocardiography. J Am Coll Cardiol. 1997;30(3):621–6.
17. Bagheri RK, Ahmadi M, Alimi H, Valaee L, Sahranavard T, Andalibi MSS. Dobutamine stress-induced ischemic right ventricular dysfunction in patients with three-vessel coronary artery disease. Electron Physician. 2018;10(5):6775–80.
18. Rambaldi R, Poldermans D, Fioretti PM, ten Cate FJ, Vletter WB, Bax JJ, et al. Usefulness of pulse-wave Doppler tissue sampling and dobutamine stress echocardiography for the diagnosis of right coronary artery narrowing. Am J Cardiol. 1998;81(12):1411–5.
19. Meimoun P, Tribouilloy C. Non-invasive assessment of coronary flow and coronary flow reserve by transthoracic Doppler echocardiography: a magic tool for the real world. Eur J Echocardiogr. 2008;9(4):449–57.

20. Matsumura Y, Hozumi T, Watanabe H, Fujimoto K, Sugioka K, Takemoto Y, et al. Cut-off value of coronary flow velocity reserve by transthoracic Doppler echocardiography for diagnosis of significant left anterior descending artery stenosis in patients with coronary risk factors. Am J Cardiol. 2003;92(12):1389–93.
21. Cortigiani L, Rigo F, Gherardi S, Bovenzi F, Molinaro S, Picano E, et al. Coronary flow reserve during dipyridamole stress echocardiography predicts mortality. JACC Cardiovasc Imaging. 2012;5(11):1079–85.
22. Meimoun P, Benali T, Elmkies F, Sayah S, Luycx-Bore A, Doutrelan L, et al. Prognostic value of transthoracic coronary flow reserve in medically treated patients with proximal left anterior descending artery stenosis of intermediate severity. Eur J Echocardiogr. 2009;10(1):127–32.
23. Djordjevic Dikic A, Tesic M, Boskovic N, Giga V, Stepanovic J, Petrovic M, et al. Prognostic value of preserved coronary flow velocity reserve by noninvasive transthoracic doppler echocardiography in patients with angiographically intermediate left main stenosis. J Am Soc Echocardiogr. 2019;32(1):74–80.
24. Gaibazzi N, Rigo F, Lorenzoni V, Molinaro S, Bartolomucci F, Reverberi C, et al. Comparative prediction of cardiac events by wall motion, wall motion plus coronary flow reserve, or myocardial perfusion analysis: a multicenter study of contrast stress echocardiography. JACC Cardiovasc Imaging. 2013;6(1):1–12.
25. Patel H, Mazur W, Williams KA Sr, Kalra DK. Myocardial viability-state of the art: is it still relevant and how to best assess it with imaging? Trends Cardiovasc Med. 2018;28(1):24–37.
26. Bax JJ, Cornel JH, Visser FC, Fioretti PM, van Lingen A, Reijs AE, et al. Prediction of recovery of myocardial dysfunction after revascularization. Comparison of fluorine-18 fluorodeoxyglucose/thallium-201 SPECT, thallium-201 stress-reinjection SPECT and dobutamine echocardiography. J Am Coll Cardiol. 1996;28(3):558–64.
27. Bax JJ, Wijns W, Cornel JH, Visser FC, Boersma E, Fioretti PM. Accuracy of currently available techniques for prediction of functional recovery after revascularization in patients with left ventricular dysfunction due to chronic coronary artery disease: comparison of pooled data. J Am Coll Cardiol. 1997;30(6):1451–60.
28. Elfigih IA, Henein MY. Non-invasive imaging in detecting myocardial viability: myocardial function versus perfusion. Int J Cardiol Heart Vasc. 2014;5:51–6.
29. Lima EG, Carvalho FPC, Linhares Filho JPP, Pitta FG, Serrano CV Jr. Ischemic left ventricle systolic dysfunction: an evidence-based approach in diagnostic tools and therapeutics. Rev Assoc Med Bras (1992). 2017;63(9):793–800.
30. Cornel JH, Bax JJ, Elhendy A, Maat AP, Kimman GJ, Geleijnse ML, et al. Biphasic response to dobutamine predicts improvement of global left ventricular function after surgical revascularization in patients with stable coronary artery disease: implications of time course of recovery on diagnostic accuracy. J Am Coll Cardiol. 1998;31(5):1002–10.
31. Chen C, Li L, Chen LL, Prada JV, Chen MH, Fallon JT, et al. Incremental doses of dobutamine induce a biphasic response in dysfunctional left ventricular regions subtending coronary stenoses. Circulation. 1995;92(4):756–66.
32. Bax JJ, Poldermans D, Elhendy A, Cornel JH, Boersma E, Rambaldi R, et al. Improvement of left ventricular ejection fraction, heart failure symptoms and prognosis after revascularization in patients with chronic coronary artery disease and viable myocardium detected by dobutamine stress echocardiography. J Am Coll Cardiol. 1999;34(1):163–9.
33. Schinkel AF, Bax JJ, Poldermans D, Elhendy A, Ferrari R, Rahimtoola SH. Hibernating myocardium: diagnosis and patient outcomes. Curr Probl Cardiol. 2007;32(7):375–410.
34. Smart SC, Sawada S, Ryan T, Segar D, Atherton L, Berkovitz K, et al. Low-dose dobutamine echocardiography detects reversible dysfunction after thrombolytic therapy of acute myocardial infarction. Circulation. 1993;88(2):405–15.

35. Bax JJ, Poldermans D, Elhendy A, Boersma E, Rahimtoola SH. Sensitivity, specificity, and predictive accuracies of various noninvasive techniques for detecting hibernating myocardium. Curr Probl Cardiol. 2001;26(2):147–86.
36. Senior R, Becher H, Monaghan M, Agati L, Zamorano J, Vanoverschelde JL, et al. Clinical practice of contrast echocardiography: recommendation by the European Association of Cardiovascular Imaging (EACVI) 2017. Eur Heart J Cardiovasc Imaging. 2017;18(11):1205-af.
37. Eskandari M, Monaghan M. Contrast echocardiography in daily clinical practice. Herz. 2017;42(3):271–8.
38. Wei K, Jayaweera AR, Firoozan S, Linka A, Skyba DM, Kaul S. Quantification of myocardial blood flow with ultrasound-induced destruction of microbubbles administered as a constant venous infusion. Circulation. 1998;97(5):473–83.
39. Gaibazzi N, Rigo F, Reverberi C. Detection of coronary artery disease by combined assessment of wall motion, myocardial perfusion and coronary flow reserve: a multiparametric contrast stress-echocardiography study. J Am Soc Echocardiogr. 2010;23(12):1242–50.
40. Shah BN, Chahal NS, Bhattacharyya S, Li W, Roussin I, Khattar RS, et al. The feasibility and clinical utility of myocardial contrast echocardiography in clinical practice: results from the incorporation of myocardial perfusion assessment into clinical testing with stress echocardiography study. J Am Soc Echocardiogr. 2014;27(5):520–30.
41. Brown AS, Calachanis M, Evdoridis C, Hancock J, Wild S, Prasan A, et al. Sonovue improves endocardial border detection and variability in assessing wall motion score and ejection fraction during stress echocardiography. Ir J Med Sci. 2004;173(1):13–7.
42. Tsutsui JM, Xie F, McGrain AC, Mahrous H, Hankins J, O'Leary EL, et al. Comparison of low-mechanical index pulse sequence schemes for detecting myocardial perfusion abnormalities during vasodilator stress echocardiography. Am J Cardiol. 2005;95(5):565–70.
43. Senior R, Lepper W, Pasquet A, Chung G, Hoffman R, Vanoverschelde JL, et al. Myocardial perfusion assessment in patients with medium probability of coronary artery disease and no prior myocardial infarction: comparison of myocardial contrast echocardiography with 99mTc single-photon emission computed tomography. Am Heart J. 2004;147(6):1100–5.
44. Masugata H, Lafitte S, Peters B, Strachan GM, DeMaria AN. Comparison of real-time and intermittent triggered myocardial contrast echocardiography for quantification of coronary stenosis severity and transmural perfusion gradient. Circulation. 2001;104(13):1550–6.
45. Yao SS, Qureshi E, Sherrid MV, Chaudhry FA. Practical applications in stress echocardiography: risk stratification and prognosis in patients with known or suspected ischemic heart disease. J Am Coll Cardiol. 2003;42(6):1084–90.
46. Metz LD, Beattie M, Hom R, Redberg RF, Grady D, Fleischmann KE. The prognostic value of normal exercise myocardial perfusion imaging and exercise echocardiography: a meta-analysis. J Am Coll Cardiol. 2007;49(2):227–37.
47. Yao SS, Qureshi E, Syed A, Chaudhry FA. Novel stress echocardiographic model incorporating the extent and severity of wall motion abnormality for risk stratification and prognosis. Am J Cardiol. 2004;94(6):715–9.
48. Sicari R, Cortigiani L, Bigi R, Landi P, Raciti M, Picano E, et al. Prognostic value of pharmacological stress echocardiography is affected by concomitant antiischemic therapy at the time of testing. Circulation. 2004;109(20):2428–31.
49. Attenhofer CH, Pellikka PA, Oh JK, Roger VL, Sohn DW, Seward JB. Comparison of ischemic response during exercise and dobutamine echocardiography in patients with left main coronary artery disease. J Am Coll Cardiol. 1996;27(5):1171–7.
50. Bangalore S, Yao SS, Chaudhry FA. Role of right ventricular wall motion abnormalities in risk stratification and prognosis of patients referred for stress echocardiography. J Am Coll Cardiol. 2007;50(20):1981–9.

51. Sitia S, Tomasoni L, Turiel M. Speckle tracking echocardiography: a new approach to myocardial function. World J Cardiol. 2010;2(1):1–5.
52. Alaika O, Jamai S, Doghmi N, Cherti M. Diagnostic accuracy of global longitudinal strain for detecting significant coronary artery disease in diabetic patients without regional wall motion abnormality. J Saudi Heart Assoc. 2020;32(3):425–33.
53. Pastore MC, Mandoli GE, Contorni F, Cavigli L, Focardi M, D'Ascenzi F, et al. Speckle tracking echocardiography: early predictor of diagnosis and prognosis in coronary artery disease. Biomed Res Int. 2021;2021:6685378.
54. Zoroufian A, Razmi T, Taghavi-Shavazi M, Lotfi-Tokaldany M, Jalali A. Evaluation of subclinical left ventricular dysfunction in diabetic patients: longitudinal strain velocities and left ventricular dyssynchrony by two-dimensional speckle tracking echocardiography study. Echocardiography. 2014;31(4):456–63.
55. Malagoli A, Fanti D, Albini A, Rossi A, Ribichini FL, Benfari G. Echocardiographic strain imaging in coronary artery disease: the added value of a quantitative approach. Cardiol Clin. 2020;38(4):517–26.
56. Anwar AM. Accuracy of two-dimensional speckle tracking echocardiography for the detection of significant coronary stenosis. J Cardiovasc Ultrasound. 2013;21(4):177–82.
57. Biering-Sorensen T, Hoffmann S, Mogelvang R, Zeeberg Iversen A, Galatius S, Fritz-Hansen T, et al. Myocardial strain analysis by 2-dimensional speckle tracking echocardiography improves diagnostics of coronary artery stenosis in stable angina pectoris. Circ Cardiovasc Imaging. 2014;7(1):58–65.
58. Rumbinaite E, Zaliaduonyte-Peksiene D, Lapinskas T, Zvirblyte R, Karuzas A, Jonauskiene I, et al. Early and late diastolic strain rate vs global longitudinal strain at rest and during dobutamine stress for the assessment of significant coronary artery stenosis in patients with a moderate and high probability of coronary artery disease. Echocardiography. 2016;33(10):1512–22.
59. Uusitalo V, Luotolahti M, Pietila M, Wendelin-Saarenhovi M, Hartiala J, Saraste M, et al. Two-dimensional speckle-tracking during dobutamine stress echocardiography in the detection of myocardial ischemia in patients with suspected coronary artery disease. J Am Soc Echocardiogr. 2016;29(5):470–9 e3.
60. Brainin P, Haahr-Pedersen S, Olsen FJ, Holm AE, Fritz-Hansen T, Jespersen T, et al. Early systolic lengthening in patients with ST-segment-elevation myocardial infarction: a novel predictor of cardiovascular events. J Am Heart Assoc. 2020;9(3):e013835.
61. Kozuma A, Asanuma T, Masuda K, Adachi H, Minami S, Nakatani S. Assessment of myocardial ischemic memory using three-dimensional speckle-tracking echocardiography: a novel integrated analysis of early systolic lengthening and postsystolic shortening. J Am Soc Echocardiogr. 2019;32(11):1477–86.
62. Brainin P, Hoffmann S, Fritz-Hansen T, Olsen FJ, Jensen JS, Biering-Sorensen T. Usefulness of postsystolic shortening to diagnose coronary artery disease and predict future cardiovascular events in stable angina pectoris. J Am Soc Echocardiogr. 2018;31(8):870–9 e3.
63. Pislaru C, Belohlavek M, Bae RY, Abraham TP, Greenleaf JF, Seward JB. Regional asynchrony during acute myocardial ischemia quantified by ultrasound strain rate imaging. J Am Coll Cardiol. 2001;37(4):1141–8.
64. Longobardo L, Suma V, Jain R, Carerj S, Zito C, Zwicke DL, et al. Role of two-dimensional speckle-tracking echocardiography strain in the assessment of right ventricular systolic function and comparison with conventional parameters. J Am Soc Echocardiogr. 2017;30(10):937–46 e6.
65. Sabatino J, De Rosa S, Leo I, Strangio A, Spaccarotella C, Polimeni A, et al. Prediction of significant coronary artery disease through advanced echocardiography: role of non-invasive myocardial work. Front Cardiovasc Med. 2021;8:719603.

66. Baldea SM, Velcea AE, Rimbas RC, Andronic A, Matei L, Calin SI, et al. 3-D echocardiography is feasible and more reproducible than 2-D echocardiography for in-training echocardiographers in follow-up of patients with heart failure with reduced ejection fraction. Ultrasound Med Biol. 2021;47(3):499–510.
67. Soliman OI, Kirschbaum SW, van Dalen BM, van der Zwaan HB, Mahdavian Delavary B, Vletter WB, et al. Accuracy and reproducibility of quantitation of left ventricular function by real-time three-dimensional echocardiography versus cardiac magnetic resonance. Am J Cardiol. 2008;102(6):778–83.
68. Berbarie RF, Dib E, Ahmad M. Stress echocardiography using real-time three-dimensional imaging. Echocardiography. 2018;35(8):1196–203.
69. Shivalkar B, De Keersmaeker A, Van Hoeck N, Belkova P, Van de Heyning CM, De Maeyer C, et al. Is 3D dobutamine stress echocardiography ready for prime time? Diagnostic and prognostic implications. Eur Heart J Cardiovasc Imaging. 2020;21(4):428–36.
70. Picano E, Ciampi Q, Cortigiani L, Arruda-Olson AM, Borguezan-Daros C, de Castro ESPJL, et al. Stress Echo 2030: the Novel ABCDE-(FGLPR) protocol to define the future of imaging. J Clin Med. 2021;10(16).
71. Ciampi Q, Zagatina A, Cortigiani L, Wierzbowska-Drabik K, Kasprzak JD, Haberka M, et al. Prognostic value of stress echocardiography assessed by the ABCDE protocol. Eur Heart J. 2021;42(37):3869–78.
72. Scali MC, Zagatina A, Ciampi Q, Cortigiani L, D'Andrea A, Daros CB, et al. Lung ultrasound and pulmonary congestion during stress echocardiography. JACC Cardiovasc Imaging. 2020;13(10):2085–95.
73. Picano E, Ciampi Q, Citro R, D'Andrea A, Scali MC, Cortigiani L, et al. Stress echo 2020: the international stress echo study in ischemic and non-ischemic heart disease. Cardiovasc Ultrasound. 2017;15(1):3.
74. Collet JP, Thiele H, Barbato E, Barthelemy O, Bauersachs J, Bhatt DL, et al. 2020 ESC guidelines for the management of acute coronary syndromes in patients presenting without persistent ST-segment elevation. Eur Heart J. 2021;42(14):1289–367.
75. Cheitlin MD, Armstrong WF, Aurigemma GP, Beller GA, Bierman FZ, Davis JL, et al. ACC/AHA/ASE 2003 guideline update for the clinical application of echocardiography: summary article: a report of the American College of Cardiology/American Heart Association Task Force on Practice Guidelines (ACC/AHA/ASE Committee to Update the 1997 Guidelines for the Clinical Application of Echocardiography). Circulation. 2003;108(9):1146–62.
76. American College of Cardiology Foundation Appropriate Use Criteria Task F, American Society of E, American Heart A, American Society of Nuclear C, Heart Failure Society of A, Heart Rhythm S, et al. ACCF/ASE/AHA/ASNC/HFSA/HRS/SCAI/SCCM/SCCT/SCMR 2011 Appropriate Use Criteria for Echocardiography. A Report of the American College of Cardiology Foundation Appropriate Use Criteria Task Force, American Society of Echocardiography, American Heart Association, American Society of Nuclear Cardiology, Heart Failure Society of America, Heart Rhythm Society, Society for Cardiovascular Angiography and Interventions, Society of Critical Care Medicine, Society of Cardiovascular Computed Tomography, Society for Cardiovascular Magnetic Resonance American College of Chest Physicians. J Am Soc Echocardiogr. 2011;24(3):229–67.
77. Ondrus T, Kanovsky J, Novotny T, Andrsova I, Spinar J, Kala P. Right ventricular myocardial infarction: from pathophysiology to prognosis. Exp Clin Cardiol. 2013;18(1):27–30.
78. Albulushi A, Giannopoulos A, Kafkas N, Dragasis S, Pavlides G, Chatzizisis YS. Acute right ventricular myocardial infarction. Expert Rev Cardiovasc Ther. 2018;16(7):455–64.
79. Damluji AA, van Diepen S, Katz JN, Menon V, Tamis-Holland JE, Bakitas M, et al. Mechanical complications of acute myocardial infarction: a scientific statement from the American Heart Association. Circulation. 2021;144(2):e16–35.

80. Valle JA, Miyasaka RL, Carroll JD. Acute mitral regurgitation secondary to papillary muscle tear: is transcatheter edge-to-edge mitral valve repair a new paradigm? Circ Cardiovasc Interv. 2017;10(6).
81. Mahmood M, Haque SS, Siddique MA, Ahmed CM, Hossain Z. Doppler evaluation of left to right shunt (Qp/Qs) in patients with isolated ventricular septal defect (Vsd). Mymensingh Med J. 2007;16(2):181–6.
82. Schlotter F, de Waha S, Eitel I, Desch S, Fuernau G, Thiele H. Interventional post-myocardial infarction ventricular septal defect closure: a systematic review of current evidence. EuroIntervention. 2016;12(1):94–102.
83. Mittle S, Makaryus AN, Mangion J. Role of contrast echocardiography in the assessment of myocardial rupture. Echocardiography. 2003;20(1):77–81.
84. McCarthy CP, Vaduganathan M, McCarthy KJ, Januzzi JL Jr, Bhatt DL, McEvoy JW. Left ventricular thrombus after acute myocardial infarction: screening, prevention, and treatment. JAMA Cardiol. 2018;3(7):642–9.
85. Weinsaft JW, Kim J, Medicherla CB, Ma CL, Codella NC, Kukar N, et al. Echocardiographic algorithm for post-myocardial infarction LV thrombus: a gatekeeper for thrombus evaluation by delayed enhancement CMR. JACC Cardiovasc Imaging. 2016;9(5):505–15.
86. Kirkpatrick JN, Wong T, Bednarz JE, Spencer KT, Sugeng L, Ward RP, et al. Differential diagnosis of cardiac masses using contrast echocardiographic perfusion imaging. J Am Coll Cardiol. 2004;43(8):1412–9.
87. Prastaro M, Pirozzi E, Gaibazzi N, Paolillo S, Santoro C, Savarese G, et al. Expert review on the prognostic role of echocardiography after acute myocardial infarction. J Am Soc Echocardiogr. 2017;30(5):431–43 e2.
88. Sutton NR, Li S, Thomas L, Wang TY, de Lemos JA, Enriquez JR, et al. The association of left ventricular ejection fraction with clinical outcomes after myocardial infarction: findings from the Acute Coronary Treatment and Intervention Outcomes Network (ACTION) Registry-Get With the Guidelines (GWTG) Medicare-linked database. Am Heart J. 2016;178:65–73.
89. Nicolosi GL, Latini R, Marino P, Maggioni AP, Barlera S, Franzosi MG, et al. The prognostic value of predischarge quantitative two-dimensional echocardiographic measurements and the effects of early lisinopril treatment on left ventricular structure and function after acute myocardial infarction in the GISSI-3 Trial. Gruppo Italiano per lo Studio della Sopravvivenza nell'Infarto Miocardico. Eur Heart J. 1996;17(11):1646–56.
90. Moller JE, Hillis GS, Oh JK, Reeder GS, Gersh BJ, Pellikka PA. Wall motion score index and ejection fraction for risk stratification after acute myocardial infarction. Am Heart J. 2006;151(2):419–25.
91. Antoni ML, Scherptong RW, Atary JZ, Boersma E, Holman ER, van der Wall EE, et al. Prognostic value of right ventricular function in patients after acute myocardial infarction treated with primary percutaneous coronary intervention. Circ Cardiovasc Imaging. 2010;3(3):264–71.
92. Munk K, Andersen NH, Terkelsen CJ, Bibby BM, Johnsen SP, Botker HE, et al. Global left ventricular longitudinal systolic strain for early risk assessment in patients with acute myocardial infarction treated with primary percutaneous intervention. J Am Soc Echocardiogr. 2012;25(6):644–51.
93. Ersboll M, Valeur N, Mogensen UM, Andersen MJ, Moller JE, Velazquez EJ, et al. Prediction of all-cause mortality and heart failure admissions from global left ventricular longitudinal strain in patients with acute myocardial infarction and preserved left ventricular ejection fraction. J Am Coll Cardiol. 2013;61(23):2365–73.
94. Haugaa KH, Grenne BL, Eek CH, Ersboll M, Valeur N, Svendsen JH, et al. Strain echocardiography improves risk prediction of ventricular arrhythmias after myocardial infarction. JACC Cardiovasc Imaging. 2013;6(8):841–50.

95. Perry R, Patil S, Marx C, Horsfall M, Chew DP, Sree Raman K, et al. Advanced echocardiographic imaging for prediction of SCD in moderate and severe LV systolic function. JACC Cardiovasc Imaging. 2020;13(2 Pt 2):604–12.
96. Gong L, Li D, Chen J, Wang X, Xu T, Li W, et al. Assessment of myocardial viability in patients with acute myocardial infarction by two-dimensional speckle tracking echocardiography combined with low-dose dobutamine stress echocardiography. Int J Cardiovasc Imaging. 2013;29(5):1017–28.
97. Hoffer EP, Dewe W, Celentano C, Pierard LA. Low-level exercise echocardiography detects contractile reserve and predicts reversible dysfunction after acute myocardial infarction: comparison with low-dose dobutamine echocardiography. J Am Coll Cardiol. 1999;34(4):989–97.
98. Galiuto L, Garramone B, Scara A, Rebuzzi AG, Crea F, La Torre G, et al. The extent of microvascular damage during myocardial contrast echocardiography is superior to other known indexes of post-infarct reperfusion in predicting left ventricular remodeling: results of the multicenter AMICI study. J Am Coll Cardiol. 2008;51(5):552–9.
99. Abate E, Hoogslag GE, Antoni ML, Nucifora G, Delgado V, Holman ER, et al. Value of three-dimensional speckle-tracking longitudinal strain for predicting improvement of left ventricular function after acute myocardial infarction. Am J Cardiol. 2012;110(7):961–7.
100. Gheorghiade M, Sopko G, De Luca L, Velazquez EJ, Parker JD, Binkley PF, et al. Navigating the crossroads of coronary artery disease and heart failure. Circulation. 2006;114(11):1202–13.
101. Bax JJ, Di Carli M, Narula J, Delgado V. Multimodality imaging in ischaemic heart failure. Lancet. 2019;393(10175):1056–70.
102. Kramer DG, Trikalinos TA, Kent DM, Antonopoulos GV, Konstam MA, Udelson JE. Quantitative evaluation of drug or device effects on ventricular remodeling as predictors of therapeutic effects on mortality in patients with heart failure and reduced ejection fraction: a meta-analytic approach. J Am Coll Cardiol. 2010;56(5):392–406.
103. Wong M, Staszewsky L, Latini R, Barlera S, Glazer R, Aknay N, et al. Severity of left ventricular remodeling defines outcomes and response to therapy in heart failure: valsartan heart failure trial (Val-HeFT) echocardiographic data. J Am Coll Cardiol. 2004;43(11):2022–7.
104. Kalam K, Otahal P, Marwick TH. Prognostic implications of global LV dysfunction: a systematic review and meta-analysis of global longitudinal strain and ejection fraction. Heart. 2014;100(21):1673–80.
105. Sengelov M, Jorgensen PG, Jensen JS, Bruun NE, Olsen FJ, Fritz-Hansen T, et al. Global longitudinal strain is a superior predictor of all-cause mortality in heart failure with reduced ejection fraction. JACC Cardiovasc Imaging. 2015;8(12):1351–9.
106. Cazeau S, Toulemont M, Ritter P, Reygner J. Statistical ranking of electromechanical dyssynchrony parameters for CRT. Open Heart. 2019;6(1):e000933.
107. Chung ES, Leon AR, Tavazzi L, Sun JP, Nihoyannopoulos P, Merlino J, et al. Results of the predictors of response to CRT (PROSPECT) trial. Circulation. 2008;117(20):2608–16.
108. Agricola E, Oppizzi M, Pisani M, Meris A, Maisano F, Margonato A. Ischemic mitral regurgitation: mechanisms and echocardiographic classification. Eur J Echocardiogr. 2008;9(2):207–21.
109. Kwon DH, Kusunose K, Obuchowski NA, Cavalcante JL, Popovic ZB, Thomas JD, et al. Predictors and prognostic impact of progressive ischemic mitral regurgitation in patients with advanced ischemic cardiomyopathy: a multimodality study. Circ Cardiovasc Imaging. 2016;9(7).
110. Baumgartner H, Falk V, Bax JJ, De Bonis M, Hamm C, Holm PJ, et al. 2017 ESC/EACTS guidelines for the management of valvular heart disease. Rev Esp Cardiol (Engl Ed). 2018;71(2):110.
111. Zoghbi WA, Adams D, Bonow RO, Enriquez-Sarano M, Foster E, Grayburn PA, et al. Recommendations for noninvasive evaluation of native valvular regurgitation: a report from

the American Society of Echocardiography Developed in Collaboration with the Society for Cardiovascular Magnetic Resonance. J Am Soc Echocardiogr. 2017;30(4):303–71.
112. Grayburn PA, Sannino A, Packer M. Proportionate and disproportionate functional mitral regurgitation: a new conceptual framework that reconciles the results of the MITRA-FR and COAPT trials. JACC Cardiovasc Imaging. 2019;12(2):353–62.
113. Bartko PE, Arfsten H, Heitzinger G, Pavo N, Toma A, Strunk G, et al. A unifying concept for the quantitative assessment of secondary mitral regurgitation. J Am Coll Cardiol. 2019;73(20):2506–17.

Cardiac Catheterization and Coronary Arteriography

Antonio Mangieri, Mauro Gitto, Sara Baggio, Guido Del Monaco, Aisha Gohar, and Bernard Reimers

1 Introduction and History of Cardiac Catheterization

Cardiac catheterization has provided indisputable improvements in the diagnostic and therapeutic management of patients with ischemic heart disease (IHD), extending our understanding of circulatory anatomy and vascular pathophysiology.

From the first cardiac catheterization performed by Claude Bernard in 1844 on a horse [1], by a retrograde approach from the jugular vein to the right ventricle and from the carotid artery to the left ventricle, we had to wait more than half a century to obtain the first cardiac catheterization on humans: in 1929, the German physician Werner Forssmann inserted a 65 cm catheter through one of his left antecubital veins, guiding it by fluoroscopy to his right atrium; he proved the successful self-catheterization with an X-ray and published it with the title "*Über die Sondierung des rechten Herzens*" (*About probing of the right heart*) [2].

Based upon these few early studies, in the 1940s, Andre Cournand and Dickinson Richards produced a remarkable series of investigations of right-heart physiology in humans [3–5]. They shared the Nobel Prize in Medicine with W. Forssmann in 1956 for their contribution of the discovery of cardiac catheterization and hemodynamic measurements.

Subsequent studies extended the application of cardiac catheterization to the study of congenital heart disease and evaluation of pulmonary pressures. In 1947, by reaching the distal pulmonary artery with a catheter, Dexter proved that pulmonary artery wedge pressure was a good estimate of pulmonary venous and left atrial pressures [6].

A. Mangieri (✉) · M. Gitto · S. Baggio · G. Del Monaco · A. Gohar · B. Reimers
Cardio Center, Humanitas Research Hospital, Milan, Italy
e-mail: guido.delmonaco@humanitas.it; aishagohar@doctors.org.uk; bernhard.reimers@humanitas.it

G. Concistrè (ed.), *Ischemic Heart Disease*,
https://doi.org/10.1007/978-3-031-25879-4_13

Selective coronary arteriography was first reported by the pediatric cardiologist Mason Sones in 1959, when he accidentally injected radiocontrast into a coronary artery instead of the left ventricle [7].

In the late 1970s, coronary catheterization was extended to therapeutic purposes, with the advent of catheter-based interventions, pioneered by Andreas Grüntzig, who introduced the technique of balloon angioplasty, generally known as percutaneous transluminal coronary angioplasty (PTCA) [8, 9]. Since then, there has been an exponential growth in cardiac catheterization, in terms of both diagnostic evaluation and therapeutic interventions, leading to a revolution in the management of patients with IHD, continually resulting in improved outcomes.

In essence, these new procedures have led to the blooming of the interventional cardiology field. In 2020, despite a significant decrease in procedural volumes due to the COVID-19 pandemic, the US interventional cardiology device market size was valued at approximately $3.2 billion, with over 1.2 million coronary stents implanted per year. The market size is expected to reach $4.1 billion by 2026 [10].

2 Indications for Cardiac Catheterization

Cardiac catheterization is a useful procedure for both diagnostic and therapeutic purposes. Nevertheless, due to its invasiveness, it is essential to carefully evaluate the balance between its risks and anticipated benefits while also involving the patient in the decision-making process. Increasing attention is being given to the rational use of invasive cardiovascular procedures, as evident by the development of Appropriate Use Criteria (AUC) [11] to assess patient selection for diagnostic coronary procedures, as summarized in Table 1.

The first step in selecting a patient to undergo cardiac catheterization is a comprehensive clinical and noninvasive evaluation in order to define the presence of an acute or chronic condition, which helps to identify the appropriate timing for intervention.

2.1 Indications for Coronary Angiography in Acute Coronary Syndromes

In the setting of acute coronary syndromes, the goal of cardiac catheterization is to identify the lesion responsible for the current event (culprit) and then to restore vessel patency, mainly with percutaneous coronary interventions (PCI).

In the setting of ST-elevation myocardial infarction (STEMI), the culprit lesion is in most cases evident on coronary angiography. However, it is usually not as simple in the case of non-ST-elevation myocardial infarction (NSTEMI): a significant portion of such patients have complex multivessel disease and more than 10% of them may not present a clear culprit lesion on angiography [12]; therefore, complementary invasive imaging is implemented in

Table 1 Summary of the main appropriate indications for diagnostic cardiac catheterization, in accordance with Appropriate Use Criteria. A detailed description of appropriate, uncertain, and inappropriate indications is reported in the consensus document by Patel et al. [11]

Diagnostic Catheterization Appropriate Use Criteria—Appropriate Indications

- *Suspected acute coronary syndrome*
- *Suspected CAD (no prior PCI, CABG, or angiogram showing > 50% stenosis)*:
  - No prior noninvasive stress imaging, but high pretest probability and symptomatic
  - Prior noninvasive testing
    - High-risk finding on ECG stress testing
    - Stress test with imaging: intermediate-risk findings in a symptomatic patient; high-risk findings; discordant or equivocal findings in a symptomatic patient; baseline resting LV dysfunction and evidence of myocardial viability in dysfunctional segment
    - Echocardiography: newly recognized LV systolic dysfunction with unknown etiology; new regional wall motion abnormality with unknown etiology and normal LV systolic function; suspected significant ischemic complication related to CAD (e.g., ischemic mitral regurgitation or VSD)
    - Coronary CTA: stenosis ≥50% or of unclear severity in a symptomatic patient; lesion of unclear severity, possibly obstructive in the left main, even in asymptomatic patients
  - Adjunctive invasive diagnostic testing in patients undergoing appropriate diagnostic coronary angiography:
    - FFR for lesion severity
    - IVUS for lesion severity and examination of lesion or artery morphology
- *Patients with known obstructive CAD*
  - Intermediate-risk noninvasive findings and worsening or limiting symptoms; high-risk noninvasive findings
- *Arrhythmias*
  - Resuscitated cardiac arrest with return of spontaneous circulation
  - VF or sustained VT
- *Valvular disease*
  - Preoperative assessment before valvular surgery
  - Pulmonary hypertension out of proportion to the severity of valvular disease
  - LV dysfunction out of proportion to the severity of valvular disease
  - Chronic valvular disease but with noninvasive imaging conflicting with clinical impression of severity
- *Pericardial diseases:*
  - Suspected pericardial tamponade
  - Suspected or clinical uncertainty between constrictive and restrictive physiology
- *Cardiomyopathies*
  - Known or suspected cardiomyopathy with or without heart failure
  - Re-evaluation of known cardiomyopathy
- *Pulmonary hypertension and intracardiac shunt evaluation*

ACS acute coronary syndrome; *CABG* coronary bypass grafting surgery; *CAD* coronary artery disease; *CTA* computed tomography angiography; *ECG* electrocardiogram; *FFR* fractional flow reserve; *IVUS* intravascular ultrasound; *LV* left ventricular; *LVEF* left ventricular ejection fraction; *MI* myocardial infarction; *PCI* percutaneous coronary intervention; *VF* ventricular fibrillation; *VSD* ventricular septal defect; *VT* ventricular tachycardia the acute setting to enhance the diagnostic accuracy of culprit lesion detection, assessing for the presence of plaque erosion, rupture, ulceration, or thrombus apposition.

Based upon the current indications for reperfusion therapy in ACS [13–16], immediate coronary angiography (within 2 h) and subsequent revascularization are recommended in the following cases:

- All patients with symptoms of ischemia of less than 12-h duration and persistent ST-segment elevation.
- In the setting of NSTEMI, the results of several RCTs and their meta-analyses highlight the role of risk stratification in the decision process and support a routine invasive strategy in very-high-risk patients, with suspected ongoing ischemic symptoms suggestive of MI and at least one high-risk feature, including hemodynamic instability or cardiogenic shock, recurrent or ongoing chest pain refractory to medical treatment, life-threatening arrhythmias or cardiac arrest, mechanical complications of MI, acute heart failure, and recurrent dynamic ST-segment or T wave changes, particularly with intermittent ST-segment elevation. An early invasive approach with angiography performed in the first 24 h is recommended in high-risk patients with NSTEMI.
- In selected STEMI patients with time from symptom onset of more than 12 h, in the presence of ongoing symptoms suggestive of ischemia, hemodynamic instability, or life-threatening arrhythmias. In asymptomatic patients, routine PCI of an occluded infarct-related artery more than 48 h after the onset of STEMI is not indicated.

2.2 Indications to Coronary Angiography in Acute Coronary Syndromes

Regarding chronic coronary syndromes (CCS) or suspected stable CAD, myocardial revascularization in stable CAD is performed to improve either prognosis in a subset of patients with high-risk characteristics or quality of life and symptoms in cases of refractory to medical therapy [17].

Two key aspects should be taken into account in this context: the improved sensibility and specificity of noninvasive diagnostic tests for the detection of myocardial ischemia and CAD and the results of several trials which placed renewed emphasis on intensive medical therapy for stable patients. From the results of the COURAGE [18] (Clinical Outcomes Utilizing Revascularization and Aggressive Drug Evaluation) trial published in 2007 to the recently released ORBITA [19] (Objective Randomized Blinded Investigation With Optimal Medical Therapy of Angioplasty in Stable Angina) and ISCHEMIA [20] (International Study of Comparative Health Effectiveness with Medical and Invasive Approaches) trials, data have tempered the expected benefits of PCI in elective cases, confirming the need of careful patient selection for myocardial revascularization in CCS, especially in the presence of mild symptoms and preserved left ventricle ejection fraction and once left main stenosis, proximal CAD, or severe multivessel CAD have been ruled out. Therefore, guidelines suggest the use of invasive coronary angiography (ICA) only in patients with suspected CAD in cases when noninvasive testing has proven inconclusive, in patients from particular professions, due to regulatory issues, or if noninvasive assessment suggests a high risk of events, in order to determine the options for revascularization.

ICA should not be performed in patients with angina who either refuse invasive procedures or prefer to avoid revascularization, or in whom revascularization is not expected to improve functional status or quality of life.

Furthermore, cardiac catheterization should be performed in:

- Patients considered for heart surgery, with the possibility of noninvasive assessment only in selected young subjects with no coronary risk factors, no history of CAD, and no evidence of ischemia or in urgent settings.
- Pulmonary hypertension, to confirm the diagnosis and to assess potential responsiveness to pharmacologic agents.
- Advanced congestive heart failure, including screening for replacement therapies.
- Symptomatic patients with suspected cardiomyopathy, to exclude concomitant ischemic disease.

Finally, cardiac catheterization may be performed for research investigations, in order to compare or test different therapeutic devices or strategies, after the prior approval of the Food and Drug Administration (FDA) in the form of an Investigational Device Exemption, of the local Committee on Human Research at the institution (Institutional Review Board, or IRB), and attainment of informed consent after the details of the risks and potential benefits of the procedure and its alternatives have been thoroughly explained.

3 Contraindications to Cardiac Catheterization

At present, the only absolute contraindication to cardiac catheterization is the refusal of a compos mentis patient to consent to the procedure. Nevertheless, several relative contraindications must be evaluated, including concomitant conditions which correcting would improve the safety of the procedure.

The possibility of hemodynamic stabilization prior to the catheterization reduces the risk of complications: for instance, hypertension, but also hypotension, predisposes to myocardial ischemia, acute decompensation, hemorrhagic stroke following anticoagulation, and bleeding and should be controlled before and during the procedure.

Especially in an elective setting, postponing catheterization should always be considered in patients with:

- Febrile illnesses or suspected infection.
- Congestive heart failure, due to the higher risk of pulmonary edema following contrast media and fluid administration during the procedure and patient's inability to lay flat during the procedure.

- Suspected active bleeding, which exposes patients to major bleeding complications after the administration of antithrombotic drugs during the procedure.
- Drug toxicity and electrolyte imbalance (e.g., hyperkalemia, hypokalemia, digitalis toxicity), since they increase the risk of arrhythmias.

Regarding vitamin K antagonists (VKA, e.g., warfarin), the general approach is to postpone elective procedures until the international normalized ratio (INR) of prothrombin time reaches values less than 2 (and in many labs less than 1.5).

Given that direct oral anticoagulants (DOACs) have become the foundation for prevention of thromboembolic complications in patients with non-valvular (NV) atrial fibrillation (AF), several protocols for their management in the periprocedural period have been developed [21, 22]. The American College of Cardiology classifies PCI via the femoral artery as a moderate-risk bleeding procedure, instructing to discontinue factor Xa inhibitors for 48 h prior to the procedure [21]; this conflicts with the American Heart Association consensus, which categorizes catheterization via the femoral artery as a high-risk procedure, but suggests a shorter hold time of at least 24 h [22].

In order to reduce bleeding risk, patients should be screened for the presence of thrombocytopenia before the procedure: a severe reduction in platelet count should be considered a relative contraindication to cardiac catheterization; the general consensus is that a platelet count of at least 40,000–50,000/mm^3 is sufficient to perform major invasive procedures with safety, in the absence of associated coagulation abnormalities [23].

Finally, allergy to radiographic contrast agent is another relative contraindication. Up to 8% of patients receiving a contrast media will develop some form of reaction; even though most of them are mild and resolve without treatment, moderate and severe life-threatening reactions are seen in 1% and 0.1% of people receiving contrast media, respectively [24]. Protocols of premedication and use of low osmolar contrast agents have both effectively reduced the risks of a major adverse reaction.

4 Cardiac Catheterization Laboratory: A Modern Setup

Contemporary cardiac catheterization laboratories must have sufficient space to house the fluoroscope, an increasing array of ancillary equipment (e.g., IVUS, IABP), work, and storage areas [25]. The angiographic room requires structural and movable radiation shielding, designed by an expert qualified medical physicist, to assure optimal protection. The centerpiece of the cardiac catheterization laboratory is the gantry that holds the X-ray tube and the image receptor in correct alignment. Its role is to provide a full range of two-dimensional rotation (left-to-right anterior oblique) and skew (cranial to caudal) in the direction with which the X-ray beam passes through the patient. The two axes of rotation meet at a single point called the isocenter. An object, such as the patient's heart, placed at isocenter will remain centered on the screen as the beam direction is changed. The patient is supported on an adjustable-height flat-top table. The tabletop can be panned in the left-right or head-foot direction to move the patient relative to the X-ray beam. Some tables feature a tilt capability to put the patient into Trendelenburg or reverse Trendelenburg positions. Robotic base systems provide further extension and integration of gantry and table motions. A second complete imaging chain is provided in some laboratories to provide simultaneous viewing from two angles. Biplane imaging can be indispensable for certain patients and procedures but is usually not required for most invasive cardiology procedures. Physiological monitors (invasive blood pressure, heart rate, ECG) and their displays are vital. These are increasingly integrated into the laboratory's clinical information system such that physiological data, event logs, and other information are time-stamped and recorded while the procedure is in progress. Such systems offer structured reporting, generating a complete report as soon as the procedure is completed. Each piece of equipment in the laboratory must meet specific patient electrical safety requirements if there is any possibility that it could come in contact with the patient under either normal or emergency circumstances. These include non-X-ray imaging devices (e.g., ultrasound), emergency equipment (e.g., defibrillator), interventional devices (e.g., rotablator), physiological monitors, etc.

5 Radiation Exposure During Cardiac Catheterization

Radiation exposure during coronary angiography in the cardiac catheterization laboratory tends to be higher than other radiologic examinations, the level of which can be potentially harmful to the patient and operator, mainly in cases of prolonged procedures [26]. Necessary images need to be obtained while protecting both patients and staff from unnecessary radiation. Clinical radiation dose measurements in the interventional fluoroscopic laboratory are used as practical indicators of patient risk. In the laboratory, dose exposure is usually described in terms of the following parameters:

1. **Fluoroscopic Time (min):** The time during a procedure in which fluoroscopy is used but does not include cine acquisition imaging. Therefore, considered alone, it tends to underestimate the total radiation dose received.
2. **Cumulative Air Kerma (Gy):** The cumulative air kerma is a measure of X-ray energy delivered to air at the interventional reference point (15 cm from the isocenter in the direction of the focal spot). This measurement has been closely associated with deterministic skin effects.
3. **Dose-Area Product (Gy cm^2):** This is the cumulative sum of the instantaneous air kerma and the X-ray field area. This monitors the patient dose burden and is a good indicator of stochastic effects.

Radiation injuries are induced by one of the two mechanisms, stochastic and deterministic. The stochastic mechanism is a non-threshold biologic effect that occurs by chance to a population whose probability is proportional to the dose and whose severity is independent of the dose. It is induced by unrepaired injury to the DNA of a single viable cell. Radiogenic cancer is the principal stochastic risk in the interventional laboratory. As clinical disease requires cellular proliferation, radiogenic cancer will take years to decades before it becomes clinically apparent. The deterministic effect is a dose-dependent damage of radiation of which a threshold is believed to exist. It occurs when the radiation dose is sufficient to result in cell death and creates organ dysfunction [27, 28]. It most commonly results in skin injury, but also bone marrow, gonadal suppression, and cataracts. Operators should make every effort to reduce radiation dose to a level that is "as low as reasonably achievable" (ALARA principle) that provides sufficient diagnostic information [29]. Therefore, it is advisable and good practice to limit radiation exposure to patients and interventional operators as much as possible, by appropriate use of angiographic systems without compromising the effectiveness of the procedures. In addition to the multiple factors affecting radiation exposure such as procedure complexity, type of radiation protection employed, patient anatomy, physician experience, and vascular access site, the type of angiography equipment and dose protocol can affect the amount of emitted radiation [30]. However, there are no specific safety guidelines that address limiting the radiation dose and there are currently no dose reduction strategies in the cardiac catheterization laboratory. A low-dose protocol (LDP) may be obtained with an inferior entrance dose rate limit value as compared to standard dose protocol (SDP), and a reduced frame rate for the cine acquisition. Recommended strategies to minimize radiation exposure are the use of radiation only when imaging is necessary with minimization of the use of cine angiography, steep angles of X-ray beam (e.g., avoiding the left anterior oblique cranial angulation, which has the highest degree of scatter exposure to the operator), magnification mode without additional radiation, and reduction of frame rate from 15 frames/second to 7.5 frames/second. Keeping the image detector close to the patient and monitoring radiation dose in real time are also useful methods to reduce radiation exposure. It is also important for the operator to have the necessary equipment (glasses, vest, safety cap) to allow protection from the radiation beams (Fig. 1).

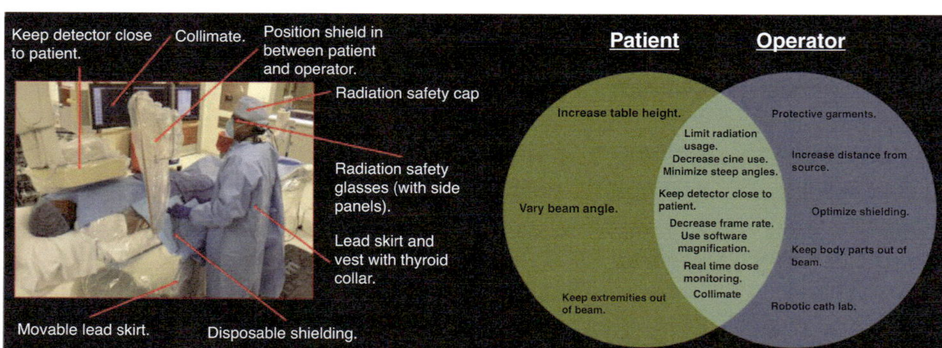

Fig. 1 Strategies to reduce patients and operator radiation exposure

6 Vascular Accesses

Thanks to the development of new catheters and advancement in vascular access techniques, nowadays coronary angiography is performed using a percutaneous approach with progressive use of radial access instead of other access sites, which carry a higher rate of complications.

7 Transfemoral Approach

Transfemoral approach was considered as the main route of arterial access for cardiac catheterization for a long time. The reason for its widespread adoption included the ability to puncture an unlimited number of times, easy access, less radiation time, and less contrast use compared to other access sites. Nowadays, femoral access is still utilized in cases of complex PCI (such as chronic total occlusions, severe calcification and tortuosity, challenging bifurcations). However, the femoral route has been abandoned over time due to the associated higher bleeding rate and vascular complications. Relative contraindications of femoral vascular access include peripheral vascular disease, marked iliac tortuosity, prior femoral arterial graft surgery, or gross obesity; however, catheter insertion and manipulation may present technical challenges even for experienced operators. Recognition of these features may favor the use of the percutaneous radial, brachial, axillary, or even translumbar aortic approaches.

Nowadays, femoral puncture should always be guided by ultrasound minimizing the risk of complications by offering a clear visualization of the vascular structure. If ultrasound-guided puncture is not possible, femoral artery puncture can be achieved under fluoroscopy, placing a radiopaque marker (generally a vascular clamp) at the site where the pulse is most palpable and adjusted until the tip of the marker is located at the inferior border of the femoral head.

7.1 Femoral Access Hemostasis

After catheterization, femoral access hemostasis can be achieved using different approaches:

- *Manual compression:* A compressive force, sufficient to obliterate pedal pulses, is applied with the fingers at the level of femoral artery. The duration of compression should be approximately 2–3 min multiplied by the sheath size. For example, for a 6-French sheath, the duration of compression should be about 12–18 min. The patient should be monitored (blood pressure, telemetry), and fluids and/or atropine need to be administered; if the patient has vasovagal reactions, they should be treated accordingly.

- *Mechanical pressure:* Devices like FemoStop-Abbott Vascular can replace manual pressure, but they are generally uncomfortable for the patients and supervision of a trained expert is required to ensure that peripheral perfusion is not compromised.
- *Percutaneous vascular closure devices:* Vascular closure devices achieve a better control of hemostasis while being more comfortable for the patient, speeding up ambulation, and reducing access-site complications. They allow sheath removal in the cardiac catheterization laboratory even in fully anticoagulated patients. Vascular closure devices can be divided into two groups according to their mechanism of action: passive and active. The passive closure devices are an aid to manual compression and enhance hemostasis by delivering material that facilitates clot formation during mechanical compression. In small randomized controlled trials (RCTs), they did not show any improvement in early ambulation or control of hemostasis at the puncture site. Active vascular closure devices have different mechanisms but usually promote hemostasis by delivering a plug or a suture, which closes the disruption in the vessel structure. Vascular closure devices can be used even when the ACT is high, although it is not recommended to use them if the ACT is >300 s. Successful hemostasis of vascular closure devices mainly depends on the precision of arterial puncture, the conditions of vascular access, as well as the training of the operator.

7.2 Radial Approach

Since 1989, when Lucien Campeau published his successful series of 100 coronary angiographies performed with minimal occurrence of complications, transradial approach (TRA) gained popularity all over the world and became the technique of choice. According to 2018 ESC Guidelines on myocardial revascularization, radial access is preferred for PCI irrespective of clinical presentation, unless there are overriding procedural considerations [11]. TRA is associated with significantly fewer access-site complications and greater patient satisfaction compared with femoral access [31] despite providing a more challenging engagement of the coronary arteries and a suboptimal support of the guide catheter. As it carries a reduction in bleeding and hematoma formation, radial access has been associated with lower mortality in STEMI patients. Radial access is also preferred in patients who receive oral anticoagulants or are at high risk of bleeding [32]. Disadvantages of TRA include a relatively steep learning curve, increased radiation exposure, incompatibility of the radial artery with sheaths larger than 6F, and higher access failure rates.

Allen's test had been routinely performed in the past to assess the patency of collateral circulation of the hand, the ulnar artery. The RADAR trial (Predictive Value of Allen's Test Result in Elective Patients Undergoing Coronary Catheterization Through Radial Approach) showed that radial access was safe and feasible independently of Allen's test results. For this reason, Allen's test is no longer recommended prior to obtaining radial access [33].

TRA can be performed via the left or right radial artery. Due to ergonomic considerations, most operators prefer using the right TRA. Left TRA should be preferred in patients with previous coronary artery bypass grafting (CABG) with a left internal mammary artery (LIMA). In the TALENT trial, left TRA was associated with a significantly shorter learning curve and progressive reductions in cannulation and fluoroscopy times as the operator volume increased, compared to right TRA [34].

Radial artery spasm is the most common TRA complication and is a frequent reason for failure and crossover to transfemoral access [35]. Prevention of spasm should be performed using a hydrophilic coated sheath with the injection of a vasodilator (verapamil, nitroglycerin—either alone or in combination—nicardipine, lidocaine, and papaverine) after obtaining access [36].

One of the consequences of the TRA is radial artery occlusion (RAO), which occurs in approximately 5–10% of transradial procedures, and in most cases, it occurs due to vessel injury and thrombosis. The clinical signs include painless loss of radial pulse. Risk factors associated with RAO are a lack of anticoagulation during the procedure, larger diameter sheaths, multiple procedures through the same radial artery, and prolonged occlusive compression for hemostasis. Spontaneous recanalization of RA is reported to be around 25–50% at 30 days [37, 38].

7.3 Distal Radial Approach

The distal transradial approach (dTRA) has been recently introduced in clinical practice to overcome the possible limitations of the TRA and involves puncturing the artery at the level of the snuffbox. As the radial artery has reached the anatomic snuffbox, it has already given rise to some branches that, in case of vessel occlusion, could avoid flow interruption. In the most recent registries and trials, success rate of dTRA has been reported to be approximately 90%. Potential advantages of this technique include a more comfortable arm position for the patient, a lower rate of distal radial artery obstruction due to maintenance of antegrade flow through the superficial palmar arch, early hemostasis, low risk for hematoma formation and compartment syndrome, low level of pain, and possibility of saving the radial artery for possible future coronary artery bypass graft. The disadvantages of dTRA are that they are technically more demanding and time consuming, especially in access time [39].

7.4 Radial Access Hemostasis

One of the advantages of TRA and dTRA is that the vascular sheath is always removed at the end of the procedure regardless of the antithrombotic therapy. Currently, a radial compression device is used for achieving hemostasis after radial catheterization. The most used compression device is the TR Band (Terumo Medical, Somerset, NJ), which allows fine adjustments of the hemostatic pressure and direct visualization of the arteriotomy site through the transparent balloon material. Dedicated closure devices are available to achieve safe hemostasis of the distal radial access.

8 Angiographic Coronary Artery Anatomy and Projections

8.1 Angiograph Views

Contrast injections in multiple views are necessary to ensure a clear visualization of all coronary segments without foreshortening or overlap. The angulation of each view is defined using two terms, with the first one denoting the degree of rotation over the anterior chest wall and the second one describing skewness, which means the degree of angulation towards the patient's head (cranial) or foot (caudal). Coronary anatomy in an angiographic view can be represented considering two orthogonal planes, the first one representing the interventricular septum and the second one representing the atrioventricular valves. To execute an adequate coronary angiography, it is not necessary to study all potential views, but a series of screening views should be performed, extending the exam with one or more additional views to complete the study according to the clinical case (Figs. 1 and 2).

- **Right Anterior Oblique (RAO) Projections:** Straight RAO projections are generally avoided due to overlapping and foreshortening of the left anterior descending (LAD) and circumflex (Cx) arteries.
- **RAO Cranial (10–30° RAO, 25–40° Cranial):** The RAO-cranial (10–30° RAO; 25–40° cranial) projection should be performed after the first view. In this projection, the mid- and distal portion of the LAD and the origin of septal and diagonal branches can be visualized. The distal right coronary artery (RCA) can also be viewed in this projection, or the Cx (in case of left dominance) at the point where these vessels give rise to the posterior descending (PDA) and posterolateral (PL) branches. This view rarely provides information about LMCA and Cx due to overlapping and foreshortening (Fig. 3).
- **LAO Straight (60° LAO):** The straight 60° LAO projection provides a good view of proximal and mid-RCA, but is very limited in evaluating the left coronary artery.
- **LAO Cranial (LAO 60°, Cranial 15-30°):** By adding a 15–30° cranial angulation, the LAO-cranial view is obtained. In this projection, ostial and distal LMCA is clearly shown together with middle and distal portion of LAD with the origin of septal and diagonal branches. Sometimes, when present, the ramus intermedius can be clearly shown. Finally, proximal Cx and obtuse marginal branch (OMB) can be seen on the extreme right of the screen. With about 25 degrees of cranial angulation, the LAO cranial projection shows the midportion of RCA and, in the case of right dominance, the origin and course of PDA. Reducing LAO angulation to 30–40° allows a better visualization of LAD between the right hemidiaphragm and the spine. With maximal inspiration, diaphragm is pulled down and X-rays better penetrate.

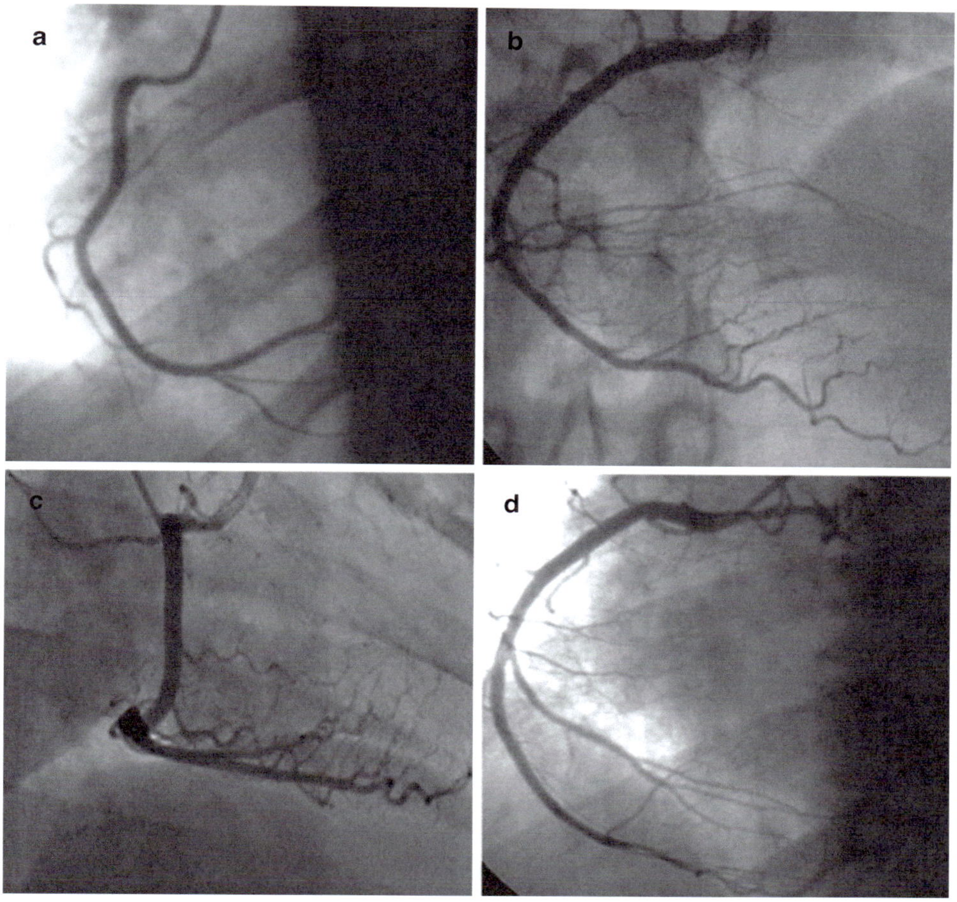

Fig. 2 Projections for the right coronary artery: (**a**) LAO 10° CRA 20° projection to better visualize the distal portion of the right coronary artery. (**b**) AP caudal offers a good evaluation of the mid-part of the right coronary artery with clear visualization of septal coming from the posterior descending artery. (**c**) RAO projection is useful to clarify the anatomy of the posterior descending artery. (**d**) LAO view is utilized as standard projection for right coronary artery cannulation and visualization of the proximal part of the vessel

- **LAO Caudal—Spider (60° LAO, 10–20° Caudal)***:* In LAO-caudal view—the so-called spider (60° LAO; 10–20° caudal)—LMCA is seen in a spiderlike appearance, giving origin to the proximal segments of LAD and Cx. Also, the distal RCA and its bifurcation in PDA and PL with their respective course are well explored in this view. With maximal expiration, the horizontal cardiac position is accentuated with a better view from below the heart and coronary branches.

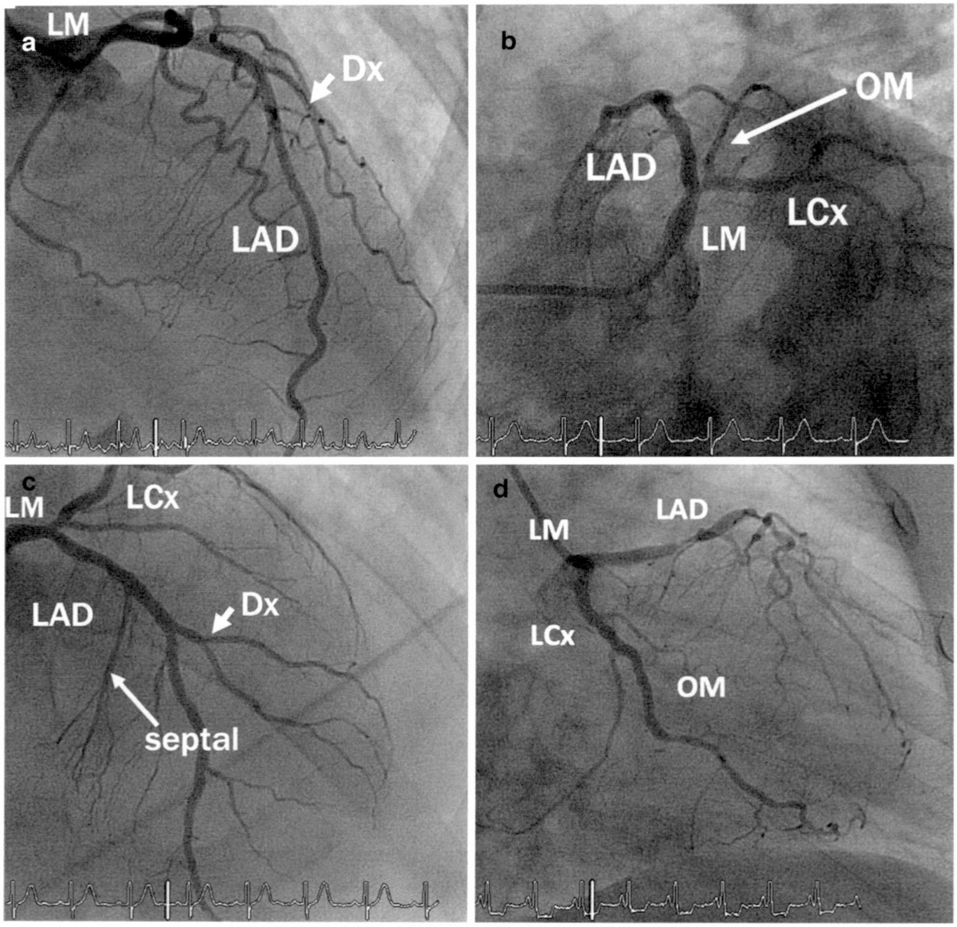

Fig. 3 Projections for the left coronary artery: (**a**) LAO 0° CRA 25° (AP cranial) is the projection to better visualize the proximal-mid-segment of the left descending artery, diagonals, and septal. (**b**) Spider view (LAO 15°, CAU 20°) caudal offers a good evaluation of the distal left main bifurcation with clear visualization of the proximal segments of the circumflex and of the left descending artery. (**c**) LAO 15° CRA 25° is useful for a clear view of the proximal left descending artery, (**d**) RAO 20 °, CAU 20° is the standard projection that should be firstly performed during the left coronary catheterization. It gives a clear visualization of the circumflex and a good vision of the mid-distal segments of the left descending artery. Abbreviations: *OM* obtuse marginal; *LM* left main; *LAD* left anterior descending; *LCx* left circumflex artery

– **Posteroanterior and Left Lateral Projections:** These projections are underused but can still provide some additional information to the exam. PA projection, for example, frequently provides the best view of the left main ostium. On the other hand, the distal LM can be better seen with RAO-caudal view.

- **Lateral Projections:** Left lateral projection, especially if combined with 10–15° cranial angulation, is useful to exam proximal Cx and proximal and distal LAD. This projection also offers an excellent look at the mid-RCA with the possibility of limiting motion comparing to the sight in straight RAO.
- **RAO Caudal (10–30° RAO, 15–20° Caudal):** The RAO-caudal projection (10–30° RAO and 15–20° caudal) should be the first view of choice as it gives an optimal view of the left main coronary artery (LMCA) bifurcation, the proximal LAD, and also the proximal and midportion of Cx.

8.2 Catheters

Catheters have multiple roles during coronary angiography, which include reaching and engaging coronary arteries for contrast injection and angiographic visualization; monitoring artery pressure during the procedure; and delivering the necessary equipment into the coronary artery. They can be divided, according to their function, into two main groups: guide and diagnostic catheters.

A guide catheter has thinner walls and a larger lumen allowing the delivery of necessary equipment during cardiac catheterization. The guide walls are made thinner through the use of a layer of metal mesh that prevents the guide catheter walls from collapsing. Guide catheters have also softer tips compared with diagnostic catheters. This allows longer coronary engagement and deep seating and also limits the risk of coronary dissection.

Diagnostic catheters have thicker walls which allow them to be more torquable. The catheter outer diameter is measured using French (1 French = 0.33 mm) and varies from 4F to 8F. Most PCIs can be performed through 6-French (2 mm) guide catheters, but guide catheters with larger diameter (7- or 8-French) provide better support and improve vessel visualization and may be required for delivery of some equipment or in cases where multiple simultaneous equipment may be necessary. The average length of most catheters is about 100 cm. Shorter guide catheters (usually 90 cm) can be utilized to deliver equipment in distal target lesions or for retrograde chronic total occlusion PCI [40]. Longer guide catheters (125 cm long) may be needed in case of tortuosity or dilation of aorta or tall patients to reach the coronary arteries.

Guiding catheters can have side holes that prevent pressure dampening in the presence of ostial plaques. Dedicated guiding catheters designed for radial access are available and allow cannulation of both coronary ostia.

8.3 Guiding Catheter Shapes

Most guide catheter shapes are specific for the right or left coronary artery or for bypass grafts, although some guide catheters can be used to engage various vessels. Guide catheters are described by the shape name and the length of their distal segment. Selecting diagnostic

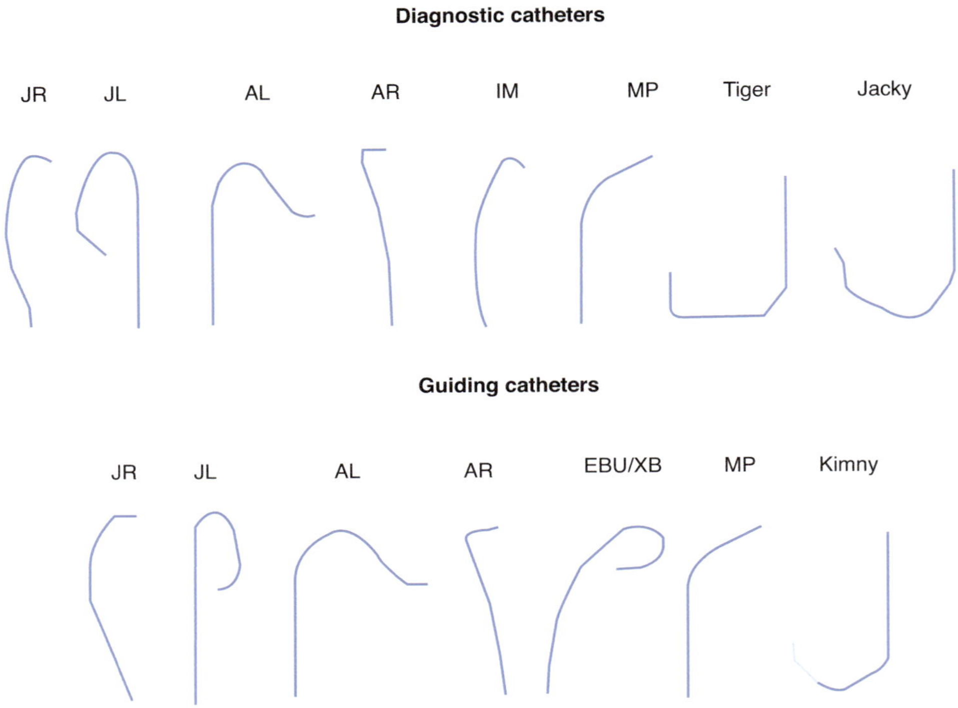

Fig. 4 Examples of diagnostic and guiding catheters most commonly utilized in the clinical practice

and guide catheter size depends on the size of the aortic root, with larger catheters needed for larger aortic root sizes. The mostly utilized diagnostic catheters are the Judkins left and right for selective cannulation of the coronary ostia. Similarly, left and right Amplatz catheters are dedicated for selective cannulation of the coronaries. Universally, Amplatz left catheter is utilized for cannulation also of the RCA providing more support.

Other specific catheters are designed to cannulate anomalous origin of the coronaries, bypass grafts, and peripheral vessels. A detailed list of the mostly available catheters is provided in Fig. 4. Some catheters (TIG and Jacky catheters) are available for cannulation of both coronary ostia through the radial access.

9 Periprocedural Drugs

9.1 Heparin

The rationale for the use of anticoagulation is 1) to mitigate the sequelae of iatrogenic plaque rupture from balloon angioplasty or stenting; 2) to prevent thrombotic occlusion of vascular access, in particular when the radial access is utilized; and 3) to reduce the risk of thrombus formation on intravascular PCI equipment. Conversely, anticoagulation can increase the risk of bleeding during cardiac catheterization, so a balance between bleeding and thrombotic complications should be evaluated.

Unfractionated heparin (UFH) remains the cornerstone of anticoagulation treatment in patients undergoing cardiac catheterization. It produces its major anticoagulant effect by inactivating thrombin and activated factor X (factor Xa) through an antithrombin (AT)-dependent mechanism. By inactivating thrombin, heparin not only prevents fibrin formation but also inhibits thrombin-induced activation of platelets and of factors V and VIII [41].

High-intensity anticoagulation should be considered in transradial diagnostic procedures for the prevention of forearm occlusion (high [100 IU/kg] versus standard [50 IU/kg] heparin dose) [42]. The intensity of anticoagulation with heparin is evaluated measuring the activated clotting time (ACT) and should be between 250 and 350 s.

Anticoagulation with UFH alone does not seem to be sufficient for protection from ischemic sequelae, such as periprocedural MI. One cause of these events is embolization of platelet aggregates that form as a result of platelet activation induced by UFH.

Another limitation of UFH is the potential risk of developing heparin-induced thrombocytopenia with or without thrombosis syndrome [HIT(TS)]. The development of HIT(TS) is associated with prolonged use of UFH and is a rare occurrence during cardiac catheterization. The development of thrombocytopenia during PCI is associated with increased mortality [43].

Despite the aforementioned limitations, several other drugs have been compared with heparin, but none of them have been proven superior.

9.2 Bivalirudin

Bivalirudin is a synthetic 20-residue peptide, which reversibly inhibits thrombin. Once bound to the active site, thrombin cannot activate fibrinogen into fibrin, the crucial step in the formation of thrombus. Bivalirudin mediates an inhibitory action on thrombin by specifically binding to both the catalytic site and anion-binding exosite of circulating and clot-bound thrombin. The action of bivalirudin is reversible because unbound thrombin cleaves the thrombin-bivalirudin complex, thus inactivating it. Due to its pharmacokinetic properties, the half-life of bivalirudin is short (25 min) and is largely dependent on the proteolysis (80%) of the thrombin-bivalirudin complex while the remaining 20% is excreted by kidneys.

Bivalirudin has been studied only in patients receiving concomitant aspirin. The recommended dose of bivalirudin is an intravenous bolus dose of 0.75 mg/kg, followed immediately by an infusion of 1.75 mg/kg/h for the duration of the procedure. Five minutes after the bolus dose has been administered, an ACT should be performed and an additional bolus of 0.3 mg/kg should be given if needed.

Bivalirudin is actually indicated as intravenous anticoagulation in patients with acute myocardial infarction, unstable angina, percutaneous coronary intervention, and thrombosis in patients with a history of HIT [44].

9.3 Enoxaparin

Low-molecular-weight heparin (LMWH) is derived from heparin by chemical or enzymatic depolymerization to yield fragments approximately one-third of the size of heparin. Compared with UFH, LMWHs have reduced ability to inactivate thrombin because the smaller fragments cannot bind simultaneously to AT and thrombin. In contrast, LMWH can easily bind AT and factor Xa, thus inhibiting its action.

Reduced binding to plasma proteins and cells is responsible for the more predictable dose-response relationship of LMWH, longer plasma half-life (compared with UFH), and lower risk of heparin-induced thrombocytopenia and osteopenia. LMWHs are principally renally cleared, so its dosage should be adjusted in patients with impaired kidney function. One of the clearest benefits of enoxaparin over heparin is that it does not require point-of-care monitoring in the cardiac catheterization laboratory. The anticoagulant effect of enoxaparin can be monitored via monitoring of anti-factor Xa levels, although this is not the standard of care and there is little clinical evidence to establish any clinical utility in measuring anti-factor Xa. LMWHs do not have an antidote, but protamine administration may be useful in an emergency; however, this does not result in the complete reversal of the anticoagulant effect. Dalteparin, another LMWH agent, has also been evaluated in ACS in several small studies, though its use is not recommended in current guidelines.

9.4 Fondaparinux

Fondaparinux is an inhibitor of the factor X. Studies have demonstrated that its use during coronary angiography is associated with a higher incidence of catheter thrombosis; its mechanism of action does not inhibit catheter-induced clotting as it does not inhibit upstream coagulation via the contact pathway nor does it inhibit downstream clotting mediated by thrombin. For this reason, the use of fondaparinux in the setting of coronary angiographies is contraindicated.

9.5 Limitations of Cardiac Catheterization for the Detection of Coronary Artery Disease Severity

Despite being the first-line diagnostic test to assess the presence and extent of coronary atherosclerosis, coronary angiography has several intrinsic limitations, which have led to the development of adjunctive intra-procedural tools in order to increase overall accuracy.

As first, evaluation of the degree of coronary stenosis during angiography is primarily based on the physician's visual assessment, which is subject to consistent inter-operator and intra-operator variability [45]. Secondly, coronary angiography provides an anatomical evaluation of CAD and does not predict the probability of a lesion to induce myocardial ischemia. Third, by means of intracoronary contrast injection, it only allows the visualization of vascular contour. While this approach might be useful to estimate the degree by which obstructive atherosclerotic plaques reduce arterial lumen, it does not allow plaque catheterization and underestimates the severity of eccentric or diffuse atherosclerotic lesions [46]. Fourth, the spatial resolution of angiography is limited to 300 um approximately, and coronary microvascular dysfunction cannot be detected [47].

9.5.1 Fractional Flow Reserve (FFR)

Coronary pressure flow measurements can be used to define the functional significance of coronary stenosis, which is the ability of a stenosis to induce myocardial ischemia. This assessment is generally required in cases of angiographically intermediate coronary lesions or in cases of diffuse CAD in order to guide revascularization. Pressure wires are sensory-tipped angioplasty guidewires, which measure the pressure and/or flow drop across a stenosis.

The simplest pressure wire-based index is the resting distal coronary artery pressure/aortic pressure (Pd/Pa), which indicates the ratio of distal coronary artery pressure to aortic pressure at rest. Since coronary flow reserve reduction associated with stable coronary artery disease becomes overt in exercise, Pd/Pa alone is not accurate for the detection of functional significance.

Fractional flow reserve (FFR) evaluates the discrepancy between the maximum blood flow in the coronary artery in the presence of a stenosis and the maximum flow in the same vessel in the theoretical absence of any stenosis. Maximum blood flow (hyperemia) is usually obtained through intravenous or intracoronary adenosine injection (at a dose of at least 40 ug IC bolus in the right coronary artery and 40–80 ug in the left coronary artery). Assuming linear relationship between perfusion pressure and coronary blood flow during hyperemia and venous pressure to be equal to zero, the ratio between distal coronary artery pressure and aortic pressure equals to the ratio of maximum flows. Therefore, FFR can be indirectly measured through Pd/Pa after hyperemic stimulus.

The theoretically normal FFR value in the absence of any coronary lesions is 1; the lower the FFR, the higher the ability of a stenosis to limit coronary blood flow. The first FFR cutoff to be validated using noninvasive stress imaging as the reference standard was 0.75 [48]. In a subsequent series of large randomized clinical trials, FFR cutoff of 0.8 has been proven to improve long-term outcomes when used to guide or defer coronary revascularization [49, 50]. Based on this evidence, angiographically intermediate (40–90%) coronary lesions with FFR $\leq$0.80 should be considered for revascularization according to 2019 ESC Guidelines [51].

While outperforming coronary angiography alone, FFR assessment in angiographically intermediate lesions presents some inherent limitations. Firstly, adenosine-related side effects such as hypotension, bradyarrhythmias, and respiratory distress are not uncommon [52]. Secondly, the key assumption behind FFR calculation is a linear relationship between flow and pressure under conditions of constant intracoronary resistance. However, even after adenosine administration, coronary resistance changes throughout the cardiac cycle and final FFR value is time averaged. In order to overcome these two limitations, a non-hyperemic pressure-derived index, the instantaneous wave-free ratio (iFR), has recently been developed [53]. The rationale of iFR is the presence of a phase in the cardiac cycle in which coronary resistance is naturally stable and coronary pressure is proportional to the flow. The so-called wave-free period, in which the ratio of trans-stenotic pressures is measured, corresponds to the end-diastolic phase. Two large randomized clinical trials have recently compared FFR with iFR to guide coronary revascularization, showing similar long-term outcomes and higher rates of periprocedural complications associated with FFR, mainly related to adenosine administration [54, 55]. iFR values below 0.89 indicate the presence of a flow-limiting stenosis.

9.5.2 Intravascular Imaging (OCT and IVUS)

Intravascular imaging techniques—intravascular ultrasound (IVUS) and optical coherence tomography (OCT)—have been developed in order to provide more detailed information of the vascular wall, as coronary angiography only indirectly provides vessel contour. Both OCT and IVUS are particularly useful in optimizing PCI in the following ways [56]:

- They guide optimal stent size and length selection, by detecting the final stent area and exploring the extent of residual atherosclerosis at the proximal and distal landing zones.
- They identify acute PCI complications, including edge dissection.
- They distinguish culprit and non-culprit coronary lesions in acute coronary syndromes.
- They are pivotal in determining the underlying etiology of revascularization failure (i.e., stent thrombosis, in-stent restenosis, neoatherosclerosis).

IVUS is performed through a catheter with a miniaturized ultrasound probe mounted at its tip. High-ultrasound frequencies are used in order to guarantee an appropriate wavelength and adequate image resolution [57].

The normal appearance of a coronary artery at IVUS examination is the so-called three-layer appearance [58] (Fig. 5a). In fact, there are two interfaces at which the ultrasounds are reflected, the first between blood and intima and the second between media and adventitia. The intima is mainly composed of endothelial cells and collagen and appears as a thin and poorly defined layer in the normal vessel. The media is composed of smooth muscle cells, which do not reflect the ultrasound and therefore result as a distinct dark layer at IVUS image. Finally, the adventitia with its high density of collagen fibers is highly reflective and appears as a very bright outer layer.

In the presence of atherosclerotic disease, IVUS allows to accurately define both the extension and the composition of coronary plaques. With regard to extension, the tomographic cross-sectional view of the artery is superior to the conventional angiographic projections in identifying those plaques with prevalent eccentric distribution [46]. Moreover, different plaques present different echogenicity patterns depending on their composition. Conversely, completely calcified lesions are bright and are associated with an acoustic shadow, as all the ultrasounds are reflected.

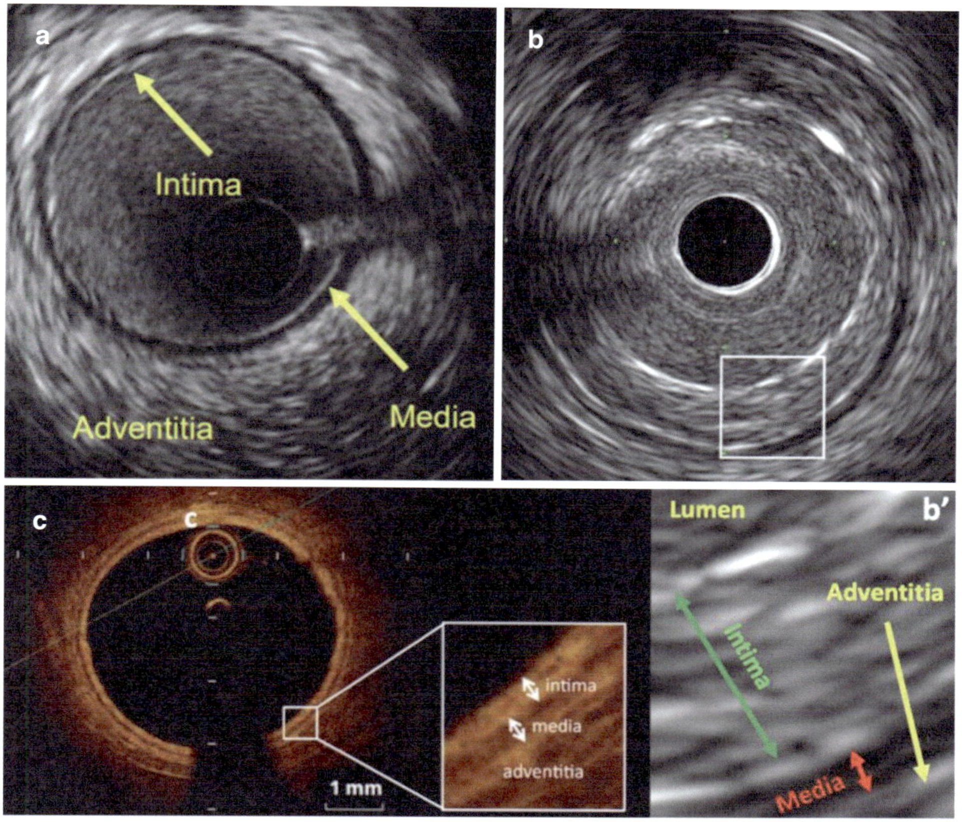

Fig. 5 Comparison between OCT and IVUS imaging. (**a**) Visualization of a normal vessel using the IVUS probe. (**b** and **b'**) Evidence of intimal proliferation at IVUS. (**c**) Normal coronary artery at the OCT evaluation

In the last decade, several trials and real-world registries have shown that IVUS guidance has improved prognosis of patients with complex coronary disease (i.e., unprotected left main disease, long LAD lesions, bifurcation lesions, chronic total occlusions), when compared with coronary angiography alone [59–61]. Current research is mainly focusing on the outcomes of IVUS-guided PCI among all-comers, and even in this setting, the results associated with this technology seem promising [62].

Being based on ultrasound, the IVUS technique has some intrinsic limitations. As first, it does not accurately distinguish tissue histology. Secondly, it is subject to several artifacts, such as the "blooming" artifact and the "ring-down" artifacts, occurring due to acoustic oscillations in the piezoelectric transducer and consisting of several layers around the catheter that compromise vessel lumen definition.

OCT uses infrared light waves, with a wavelength of approximately 1300 nm (while ultrasound provides an ~40 um wavelength at 40 MHz). This implies that OCT has a much higher spatial resolution compared to IVUS, at the cost of reduced tissue penetration. Another key difference between the two imaging techniques is that OCT requires blood clearance, while IVUS does not. In fact, OCT wavelength is even shorter than blood cell diameter, so that backscattering from blood would occur in the absence of blood clearance. Blood clearance is obtained through contrast injection for the whole duration of the pullback. As a consequence, OCT provides better determination of tissue characteristics (i.e., difference between calcium, thrombus, and neointimal tissue) and more accurate assessment of stent positioning, while IVUS is better suited for large vessels and bifurcation lesions.

A normal coronary artery has a bright-dark-bright (three-layer) appearance on OCT. In fact, light signal is highly reflected by the intima and the adventitia (Fig. 5b).

Given its excellent resolution, OCT is the most accurate technique to discriminate plaque morphology. Here are some examples of how atherosclerotic lesions should be interpreted at OCT images [56, 63]:

- Fibrous plaques, composed of collagen fibers and muscular cells, provide a homogeneous and bright signal.
- Calcific plaques are heterogeneous, signal-poor, and with well-delineated borders.
- Lipid-rich plaques are signal-poor and with undefined borders. The media beyond the plaque is usually not visible because of high signal attenuation and, in some cases, an external signal-rich band might be present, corresponding to the fibrous cap.
- Thrombus usually appears as masses floating into the vessel lumen. White thrombus (mainly composed of platelets and white blood cells) provides a very low signal attenuation, while red thrombus (with high density of red blood cells) is closer to the vessel wall and provides high signal attenuation.

9.6 Complications of Cardiac Catheterization

The risk of major complications related to diagnostic cardiac catheterization has progressively decreased over time owing to more advanced technical equipment, increased operators' experience, and improved patient's periprocedural management. However, a variety of adverse events might occur after coronary angiography, mainly including access-site complications, peripheral vascular or ostial coronary dissections, contrast-induced nephropathy, and arrythmias.

9.6.1 Ostial Coronary Dissections

Catheter-induced coronary dissections following a diagnostic coronary angiography are currently very rare but associated with potentially catastrophic outcomes. They occur when the tip of the guiding catheter disrupts the endothelial cells of the intima and causes blood extravasation into the subintimal space, thereby creating a false lumen. Their entry site is usually located at the ostium of major epicardial vessels, mainly left main and left anterior descending. In such cases, the mechanical compression exerted by the false lumen on the true vessel lumen can limit coronary perfusion and lead to extensive periprocedural acute myocardial infarctions. Furthermore, if the mechanical injury involves the whole vessel wall, a dissection can rapidly evolve into a perforation, presenting with pericardial effusion and cardiac tamponade.

The management of catheter-induced coronary dissections therefore requires an immediate evaluation of hemodynamic compromise, eventually considering mechanical circulatory support or inotropes. Another cornerstone of their treatment is avoiding further anterograde contrast injection, which might increase pressure inside the false lumen and cause the dissection to extend both proximally towards the aorta and distally. IVUS might be useful to confirm the entry point and to evaluate whether the guidewire is in the true or in the false lumen. Several treatment strategies might be considered, with covered stents being usually preferred [64].

9.6.2 Vascular Complications

Vascular complications at the site of catheter insertion are among the most common adverse events occurring in the peri- and immediate post-procedural phase of a cardiac catheterization. Most of them (i.e., hematomas, small pseudoaneurysm) are self-limiting and can be conservatively managed, while a surgical intervention must be considered in other cases.

The rate of local vascular complications following coronary angiography has substantially decreased in the last years owing to the progressively higher use of radial over femoral arterial access [31].

The most common vascular complications of coronary angiography are the following:

- *Hematomas*, which are due to blood swelling and extravasation in the surrounding soft tissues. Predisposing factors for hematoma occurrence include multiple puncture attempts, tortuous arterial anatomy, and inadequate compression (i.e., misplacement of a compression device). Most hematomas developing both at the radial and at the femoral access site resolve within a few days and can be treated conservatively. More severe complications of hematomas might include compartment syndromes and nerve compression with paresthesia.
- *Pseudoaneurysms* are a collection of blood between the two outer layers of the artery, the media and the adventitia. The pseudoaneurysm presents as a tender and most times painful pulsatile mass, and final diagnosis is made with Doppler ultrasound showing an arterial flow directed from the artery to the hematoma. Key risk factors for its formation include anticoagulation, inadequate manual compression, and large-bore sheaths. Treatment options might include:
  - Manual or ultrasound-guided compression, indicated in cases of small pseudoaneurysms.
  - Ultrasound-guided thrombin injection, which is highly effective but limited by a not negligible risk of distal ischemia.

   - Surgical repair, which should be considered in cases of large and painful pseudoaneurysms for which conservative management is not effective.
- *Arteriovenous (AV) fistula* is extremely rare, especially after transradial access [65], while it might complicate transfemoral access when arterial puncture is performed below the common femoral artery. AV fistula does in fact develop if venous side branches are punctured during access positioning due to erroneous needle deviation. If AV fistula is recognized early during angiography, it can be immediately treated by sealing the connection between the artery and vein. If this is not the case, surgical treatment is usually required.
- *Radial artery spasm* is currently the most common complication of radial access. It should be suspected when a resistance suddenly develops as the catheters pass up the arm. Predisposing factors are related both to the patient, including anxiety and lower BMI, and to the procedure, especially if large sheaths are used or multiple catheters are exchanged. In case of radial spasm, a crossover to femoral access may be required. Patient sedation during the procedure is probably the most effective strategy to prevent radial spasm; other therapeutic options such as intra-arterial nitrate or calcium channel blocker (verapamil or diltiazem) injection can be useful to reduce the rate of spasm.
- ***Radial artery occlusion*** after cardiac catheterization has an estimated prevalence ranging from 1 to 10% [66] and is usually asymptomatic and unrecognized owing to the several collaterals arising from the ulnar artery and perfusing the whole hand. When symptomatic, it can present with pain, discoloration, and paresthesia of the hand and the fingers, and the radial pulse is not palpable. A common risk factor for radial arterial occlusion is prolonged manual compression at the access site. Other causes include large sheaths and multiple catheter exchange, as well as non-ultrasound-guided puncture. Of note, distal radial access at the level of the anatomical snuffbox or of the dorsum of the hand has recently been proved to reduce the rate of radial occlusion [67].

9.6.3 Stroke

Cerebrovascular accidents during diagnostic coronary angiography might occur due to several mechanisms, even though the overall incidence is low.

Ischemic stroke is a direct complication of catheterization, which involves catheter advancement towards large arteries and contrast injection. Wire manipulation in the aorta might cause debris, thrombi, or cholesterol dislocation over the aortic arch and the carotid arteries; indeed, patients with a history of CAD have a higher risk of periprocedural stroke compared to those with no history. Another source of embolization is represented by contrast injection which mostly leads to air bubble embolization [68]. The latter mechanism seems to be more frequently associated with asymptomatic cerebral embolism rather than overt ischemic stroke.

Hemorrhagic strokes, on the other hand, are mainly associated with periprocedural anticoagulation and antiplatelet therapies, potentially contributing to hemostasis dysregulation.

9.7 Arrythmias

Ventricular arrythmias, such as ventricular tachycardia (VT) and ventricular fibrillation (VF), have been described, being caused by the guiding catheter irritating the myocardium especially when the right coronary artery is cannulated. The prevalence of this complication was much higher when high osmolar ionic contrast was used [69]. When a run of VT/VF is observed on the EKG monitor, the guiding catheter should be immediately removed and, based on the hemodynamic compromise, intravenous antiarrhythmic drug administration (amiodarone or lidocaine) or electric cardioversion should be considered.

Atrial arrythmias are more frequently associated with left- or right-heart catheterization rather than with coronary angiography alone.

Conversely, bradycardia is not an uncommon complication of coronary angiography that may occur after contrast injection in the right coronary artery. Also, it may be related to a vasovagal reaction, potentially starting even before local anesthesia. Sustained bradycardias are treated with fluid administration and eventual intravenous atropine infusion, depending on their severity.

9.8 Contrast-Induced Nephropathy

Contrast-induced nephropathy (CIN) is a type of acute kidney injury (AKI), defined by a 25% relative increase or a 0.5 mg/dL (44 umol/L) absolute increase in serum creatinine occurring within the first 2–3 days following intravenous contrast administration [70]. Since no diagnostic test can confirm the causal relation between contrast injection and subsequent AKI, the exclusion of any other causes of kidney impairment through a comprehensive clinical evaluation is pivotal for CIN diagnosis.

The pathogenic substrate of CIN is represented by acute tubular necrosis, even though the exact mechanisms underlying this damage are unclear. A combination of vasoconstriction, hypoxia, ischemia, and direct damage on tubular cells is probably at the core of its pathogenesis.

The most common risk factor for CIN is preexistent chronic kidney disease (CKD), with lower glomerular filtration rate at baseline being associated with higher risk of developing this complication [71]. Other predisposing factors include comorbidities, such as diabetes mellitus and congestive heart failure, and procedural characteristics, such as contrast volume. Indeed, a clinical score (the Roxana Mehran score) has been developed to predict the pretest probability to develop CIN [72].

Differently than other types of AKI, CIN does not lead to oligo-anuria and is detected only through an increase in serum creatinine in the majority of cases. However, it represents the third cause of iatrogenic kidney injury after cardiac intervention, with an estimated prevalence of up to 15% [73]. Serum creatinine usually goes back to baseline values after one or two weeks after contrast injection. A minority of patients, especially those with preexisting comorbidities and chronic kidney disease, require renal replacement therapy and present worse prognosis.

The differential diagnosis of a creatinine rise following cardiac catheterization should at first include prerenal injury due to hypoperfusion, especially in those patients who are predisposed to volume depletion. Blood urea nitrogen/creatinine ratio > 15 and a fractional excretion of sodium >2% should raise the suspicion of CIN.

The management of CIN is basically supportive and includes hydration, avoidance of any potential kidney insult and serial urinary output, and electrolyte monitoring. Nonetheless, CIN should be prevented in patients with high baseline risk through peri- and post-procedural hydration with saline solution. Acetylcysteine and bicarbonate have been suggested to be effective for the prevention of CIN, but clinical trials did not show a superiority over standard intravenous hydration [74].

9.9 Infections

Catheter-related bacteremia and sepsis are extremely rare since catheterization has to be performed under sterile conditions. The most common source of infection is usually represented by the vascular access, especially in case of hematomas or other vascular complications.

Endocarditis prophylaxis is therefore not recommended, while coronary angiography should preferably not be performed in patients with fever and/or ongoing infections.

References

1. Cournand A, Cardiac catheterization. Development of the technique, its contributions to experimental medicine, and its initial application in man. Acta Med Scand Suppl. 1975;579:1–32.
2. Forssmann W. Die Sondierung des rechten Herzens. Klin Wochenschr. 1929;8:2085.
3. Cournand AF, Ranges HS. Catheterization of the right auricle in man. Proc Soc Exp Biol Med. 1941;46:462.
4. Cournand AF. Measurement of cardiac output in man using the technique of catheterization of the right auricle or ventricle. Clin Invest. 1945;24:106.
5. Richards D. Cardiac output by the catheterization technique in various clinical conditions. Fed Proc. 1945;4:215–20.
6. Dexter L. Studies of congenital heart disease. The pressure and oxygen content of blood in the right auricle, right ventricle, and pulmonary artery in control patients, with observations on the oxygen saturation and source of pulmonary "capillary" blood. Clin Invest. 1947;26:554.
7. Sones F. Cinecoronary arteriography. Circulation. 1959;20:773.
8. Grüntzig A. Coronary transluminal angioplasty. Circulation. 1977;56(II):319.
9. Gruntzig A, Senning A, Siegenthaler W. Non operative dilatation of coronary artery stenoses. Percutaneous transluminal coronary angioplasty. N Eng Jou Med. 1979;301:61.
10. MedSuite. Interventional Cardiology Market Size, Share & COVID19 Impact Analysis | United States | 2020–2026. 2020.

11. Patel MR, Bailey SR, Bonow RO, et al. ACCF/SCAI/AATS/AHA/ASE/ASNC/HFSA/HRS/SCCM/SCCT/SCMR/STS 2012 appropriate use criteria for diagnostic catheterization. J Am Coll Cardiol. 2012;59(22):1995–2027. https://doi.org/10.1016/j.jacc.2012.03.003.
12. Balbi MM, Scarparo P, Tovar MN, et al. Culprit lesion detection in patients presenting with non-ST elevation acute coronary syndrome and multivessel disease. Cardiovasc Revascularization Med. 2021:5(30-453). https://doi.org/10.1016/j.carrev.2021.03.019.
13. Amsterdam EA, Wenger NK, Brindis RG, et al. 2014 AHA/acc guideline for the management of patients with Non-ST-Elevation acute coronary syndromes: a report of the American College of Cardiology/American Heart Association Task Force on Practice Guidelines. J Am Coll Cardiol. 2014;64(24):e139–228. https://doi.org/10.1016/j.jacc.2014.09.017.
14. O'Gara PT, Kushner FG, Ascheim DD, et al. 2013 ACCF/AHA guideline for the management of st-elevation myocardial infarction: a report of the American College of Cardiology Foundation/American Heart Association task force on practice guidelines. J Am Coll Cardiol. 2013;61(4):78–140. https://doi.org/10.1016/j.jacc.2012.11.019.
15. Ibanez B, James S, Agewall S, et al. 2017 ESC Guidelines for the management of acute myocardial infarction in patients presenting with ST-segment elevation. Eur Heart J. 2018;39(2):119–77. https://doi.org/10.1093/eurheartj/ehx393.
16. Collet JP, Thiele H, Barbato E, et al. 2020 ESC Guidelines for the management of acute coronary syndromes in patients presenting without persistent ST-segment elevation. Eur Heart J. 2021;42(14):1289–367. https://doi.org/10.1093/eurheartj/ehaa575.
17. Neumann FJ, Sechtem U, Banning AP, et al. 2019 ESC Guidelines for the diagnosis and management of chronic coronary syndromes. Eur Heart J. 2020;41(3):407–77. https://doi.org/10.1093/eurheartj/ehz425.
18. Boden W, O'Rourke R, Teo K, et al. Optimal medical therapy with or without PCI for stable coronary disease. N Engl J Med. 2007;356:1503–1.
19. Al-Lamee R, Thompson D, Dehbi H, Sen S. Percutaneous coronary intervention in stable angina (ORBITA): a double-blind, randomised controlled trial. Lancet. 2018;391(10115):31–40.
20. Maron D, Hochman J, Reynolds H, Bangalore S. Initial invasive or conservative strategy for stable coronary disease. N Engl J Med. 2020;382:1395–1.
21. Doherty J, Gluckman T, Hucker W. 2017 ACC expert consensus decision pathway for periprocedural management of anticoagulation in patients with nonvalvular atrial fibrillation: a report of the American College of Cardiology Clinical Expert Consensus Document Task Force. J Am Coll Cardiol. 2017;69:871–98.
22. Raval A, Cigarroa J, Chung M. Management of patients on non-vitamin K antagonist oral anticoagulants in the acute care and periprocedural setting: a scientific statement from the American Heart Association. Circulation. 2017;135:e604-e.
23. Schiffer A, Andersonm K, Bennett C. Platelet transfusion for patients with cancer: clinical practice guidelies of the American Society of Clinical Oncology. J Clin Oncol. 2001;19:1519–5.
24. Manouchehr S. Intravenous radiocontrast media: a review of allergic reactions. US Pharm. 2012;37(5):HS-1.
25. Klein LW, Miller DL, Goldstein J, et al. The catheterization laboratory and interventional vascular suite of the future: anticipating innovations in design and function. Catheter Cardiovasc Interv. 2011;77(3):447–55. https://doi.org/10.1002/ccd.22872.
26. Hirshfeld JW, Balter S, Brinker JA, et al. ACCF/AHA/HRS/SCAI clinical competence statement on physician knowledge to optimize patient safety and image quality in fluoroscopically guided invasive cardiovascular procedures: a report of the American College of Cardiology Foundation/American Heart Association/American College of Physicians Task Force on Clinical Competence and Training. J Am Coll Cardiol. 2004;44(11):2259–82. https://doi.org/10.1016/j.jacc.2004.10.014.

27. Bashore TM, Balter S, Barac A, et al. American college of cardiology foundation/society for cardiovascular angiography and interventions expert consensus document on cardiac catheterization laboratory standards update: American College of Cardiology Foundation Task Force on expert consensus documents society of thoracic surgeons society for vascular medicine. Catheter Cardiovasc Interv. 2012;2012:80(3). https://doi.org/10.1002/ccd.24466.
28. Chambers CE, Fetterly KA, Holzer R, et al. Radiation safety program for the cardiac catheterization laboratory. Catheter Cardiovasc Interv. 2011;77(4):546–56. https://doi.org/10.1002/ccd.22867.
29. Prasad KN, Cole WC, Haase GM. Radiation protection in humans: extending the concept of as low as reasonably achievable (ALARA) from dose to biological damage. Br J Radiol. 2004;77(914):97–9. https://doi.org/10.1259/bjr/88081058.
30. Georges JL, Livarek B, Gibault-Genty G, et al. Reduction of radiation delivered to patients undergoing invasive coronary procedures. Effect of a programme for dose reduction based on radiation-protection training. Arch Cardiovasc Dis. 2009;102(12):821–7. https://doi.org/10.1016/j.acvd.2009.09.007.
31. Ferrante G, Rao SV, Jüni P, et al. Radial versus femoral access for coronary interventions across the entire spectrum of patients with coronary artery disease: a meta-analysis of randomized trials. JACC Cardiovasc Interv. 2016;9(14):1419–34. https://doi.org/10.1016/j.jcin.2016.04.014.
32. Urban P, Mehran R, Colleran R, et al. Defining high bleeding risk in patients undergoing percutaneous coronary intervention. Circulation. 2019;140(3):240–61. https://doi.org/10.1161/CIRCULATIONAHA.119.040167.
33. Valgimigli M, Campo G, Penzo C, Tebaldi M, Biscaglia S, Ferrari R. Transradial coronary catheterization and intervention across the whole spectrum of allen test results. J Am Coll Cardiol. 2014;63(18):1833–41. https://doi.org/10.1016/j.jacc.2013.12.043.
34. Sciahbasi A, Romagnoli E, Trani C, et al. Evaluation of the "learning Curve" for left and right radial approach during percutaneous coronary procedures. Am J Cardiol. 2011;108(2):185–8. https://doi.org/10.1016/j.amjcard.2011.03.022.
35. He GW, Yang CQ. Radial artery has higher receptor-mediated contractility but similar endothelial function compared with mammary artery. Ann Thorac Surg. 1997;63(5):1346–52. https://doi.org/10.1016/S0003-4975(97)00106-9.
36. Khan MZ, Patel K, Franklin S, et al. Radial artery spasm: reviews and updates. Ir J Med Sci. 2020;189(4):1253–58.
37. Tuncez A, Kaya Z, Aras D, et al. Incidence and predictors of radial artery occlusion associated transradial catheterization. Int J Med Sci. 2013;10(12):1715–9. https://doi.org/10.7150/ijms.7087.
38. Rashid M, Kwok CS, Pancholy S, et al. Radial artery occlusion after transradial interventions: a systematic review and meta-analysis. J Am Heart Assoc. 2016;5(1):1–22. https://doi.org/10.1161/JAHA.115.002686.
39. Nairoukh Z, Jahangir S, Adjepong D, Malik BH. Distal radial artery access: the future of cardiovascular intervention. Cureus. 2020;12(3) https://doi.org/10.7759/cureus.7201.
40. Tajti P, Sandoval Y, Brilakis ES. "Around the world"—how to reach native coronary artery lesions through long and tortuous aortocoronary bypass grafts. Hell J Cardiol. 2018;59(6):354–7. https://doi.org/10.1016/j.hjc.2017.12.002.
41. Hirsh J, Anand SS, Halperin JL, Fuster V. Mechanism of action and pharmacology of unfractionated heparin. Arterioscler Thromb Vasc Biol. 2001;21(7):1094–6. https://doi.org/10.1161/HQ0701.093686.
42. Bossard M, Lavi S, Rao SV, et al. Heparin use for diagnostic cardiac catheterization with a radial artery approach: an international survey of practice patterns. Catheter Cardiovasc Interv. 2018;92(5):854–9. https://doi.org/10.1002/CCD.27530.

43. Dewilde WJM, Oirbans T, Verheugt FWA, et al. Use of clopidogrel with or without aspirin in patients taking oral anticoagulant therapy and undergoing percutaneous coronary intervention: an open-label, randomised, controlled trial. Lancet. 2013;381(9872):1107–15. https://doi.org/10.1016/S0140-6736(12)62177-1.
44. Hamdi AHA, Dali AF, Nuri THM, et al. Safety and effectiveness of bivalirudin in patients undergoing percutaneous coronary intervention: a systematic review and meta-analysis. Front Pharmacol. 2017;8:410. https://doi.org/10.3389/FPHAR.2017.00410.
45. Nallamothu BK, Spertus JA, Lansky AJ, et al. Comparison of clinical interpretation with visual assessment and quantitative coronary angiography in patients undergoing percutaneous coronary intervention in contemporary practice: the assessing angiography (A2) project. Circulation. 2013;127(17):1793–800. https://doi.org/10.1161/CIRCULATIONAHA.113.001952.Comparison.
46. Mintz GS, Popma JJ, Pichard AD, et al. Limitations of angiography in the assessment of plaque distribution in coronary artery disease: a systematic study of target lesion eccentricity in 1446 lesions. Circulation. 1996;93(5):924–31. https://doi.org/10.1161/01.cir.93.5.924.
47. Camici PG, Crea F. Coronary microvascular dysfunction. N Engl J Med. 2007;356(8):830–40. https://doi.org/10.1056/NEJMra061889.
48. Pijls NH, De Bruyne B, Peels K, et al. Measurement of fractional flow reserve to assess the functional severity of coronary-artery stenoses. N Engl J Med. 1996;334(26):1703–8. https://doi.org/10.1056/NEJM199606273342604.
49. Tonino PAL, De Bruyne B, Pijls NHJ, et al. Fractional flow reserve versus angiography for guiding percutaneous coronary intervention. N Engl J Med. 2009;360(3):213–24. https://doi.org/10.1056/NEJMoa0807611.
50. Zhang D, Lv S, Song X, et al. Fractional flow reserve versus angiography for guiding percutaneous coronary intervention: a meta-analysis. Heart. 2015;101(6):455–62. https://doi.org/10.1136/heartjnl-2014-306578.
51. Knuuti J, Wijns W, Saraste A, et al. ESC Guidelines for the diagnosis and management of chronic coronary syndromes. Eur Heart J. 2019;2019:1–71. https://doi.org/10.1093/eurheartj/ehz425.
52. Rudzinski W, Waller AH, Rusovici A, et al. Comparison of efficacy and safety of intracoronary sodium nitroprusside and intravenous adenosine for assessing fractional flow reserve. Catheter Cardiovasc Interv Off J Soc Card Angiogr Interv. 2013;81(3):540–4. https://doi.org/10.1002/ccd.24652.
53. Sen S, Escaned J, Malik IS, et al. Development and validation of a new adenosine-independent index of stenosis severity from coronary wave-intensity analysis: results of the ADVISE (ADenosine Vasodilator Independent Stenosis Evaluation) study. J Am Coll Cardiol. 2012;59(15):1392–402. https://doi.org/10.1016/j.jacc.2011.11.003.
54. Davies JE, Sen S, Dehbi H-M, et al. Use of the Instantaneous Wave-free Ratio or Fractional Flow Reserve in PCI. N Engl J Med. 2017;376(19):1824–34. https://doi.org/10.1056/NEJMoa1700445.
55. Götberg M, Christiansen EH, Gudmundsdottir IJ, et al. Instantaneous wave-free ratio versus fractional flow reserve to guide PCI. N Engl J Med. 2017;376(19):1813–23. https://doi.org/10.1056/NEJMoa1616540.
56. Maehara A, Matsumura M, Ali ZA, Mintz GS, Stone GW. IVUS-guided versus OCT-guided coronary stent implantation: a critical appraisal. JACC Cardiovasc Imaging. 2017;10(12):1487–503. https://doi.org/10.1016/j.jcmg.2017.09.008.
57. Nissen SE, Yock P. Intravascular ultrasound: novel pathophysiological insights and current clinical applications. Circulation. 2001;103(4):604–16. https://doi.org/10.1161/01.cir.103.4.604.
58. Fitzgerald PJ, St Goar FG, Connolly AJ, et al. Intravascular ultrasound imaging of coronary arteries. Is three layers the norm? Circulation. 1992;86(1):154–8. https://doi.org/10.1161/01.cir.86.1.154.

59. Hong S-J, Kim B-K, Shin D-H, et al. Effect of intravascular ultrasound-guided vs angiography-guided everolimus-eluting stent implantation: the IVUS-XPL randomized clinical trial. JAMA. 2015;314(20):2155–63. https://doi.org/10.1001/jama.2015.15454.
60. Kim J-S, Kang T-S, Mintz GS, et al. Randomized comparison of clinical outcomes between intravascular ultrasound and angiography-guided drug-eluting stent implantation for long coronary artery stenoses. JACC Cardiovasc Interv. 2013;6(4):369–76. https://doi.org/10.1016/j.jcin.2012.11.009.
61. Kim B-K, Shin D-H, Hong M-K, et al. Clinical impact of intravascular ultrasound-guided chronic total occlusion intervention with zotarolimus-eluting versus biolimus-eluting stent implantation: randomized study. Circ Cardiovasc Interv. 2015;8(7):e002592. https://doi.org/10.1161/CIRCINTERVENTIONS.115.002592.
62. Gao X-F, Ge Z, Kong X-Q, et al. 3-year outcomes of the ULTIMATE trial comparing intravascular ultrasound versus angiography-guided drug-eluting stent implantation. JACC Cardiovasc Interv. 2021;14(3):247–57. https://doi.org/10.1016/j.jcin.2020.10.001.
63. Ali ZA, Karimi Galougahi K, Maehara A, et al. Intracoronary optical coherence tomography 2018: current status and future directions. JACC Cardiovasc Interv. 2017;10(24):2473–87. https://doi.org/10.1016/j.jcin.2017.09.042.
64. Harding SA, Fairley SL. Catheter-induced coronary dissection: keep calm and don't inject. JACC Case reports. 2019;1(2):113–5. https://doi.org/10.1016/j.jaccas.2019.07.002.
65. Spence MS, Byrne J, Haegeli L, Mildenberger R, Kinloch D. Rare access site complications following transradial coronary intervention. Can J Cardiol. 2009;25(6):e206. https://doi.org/10.1016/s0828-282x(09)70105-9.
66. Kotowycz MA, Dzavík V. Radial artery patency after transradial catheterization. Circ Cardiovasc Interv. 2012;5(1):127–33. https://doi.org/10.1161/CIRCINTERVENTIONS.111.965871.
67. Corcos T. Distal radial access for coronary angiography and percutaneous coronary intervention: a state-of-the-art review. Catheter Cardiovasc Interv Off J Soc Card Angiogr Interv. 2019;93(4):639–44. https://doi.org/10.1002/ccd.28016.
68. Bladin CF, Bingham L, Grigg L, Yapanis AG, Gerraty R, Davis SM. Transcranial Doppler detection of microemboli during percutaneous transluminal coronary angioplasty. Stroke. 1998;29(11):2367–70. https://doi.org/10.1161/01.str.29.11.2367.
69. Zukerman LS, Friehling TD, Wolf NM, Meister SG, Nahass G, Kowey PR. Effect of calcium-binding additives on ventricular fibrillation and repolarization changes during coronary angiography. J Am Coll Cardiol. 1987;10(6):1249–53. https://doi.org/10.1016/s0735-1097(87)80126-2.
70. Mehran R, Dangas GD, Weisbord SD. Contrast-associated acute kidney injury. N Engl J Med. 2019;380(22):2146–55. https://doi.org/10.1056/NEJMra1805256.
71. McDonald JS, McDonald RJ, Tran CL, Kolbe AB, Williamson EE, Kallmes DF. Postcontrast acute kidney injury in pediatric patients: a cohort study. Am J kidney Dis Off J Natl Kidney Found. 2018;72(6):811–8. https://doi.org/10.1053/j.ajkd.2018.05.014.
72. Mehran R, Aymong ED, Nikolsky E, et al. A simple risk score for prediction of contrast-induced nephropathy after percutaneous coronary intervention: development and initial validation. J Am Coll Cardiol. 2004;44(7):1393–9. https://doi.org/10.1016/j.jacc.2004.06.068.
73. McCullough PA, Wolyn R, Rocher LL, Levin RN, O'Neill WW. Acute renal failure after coronary intervention: incidence, risk factors, and relationship to mortality. Am J Med. 1997;103(5):368–75. https://doi.org/10.1016/s0002-9343(97)00150-2.
74. Acetylcysteine for prevention of renal outcomes in patients undergoing coronary and peripheral vascular angiography: main results from the randomized Acetylcysteine for Contrast-induced nephropathy Trial (ACT). Circulation. 2011;124(11):1250–59. https://doi.org/10.1161/CIRCULATIONAHA.111.038943.

Computed Tomography Cardiac Imaging: Coronary Artery Disease and Ischemia

Alberto Clemente

Abbreviations

ACR	American College of Radiology
ACS	Acute coronary syndrome
AHA	American Heart Association
CACS	Coronary artery calcium score
CAD	Coronary artery disease
CCT	Coronary CT angiography
CFD	Computational fluid dynamics
CT	Computed tomography
CTP	CT perfusion
DECT	Dual-energy CT
FFR-CT	CT-derived fractional flow reserve
GUCH	Grown-up congenital heart disease
ICA	Invasive coronary angiography
IVUS	Intravascular ultrasound
NASCI	North American Society for Cardiovascular Imaging
PCD	Photon counting detector
SCCT	Society of Cardiovascular Computed Tomography
STR	Society of Thoracic Radiology

A. Clemente (✉)
Fondazione Toscana G. Monasterio - Ospedale del cuore "G. Pasquinucci", Massa, Italy
e-mail: alberto.clemente@ftgm.it

G. Concistrè (ed.), *Ischemic Heart Disease*,
https://doi.org/10.1007/978-3-031-25879-4_14

1 Introduction

The execution and interpretation of CCT by highly experienced specialists allow to understand in depth the normal and pathological cardiac anatomy: the normal coronary tree (Fig. 1) and CAD; the morphological and functional characteristics of the cardiac chambers and valves; congenital anomalies; and the characteristic appearance of the heart linked to aging or pathogens.

Particular attention must be paid to the knowledge of the technical and technological part, which is an indispensable requirement in order to obtain sophisticated diagnoses. The planning of the acquisition phases without and with contrast medium, the use of three-dimensional cardiac-specific interpretation software, and the ability to identify and overcome image artifacts in the available image dataset [1, 2] provide the basis of the training process currently recommended to achieve the appropriate proficiency [3].

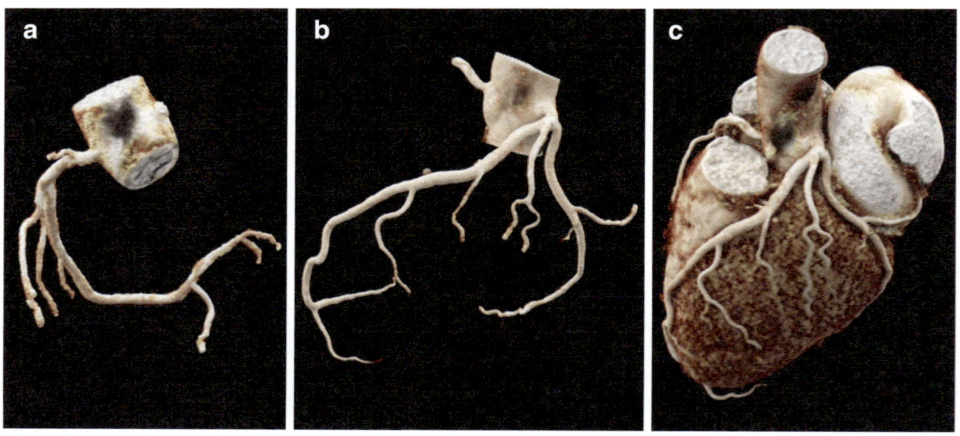

Fig. 1 Coronary CT angiography curved multiplanar reconstruction of the left anterior descending artery (LAD) showing a critical >70% luminal narrowing at the proximal segment due to a mixed plaque with spotty calcium (**a**). CT angiography dual-energy iodine color map in short-axis view showing the myocardial perfusion defect at the anteroseptal and anterior wall. Note the reduction of iodine content (iodine density: −0.9 mg/mL, −26%) with respect to the remote myocardium (**b**), Complete view on the heart (**c**)

2 Coronary Anatomy Segmentation

The AHA recommended a schematic coronary tree segmentation classification that can be used to create a schematic CCT scoring system similarly to that used in conventional coronary angiography [4]. The coronary tree should be initially examined for the course and branching of the main coronary vessels and secondary branches following the 15- or 16-segment pattern.

The SCCT guidelines recommend an axial model of coronary segmentation, adapted for CCT [3]. This pattern varies from standard AHA segmentation in the following ways: an intermediate branch has been added as segment 17, and a left posterolateral branch is identified as segment 18.

Attention should initially be focused on the axial plane on the aortic root to confirm the normal origin of the coronaries. Any anomalies of origin and course and the relationship with surrounding structures such as the heart chambers, the aorta, the pulmonary artery, the cardiac veins, and the interventricular septum may require the use of evaluation plans other than the axial plane up to the need for unusual planes generated by the stretched centerline of the vessels.

3 Congenital Coronary Artery Anomalies

Coronary CT is considered an important and appropriate imaging modality for the evaluation of adult congenital heart disease, particularly of the coronary arteries. Congenital coronary anomalies are of great importance in clinical cardiology and cardiac surgery due to their association with myocardial ischemia and sudden death. These anomalies are detectable noninvasively by CCT and, according to various definitions, their prevalence ranges from 0.21% to 5.79%. The most commonly used classification is based solely on anatomical considerations [5, 6]. The working group of Anatomy and Pathology of the European Society of Cardiology has published a position statement (2016) in order to provide a classification linked to the mechanisms of coronary embryonic development and to congenital coronary anomalies [7].

The high spatial resolution of CCT allows us to evaluate the intrinsic mechanisms of the coronary artery anomalies generating dysfunction (stenosis) and clinical or prognostic relevance.

The correct knowledge of the normal coronary origin and course and the coronary anomalies related to ischemia represents a key role in the operative planning, and highly detailed anatomical images are crucial to define the surgical indication. Consequently, CCT allows us to verify the surgical result by highlighting all anatomical details of the surgical techniques employed [8].

Angelini P. (2019) pointed out that among all coronary anomalies, the intramural course of an anomalous coronary artery from the opposite sinus of Valsalva (ACAOS-IM) can cause coronary insufficiency (i.e., myocardial ischemia) in young adults involved in strenuous exertion [9].

The main cause of ischemia in these patients is generally the narrowing of the initial segment of the coronary artery as it enters or exits the aortic wall, at an intramural course by compression in between the inner and outer layers of the aortic tunica media [10, 11]. This morphologic variation during the cardiac cycle of the coronary morphology at the level of the intramural course is usually seen by IVUS, but nowadays a retrospective CCT acquisition permits a noninvasive evaluation of systolic to diastolic variations in terms of both morphology and degree of stenosis (Fig. 2).

In recent years, CCT has also acquired a role of increasing importance in the diagnosis and preoperative planning of congenital heart defects [12], allowing the study of the coronary tree together with structural abnormalities. In adult GUCH undergoing multiple surgical procedures during their life, the role of CCT becomes crucial in defining the relationship between cardiac structures, the coronary distribution, and the anterior chest wall in order to plan the surgical approach and avoid complications. In this scenario, the development of tenacious cardio-sternal adhesions represents an element of considerable bleeding risk during the chest reopening phase. Therefore, CCT imaging becomes a fundamental aid in guiding the reopening procedure allowing the adoption of the strategy with less surgical risk [13].

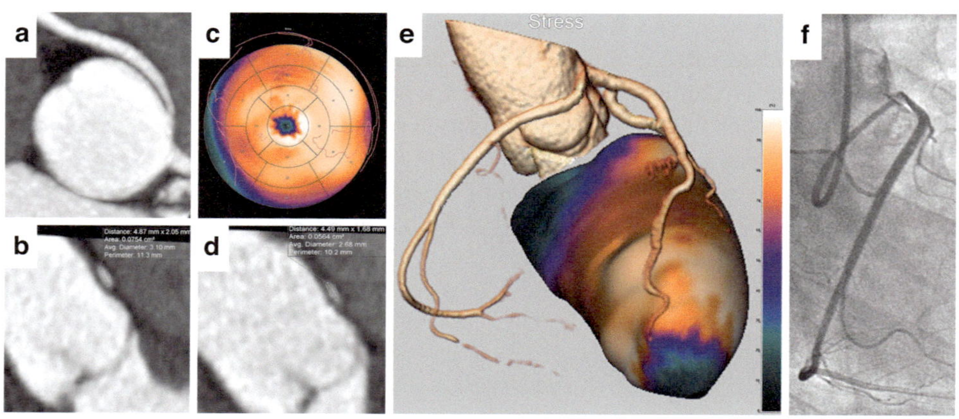

Fig. 2 Anomalous origin of the right coronary artery (RCA) from the left sinus of Valsalva with interarterial course and "slit-like ostium" (**a**) showing oval shape during diastole (**b**) and compression during systole (**d**). Hybrid SPECT/CCT volume rendering (**e**) and bull's eye (**c**) showing the segmental ischemia and its relationship with the anomalous coronary origin. The conventional angiography (**f**) confirms the "slit-like ostium"

Another field of application is represented by the group of congenital anomalies concerning systemic and pulmonary venous returns. In particular, for the correct preoperative diagnostic definition of partial and total anomalous pulmonary venous connections, echocardiography is often insufficient to guide surgical planning, and a second-level imaging examination such as CCT becomes essential. Especially in the total and mixed forms of anomalous pulmonary venous connection, the questions that CCT must answer are the anatomy of the vein confluence and the course and draining site of the venous collector [14].

The choice of the best surgical technique is the consequence of a perfect and exhaustive preoperative anatomical definition.

4 Coronary Atherosclerosis

The SCCT recommends performing preliminary non-contrast CT examination for coronary artery and other cardiac structural calcifications [3, 15].

Calcified lesions are usually quantified using the "Agatston score" [16, 17].

The SCCT and the STR have produced a consensus document regarding the prognostic value of CACS [18] because the coronary calcium quantification has been shown to be the best predictor of future cardiovascular events in the general population, in the elderly, and in the diabetics.

After intravenous injection of contrast agent, CCT can visualize the coronary artery lumen and the lesions involved in the stenosis [19, 20].

Atherosclerotic lesions should be considered in relationship to their segmental position to determine the overall myocardium risk [21, 22]. The impact of luminal plaque should be evaluated in terms of resultant maximal diameter stenosis [3]. CCT can visualize the coronary wall alterations related to CAD and plaque remodeling, and it can differentiate the calcified and noncalcified components of the plaque (mixed) [18].

Maurovich-Horvat et al. [23] proposed a qualitative assessment of plaque features related to histopathologic findings. Plaque attenuation pattern-based classification has been proposed distinguishing noncalcified plaque with or without "napkin-ring" sign.

SCOT-Heart Study [22] assessed the association between coronary plaque features and clinical outcome defining four types of adverse plaque: positive remodeling, low-attenuation plaque, spotty calcification, and "napkin-ring" sign. These specific plaque features are detectable and should be annotated because of their prognostic significance [24, 25].

The qualitative and quantitative grading of the coronary stenosis severity and the plaque features along the vessel are the main information to be reported [26, 27]. The SCOT-Heart study modified SCCT Guidelines stenosis grading defining as normal coronary segment with or without nonobstructive plaque; moreover, obstructive disease was defined as >70% stenosis in one or more epicardial vessels or 50% stenosis in the LM.

On the basis of clinical trials [21, 22], the SCCT, the ACR, and the NASCI have evaluated the clinical utility and the relevance of CCT findings in the context of suspected stable CAD and in patients with acute chest pain. In order to describe a standardized reporting system for patients undergoing CCT, CAD-RADS (Coronary Artery Disease Reporting and Data

System) was proposed with the aim to improve the communication between interpreting and referring physicians, facilitate research, and offer mechanisms to contribute to peer review and quality assurance, ultimately resulting in improvements to the quality of care [28].

The current European Guidelines advocate the use of CCT in patients with suspected CAD with a Class I recommendation (Level of Evidence B) due to its diagnostic and prognostic performance [29]. CCT is considered a first-line tool for all patients presenting with chest pain of suspected cardiac origin and the most cost-effective imaging-based strategy [30].

From the 64-slice CCT systems which have a temporal resolution of 175 ms, nowadays the temporal resolution has increased up to 66 ms; the spatial resolution reaches isotropic dimensions of ~0.2–0.3 mm, which allow a good assessment of significant coronary artery stenosis and plaque characterization [31].

The last-generation CCT scanners allow a spatial resolution of up to 0.1 mm combined with photon counting technology [32].

A strength of CCT is the exclusion of the presence of CAD or the identification of patients with nonobstructive CAD, in order to restratify the clinical risk stratification (an intermediate risk of hard events and may represent the target population) [33, 34].

The prognosis related to CAD is related to the presence, extent, and severity of the lesions. The anatomical coronary evaluation can nowadays be supported by myocardial CT perfusion, FFR-CT, and high-risk plaque feature quantification in order to refine and improve risk assessment for future cardiac events [35–38].

5 CCT Prognostic Value

Several longitudinal studies demonstrated that CCT holds important prognostic value in both patients with known and suspected CAD [39–44].

In a meta-analysis including 29,243 patients (median follow-up of 25 months), adverse cardiovascular events among patients with normal findings on CCT were demonstrated to be rare (annual MACE rate of 0.21%) [45].

Nonobstructive (<50% stenosis) or obstructive (≥50% stenosis) CAD was demonstrated to predict increasing future MACE (annualized event rates of 1.24–6.21%, respectively, $p < 0.05$) [45]. Most of the key answers on the prognostic utility of CCT are derived from the CONFIRM registry that includes more than 32,000 consecutive adults with suspected CAD who underwent ≥64-slice CCT at 12 centers in 6 countries between 2005 and 2009, investigating the link between cardiovascular risk factors, symptoms, coronary atherosclerotic plaque burden, and outcome. Some studies from this registry have demonstrated that the presence, extent, and severity of CAD on CCT result in increased future risk to the patient, across age, gender, and other several clinical sub-analyses [46–48].

A very low annual event rate for those with normal CCT findings has been consistently demonstrated, which is comparable to the background event rate among healthy low-risk individuals (<1%). In risk-adjusted analysis, both per-patient nonobstructive (hazard ratio

[HR]: 1.60; 95% confidence interval [CI]: 1.18–2.16; p = 0.002) and obstructive (>50% stenosis) (HR: 2.60; 95% CI: 1.94–3.49; p < 0.0001) CAD conferred increased risk of mortality compared with patients without evidence of CAD [46]. The clinical importance of nonobstructive CAD and its strong relationship with all-cause mortality were evidenced. Moreover, the total coronary plaque burden has emerged as an important predictor of outcomes (Fig. 3).

The CT screening can be used cost effectively to reduce morbidity and mortality from CHD in symptomatic patients [47].

Moreover, as the definition of clinically significant atherosclerosis includes asymptomatic disease, the identification of individuals at risk requires a screening strategy and CCT seems to express adequate characteristics to be used for this purpose in this area also in order to evaluate the drug therapy efficacy (Fig. 4) [48].

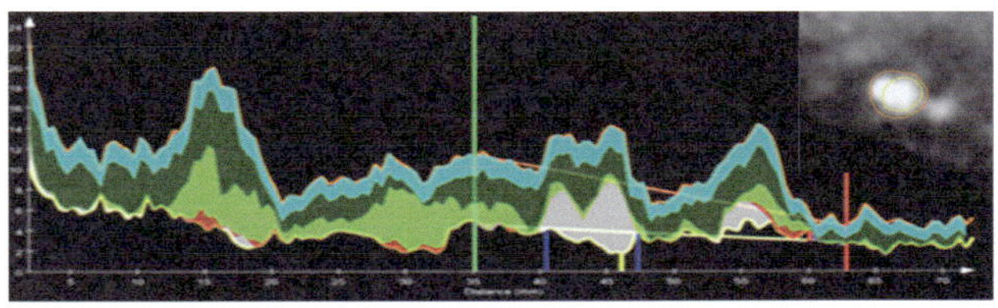

Fig. 3 Example of semiautomatic coronary plaque burden quantification

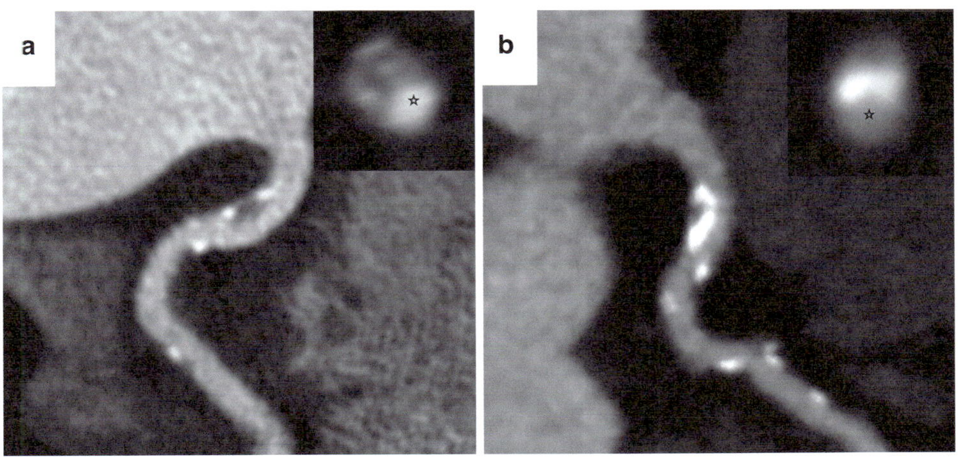

Fig. 4 Proximal right coronary artery mixed heterogeneous plaque with positive remodeling at baseline (**a**) and calcification after 7 years of statin and acetylic salicylic acid (ASA) treatment (**b**). (☆: coronary lumen)

6 CCT Plaque Characterization

Some features of the coronary plaque seen at CCT have been demonstrated to be correlated with the risk of rupture and subsequent risk of ACS [35]. These high-risk features include the low-attenuation plaque, positive remodeling, spotty calcification, "napkin-ring" sign, and dishomogeneity of the plaque components [35–51].

Low-attenuation plaque features (<60 HU) and "napkin-ring" sign were the most powerful MACE predictors (HR 4.96; 95% CI: 2.0–12.2 and HR 3.85; 95% CI: 1.7–8.6; $p < 0.0001$) in a study by Feuchtner et al. (mean follow-up of 7.8 years) [52].

Adverse features such as positive remodeling, low-attenuation plaque, or "napkin ring" were demonstrated to be associated with increased risk of death, MI, or hospitalization for unstable angina at 2 years (HR 2.73, 95% CI 1.89–3.93) [53].

Accordingly, the low-attenuation plaque burden (i.e., % plaque to vessel volume) was demonstrated to be the strongest predictor of fatal or nonfatal MI irrespective of cardiovascular risk score, CACS, or coronary artery area stenosis (HR 1.60, 95% CI: 1.10–2.34 per doubling; $p = 0.014$) [54].

7 Myocardial CT Perfusion and FFR-CT

The new-generation CT scanners permit both the static (single-phase) and the dynamic (multiphase) myocardial CTP acquisition. The qualitative and quantitative evaluation with the assessment of perfusion parameters of ischemia, such as the myocardial blood flow and volume [55], is evaluable together with coronary anatomy evaluation. CFD algorithms could enable prediction of changes in coronary flow and pressure for the noninvasive estimation of FFR (FFR-CT) [55, 56].

The inability of the traditional ICA to assess the functional significance of coronary stenosis and determine the need of revascularization [52] has led to the development of techniques that are able to assess the functional severity of coronary stenoses. FFR was introduced to the clinical setting in the mid-1990s and was established as a crucial enhancement to ICA for clinical decision-making in CAD [53] based on a linear relationship between flow and pressure. The FFR was initially presented as a pressure-derived assessment index of the impairment of coronary flow due to the presence of arterial stenoses. When the FFR value is close to 1, a normal coronary physiology is assumed with no need for revascularization. The well-accepted FFR cutoff value has been set to 0.75, under which myocardial ischemia occurs with an overall accuracy that reaches 97% [57]. However, there is a so-called gray zone which ranges from 0.75 to 0.80, at which the clinician has to assess every parameter in order to decide on a possible revascularization procedure. Due to the noninvasive nature of CCT, the application of CFD algorithms on CCT-derived 3D arterial models has received wide clinical interest regarding the noninvasive FFR assessment. According to this approach, hemodynamic factors such as flow and pressure are not known a priori, so lumped parameter models regarding the cardiac output, the resistance of the coronary microcirculation, and the pressure of the systemic circulation are coupled with the flow domain of the aortic root and the epicardial arteries, where the governing equations of flow dynamics are solved and can consequently provide FFR calculations. DISCOVER-FLOW, DeFACTO, and HeartFlow NXT studies compared their computational FFR results to the measured FFR values, producing promising results and making the method a valuable tool in the clinical settings [58–60].

The DISCOVER-FLOW study exhibited a good correlation between FFR-CT and FFR ($r = 0.68$) with the respective diagnostic accuracy, sensitivity, specificity, positive predictive value, and negative predictive value for predicting hemodynamically significant stenoses (FFR $\leq$0.8) being 84, 88, 82, 74, and 92% [60]. Furthermore, when compared to cases of $\geq$50% stenosis detected solely by CCT, FFR-CT showed superior discrimination (AUC: 0.90 vs. 0.75, $p = 0.001$). In the DeFACTO study, stable CAD patients underwent CCT, FFR-CT, and invasive coronary angiography with FFR measurement [58]. The per patient diagnostic accuracy, sensitivity, specificity, positive predictive value, and negative predictive value for predicting an FFR $\leq$0.8 were 73, 90, 54, 67, and 84%, respectively. Good correlation was also found between the two methods ($r = 0.68$). The most recent HeartFlow NXT further validated FFR-CT, by making use of updated proprietary software which included refined mathematical models and further increased automation, image quality assessment, and better image segmentation [59]. Diagnostic accuracy, sensitivity, specificity, positive predictive value, and negative predictive value for predicting an FFR $\leq$0.8 were 81, 86, 79, 65, and 93%, respectively, on a per-patient basis and 86, 84, 86, 61, and 95%, respectively, on a per-vessel basis. Finally, good correlation was found between FFR-CT and FFR ($r = 0.82$). The PLATFORM study focused on the clinical outcomes of FFR by CCT-guided diagnostic strategies compared to the common care in CAD-suspected patients, providing insight on the clinical utilization of FFR-CT [61]. Following the findings of the PLATFORM trial, the PROMISE study concluded that if ICA is performed only in patients with FFR-CT $\leq$0.8, then selected ICA with obstructive stenosis could decrease by 44% and the total number of patients with ICA requiring appropriate revascularization would increase by 24% [57]. Sensitivity and specificity have been shown to vary through different cohorts (DISCOVER-FLOW, DeFACTO, NXT [58–60], Kim et al. [62], Renker et al. [63], Coenen et al. [64], Kruk et al. [65], Ko et al. [66]) due to differences in sample sizes and study population characteristics [67]. Nowadays, there are four approaches in noninvasive, in silico CCT-derived FFR estimation: full-order model computations, reduced-order/steady-state modeling, hybrid models, and deep machine learning algorithms, including commercially available solutions and technologies still in progress [68]. These techniques are applied to a patient-specific anatomic coronary artery 3D model, obtained via a preliminary segmentation and contouring of the vessels. The full-order approaches require a complete model of the entire coronary tree, and an additional physiology model of the coronary microcirculation fluid dynamics (derived from patient-specific boundary conditions), from which a coronary blood flow model is computed. This process is computationally demanding, requiring off-site supercomputers in core laboratories. In order to simplify the processes, lean models have been introduced, which are either segment specific and/or rely on a generalized (nonpatient-specific) hemodynamic model. For these reasons, CCT together with CTP or FFR-CT potentially should be the method to combinedly evaluate CAD phenotype and ischemic functional significance of the stenosis. Initial evidence on the prognostic value and improvement in risk stratification of CTP has been shown in the CORE-320 trial demonstrating that a combined approach with coronary CCT and CTP enables similar prediction of 2-year major adverse cardiac events and event-free survival, when compared to invasive coronary angiography and SPECT combined [55]. Moreover, stress dynamic CTP has incremental predictive value for future major adverse cardiac events over clinical risk factors and detection of coronary stenosis at CCT [56, 69–71]. On the other side, FFR-CT, besides an improved accuracy for the detection of hemodynamically relevant lesions, may have favorable clinical outcomes, similar quality of life, and lower costs and radiation exposure, when compared with usual care over 1-year follow-up [69, 72, 73]. However, despite efforts to create an artificial score similar to the useful value of FFR but through noninvasive imaging of the CCT to decide which stenosis should be revascularized, the inherent limitation of this method remains its inability to discriminate whether a stenosis is severe, that is, if it is flow limiting, around the value 0.8, which is exactly in the gray zone around the value of 0.8, which corresponds to the uncertainty value of the CCT (i.e., stenosis between 50 and 70%). So, these models may have a clinical role as their performance improves along with technology. On the other hand, motion or beam hardening artifacts that may occur during CTP acquisition can create erroneous signals of ischemia; therefore, in the near future, the technology will improve its performance in this regard.

8 Dual-Energy CT and Multi-Energy CT

Rapid advances in CT hardware and software technology have occurred and have been applied to last-generation scanners DECT and multi-energy CT imaging [74–76].

Four different technical approaches have been used to develop DECT technology: 1) two X-ray tubes operating at two different energy levels (70–80–90/140–150 kVp); 2) fast switching of kVp between low- and high-energy spectra; 3) two temporally sequential scans (not applied in cardiac imaging); and 4) multilayer detector for spectral separation [74].

DECT systems allow the signal differentiation of different materials by evaluating the attenuation characteristics at two different energy levels of the photons.

DECT can improve the diagnostic performance of CT in myocardial perfusion and scar imaging by improving iodine contrast-to-noise ratio (CNR) (Fig. 5) [76].

DECT allows the quantification of iodine distribution within the myocardium through the direct correlation with myocardial blood flow, thus being useful for dif-

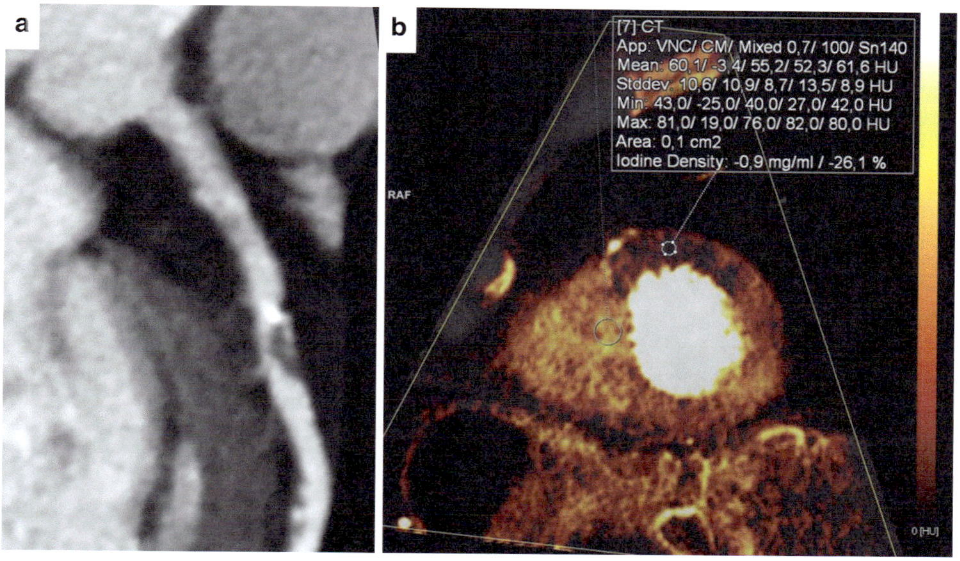

Fig. 5 Coronary CT angiography curved multiplanar reconstruction of the left anterior descending artery (LAD) showing a critical >70% luminal narrowing at the proximal segment due to a mixed plaque with spotty calcium (**a**). CT angiography dual-energy iodine color map in short-axis view showing the myocardial perfusion defect at the anteroseptal and anterior wall. Note the reduction of iodine content (iodine density: −0.9 mg/mL, −26%) with respect to the remote myocardium (**b**)

ferentiating between normal, ischemic, and necrotic myocardium providing color-coded iodine images. In this way, a measurement of myocardial per-voxel iodine concentration expressed in mg/mL is provided, improving accuracy over the standard visual analysis.

Furthermore, DECT acquisition can reduce artifacts such as beam hardening and blooming artifacts usually present in single-energy CT acquisitions, without increasing the radiation dose [75, 76].

More recently, new energy-sensitive PCD has been developed allowing to directly count the number of incident photons and measure their photon energies separately. Multi-energy CT with PCD can provide more spectral information than DECT systems, but they are the subject of ongoing research and their commercialization is only now starting. A recent preclinical experimental model demonstrated the feasibility and accuracy of PCDs with respect to MRI and histology as the gold standard for quantitative separation of blood pool, scar, and remote myocardium using a simultaneous protocol of multi-contrast agents [77].

9 Conclusions

CCT has been shown to provide diagnostic and prognostic information regarding CAD and ischemia. CCT, if used with the most advanced technology by expert operators, is able to offer at the same time the accurate anatomical evaluation of the heart and coronaries and the phenotype of the coronary plaque, quantify the atherosclerotic plaque burden, simulate the coronary flow alterations, and guide revascularization. CCT is therefore a useful tool to stratify the risk of CAD in the population as suggested by international guidelines and to study the pathophysiology of human atherosclerosis with a noninvasive method that is well accepted by patients. The certain exclusion of CAD, the main prerogative of CCT, and the characterization of the nonobstructive disease are certainly a necessary aid to guide preventive therapy and modify the risk of events. The evaluation of CAD using advanced imaging and with the help of radiomics, machine learning, and deep learning features [78] is being proposed as an integrated system that generates new knowledge to be used in the near future.

References

1. Kramer CM, Budoff MJ, Fayad ZA, et al. ACCF/AHA 2007 clinical competence statement on vascular imaging with computed tomography and magnetic resonance. A report of the American College of Cardiology Foundation/American Heart Association/American College of Physicians Task Force on Clinical Competence and Training. J Am Coll Cardiol. 2007;50:1097–114.
2. Beller GA, Bonow RO, Fuster V. ACCF 2008 recommendations for training in adult cardiovascular medicine core cardiology training (COCATS 3) (revision of the 2002 COCATS Training Statement). J Am Coll Cardiol. 2008;51:335–8.
3. Leipsic J, Abbara S, Achenbach S, et al. SCCT guidelines for the interpretation and reporting of coronary CT angiography: a report of the Society of Cardiovascular Computed Tomography guidelines committee. J Cardiovasc Comput Tomogr. 2014;8:342–58.
4. Austen WG, Edwards JE, Frye RL, et al. A reporting system on patients evaluated for coronary artery disease. Report of the Ad Hoc Committee for Grading of Coronary Artery Disease, Council on Cardiovascular Surgery, American Heart Association. Circulation. 1975;51(4 suppl):5–40.
5. Angelini P, Villason S, Chan AV Jr, Diez JG. Normal and anomalous coronary arteries in humans. In: Angelini P, editor. Coronary artery anomalies: a comprehensive approach. Philadelphia: Lippincott Williams & Wilkins; 1999. p. 27–150.
6. Angelini P. Coronary artery anomalies—current clinical issues: definitions, classification, incidence, clinical relevance, and treatment guidelines. Tex Heart Inst J. 2002;29(4):271–8. Review
7. Pérez-Pomares JM, de la Pompa JL, Franco D, et al. Congenital coronary artery anomalies: a bridge from embryology to anatomy and pathophysiology—a position statement of the development, anatomy, and pathology ESC Working Group. Cardiovasc Res. 2016;109:204–16. https://doi.org/10.1093/cvr/cvv251.
8. Mery CM, De Leòn LE, Molossi S, Sexson-Tejtel SK, Agrawal H, Krishnamurthy R, Masand P, Qureshi AM, McKenzie ED, Fraser CD, jr. Outcomes of surgical intervention for anomalous aortic origin of a coronary artery: a large contemporary prospective cohort study. J Thorac Cardiovasc Surg. 2018;155(1):305–19.

9. Angelini P. Imaging approaches for coronary artery anomalies: purpose and techniques. Curr Cardiol Rep. 2019;21(9):101.
10. Angelini P, Uribe C. Anatomic spectrum of left coronary artery anomalies and associated mechanisms of coronary insufficiency. Catheter Cardiovasc Interv. 2018;92:313–21.
11. Angelini P, Uribe C, Monge J, et al. Origin of the right coronary artery from the opposite sinus of Valsalva in adults: characterization by intravascular ultrasonography at baseline and after stent angio-plasty. Catheter Cardiovasc Interv. 2015;86:199–208.
12. Ou P, Celermajer DS, Calcagni G, Brunelle F, Bonnet D, Sidi D. Three-dimensional CT-scanning: a new diagnostic modality in congenital heart disease. Heart 2007; 93(8): 908–13.).
13. Hamid IU, Digney R, Soo L, Leung S, Graham AN. Incidence and outcome of re-entry injury in redo cardiac surgery: benefits of preoperative planning. Eur J Cardiothorac Surg. 2015;47(5):819–23.
14. Shi G, Zhu Z, Chen J, Ou Y, Hong H, Nie Z, Zhang H, Liu X, Zheng J, Sun Q, Liu J, Chen H, Zhuang J. Total anomalous pulmonary venous connection: the current management strategies INA pediatric cohort of 768 patients. Circulation. 2017;135(1):48–58.
15. Mantini C, Maffei E, Toia P, Ricci F, Seitun S, Clemente A, Malagò R, Runza G, La Grutta L, Midiri M, Cotroneo AR, Forte E, Cademartiri F. Influence of image reconstruction parameters on cardiovascular risk reclassification by Computed Tomography Coronary Artery Calcium Score. Eur J Radiol. 2018;101:1–7. https://doi.org/10.1016/j.ejrad.2018.01.005.
16. Agatston AS, Janowitz WR, Hildner FJ, Zusmer NR, Viamonte M Jr, Detrano R. Quantification of coronary artery calcium using ultrafast computed tomography. J Am Coll Cardiol. 1990;15:827–32.
17. Yaghoubi S, Tang W, Wang S, et al. Offline assessment of atherosclerotic coronary calcium from electron beam tomograms. Am J Card Imaging. 1995;9:231–6.
18. Hecht et al. 2016 SCCT/STR guidelines for coronary artery calcium scoring of noncontrast noncardiac chest CT scans: a report of the Society of Cardiovascular Computed Tomography and Society of Thoracic Radiology. J Thorac Imaging 2017;32(5).
19. Maffei E, Martini C, Arcadi T, Clemente A, Seitun S, Zuccarelli A, Torri T, Mollet NR, Rossi A, Catalano O, Messalli G, Cademartiri F. Plaque imaging with CT coronary angiography: effect of intra-vascular attenuation on plaque type classification. World J Radiol. 2012;4(6):265–72. https://doi.org/10.4329/wjr.v4.i6.265.
20. Maffei E, Martini C, Rossi A, Mollet N, Lario C, Castiglione Morelli M, Clemente A, Gentile G, Arcadi T, Seitun S, Catalano O, Aldrovandi A, Cademartiri F. Diagnostic accuracy of second-generation dual-source computed tomography coronary angiography with iterative reconstructions: a real-world experience. Radiol Med. 2012;117(5):725–38. https://doi.org/10.1007/s11547-011-0754-x. Epub 2011 Nov 17
21. Douglas PS, Hoffmann U, Patel MR, et al. PROMISE Investigators. Outcomes of anatomical versus functional testing for coronary artery disease. N Engl J Med. 2015;372:1291–300.
22. SCOT-HEART Investigators. CT coronary angiography in patients with suspected angina due to coronary heart disease (SCOT-HEART): an open-label, parallel-group, multicentre trial. Lancet. 2015;6736:60291–4.
23. Maurovich-Horvat P, Schlett CL, Alkadhi H, et al. The napkin-ring sign indicates advanced atherosclerotic lesions in coronary CT angiography. J Am Coll Cardiol Img. 2012;5:1243–52.
24. Maffei E, Nieman K, Martini C, Catalano O, Seitun S, Arcadi T, Malagò R, Rossi A, Clemente A, Mollet NR, Cademartiri F. Classification of noncalcified coronary atherosclerotic plaque components on CT coronary angiography: impact of vascular attenuation and density thresholds. Radiol Med. 2012;117(2):230–41. https://doi.org/10.1007/s11547-011-0744-z.
25. Maffei E, Seitun S, Martini C, Aldrovandi A, Arcadi T, Clemente A, Messalli G, Malagò R, Weustink A, Mollet N, Nieman K, Ardissino D, de Feyter P, Krestin G, Cademartiri F. Prognostic

value of CT coronary angiography: focus on obstructive vs. nonobstructive disease and on the presence of left main disease. Radiol Med. 2011;116(1):15–31. https://doi.org/10.1007/s11547-010-0592-2.
26. Miller JM, Rochitte CE, Dewey M, et al. Diagnostic performance of coronary angiography by 64-row CT. N Engl J Med. 2008;359:2324–36.
27. Cheng V, Gutstein A, Wolak A, et al. Moving beyond binary grading of coronary arterial stenoses on coronary computed tomographic angiography: insights for the imager and referring clinician. J Am Coll Cardiol Img. 2008;1:460–71.
28. Cury RC, Abbara S, Achenbach S, et al. CAD-RADS(TM) Coronary Artery Disease—reporting and Data System. An expert consensus document of the Society of Cardiovascular Computed Tomography (SCCT), the American College of Radiology (ACR) and the North American Society for Cardiovascular Imaging (NASCI). Endorsed by the American College of Cardiology. J Cardiovasc Comput Tomogr. 2016;10(4):269–81. https://doi.org/10.1016/j.jcct.2016.04.005. Epub 2016 Jun 15
29. Knuuti J, Wijns W, Saraste A, et al. ESC Scientific Document Group. 2019 ESC Guidelines for the diagnosis and management of chronic coronary syndromes. Eur Heart J. 2020;41:407–77.
30. National Institute for Health and Clinical Excellence. Chest pain of recent onset: assessment and diagnosis of recent onset chest pain or discomfort of suspected cardiac origin (update). CG95. London: National Institute for Health and Clinical Excellence; 2016. http://www.nice.org.uk/guidance/CG95.
31. Maffei E, Martini C, De Crescenzo S, et al. Low dose CT of the heart: a quantum leap into a new era of cardiovascular imaging. Radiol Med. 2010;115:1179–207.
32. Boussel L, Coulon P, Thran A, Roessl E, Martens G, Sigovan M, Douek P. Photon counting spectral CT component analysis of coronary artery atherosclerotic plaque samples. Br J Radiol. 2014;87(1040):20130798.
33. Adamson PD, Williams MC, Dweck MR, et al. Guiding therapy by coronary CT angiography improves outcomes in patients with stable chest pain. J Am Coll Cardiol. 2019;74:2058–70.
34. Chow BJ, Small G, Yam Y, et al. Prognostic and therapeutic implications of statin and aspirin therapy in individuals with nonobstructive coronary artery disease: results from the CONFIRM (COronary CT Angiography EvaluatioN For Clinical Outcomes: An InteRnational Multicenter registry) registry. Arterioscler Thromb Vasc Biol. 2015;35:981–9.
35. Rosa GM, Bauckneht M, Masoero G, et al. The vulnerable coronary plaque: update on imaging technologies. Thromb Haemost. 2013;110:706–22.
36. Seitun S, De Lorenzi C, Cademartiri F, et al. CT myocardial perfusion imaging: a new frontier in cardiac imaging. Biomed Res Int. 2018;2018:7295460.
37. Cademartiri F, Seitun S, Clemente A, et al. Myocardial blood flow quantification for evaluation of coronary artery disease by computed tomography. Cardiovasc Diagn Ther. 2017;7:129–50.
38. Seitun S, Castiglione Morelli M, Budaj I, et al. Stress computed tomography myocardial perfusion imaging: a new topic in cardiology. Rev Esp Cardiol (Engl Ed). 2016;69:188–200.
39. Maffei E, Seitun S, Palumbo A, et al. Prognostic value of Morise clinical score, calcium score and computed tomography coronary angiography in patients with suspected or known coronary artery disease. Radiol Med. 2011;116:1188–202.
40. Cademartiri F, Seitun S, Romano M, et al. Prognostic value of 64-slice coronary angiography in diabetes mellitus patients with known or suspected coronary artery disease compared with a non-diabetic population. Radiol Med. 2008;113:627–43. https://doi.org/10.1007/s11547-008-0268-3.
41. Maffei E, Seitun S, Martini C, et al. Prognostic value of computed tomography coronary angiography in patients with chest pain of suspected cardiac origin. Radiol Med. 2011;116:690–705. https://doi.org/10.1007/s11547-011-0647-z.

42. Aldrovandi A, Maffei E, Palumbo A, et al. Prognostic value of computed tomography coronary angiography in patients with suspected coronary artery disease: a 24-month follow-up study. Eur Radiol. 2009;19:1653–60. https://doi.org/10.1007/s00330-009-1344-3.
43. Van Werkhoven JM, Cademartiri F, Seitun S, et al. Diabetes: prognostic value of CT coronary angiography—comparison with a nondiabetic population. Radiology. 2010;256(1):83–92.
44. Andreini D, Pontone G, Mushtaq S, et al. A long-term prognostic value of coronary CT angiography in suspected coronary artery disease. JACC Cardiovasc Imaging. 2012;5:690–701.
45. Jiang B, Wang J, Lv X, Cai W. Prognostic value of cardiac computed tomography angiography in patients with suspected coronary artery disease: a meta-analysis. Cardiology. 2014;128:304–12.
46. Min JK, Dunning A, Lin FY, et al. Age- and sex-related differences in all-cause mortality risk based on coronary computed tomography angiography findings: results from the International Multicenter CONFIRM (Coronary CT Angiography Evaluation for Clinical Outcomes: An International Multicenter Registry) of 23,854 Patients Without Known Coronary Artery Disease. J Am Coll Cardiol. 2011;58:849–60.
47. Rubin GD. Emerging and evolving roles for CT in screening for coronary heart disease. J Am Coll Radiol. 2013;10(12):943–8.
48. Lee JH, Han D, Hartaigh BÓ, et al. Influence of symptom typicality for predicting MACE in patients without obstructive coronary artery disease: from the CONFIRM registry (Coronary Computed Tomography Angiography Evaluation for Clinical Outcomes: An International Multicenter Registry). Clin Cardiol. 2018;41:586–93.
49. Libby P, Buring JE, Badimon L, Hansson GK, Deanfield J, Bittencourt MS, Tokgözoğlu L, Lewis EF. Atherosclerosis Nat Rev Dis Primers. 2019;5(1):56.
50. Blanke P, Naoum C, Ahmadi A, et al. Long-term prognostic utility of coronary CT angiography in stable patients with diabetes mellitus. JACC Cardiovasc Imaging. 2016;9:1280–8.
51. Nadjiri J, Hausleiter J, Jähnichen C, et al. Incremental prognostic value of quantitative plaque assessment in coronary CT angiography during 5 years of follow up. J Cardiovasc Comput Tomogr. 2016;10:97–104.
52. Feuchtner G, Kerber J, Burghard P, et al. The high-risk criteria low-attenuation plaque < 60 HU and the napkin-ring sign are the most powerful predictors of MACE: a long-term follow-up study. Eur Heart J Cardiovasc Imaging. 2017;18:772–9.
53. Seitun S, Clemente A, De Lorenzi C, Benenati S, Chiappino D, Mantini C, Sakellarios AI, Cademartiri F, Bezante GP, Porto I. Cardiac CT perfusion and FFRCTA: pathophysiological features in ischemic heart disease. Cardiovasc Diagn Ther. 2020;10(6):1954–78. https://doi.org/10.21037/cdt-20-414.
54. Sakellarios A, Correia J, Kyriakidis S et al. A cloud-based platform for the non-invasive management of coronary artery disease. Enterprise Inf Syst. 2020. ([Epub ahead of print]). https://doi.org/10.1080/17517575.2020.1746975.
55. Chen MY, Rochitte CE, Arbab-Zadeh A, et al. Prognostic value of combined CT angiography and myocardial perfusion imaging versus invasive coronary angiography and nuclear stress perfusion imaging in the prediction of major adverse cardiovascular events: the CORE320 multicenter study. Radiology. 2017;284:55–65.
56. Meinel FG, Pugliese F, Schoepf UJ, et al. Prognostic value of stress dynamic myocardial perfusion CT in a multicenter population with known or suspected coronary artery disease. AJR Am J Roentgenol. 2017;208:761–9.
57. Pijls NH, De Bruyne B, Peels K, Van Der Voort PH, Bonnier HJ, Bartunek JKJJ, et al. Measurement of fractional flow reserve to assess the functional severity of coronary-artery stenoses. N Engl J Med. 1996;334:1703–8.
58. Min JK, Leipsic J, Pencina MJ, et al. Diagnostic accuracy of fractional flow reserve from anatomic CT angiography. JAMA. 2012;308(12):1237–45.

59. Norgaard BL, Leipsic J, Gaur S, Seneviratne S, Ko BS, Ito H, et al. Diagnostic performance of noninvasive fractional flow reserve derived from coronary computed tomography angiography in suspected coronary artery disease: the NXT trial (Analysis of Coronary Blood Flow Using CT Angiography: Next Steps). J Am Coll Cardiol. 2014;63:1145–55.
60. Koo BK, Erglis A, Doh JH, Daniels DV, Jegere S, Kim HS, et al. Diagnosis of ischemia-causing coronary stenoses by noninvasive fractional flow reserve computed from coronary computed tomographic angiograms. Results from the prospective multicenter DISCOVER-FLOW (Diagnosis of Ischemia-Causing Stenoses Obtained Via Noninvasive Fractional Flow Reserve) study. J Am Coll Cardiol. 2011;58:1989–97.
61. Douglas PS, De Bruyne B, Pontone G, Patel MR, Norgaard BL, Byrne RA, et al. 1-year outcomes of FFRCT-guided care in patients with suspected coronary disease: the PLATFORM study. J Am Coll Cardiol. 2016;68:435–45.
62. Kim HL, Kim YJ, Lee SP, et al. Incremental prognostic value of sequential imaging of single-photon emission computed tomography and coronary computed tomography angiography in patients with suspected coronary artery disease. Eur Heart J Cardiovasc Imaging. 2014;15:878–85.
63. Renker M, Schoepf UJ, Wang R, et al. Comparison of diagnostic value of a novel noninvasive coronary computed tomography angiography method versus standard coronary angiography for assessing fractional flow reserve. Am J Cardiol. 2014;114(9):1303–8.
64. Coenen A, Lubbers MM, Kurata A, et al. Fractional flow reserve computed from noninvasive CT angiography data: diagnostic performance of an on-site clinician-operated computational fluid dynamics algorithm. Radiology. 2015;274:674–83.
65. Kruk M, Wardziak Ł, Demkow M, et al. Workstation-based calculation of CTA-based FFR for intermediate stenosis. JACC Cardiovasc Imaging. 2016;9:690–9.
66. Ko BS, Cameron JD, Munnur RK, et al. Noninvasive CT-derived FFR based on structural and fluid analysis: a comparison with invasive FFR for detection of functionally significant stenosis. JACC Cardiovasc Imaging. 2017;10:663–73.
67. Papafaklis MI, Mavrogiannis MC, Siogkas PK, Lakkas LS, Katsouras, Fotiadis DI, Michalis LK. Functional assessment of lesion severity without using the pressure wire: coronary imaging and blood flow simulation. Expert Rev Cardiovasc Ther. 2017;15(11):863–77.
68. Tesche C, De Cecco CN, Albrecht MH, Duguay TM, Bayer RR 2nd, Litwin SE, Steinberg DH, Schoepf UJ. Coronary CT angiography-derived fractional flow reserve. Radiology. 2017;285(1):17–33.
69. Seitun S, Clemente A, De Lorenzi C et al. Cardiac CT perfusion and FFRCTA: pathophysiological features in ischemic heart disease. Cardiovasc Diagn Ther. 2020. https://doi.org/10.21037/cdt-20-414.
70. Nakamura S, Kitagawa K, Goto Y, et al. Incremental prognostic value of myocardial blood flow quantified with stress dynamic computed tomography perfusion imaging. JACC Cardiovasc Imaging. 2019;12(7 Pt 2):1379–87.
71. van Assen M, De Cecco CN, Eid M, et al. Prognostic value of CT myocardial perfusion imaging and CT-derived fractional flow reserve for major adverse cardiac events in patients with coronary artery disease. J Cardiovasc Comput Tomogr. 2019;13:26–33.
72. Bilbey N, Blanke P, Naoum C, et al. Potential impact of clinical use of noninvasive FFRCT on radiation dose exposure and downstream clinical event rate. Clin Imaging. 2016;40:1055–60.
73. Douglas PS, De Bruyne B, Pontone G, et al. PLATFORM investigators. 1-Year outcomes of FFRCT-guided care in patients with suspected coronary disease: the PLATFORM study. J Am Coll Cardiol. 2016;68:435–45.
74. McCollough CH, Leng S, Yu L, Fletcher JG. Dual- and multi-energy CT: principles, technical approaches, and clinical applications. Radiology. 2015;276:637–53. https://doi.org/10.1148/radiol.2015142631.

75. Danad I, Fayad ZA, Willemink MJ, et al. New applications of cardiac computed tomography: dual-energy, spectral, and molecular CT imaging. JACC Cardiovasc Imaging. 2015;8:710–23. https://doi.org/10.1016/j.jcmg.2015.03.005.
76. Danad I, Hartaigh Ó, B, Min JK. Dual-energy computed tomography for detection of coronary artery disease. Expert Rev Cardiovasc Ther. 2015;13:1345–56. https://doi.org/10.1586/14779072.2015.1102055.
77. Symons R, Cork TE, Lakshmanan MN, et al. Dual-contrast agent photon-counting computed tomography of the heart: initial experience. Int J Cardiovasc Imaging. 2017;33:1253–61. https://doi.org/10.1007/s10554-017-1104-4.
78. Kolossváry M, De Cecco CN, Feuchtner G, Maurovich-Horvat P. Advanced atherosclerosis imaging by CT: radiomics, machine learning and deep learning. J Cardiovasc Comput Tomogr. 2019;13:274–80.

Magnetic Resonance Imaging of the Myocardium, Coronary Arteries, and Anomalous Origin of Coronary Arteries

Andrea Barison and Francesco Bianco

Abbreviations

CMR	Cardiovascular magnetic resonance
SSFP	Steady-state free precession
LGE	Late Gd accumulation
ECV	Extracellular volume
CT	Computed tomography
AVB	Atrioventricular block
MACE	Major adverse cardiovascular events
LM	Left main

1 Introduction

CMR has become a versatile noninvasive imaging tool in various forms of ischemic heart disease [1]. Biventricular morphology, volumes, and systolic function are assessed with SSFP cine sequences, acquired in two-, three-, and four-chamber long-axis views and in a short-axis cine stack. Myocardial tissue characterization is then performed using T1- and T2-weighted pre-contrast sequences (to assess fatty infiltration and edema, respectively);

A. Barison (✉)
Fondazione Toscana Gabriele Monasterio, Pisa, Italy

Scuola Superiore Sant'Anna, Pisa, Italy
e-mail: barison@ftgm.it

F. Bianco
AOU Ospedali Riuniti, Ancona, Italy
e-mail: francesco.bianco@ospedaliriuniti.marche.it

G. Concistrè (ed.), *Ischemic Heart Disease*,
https://doi.org/10.1007/978-3-031-25879-4_15

in particular, T2-weighted short-tau inversion recovery (T2-STIR) sequences are able to detect myocardial edema occurring during an acute ischemic event. Novel T1 and T2 mapping techniques allow to directly measure the absolute values of T1 and T2 of tissues (quantitative imaging) and not simply the signal intensity (qualitative imaging): myocardial edema lengthens both T1 and T2, while myocardial scars lengthen T1 only. After gadolinium (Gd)-based contrast agent injection, first-pass perfusion (FPP, acquired during Gd injection to assess myocardial perfusion) and late gadolinium enhancement sequences (LGE, acquired 10–20 min after Gd injection to assess myocardial necrosis and scars) complete a standard exam. The acquisition of T1 maps after Gd administration allows to calculate the myocardial ECV, i.e., the noncellular component of the myocardium corresponding to the extracellular matrix: it represents a finer analysis than simple LGE, allowing to quantify necrosis/fibrosis compared to the simple dichotomous distinction between areas with and without LGE.

In patients referred for stable angina, similarly to other imaging modalities, a stress CMR scan can be run by acquiring perfusion and/or cine sequences during infusion of a vasodilator or an inotropic agent, to assess myocardial changes under ischemic conditions. Besides conventional perfusion sequences, novel quantitative sequences have been recently developed to calculate absolute myocardial perfusion.

Finally, tridimensional sequences have been developed to assess the coronary artery tree. Despite a lower spatial resolution than CT, CMR represents a radiation-free imaging technique to study the origin and proximal course of major coronary arteries, particularly useful for young patients to rule out congenital anomalies and as a screening tool for coronary artery abnormalities in this population [2].

2 CMR in Acute Coronary Syndrome

2.1 Imaging Myocardial Edema, Necrosis, and Fibrosis

Cardiovascular imaging is of crucial importance in the diagnosis and risk stratification of patients with suspected acute coronary syndrome. In general, myocardial edema corresponds to the area at risk, i.e., the area of myocardium suffering an ischemic insult (both reversible and irreversible), characterized by intracellular and extracellular water content increase; it appears hyperintense in T2-STIR sequences [3, 4] (Fig. 1a) and presents increased native (pre-contrast) T1 and T2 values in mapping sequences [5, 6]. Myocardial necrosis, i.e., the area of myocardium suffering an irreversible ischemic damage, is characterized by sarcoplasmic membrane rupture, allowing Gd entry (expansion of the extracellular volume); it presents a variable hypointensity in first-pass perfusion images (Fig. 1b) and a typical hyperintensity in LGE sequences compared to the healthy (viable) myocardium (Fig. 1C). During myocardial healing, necrotic cells are progressively replaced by collagen scar: similarly to necrosis, myocardial scars cause expansion of the extracellular volume and Gd accumulation and appear hyperintense in LGE sequences.

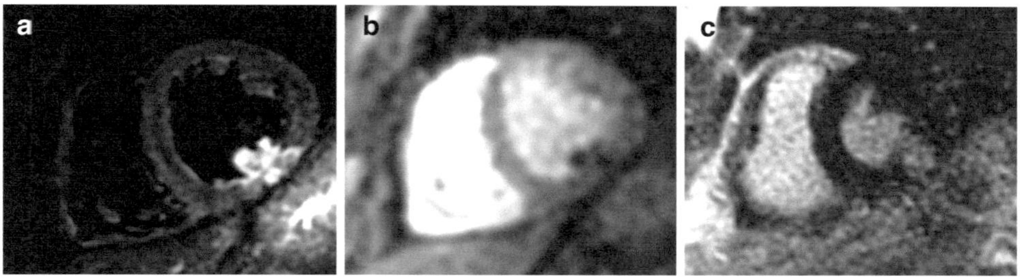

Fig. 1 (**a**) T2-weighted short-tau inversion recovery (T2-STIR) midventricular short-axis slice in a 49-year-old man with acute myocardial infarction, showing transmural hyperintensity (edema) in the inferolateral wall involving the posterior papillary muscle. (**b**) First-pass perfusion imaging, showing hypointensity (delayed contrast wash-in) in the same inferolateral wall. (**c**) Late-enhancement imaging, showing transmural hyperintensity (necrosis) in the same inferolateral wall. Please note that myocardial edema (panel A) is slightly larger than necrosis (panel B); this difference corresponds to the myocardial salvage area of the border zone (i.e., the reversibly ischemic myocardium, not subject to irreversible necrosis)

CMR has a greater sensitivity than SPECT [7] and PET [8] in detecting myocardial necrosis, especially if confined to the subendocardium, thanks to its higher spatial resolution and higher contrast difference between necrotic tissue and healthy myocardium. In experimental studies, the areas of LGE correspond to the areas of necrosis, with a spatial resolution so high that they can identify necrosis <1 g [7, 9]. Moreover, LGE extension presents a close correlation with myocardial necrosis at histology [10], with biohumoral markers of myocyte necrosis [11], and with post-infarct remodeling [12]. By subtracting the necrotic area (hyperintense in the LGE images) from the area at risk (hyperintense in T2-STIR images), the myocardial salvage index can be calculated, which presents an inverse correlation with myocardial reperfusion time in patients with acute myocardial infarction [13]. Although of limited clinical applicability, CMR might be useful in patients with acute chest pain assessed in emergency departments: in a study on patients with persistent chest pain without ischemic electrocardiographic changes, CMR with cine and LGE sequences yielded a 100% sensitivity and a 79% specificity in the diagnosis of myocardial infarction [14]; adding T2-STIR sequences, which are able to detect reversible ischemic changes, CMR yielded an overall 85% sensitivity and 96% specificity in the diagnosis of unstable angina [15].

2.2 Complications of Acute Myocardial Infarction

CMR allows to accurately diagnose possible postinfarction complications such as intramyocardial thrombosis, microvascular obstruction, and intramural hemorrhage. Intracardiac thrombosis appears hypointense in early (2–3 min) and late (8–15 min) images after Gd, as thrombotic formations typically do not take contrast (Fig. 2); while transesophageal echocardiography is the reference modality to detect intra-atrial thrombi,

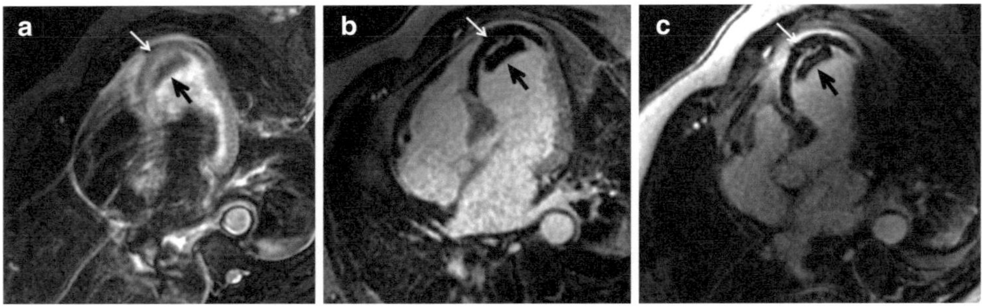

Fig. 2 (**a**) T2-weighted short-tau inversion recovery (T2-STIR) four-chamber view in a 60-year-old man with acute myocardial infarction, showing transmural hyperintensity (edema) in the anteroseptal and apical segments, with a large hypointense intramural hemorrhage (*white arrow*) and a hypointense intracardiac thrombus (*black arrow*). (**b**) Early post-contrast imaging (early enhancement), showing anteroseptal and apical hyperintensity with a large intramural hypointensity (microvascular obstruction, *white arrow*) and a hypointense intracardiac thrombus (*black arrow*). (**c**) Late-enhancement imaging, confirming the hyperintensity (necrosis) in the anteroseptal and apical wall, with a large hypointense microvascular obstruction (*white arrow*) and a hypointense intracardiac thrombus (*black arrow*)

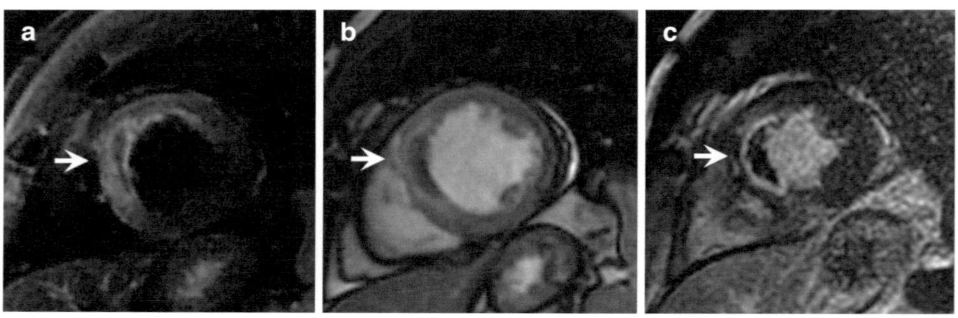

Fig. 3 (**a**) T2-weighted short-tau inversion recovery (T2-STIR) midventricular short-axis slice in a 56-year-old man with acute myocardial infarction, showing transmural hyperintensity (edema) in the anteroseptal wall (*arrow*), with a hypointense subendocardial core (intramural hemorrhage). (**b**) Post-contrast steady-state free precession (SSFP) cine imaging, showing hyperintensity (early enhancement) in the anteroseptal wall, with a hypointense subendocardial core (microvascular obstruction). (**c**) Late-enhancement imaging, confirming the hyperintensity (necrosis) in the anteroseptal wall, with a hypointense subendocardial core (microvascular obstruction)

CMR has superior diagnostic accuracy in detecting intraventricular thrombi [16]. Intramural hemorrhage appears as a hypointense core in T2-STIR sequences within the hyperintense ischemic (i.e., edematous) area [17]; this signal loss is due to paramagnetic properties of hemoglobin breakdown products, which act as a natural "negative" contrast reducing T2 and T2* (a parameter derived from T2) relaxation times (Figs. 2a and 3a).

Postinfarction hemorrhage is an independent predictor of adverse left ventricular remodeling and worse prognosis [18]. Intramural hemorrhage is often associated with microvascular obstruction, which is typically a hypoperfused (hypointense) core within the hyperintense infarcted myocardium in LGE images (Figs. 2b,c and 3b,c), because of the ischemic disruption of the coronary microcirculation; it represents an independent predictor of adverse ventricular remodeling and worse prognosis [19]. Other complications easily detectable with CMR include postinfarction pericarditis, pericardial effusion, right ventricular infarction, myocardial wall rupture, myocardial aneurysms, or pseudoaneurysms.

2.3 Differential Diagnosis of MINOCAs

CMR is currently the gold standard imaging technique for a differential and etiological diagnosis in patients with suspected acute coronary syndrome and unobstructed coronary arteries (MINOCAs) [20–22]: this is the case not only of myocarditis, pericarditis, vasospastic angina, takotsubo, nonischemic cardiomyopathies, and amyloidosis, but also of acute and subacute aortic syndromes like aneurysms, pseudoaneurysms, dissections, intramural hematomas, penetrating ulcers, and vasculitis affecting the main thoracic vessels. In patients with chest pain, negative electrocardiographic, imaging, and biohumoral findings, and low or intermediate risk of acute coronary syndrome, stress CMR is a valuable technique to stratify patients to early discharge [23].

2.4 Postinfarction Myocardial Remodeling

Following an acute coronary syndrome, echocardiography is the first-line recommended tool to track myocardial volume and function changes during follow-up. In particular, in patients with initial LV systolic dysfunction, four trajectories may be observed: a deterioration of LV geometry and function (adverse remodeling), a substantial stability over time, a trend toward recovery (reverse remodeling), or even a substantial normalization (remission). These processes correlate with prognosis, with adverse remodeling predicting worsening clinical status including hospitalization, pump failure or death, and reverse remodeling or remission predicting better prognosis. Clinical trials have considered different definitions for adverse/reverse remodeling, including changes in LV end-systolic volume, end-diastolic diameter or volume, or ejection fraction (either alone or in combination), over different times with different cutoffs [24]. Besides volumetric changes, cardiac remodeling may manifest as an increased LV mass (hypertrophy): in the adult heart, cardiomyocytes are terminally differentiated cells and, even if they do not increase in number, they may increase in size to reduce ventricular wall stress in response to an increased workload.

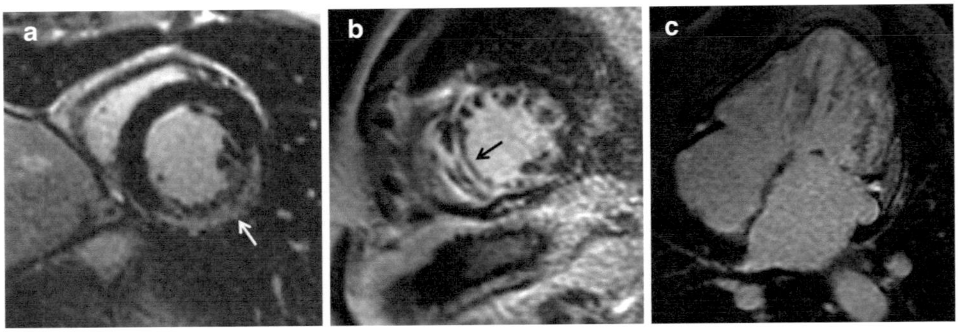

Fig. 4 Late-enhancement patterns in nonischemic cardiomyopathies. (**a**) Subepicardial pattern, involving the left ventricular lateral wall (*white arrow*) in a patient with previous myocarditis; (**b**) midwall pattern, involving the interventricular septum (*black arrow*) in a patient with primary dilated cardiomyopathy; (**c**) diffuse pattern, in a patient with cardiac amyloidosis

Compared to echocardiography, CMR allows a more accurate assessment of biventricular volumes, mass, and systolic function, but also superior tissue characterization with LGE sequences. Thanks to their peculiar subendocardial or transmural pattern, postinfarction scars can be distinguished from nonischemic scars, such as those occurring in nonischemic cardiomyopathies, myocarditis, and amyloidosis (Fig. 4) [25]. Moreover, LGE location, extent, and transmurality can be easily characterized with CMR and have clinical implications. For example, the higher is the degree of LGE transmurality, the lower is the likelihood of function recovery after myocardial revascularization [12], making LGE a unique tool to assess myocardial viability and to predict functional recovery after an acute coronary syndrome. Similarly, the presence, extent, heterogeneity, and qualitative distribution of myocardial scar have been demonstrated to predict major ventricular arrhythmias and sudden cardiac death in postinfarction cardiomyopathy [26, 27].

A postnecrotic myocardial scar can sometimes undergo fatty metaplasia, a phenomenon likely related to the transdifferentiation of multipotential interstitial cells to adipocytes. Fatty infiltration can be seen in CMR as a dark banding artifact (also named “India ink” sign) in SSFP images or as a hyperintense area in T1- or PD-weighted fast spin echo sequences [28] (Fig. 5). On the one hand, it is unclear whether different stimuli may promote cell transdifferentiation into an adipocyte phenotype, compared to a fibroblast phenotype. On the other hand, it is unclear whether fatty metaplasia plays a role in postinfarction arrhythmogenesis, because the presence of fat within the myocardium may alter the propagation of the electrical impulse and/or cause reentry circuits.

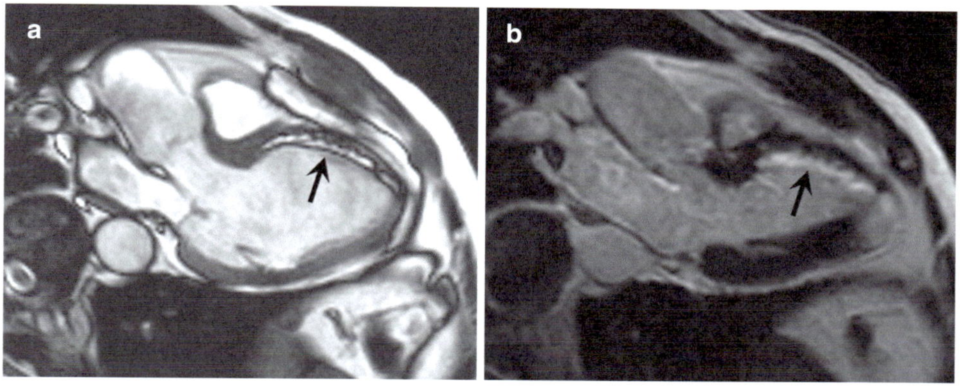

Fig. 5 Three-chamber view in a patient with previous anterior myocardial infarction and fibro-fatty metaplasia. (**a**) In cine steady-state free-precession imaging, the anteroseptal wall (*black arrow*) appears hyperintense with a peripheral banding (India ink) artifact, indicating fatty metaplasia. (**b**) In late-enhancement imaging, the anteroseptal wall (*black arrow*) appears hyperintense, indicating a subendocardial scar in the same region

3 CMR in Stable Coronary Syndromes

3.1 Imaging Myocardial Ischemia

Stress CMR is one of the currently recommended imaging methods for the diagnosis and prognostic stratification of patients with chronic stable angina. Similarly to other imaging methods, ischemia can be studied by evaluating myocardial perfusion and kinetics under maximal pharmacological vasodilation (adenosine, dipyridamole, or regadenoson) or an inotropic/chronotropic stress (dobutamine). The stress acquisitions are then complemented with rest acquisitions: rest perfusion imaging is commonly used as a reference to detect "fixed" perfusion defects (either due to a previous scar or due to an artifact); rest cine imaging as a reference for assessing wall motion abnormalities; and LGE for assessing myocardial viability.

Common contraindications to both vasodilator and inotropic stressors include unstable angina, acute myocardial infarction, severe systemic arterial hypertension (>220/120 mmHg), and other serious acute clinical conditions. Even though most adverse effects are self-limiting, i.v. aminophylline can act as an antidote for vasodilator stress testing, while i.v. beta-blockers are used for reversing the effects of dobutamine. Due to the possibility to observe clinically relevant side effects or to induce severe myocardial ischemia during a stress test, all MR staff should continuously monitor heart rhythm, blood pressure, and symptoms and should be regularly trained in the recognition and management of acute cardiovascular emergencies [29], according to the international guidelines on basic and advanced life support [30].

3.2 Stress CMR with Vasodilators

Vasodilator drugs share a common capability to bind the adenosine receptors, but differ by receptor selectivity, half-life, and duration of action [29]. *Adenosine* is administered intravenously (i.v.) at a dose of 140–210 μg/Kg min for 4–6 min and has a half-life of <10 s and short duration of action (few seconds); while the selective activation of A_{2A} receptors leads to coronary vasodilation, additional activity on A_1 and A_{2B} receptors can induce side effects such as AVB and bronchospasm, respectively. *Dipyridamole* is administered at a dose of 0.56–0.84 mg/Kg i.v. for 6 min and has longer half-life (11 h) and duration of action (about 30 min) when compared to adenosine, with similar selectivity issues and side effects (AVBs, breathlessness, bronchospasm, hypotension, headache, and flushing). Accordingly, adenosine and dipyridamole should not be used in patients with severe sinus bradycardia (<40 bpm), advanced AVB, asthma, or severe reactive pulmonary disease requiring chronic treatment with inhalers. *Regadenoson* is administered at a fixed dose of 400 μg, as a single 10-s bolus followed by a 10-s saline push, and has a relatively short half-life (30 min) and duration of action (2.3 min); its A_{2A} receptor selectivity warrants effective coronary vasodilation while limiting side effects with significantly improved patient tolerability; in particular, regadenoson can be administered in patients with asthma/reactive airway disease and is associated with lower incidence of AVB.

During intense vasodilation, myocardial regions supplied by stenotic coronary arteries show relative hypoperfusion (hypointensity during first-pass perfusion), while wall motion abnormalities appear only when the coronary stenosis is so severe to cause ischemia (an absolute blood flow reduction due to the "coronary steal" phenomenon) [31]. To preserve the diagnostic sensitivity of the test, patients should refrain from assuming coffee, tea, or other caffeine-containing beverages (including some "decaffeinated" drinks that might still contain some caffein) for at least 24 h prior to CMR, as they can block the effects of this class of vasodilators. Besides qualitative analysis, a semiquantitative method to calculate myocardial perfusion reserve is based on the ratio between myocardial signal intensity maximal upslope at peak stress and at rest, both normalized for the blood pool signal intensity. A quantitative estimation of myocardial perfusion is also feasible with very recent sequences, based either on the dual-Gd bolus technique or on the dual-sequence (myocardial/arterial input function) technique [32].

The sensitivity and specificity of adenosine stress CMR are 85–91% and 67–94%, respectively, using an anatomical gold standard such as coronary angiography [1]. A large multicenter trial (MR-IMPACT) on 241 patients reported high sensitivity (86%) and specificity (67%) and greater diagnostic accuracy compared to myocardial scintigraphy [33];

similar results were confirmed by the MR-IMPACT II study (533 patients) [34] and from the CE-MARC study (752 patients) [35]. In the recent GADA-CAD study on 764 patients undergoing both stress (adenosine or regadenoson) CMR and either coronary angiography or coronary CT as a reference, the sensitivity of CMR was 78.9%, specificity was 86.8%, and area under the curve was 0.871 for detection of a ≥70% stenosis. The sensitivity and specificity for multivessel CAD were 87.4% and 73.0%. For detection of a 50% stenosis, sensitivity was 64.6% and specificity was 86.6% [36].

Several studies have also investigated the prognostic impact of stress CMR. In the recent SPINS trial on 2349 patients with stable angina followed for a median of 5.4 years, stress CMR offered an effective cardiac prognostication: patients without ischemia or LGE experienced a low incidence of cardiac events, little need for coronary revascularization, and low spending on subsequent ischemia testing [37]. Based on the SPINS registry, in the USA, stress perfusion CMR is more cost effective than single photon emission computed tomography, CT with selective CT-FFR, and invasive FFR-based strategies [38]. In another study on 3664 patients referred for stress CMR, inducible ischemia and LGE were associated with the occurrence of MACE, defined by cardiovascular mortality or recurrent nonfatal myocardial infarction, over a median follow-up of 8.8 (IQR 6.9–9.5) years [39]. Stress CMR has a good prognostic value also in patients after coronary artery bypass graft, with a higher incidence of cardiovascular death and/or nonfatal myocardial infarction in patients with inducible ischemia and/or LGE [40]. In the MR-INFORM study, 918 patients with typical angina and either two or more cardiovascular risk factors or a positive exercise treadmill test were randomized to either adenosine stress CMR or invasive fractional flow reserve (FFR). Stress CMR led to a lower incidence of coronary revascularization (35.7%) than FFR (45.0%), but the occurrence of the primary outcome (death, nonfatal myocardial infarction, or target-vessel revascularization within 1 year) was not different (3.6% in the stress CMR group, 3.7% in the FFR group) [41]. This study seems to confirm that many if not most of the "missed" intermediate lesions may indeed be "true negative" in their hemodynamic significance rather than "false negative," a fundamental challenge in comparing physiological perfusion significance (stress CMR) versus luminal stenosis (coronary angiography or CT).

3.3 Stress CMR with Dobutamine

Functional stress cardiac MR is generally based on the administration of *dobutamine*, a synthetic catecholamine with predominant affinity for β_1-adrenergic receptors [29]. Demonstration of myocardial ischemia with dobutamine stress test relies on the increase in myocardial oxygen demand caused by positive inotropic and chronotropic effects. Dobutamine is administered at increasing doses, to a maximum of 40 μg/Kg min i.v. (±atropine) and has a half-life of 1–2 min. Cine images are acquired during each step; perfusion imaging can also be acquired at peak stress and compared with rest perfusion. Potential side effects include palpitations, shortness of breath, headache, and supraventricular and ventricular arrhythmias. Dobutamine stress MR should not be performed in case of severe aortic stenosis, obstructive hypertrophic cardiomyopathy, and complex arrhythmias. Beta-blockers should be withdrawn 48 h prior to dobutamine administration because of their competing action.

Dobutamine CMR has been shown to be superior to dobutamine echocardiography [42], mainly due to better image quality and greater reproducibility, with 78–89% sensitivity and 75–86% specificity compared to coronary angiography [1]. Other studies have shown a comparable prognostic value for adenosine and dobutamine stress CMR [43]. Although technically more complicated than other imaging methods, CMR-compatible cycloergometers have been devised for the study of kinetics and myocardial perfusion under physiological stress conditions; nevertheless, their clinical use is currently limited to experimental settings.

3.4 Ischemia with Nonobstructive Coronary Arteries (INOCAs)

Many patients with stable angina do not have obstructive coronary artery disease at invasive angiography, more common in women than in men: INOCA can result from heterogeneous mechanisms including coronary vasospasm and microvascular dysfunction and, compared to asymptomatic individuals, is associated with increased incidence of cardiovascular events, repeated hospital admissions, and impaired quality of life [44]. Diseases that affect the myocardial microvasculature (e.g., diabetes mellitus, systemic hypertension) may lead to a global subendocardial reduction in perfusion under a vasodilatory stress, typically associated with intense chest pain [45, 46]. Stress CMR is therefore able to detect true myocardial ischemia occurring despite normal coronary arteries, which can be missed by a pure anatomic diagnostic approach such as coronary CT. Nevertheless, differentiating INOCA from multivessel coronary artery disease can be challenging, because even the presence of balanced multivessel disease can result in most or all of the imaged segments appearing hypoperfused. The novel perfusion mapping sequences will allow a quantitative assessment of absolute myocardial perfusion and will help detect and grade myocardial ischemia even in patients with normal coronary arteries but underlying microvascular disease.

4 Imaging the Coronary Arteries with CMR

4.1 Sequences for Coronary Imaging

Several CMR sequences have been developed to assess the coronary tree. In particular, free-breathing 3D SSFP sequences are ECG gated, respiratory navigator gated, triggered to a single cardiac phase, and designed to directly visualize the coronary arteries with CMR. However, despite the theoretical advantage of CMR in avoiding the use of ionizing radiations and potentially nephrotoxic contrast agents, coronary imaging with CMR is still significantly inferior to CT in the diagnostic accuracy of coronary stenoses. In particular, these sequences are still limited by a long acquisition time (4–5 min), breathing/arrhythmia artifacts, and a lower spatial resolution compared to coronary CT.

Multicenter studies have shown good diagnostic accuracy of coronary CMR imaging, reporting a negative sensitivity, specificity, and predictive value of 88%, 72%, and 88%, respectively, in an analysis per patient [47]. While the assessment of coronary artery stenosis is currently performed with cardiac CT, coronary CMR angiography plays a role in the screening and assessment of congenital anomalies of coronary arteries [2, 48]. In particular, in a single-center prospective blinded study, a cardiac-gated 3D gradient-echo sequence with fat suppression demonstrated an accurate identification of the proximal coronary arteries, with a specificity of 95% [49], suggesting that respiratory-gated 3D CMR angiography is an accurate tool for the identification of proximal coronary arteries' origins and course.

4.2 Anomalies of Coronary Artery Origin

In the normal heart, the right and left coronary arteries arise from the aortic valvar sinuses adjacent to the pulmonary trunk. The right coronary artery then directly enters the right atrioventricular groove, whereas the main stem of the left coronary artery runs a short course before dividing to become the left anterior descending and circumflex arteries [50]. These arteries can have an anomalous origin from either the aorta or the pulmonary trunk; their branches can have various anomalous origins relative to arterial pedicles. Understanding of these variations is key to determining those anomalous patterns associated with sudden cardiac death [51].

Isolated congenital coronary artery anomalies have been reported in approximately 1.3% (ranging from 0.2 to 5.6%) of patients undergoing coronary angiography (CMR, CT, or invasive angiography) and approximately 0.3% of patients at autopsy [52]. About 80% of coronary anomalies are considered benign without significant clinical sequelae, with the remaining 20% potentially responsible for significant symptoms such as myocardial ischemia and sudden death [53].

Most clinically significant coronary artery anomalies are within the anomalies of origin and course. There are three main subcategories within this group including (A) absent LM artery, (B) anomalous ostium outside the aortic sinuses, and (C) anomalous ostium at an inappropriate sinus of Valsalva (Fig. 6). The latter is often associated with an interarterial course, and the most common anatomical variants recognized at the postmortem of SCD victims. Abnormalities of the left coronary artery are more commonly associated with death during exercise; when the right coronary artery is affected, SCD can occur at rest, after efforts [53].

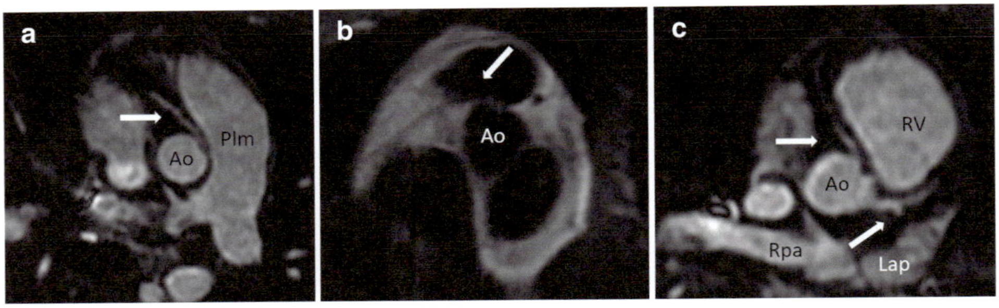

Fig. 6 A 12-year-old soccer player referred for ventricular tachycardia at the treadmill stress test. The CMR exam revealed a right coronary artery from the left coronary sinus with intramural and interarterial course (the right and left coronary arteries are indicated by *white arrows*). Panels A and C: 3D balanced steady-state free-precession sequences. Panel B: T1-double-IR fast spin echo sequence. Right coronary artery (RCA), aorta (Ao), pulmonary artery (Plm), right ventricle (Rv), right pulmonary artery (Rpa), left atrial appendage (Lap)

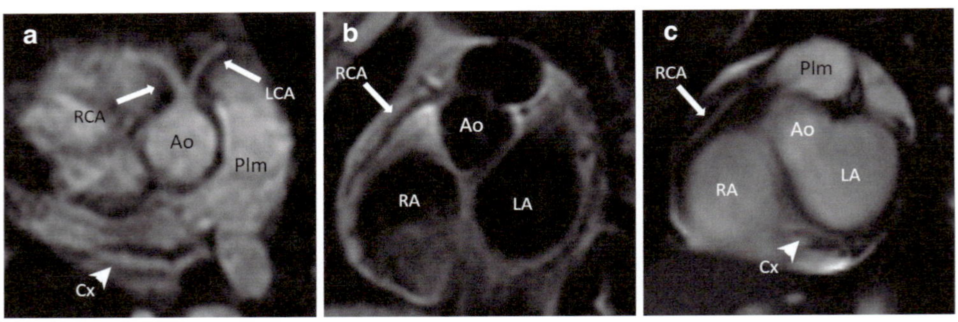

Fig. 7 A 7-year-old male referred for syncope during a karate match. The CMR exam revealed a coronary artery abnormality: single coronary artery with pre-pulmonary course of the left coronary artery (the right and left coronary arteries are indicated by *white arrows*), associated with an anomalous origin of the left circumflex from the right pulmonary artery (ALCAPA, anomalous left coronary artery from the pulmonary artery; arrowhead). Panels A and B: 3D balanced steady-state free-precession sequences. Panel C: T1-double-IR fast spin echo sequence. Left coronary artery (LCA), aorta (Ao), pulmonary artery (Plm), right atrium (RA), left atrium (LA), right pulmonary artery (Rpa)

Anomalous origins of coronary arteries from the pulmonary trunk are rare. In a contemporary cohort of 5998 outpatients (median age 16 years (Q1–Q3: 11, 36)), referred for routine echocardiography, $n = 5$, anomalous origin from the pulmonary artery was diagnosed, both right and left [54]. Their diagnosis strictly depends on clinical presentations, physician expertise and suspicion, and diagnostic methods utilized. In fact, they can originate at literally any level of the pulmonary artery: the valve, the trunk, and the right or left pulmonary arteries (Fig. 7).

4.3 Anomalies of Coronary Artery Course

The course of coronary arteries is of clinical importance especially when dealing with anomalous origin from the opposite sinus, which should be further classified, in order of frequency, as retroaortic, interarterial, subpulmonic (intraconal or intraseptal), prepulmonic, or retrocardiac (Fig. 8).

The main cause of ischemia, and potential SCD, is generally sustained by the narrowing of the initial segment of the coronary artery, as it enters or exits the aortic wall, at an intramural course by compression in between the inner and outer layers of the aortic tunica media [55]. This often happens in the case of anomalous aortic origin from the opposite sinus of Valsalva, with an intramural/interaterial course. This narrowing is not present in any others: intraseptal or infundibular, retroaortic, wraparound the apex, or retrocardiac [55, 56]. Therefore, it is evident that a prompt and accurate evaluation is crucial within a CMR scan of the origin and proximal course of the coronary arteries.

In this sense, a recent report by Angelini P. and colleagues documented coronary artery abnormalities (6 left and 17 right) from 5169 CMR studies (mean participant age, 13 ± 2 years), $n = 23$. The screening program was CMR based and implemented with a cardiac-gated MR imaging, without sedation or contrast agents. Multiple-axis images were obtained in a steady-state free precession sequence (cine SSFP) evaluating the left ventricular structure and function and the coronary artery origins and proximal courses [57].

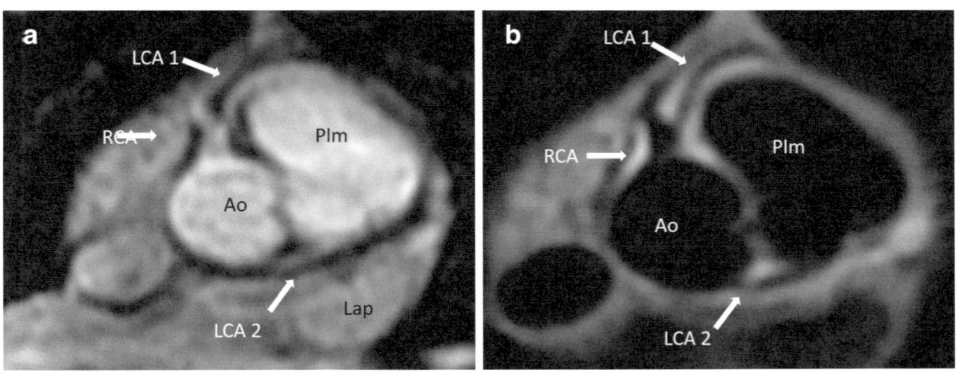

Fig. 8 Magnetic resonance imaging in a 16-year-old male referred for chest pain/discomfort after sports activities, showing duplication of the left circumflex artery (LCA) with pre-pulmonary course of one branch (LCA1) and normal course of the other branch (LCA2); the right and left coronary arteries are indicated by *white arrows*. Panel A: 3D balanced steady-state free-precession sequence. Panel B: T1-double-IR fast spin echo sequence. Left coronary artery (LCA), aorta (Ao), pulmonary artery (Plm), right atrium (RA), left atrium (LA)

5 Technical Limitations

Nowadays, advanced imaging is essential for a correct evaluation of the patient presenting with ischemic heart disease; however, CMR requires a dedicated cardiac scanner and precise local skills, with higher costs compared with echocardiography. Technical limitations including tachyarrhythmias or breathing artifacts can be considered limited and relative contraindications together with claustrophobia. Selected patients may undergo a CMR scan under general anesthesia. Several metallic devices (including pacemakers and defibrillators) represent a limitation for CMR, but patients with newer CMR-conditional devices may safely undergo a CMR scan after device reprogramming [58]. Gadolinium-based contrast agents are generally contraindicated in individuals with a glomerular filtration rate <30 mL/min/1.73 m^2, even if the risk of nephrogenic systemic fibrosis is extremely low with newer cyclic gadolinium-based contrast agents [59].

6 Future Perspectives

Several novel experimental CMR sequences are under investigation, but still not used in clinical practice. Oxygenation-sensitive CMR is a technique that allows in vivo noninvasive evaluation of tissue oxygenation thanks to the paramagnetic properties of deoxyhemoglobin: an increase in hemoglobin saturation causes an analogous increase in the BOLD (blood oxygenation level dependent) signal in specific T2 or T2* sequences [60].

Hyperpolarized contrast agents have been used for magnetic resonance spectroscopy (to assess cardiac metabolism) and imaging (as an alternative to Gd-based contrast agents). In particular, carbon-13 CMR [61] and fluoro-19 CMR [62] are the most promising techniques on the horizon. Instead of exploiting the magnetic properties of hydrogen nuclei (present in abundance especially in water and in lipids), these new techniques exploit the magnetic properties of some specific carbon or fluorine isotopes, with dedicated coils and sequences. In particular, the development of a recent hyperpolarization technique for signal enhancement, applied to the pyruvate-[1-(13) C] and pyruvate-[2-(13) C] tracers, allows to study the myocardial metabolism in vivo under different pathophysiological conditions [63].

Further advancements in CMR imaging techniques have led to the development of various 3D whole-heart coronary CMR techniques with further improvements in tissue contrast for improved delineation of the coronary arteries. 3D coronary CMR offers several advantages over 2D techniques. With 3D techniques, a volumetric acquisition of thin, truly contiguous partition images that encompass the complete coronary arterial tree can be acquired in one acquisition, minimizing the reliance on slice orientation. Other experimental sequences and coils have been tested in animal models for high-resolution intravascular coronary imaging [64].

7 Conclusions

CMR is currently one of the cornerstones of cardiac imaging for the evaluation of patients with ischemic heart disease. It allows an accurate and reproducible evaluation of morphology, function, ischemia, and myocardial viability, with a wide application across different clinical scenarios: from the diagnosis of ischemia to the evaluation of patients with chest pain and suspected acute coronary syndrome and from the differential diagnosis in patients with acute coronary syndrome and normal coronary angiograms to the study of viability in subjects with chronic ischemic heart disease and systolic ventricular dysfunction. Congenital anomalies of the coronary artery origin and course can be assessed with dedicated tridimensional angiographic sequences. The added value of CMR lies in its unique ability to combine morphological and functional assessment together with an extremely accurate in vivo myocardial tissue characterization.

References

1. Schwitter J, Arai AE. Assessment of cardiac ischaemia and viability: role of cardiovascular magnetic resonance. Eur Heart J. 2011;32:799–809. https://doi.org/10.1093/eurheartj/ehq481.
2. Angelini P, Cheong BY, Lenge De Rosen VV, Lopez A, Uribe C, Masso AH, Ali SW, Davis BR, Muthupillai R, Willerson JT. High-risk cardiovascular conditions in sports-related sudden death: prevalence in 5,169 schoolchildren screened via cardiac magnetic resonance. Texas Hear Inst J. 2018;45:205. https://doi.org/10.14503/THIJ-18-6645.
3. Walls MC, Verhaert D, Min JK, Raman SV. Myocardial edema imaging in acute coronary syndromes. J Magn Reson Imaging. 2011;34:1243–50. https://doi.org/10.1002/jmri.22737.
4. Aletras AH, Tilak GS, Natanzon A, Hsu L-Y, Gonzalez FM, Hoyt RF, Arai AE. Retrospective determination of the area at risk for reperfused acute myocardial infarction with T2-weighted cardiac magnetic resonance imaging: histopathological and displacement encoding with stimulated echoes (DENSE) functional validations. Circulation. 2006;113:1865–70. https://doi.org/10.1161/CIRCULATIONAHA.105.576025.
5. Dall'Armellina E, Ferreira VM, Kharbanda RK, Prendergast B, Piechnik SK, Robson MD, Jones M, Francis JM, Choudhury RP, Neubauer S. Diagnostic value of pre-contrast T1 mapping in acute and chronic myocardial infarction. JACC Cardiovasc Imaging. 2013;6:739–42. https://doi.org/10.1016/j.jcmg.2012.11.020.
6. Hammer-Hansen S, Ugander M, Hsu L-Y, Taylor J, Thune JJ, Køber L, Kellman P, Arai AE. Distinction of salvaged and infarcted myocardium within the ischaemic area-at-risk with T2 mapping. Eur Heart J Cardiovasc Imaging. 2014; https://doi.org/10.1093/ehjci/jeu073.
7. Wagner A, Mahrholdt H, Holly TA, Elliott MD, Regenfus M, Parker M, Klocke FJ, Bonow RO, Kim RJ, Judd RM. Contrast-enhanced MRI and routine single photon emission computed tomography (SPECT) perfusion imaging for detection of subendocardial myocardial infarcts: an imaging study. Lancet (London, England). 2003;361:374–9. https://doi.org/10.1016/S0140-6736(03)12389-6.
8. Klein C, Nekolla SG, Bengel FM, Momose M, Sammer A, Haas F, Schnackenburg B, Delius W, Mudra H, Wolfram D, Schwaiger M. Assessment of myocardial viability with contrast-enhanced magnetic resonance imaging: comparison with positron emission tomography. Circulation. 2002;105:162–7. http://www.ncbi.nlm.nih.gov/pubmed/11790695. Accessed 22 Jan 2016.

9. Ricciardi MJ, Wu E, Davidson CJ, Choi KM, Klocke FJ, Bonow RO, Judd RM, Kim RJ. Visualization of discrete microinfarction after percutaneous coronary intervention associated with mild creatine kinase-MB elevation., Circulation. 2001;103:2780–3. http://www.ncbi.nlm.nih.gov/pubmed/11401931. Accessed 22 Jan 2016.
10. Kim RJ, Fieno DS, Parrish TB, Harris K, Chen EL, Simonetti O, Bundy J, Finn JP, Klocke FJ, Judd RM. Relationship of MRI delayed contrast enhancement to irreversible injury, infarct age, and contractile function. Circulation. 1999;100:1992–2002. http://www.ncbi.nlm.nih.gov/pubmed/10556226. Accessed 4 Aug 2013.
11. Ingkanisorn WP, Rhoads KL, Aletras AH, Kellman P, Arai AE. Gadolinium delayed enhancement cardiovascular magnetic resonance correlates with clinical measures of myocardial infarction. J Am Coll Cardiol. 2004;43:2253–9. https://doi.org/10.1016/j.jacc.2004.02.046.
12. Kim RJ, Wu E, Rafael A, Chen EL, Parker MA, Simonetti O, Klocke FJ, Bonow RO, Judd RM. The use of contrast-enhanced magnetic resonance imaging to identify reversible myocardial dysfunction. N Engl J Med. 2000;343:1445–53. https://doi.org/10.1056/NEJM200011163432003.
13. Francone M, Bucciarelli-Ducci C, Carbone I, Canali E, Scardala R, Calabrese FA, Sardella G, Mancone M, Catalano C, Fedele F, Passariello R, Bogaert J, Agati L. Impact of primary coronary angioplasty delay on myocardial salvage, infarct size, and microvascular damage in patients with ST-segment elevation myocardial infarction: insight from cardiovascular magnetic resonance. J Am Coll Cardiol. 2009;54:2145–53. https://doi.org/10.1016/j.jacc.2009.08.024.
14. Kwong RY, Schussheim AE, Rekhraj S, Aletras AH, Geller N, Davis J, Christian TF, Balaban RS, Arai AE. Detecting acute coronary syndrome in the emergency department with cardiac magnetic resonance imaging., Circulation. 2003;107:531–7. http://www.ncbi.nlm.nih.gov/pubmed/12566362. Accessed 22 Jan 2016.
15. Cury RC, Shash K, Nagurney JT, Rosito G, Shapiro MD, Nomura CH, Abbara S, Bamberg F, Ferencik M, Schmidt EJ, Brown DF, Hoffmann U, Brady TJ. Cardiac magnetic resonance with T2-weighted imaging improves detection of patients with acute coronary syndrome in the emergency department. Circulation. 2008;118:837–44. https://doi.org/10.1161/CIRCULATIONAHA.107.740597.
16. Srichai MB, Junor C, Rodriguez LL, Stillman AE, Grimm RA, Lieber ML, Weaver JA, Smedira NG, White RD. Clinical, imaging, and pathological characteristics of left ventricular thrombus: a comparison of contrast-enhanced magnetic resonance imaging, transthoracic echocardiography, and transesophageal echocardiography with surgical or pathological validation. Am Heart J. 2006;152:75–84. https://doi.org/10.1016/j.ahj.2005.08.021.
17. Lotan CS, Bouchard A, Cranney GB, Bishop SP, Pohost GM. Assessment of postreperfusion myocardial hemorrhage using proton NMR imaging at 1.5 T.Circulation. 1992;86:1018–25. http://www.ncbi.nlm.nih.gov/pubmed/1516171. Accessed 25 Jan 2016.
18. Ganame J, Messalli G, Dymarkowski S, Rademakers FE, Desmet W, Van de Werf F, Bogaert J. Impact of myocardial haemorrhage on left ventricular function and remodelling in patients with reperfused acute myocardial infarction. Eur Heart J. 2009;30:1440–9. https://doi.org/10.1093/eurheartj/ehp093.
19. Wu KC. CMR of microvascular obstruction and hemorrhage in myocardial infarction. J Cardiovasc Magn Reson. 2012;14:68. https://doi.org/10.1186/1532-429X-14-68.
20. Laissy J-P, Hyafil F, Feldman LJ, Juliard J-M, Schouman-Claeys E, Steg PG, Faraggi M. Differentiating acute myocardial infarction from myocarditis: diagnostic value of early- and delayed-perfusion cardiac MR imaging. Radiology. 2005;237:75–82. https://doi.org/10.1148/radiol.2371041322.
21. Quarta G, Sado DM, J.C. Moon, cardiomyopathies: focus on cardiovascular magnetic resonance. Br J Radiol. 2011;84:S296–305. https://doi.org/10.1259/bjr/67212179.

22. Baliga RR, Nienaber CA, Bossone E, Oh JK, Isselbacher EM, Sechtem U, Fattori R, Raman SV, Eagle KA. The role of imaging in aortic dissection and related syndromes. JACC Cardiovasc Imaging. 2014;7:406–24. https://doi.org/10.1016/j.jcmg.2013.10.015.
23. Miller CD, Hwang W, Case D, Hoekstra JW, Lefebvre C, Blumstein H, Hamilton CA, Harper EN, Hundley WG. Stress CMR imaging observation unit in the emergency department reduces 1-year medical care costs in patients with acute chest pain: a randomized study for comparison with inpatient care. JACC Cardiovasc Imaging. 2011;4:862–70. https://doi.org/10.1016/j.jcmg.2011.04.016.
24. Aimo A, Gaggin HK, Barison A, Emdin M, Januzzi JL. Imaging, biomarker, and clinical predictors of cardiac Remodeling in heart failure with reduced ejection fraction. JACC Hear Fail. 2019;7 https://doi.org/10.1016/j.jchf.2019.06.004.
25. Vöhringer M, Mahrholdt H, Yilmaz A, Sechtem U. Significance of late gadolinium enhancement in cardiovascular magnetic resonance imaging (CMR). Herz. 2007;32:129–37. https://doi.org/10.1007/s00059-007-2972-5.
26. Acosta J, Fernández-Armenta J, Borràs R, Anguera I, Bisbal F, Martí-Almor J, Tolosana JM, Penela D, Andreu D, Soto-Iglesias D, Evertz R, Matiello M, Alonso C, Villuendas R, de Caralt TM, Perea RJ, Ortiz JT, Bosch X, Serra L, Planes X, Greiser A, Ekinci O, Lasalvia L, Mont L, Berruezo A. Scar characterization to predict life-threatening arrhythmic events and sudden cardiac death in patients with cardiac resynchronization therapy. JACC Cardiovasc Imaging. 2018;11:561–72. https://doi.org/10.1016/j.jcmg.2017.04.021.
27. Disertori M, Rigoni M, Pace N, Casolo G, Masè M, Gonzini L, Lucci D, Nollo G, Ravelli F. Myocardial fibrosis assessment by LGE is a powerful predictor of ventricular tachyarrhythmias in ischemic and nonischemic LV dysfunction: a meta-analysis. JACC Cardiovasc Imaging. 2016;9:1046–55. https://doi.org/10.1016/J.JCMG.2016.01.033.
28. Nucifora G, Aquaro GDGD, Masci PGPG, Barison A, Todiere G, Pingitore A, Lombardi M. Lipomatous metaplasia in ischemic cardiomyopathy: current knowledge and clinical perspective. Int J Cardiol. 2011;146:120–2. https://doi.org/10.1016/j.ijcard.2010.09.090.
29. Kramer CM, Barkhausen J, Bucciarelli-Ducci C, Flamm SD, Kim RJ, Nagel E. Standardized cardiovascular magnetic resonance imaging (CMR) protocols: 2020 update. J Cardiovasc Magn Reson. 2020;22:17. https://doi.org/10.1186/s12968-020-00607-1.
30. Nolan JP, Maconochie I, Soar J, Olasveengen TM, Greif R, Wyckoff MH, Singletary EM, Aickin R, Berg KM, Mancini ME, Bhanji F, Wyllie J, Zideman D, Neumar RW, Perkins GD, Castrén M, Morley PT, Montgomery WH, Nadkarni VM, Billi JE, Merchant RM, de Caen A, Escalante-Kanashiro R, Kloeck D, Wang TL, Hazinski MF, Executive Summary. International consensus on cardiopulmonary resuscitation and emergency cardiovascular care science with treatment recommendations. Circulation. 2020;142(2020):S2–S27. https://doi.org/10.1161/CIR.0000000000000890.
31. Pingitore A, Lombardi M, Scattini B, De Marchi D, Aquaro GD, Positano V, Picano E. Head to head comparison between perfusion and function during accelerated high-dose dipyridamole magnetic resonance stress for the detection of coronary artery disease. Am J Cardiol. 2008;101:8–14. https://doi.org/10.1016/j.amjcard.2007.07.076.
32. Lee DC, Johnson NP. Quantification of absolute myocardial blood flow by magnetic resonance perfusion imaging. JACC Cardiovasc Imaging. 2009;2:761–70. https://doi.org/10.1016/j.jcmg.2009.04.003.
33. Schwitter J, Wacker CM, van Rossum AC, Lombardi M, Al-Saadi N, Ahlstrom H, Dill T, Larsson HBW, Flamm SD, Marquardt M, Johansson L. MR-IMPACT: comparison of perfusion-cardiac magnetic resonance with single-photon emission computed tomography for the detection of coronary artery disease in a multicentre, multivendor, randomized trial. Eur Heart J. 2008;29:480–9. https://doi.org/10.1093/eurheartj/ehm617.

34. Schwitter J, Wacker CM, Wilke N, Al-Saadi N, Sauer E, Huettle K, Schönberg SO, Luchner A, Strohm O, Ahlstrom H, Dill T, Hoebel N, Simor T. MR-IMPACT II: magnetic resonance imaging for myocardial perfusion assessment in coronary artery disease trial: perfusion-cardiac magnetic resonance vs. single-photon emission computed tomography for the detection of coronary artery disease: a comparative. Eur Heart J. 2013;34:775–81. https://doi.org/10.1093/eurheartj/ehs022.
35. Greenwood JP, Maredia N, Younger JF, Brown JM, Nixon J, Everett CC, Bijsterveld P, Ridgway JP, Radjenovic A, Dickinson CJ, Ball SG, Plein S. Cardiovascular magnetic resonance and single-photon emission computed tomography for diagnosis of coronary heart disease (CE-MARC): a prospective trial. Lancet (London, England). 2012;379:453–60. https://doi.org/10.1016/S0140-6736(11)61335-4.
36. Arai AE, Schulz-Menger J, Berman D, Mahrholdt H, Han Y, Bandettini WP, Gutberlet M, Abraham A, Woodard PK, Selvanayagam JB, McCann GP, Hamilton-Craig C, Schoepf UJ, Tan RS, Kramer CM, Friedrich M, Haverstock D, Liu Z, Brueggenwerth G, Bacher-Stier C, Santiuste M, Pennell DJ, Pennell D, Kramer U, von der Recke G, Nassenstein K, Tillmanns C, Taupitz M, Pache G, Mohrs O, Lotz J, Ko SM, Choo KS, Sung YM, Kang JW, Muzzarelli S, Valeti U, McCann G, Binukrishnam S, Croisille P, Jacquier A, Cowan B, Arai A, Shah D, Avery R, Schoepf J, Carr J, Kramer C, Flamm S, Harsinghani M, Lerakis S, Kim R, Raman S, Marcotte F, Islam A, Selvanayagam J, Chong WK, San Lynette Teo L. Gadobutrol-enhanced cardiac magnetic resonance imaging for detection of coronary artery disease. J Am Coll Cardiol. 2020;76:1536–47. https://doi.org/10.1016/J.JACC.2020.07.060.
37. Kwong RY, Ge Y, Steel K, Bingham S, Abdullah S, Fujikura K, Wang W, Pandya A, Chen Y-Y, Mikolich JR, Boland S, Arai AE, Bandettini WP, Shanbhag SM, Patel AR, Narang A, Farzaneh-Far A, Romer B, Heitner JF, Ho JY, Singh J, Shenoy C, Hughes A, Leung SW, Marji M, Gonzalez JA, Mehta S, Shah DJ, Debs D, Raman SV, Guha A, Ferrari VA, Schulz-Menger J, Hachamovitch R, Stuber M, Simonetti OP. Cardiac magnetic resonance stress perfusion imaging for evaluation of patients with chest pain. J Am Coll Cardiol. 2019;74:1741–55. https://doi.org/10.1016/j.jacc.2019.07.074.
38. Ge Y, Pandya A, Steel K, Bingham S, Jerosch-Herold M, Chen YY, Mikolich JR, Arai AE, Bandettini WP, Patel AR, Farzaneh-Far A, Heitner JF, Shenoy C, Leung SW, Gonzalez JA, Shah DJ, Raman SV, Ferrari VA, Schulz-Menger J, Hachamovitch R, Stuber M, Simonetti OP, Kwong RY. Cost-effectiveness analysis of stress cardiovascular magnetic resonance imaging for stable chest pain syndromes. JACC Cardiovasc Imaging. 2020;13:1505–17. https://doi.org/10.1016/J.JCMG.2020.02.029.
39. Pezel T, Garot P, Kinnel M, Hovasse T, Champagne S, Sanguineti F, Toupin S, Unterseeh T, Garot J. Long-term prognostic value of ischaemia and cardiovascular magnetic resonance-related revascularization for stable coronary disease, irrespective of patient's sex: a large retrospective study. Eur Hear J—Cardiovasc Imaging. 2021;22:1321–31. https://doi.org/10.1093/EHJCI/JEAB186.
40. Kinnel M, Sanguineti F, Pezel T, Unterseeh T, Hovasse T, Toupin S, Landon V, Champagne S, Morice MC, Garot P, Louvard Y, Garot J. Prognostic value of vasodilator stress perfusion CMR in patients with previous coronary artery bypass graft. Eur. Hear. J.—Cardiovasc. Imaging. 2021;22:1264–72. https://doi.org/10.1093/EHJCI/JEAA316.
41. Nagel E, Greenwood JP, McCann GP, Bettencourt N, Shah AM, Hussain ST, Perera D, Plein S, Bucciarelli-Ducci C, Paul M, Westwood MA, Marber M, Richter W-S, Puntmann VO, Schwenke C, Schulz-Menger J, Das R, Wong J, Hausenloy DJ, Steen H, Berry C. Magnetic resonance perfusion or fractional flow Reserve in Coronary Disease. N Engl J Med. 2019;380:2418–28. https://doi.org/10.1056/NEJMOA1716734.
42. Nagel E, Lehmkuhl HB, Bocksch W, Klein C, Vogel U, Frantz E, Ellmer A, Dreysse S, Fleck E. Noninvasive diagnosis of ischemia-induced wall motion abnormalities with the use of

high-dose dobutamine stress MRI: comparison with dobutamine stress echocardiography. Circulation.;199999:763–70. http://www.ncbi.nlm.nih.gov/pubmed/9989961. Accessed 22 Jan 2016.
43. Jahnke C, Nagel E, Gebker R, Kokocinski T, Kelle S, Manka R, Fleck E, Paetsch I. Prognostic value of cardiac magnetic resonance stress tests: adenosine stress perfusion and dobutamine stress wall motion imaging. Circulation. 2007;115:1769–76. https://doi.org/10.1161/CIRCULATIONAHA.106.652016.
44. Kunadian V, Chieffo A, Camici PG, Berry C, Escaned J, Maas AHEM, Prescott E, Karam N, Appelman Y, Fraccaro C, Buchanan GL, Manzo-Silberman S, Al-Lamee R, Regar E, Lansky A, Abbott JD, Badimon L, Duncker DJ, Mehran R, Capodanno D, Baumbach A. An EAPCI expert consensus document on ischaemia with non-obstructive coronary arteries in collaboration with European Society of Cardiology Working Group on Coronary Pathophysiology & Microcirculation Endorsed by coronary vasomotor disorders international study group. Eur Heart J. 2020;41:3504–20. https://doi.org/10.1093/EURHEARTJ/EHAA503.
45. Bernhardt P, Levenson B, Albrecht A, Engels T, Strohm O. Detection of cardiac small vessel disease by adenosine-stress magnetic resonance. Int J Cardiol. 2007;121:261–6. https://doi.org/10.1016/J.IJCARD.2006.11.008.
46. Panting JR, Gatehouse PD, Yang G-Z, Grothues F, Firmin DN, Collins P, Pennell DJ. Abnormal subendocardial perfusion in cardiac syndrome X detected by cardiovascular magnetic resonance imaging. N Engl J Med. 2002;346:1948–53. https://doi.org/10.1056/nejmoa012369.
47. Di Leo G, Fisci E, Secchi F, Alì M, Ambrogi F, Sconfienza LM, Sardanelli F. Diagnostic accuracy of magnetic resonance angiography for detection of coronary artery disease: a systematic review and meta-analysis. Eur Radiol. 2015; https://doi.org/10.1007/s00330-015-4134-0.
48. Duerinckx AJ, Bogaert J, Jiang H, Lewis BS. Anomalous origin of the left coronary artery: diagnosis by coronary MR angiography. 2013;164:1095–7. https://doi.org/10.2214/AJR.164.5.7717210.
49. Post JC, Van Possum AC, Hofman MBM, Valk J, Visser GA. Three-dimensional respiratory-gated MR angiography of coronary arteries: comparison with conventional coronary angiography. AJR Am J Roentgenol. 1996;166:1399–404. https://doi.org/10.2214/AJR.166.6.8633453.
50. Angelini P. Normal and anomalous coronary arteries: definitions and classification. Am Heart J. 1989;117:418–34. https://doi.org/10.1016/0002-8703(89)90789-8.
51. Gentile F, Castiglione V, De Caterina R. Coronary artery anomalies. Circulation. 2021;144:983–96. https://doi.org/10.1161/CIRCULATIONAHA.121.055347.
52. Cheezum MK, Liberthson RR, Shah NR, Villines TC, O'Gara PT, Landzberg MJ, Blankstein R. Anomalous aortic origin of a coronary artery from the inappropriate sinus of Valsalva. J Am Coll Cardiol. 2017;69:1592–608. https://doi.org/10.1016/J.JACC.2017.01.031.
53. Finocchiaro G, Behr ER, Tanzarella G, Papadakis M, Malhotra A, Dhutia H, Miles C, Diemberger I, Sharma S, Sheppard MN. Anomalous coronary artery origin and sudden cardiac death: clinical and pathological insights from a National Pathology Registry. JACC Clin Electrophysiol. 2019;5:516–22. https://doi.org/10.1016/J.JACEP.2018.11.015.
54. Bianco F, Colaneri M, Bucciarelli V, Surace FC, Iezzi FV, Primavera M, Biasi A, Giusti G, Berton E, Baldoni M, Renda G, Baldinelli A, Gallina S, Pozzi M. Echocardiographic screening for the anomalous aortic origin of coronary arteries. Open Hear. 2021;8:e001495. https://doi.org/10.1136/OPENHRT-2020-001495.
55. Angelini P. Imaging approaches for coronary artery anomalies: purpose and techniques. Curr Cardiol Reports. 2019;219(21):1–6. https://doi.org/10.1007/S11886-019-1188-7.
56. Angelini P, Uribe C, Monge J, Tobis JM, Elayda MA, Willerson JT. Origin of the right coronary artery from the opposite sinus of Valsalva in adults: characterization by intravascular ultrasonography at baseline and after stent angioplasty. Catheter Cardiovasc Interv. 2015;86:199–208. https://doi.org/10.1002/CCD.26069.

57. Angelini P, Muthupillai R, Cheong B, Paisley R. We have plenty of reasons to propose new, updated policies for preventing sudden cardiac death in young athletes. J Am Heart Assoc. 2020;9 https://doi.org/10.1161/JAHA.119.014368.
58. Barison A, Baritussio A, Cipriani A, De Lazzari M, Aquaro GD, Guaricci AI, Pica S, Pontone G, Todiere G, Indolfi C, Dellegrottaglie S. Cardiovascular magnetic resonance: what clinicians should know about safety and contraindications. Int J Cardiol. 2021;331:322–8. https://doi.org/10.1016/J.IJCARD.2021.02.003.
59. Woolen SA, Shankar PR, Gagnier JJ, MacEachern MP, Singer L, Davenport MS. Risk of nephrogenic systemic fibrosis in patients with stage 4 or 5 chronic kidney disease receiving a group II gadolinium-based contrast agent: a systematic review and meta-analysis. JAMA Intern Med. 2020;180:223–30. https://doi.org/10.1001/jamainternmed.2019.5284.
60. Friedrich MG, Karamitsos TD. Oxygenation-sensitive cardiovascular magnetic resonance. J Cardiovasc Magn Reson. 2013;15:43. https://doi.org/10.1186/1532-429X-15-43.
61. Aquaro GD, Frijia F, Positano V, Menichetti L, Santarelli MF, Ardenkjaer-Larsen JH, Wiesinger F, Lionetti V, Romano SL, Bianchi G, Neglia D, Giovannetti G, Schulte RF, Recchia FA, Landini L, Lombardi M. 3D CMR mapping of metabolism by hyperpolarized 13C-pyruvate in ischemia-reperfusion. JACC Cardiovasc Imaging. 2013;6:743–4. https://doi.org/10.1016/j.jcmg.2012.11.023.
62. Flögel U, Ding Z, Hardung H, Jander S, Reichmann G, Jacoby C, Schubert R, Schrader J. In vivo monitoring of inflammation after cardiac and cerebral ischemia by fluorine magnetic resonance imaging. Circulation. 2008;118:140–8. https://doi.org/10.1161/CIRCULATIONAHA.107.737890.
63. Giovannetti G, Flori A, Santarelli MF, Positano V, Martini N, Francischello R, Schulte RF, Ardenkjaer-Larsen JH, Menichetti L, Aquaro GD, Barison A, Frijia F. Radio frequency coils for hyperpolarized^{13} c magnetic resonance experiments with a 3t mr clinical scanner: experience from a cardiovascular lab. Electron. 2021;10 https://doi.org/10.3390/electronics10040366.
64. Meng Y, Mo Z, Hao J, Peng Y, Yan H, Mu J, Ma D, Zhang X, Li Y. High-resolution intravascular magnetic resonance imaging of the coronary artery wall at 3.0 tesla: toward evaluation of atherosclerotic plaque vulnerability. Quant Imaging Med Surg. 2021;11:4522–9. https://doi.org/10.21037/QIMS-21-286.

Diagnosis of Acute Myocardial Infarction

Annamaria Mazzone and Monica Baroni

...the scientist is not a person who gives the right answers,
...... he is the one who asks the right questions.

—*Claude Levi-Strauss*

1 Definitions of Acute Myocardial Infarction

The term acute myocardial infarction (MI) should be used in the presence of myocardial injury (at least one cardiac troponin (cTn) value above the 99th percentile upper reference limit) associated with acute myocardial ischemia [1, 2], while without myocardial ischemia, we refer to nonischemic myocardial injury.

For the goal of immediate myocardial reperfusion by primary PCI or if not available, by fibrinolytic therapy, it is a usual practice to designate patients with 1) typical (chest discomfort) or atypical symptoms, suggestive of ischemia, and 2) ST-segment elevation in at least two contiguous leads or new left bundle branch block as **ST-segment-elevation myocardial infarction (STEMI)**. Symptomatic patients without persistent ST-segment elevation are designated as **non-ST-segment elevation myocardial infarction (NSTEMI)**. They do not always need a prompt reperfusion, and treatment follows specific distinguished guidelines [3]. STEMI, NSTEMI, and unstable angina account for acute coronary syndromes (ACSs).

The **diagnosis** of MI is reserved to patients with myocardial injury due to myocardial ischemia, while in the absence of ischemia, we refer to nonischemic myocardial injury.

A. Mazzone (✉) · M. Baroni
Department of Cardiologist, Fondazione Monasterio- Ospedale del Cuore, Massa, Italy
e-mail: mazzone@ftgm.it; baroni@ftgm.it

G. Concistrè (ed.), *Ischemic Heart Disease*,
https://doi.org/10.1007/978-3-031-25879-4_16

Optimal evaluation and treatment strategies for these etiologically distinct diagnoses have yet to be defined. Myocardial infarction may be classified into various types, based on pathological, clinical, and prognostic differences, along with different treatment strategies as reported in the "Fourth Universal Definition of Myocardial Infarction," which provides a taxonomy for acute myocardial injury [2] including five subtypes of MI and nonischemic myocardial injury:

Type 1: Spontaneous MI caused by ischemia due to a primary coronary event (e.g., plaque rupture, erosion, or fissuring; coronary dissection)
Type 2: Ischemia due to increased oxygen demand (i.e., hypertension), or decreased supply (e.g., coronary artery spasm or embolism, arrhythmia, hypotension)
Type 3: Related to sudden unexpected cardiac death
Type 4a: Associated with percutaneous coronary intervention (signs and symptoms of myocardial infarction with cTn values >5 × 99th percentile URL)
Type 4b: Associated with documented stent thrombosis
Type 5: Associated with coronary artery bypass grafting (signs and symptoms of myocardial infarction with cTn values >10 × 99th percentile URL) [3, 4]

2 Diagnosis

STEMI diagnosis can be very easily based on a good clinical history, physical examination, and 12-lead ECG.

A quick diagnosis of STEMI facilitates rapid decision-making and treatment and therefore improves outcome in patients presenting with symptoms of chest pain [1]. Necrosis markers are a pivotal point in the diagnostic workup of chest pain, but routine sampling for serum markers should not delay diagnosis and therefore reperfusion treatment in STEMI. Biomarkers will subsequently be used for documentation and risk stratification. Guidelines recommend the measurement of **cardiac troponin levels** for NSTEMI diagnosis and risk stratification [1], guiding therefore therapeutic strategy.

3 Emergency Care: Strategy Room

3.1 Initial Diagnosis

First medical contact (FMC) is time 0 in the diagnosis and management of ACS. Countdown begins at FMC in order to maximize efficiency to obtain regional reperfusion (time delay ≤120' PCI or time delay ≥120' fibrinolysis) in case of STEMI. In the presence of typical chest pain and/or less typical symptoms, a rapid diagnostic workup for STEMI can be obtained by acquiring and interpreting a 12-lead ECG within the first 10 min from FMC. Prehospital ECG reduces time to diagnosis and treatment and can facilitate time to reperfusion.

3.2 Clinical Presentation

Symptoms consistent with acute myocardial ischemia (MI) include tight chest pain, upper extremity, mandibular, or epigastric often with radiation to the neck, lower jaw, or left arm. Sometimes sweating is present. Chest pain reduction after nitroglycerin administration can be misleading and is not recommended as a diagnostic tool [4], while a complete normalization of the ST-segment elevation after nitroglycerin administration, along with complete relief of symptoms, is suggestive of coronary spasm, with or without associated MI and an early coronary angiography (within 24 h).

Less typical symptoms such as shortness of breath, nausea/vomiting, fatigue, palpitations, or syncope can be present alone or in various combinations. Presence and duration of symptoms are not specific for myocardial ischemia, and MI may occur with atypical symptoms or even without symptoms at all. In a recent review of more than 4 million patients with MI, almost 33% did not report typical chest pain on presentation [1].

Atypical symptoms of myocardial ischemia are more common in diabetic patients, the elderly, and women [5, 6]. Prevalence of chest pain ranges significantly from 49% to 93% STEMI, 9% to 62% NSTEMI, 0% to 27% for nonischemic myocardial injury, and 13% for patients with multifactorial or indeterminate causes of elevated cTn [4].

Dyspnea is more prevalent in NSTEMI (12–46%) and nonischemic myocardial injury (33%) than in STEMI (4–10%) [4]. However, signs and symptoms can vary according to the kind of myocardial injury and none of them is diagnostic of acute ischemia, and therefore they cannot reliably differentiate types of myocardial injury/infarction.

Relief of pain, breathlessness, and anxiety: Relief of pain is of paramount importance, not only for comfort reasons but also because the pain is associated with sympathetic activation, which causes vasoconstriction and increases the workload of the heart. Titrated intravenous (i.v.) opioids (e.g., morphine) are the analgesics most commonly used in this context. Oxygen is indicated in hypoxic patients with arterial oxygen saturation (SaO2) <90%. Anxiety is a natural response to the pain and the circumstances surrounding an MI. A mild tranquillizer (benzodiazepine) should be considered in anxious patients [1].

3.3 12-Lead Electrocardiogram (ECG)

A 12-lead ECG should be obtained within the first (10) minutes from FMC. For the sake of immediate reperfusion treatment strategies, new ST-segment elevations in two contiguous leads or new bundle branch block with ischemic repolarization patterns define ST-segment-elevation MI (STEMI). In contrast, symptomatic patients without ST-segment elevation at presentation are usually designated non-ST-segment-elevation MI (NSTEMI). In cases of symptom relief after nitroglycerin administration, another 12-lead ECG should be obtained. A complete normalization of the ST-segment elevation after nitroglycerin administration, along with complete relief of symptoms, is suggestive of coronary spasm, with or without associated MI. In these cases, an early coronary angiography (within 24 h) is recommended. In cases of recurrent episodes of ST-segment elevation or chest pain, immediate angiography is required. All patients with suspected ACS should be provided with ECG monitoring, as soon as possible, in order to detect life-threatening arrhythmias and allow prompt defibrillation if indicated. Acute myocardial ischemia is often associated with dynamic changes in ECG waveform and serial ECG acquisition can provide critical information, particularly if the ECG at presentation is nondiagnostic.

Dynamic ST-segment changes are indicative of significant ongoing, acute myocardial ischemia and can identify patients who may benefit from urgent invasive evaluation. However, dynamic ST-segment changes are found in only a minority of patients with MI.

Other **ECG signs** associated with acute myocardial ischemia include cardiac arrhythmias and several degrees of conduction delays and blocks. The ECG itself is often insufficient to diagnose acute myocardial ischemia or infarction since ST deviation may be observed in other conditions such as acute pericarditis, LVH, and LBBB. A prior ECG is often helpful in distinguishing a new from a chronic finding, but it should never delay treatment decision in the clinical suspicion of MI.

When is STEMI suspected: A prolonged new convex ST-segment elevation at the J point in two contiguous leads, particularly when associated with reciprocal ST-segment depression, usually reflects a coronary occlusion which needs a prompt reperfusion. Reciprocal changes of repolarization can help to differentiate STEMI from pericarditis or early repolarization changes.

ECG must be acquired and interpreted as soon as possible at the time of FMC to facilitate early STEMI diagnosis and triage [1, 7], in order to achieve early reperfusion and therefore to save myocytes and ventricular function [8]. If the ECG is equivocal or does not show evidence to support the clinical suspicion of MI, ECG should be repeated and, when possible, compared with previous recordings. If interpretation of prehospital ECG is not possible on-site, field transmission of the ECG is recommended [8].

ECG diagnostic criteria for STEMI: ECG must be recorded with standard calibration of the ECG as 10 mm/mV. Therefore, 0.1 mV equals to 1 mm square on the vertical axis. In the clinical context of suspicious ACS, ST-segment elevation (measured at the J point) is considered suggestive of STEM and therefore ongoing coronary artery acute occlusion, in the following cases: (1) at least two contiguous leads with ST-segment elevation 1 mm in all leads other than V2–V3 where the following cut points apply: $\geq$2 mm in men $\geq$40 years, $\geq$2.5 mm in men <40 years, and ≥ -1.5 mm in women regardless of age, and (2) in patients with inferior MI, it is recommended to record right precordial leads (V3R and V4R) seeking ST-segment elevation, to identify concomitant right ventricular (RV) infarction [1]. Likewise, ST-segment depression in leads V1–V3 suggests myocardial ischemia, especially when the terminal T-wave is positive (ST-segment elevation equivalent), and confirmation by concomitant ST-segment elevation 0.5 mm recorded in leads V7–V9 should be considered as a means to identify posterior MI. The presence of a Q-wave on the ECG should not necessarily change the reperfusion strategy decision.

3.4 ECG Special Situations

Diagnosis of MI by means of ECG may be more difficult in some cases, which nevertheless deserve prompt management and triage.

1. In the presence of **left bundle branch block (LBBB)**, the ECG diagnosis of AMI is difficult but often possible if marked ST-segment abnormalities are present. Somewhat complex algorithms have been offered to assist the diagnosis, but they do not provide diagnostic certainty; the presence of concordant ST-segment elevation (i.e., in leads with positive QRS deflections) appears to be one of the best indicators of ongoing MI with an occluded infarct artery. Patients with a clinical suspicion of ongoing myocardial ischemia and LBBB should be managed in a way similar to STEMI patients: it is important to remark that the presence of a (presumed) new LBBB does not predict an MI per se [1, 9].
2. **Right bundle branch block (RBBB)** in the setting of MI means poor prognosis. It may be difficult to detect transmural ischemia in patients with chest pain and RBBB. Therefore, a primary PCI strategy (emergent coronary angiography and PCI if indicated) should be considered when persistent ischemic symptoms occur in the presence of RBBB.
3. **Ventricular pacing:** Pacemaker rhythm often prevents ST-T interpretation, and an urgent angiography may be needed to confirm diagnosis. Reprogramming the pacemaker—allowing an evaluation of ECG changes during intrinsic heart rhythm—may be considered in patients who are not dependent on ventricular pacing, without delaying invasive investigation [10].
4. **Atrial arrhythmias,** as well as new-onset atrial fibrillation, associated or not with chest pain, may be an ischemic equivalent sign of AMI.

4 Nondiagnostic ECG

Some patients with MI may have an initial ECG without ST-segment elevation. In the very early phase, hyper-acute T-waves preceding ST-segment elevation may be detected. It is important to repeat ECG or monitor for dynamic ST-segment changes, because in particular situations (i.e., acute occlusion of a vein graft, or left main disease), ST-segment elevation may be absent, delaying prompt reperfusion with subsequent larger infarct size and worse outcomes. Extending the standard 12-lead ECG with V7–V9 leads may help in MI identification. Any clinical presentation suspicious of ongoing myocardial ischemia is an indication for a primary PCI strategy even in patients without diagnostic ST-segment elevation [11].

- **Isolated posterior MI:** When ischemia affects inferior and basal portion of the heart, often corresponding to the left circumflex territory, isolated ST-segment depression of 0.5 mm in leads V1–V3 may represent the dominant finding. These patients should be managed as STEMI patients. The use of additional posterior chest wall leads [elevation V7–V9 0.5 mm (1 mm in men, 40 years old)] is recommended to detect ST-segment elevation consistent with inferior and basal MI [1].

- **Left main coronary obstruction:** The presence of ST depression (≥1 mm) on surface leads (inferior lateral ST depression), coupled with ST-segment elevation in aVR and/or V1, suggests multivessel ischemia or left main coronary artery obstruction, particularly if patients have signs or symptoms of cardiogenic shock [12]. Blood sampling for serum markers is routinely carried out in the acute phase but should never delay the reperfusion strategy/treatment. Emergency imaging aids the provision of timely reperfusion therapy to these patients.

5 Echocardiography in Emergency for Initial Diagnosis

Noninvasive imaging in management and risk stratification of LV dysfunction is a key prognostic factor. Therefore, it is recommended that the LVEF is determined before hospital discharge in all STEMI patients. **Emergency echocardiography** at presentation is indicated in patients with cardiac arrest, cardiogenic shock, hemodynamic instability, or suspected mechanical complications, and if the diagnosis of STEMI is uncertain. **Cardiac magnetic resonance (CMR)** may be a good alternative. If echocardiography is not available or if doubts persist after echo, a primary PCI strategy is indicated (including immediate transfer to a PCI center if the patient is being treated in a non-PCI center). In the STEMI emergency setting, the use of **cardiac tomography (CT)** should be confined to selected cases where acute aortic dissection or pulmonary embolism is suspected, but CT is not recommended if STEMI diagnosis is likely.

6 Cardiac Arrest

Many deaths occur very early after STEMI onset due to ventricular fibrillation (VF) [13]. As this arrhythmia frequently occurs at an early stage, these deaths usually happen out of hospital (out-of-hospital cardiac arrest: OHCA). This means that all personnel caring for patients with suspected MI should be trained in CPR and defibrillation and that ECG monitoring should be applied in all patients in the suspicion of MI. In OHCA survivors with ECG showing potential STEMI, primary PCI is the strategy of choice. Given the high prevalence of coronary occlusions and the potential difficulties in interpreting ECG in patients after cardiac arrest, urgent angiography (within 2 h) should be considered in survivors of cardiac arrest, including unresponsive survivors, when there is a high index of suspicion of ongoing MI. In patients without ST-segment elevation, a quick evaluation at the emergency department or intensive cardiac care unit to exclude noncoronary causes is reasonable. The decision to perform urgent coronary angiography and PCI if indicated should also consider factors associated with poor neurological outcome. Unfavorable pre-hospital settings indicating a remote likelihood for neurological recovery [i.e., unwitnessed cardiac arrest, late arrival of a prehospital team without any basic life support (>10 min), presence of an initial non-shockable rhythm, or more than 20 min of advanced life support without return to spontaneous circulation] should be taken strongly into consideration to argue against an invasive coronary strategy. Unconscious patients admitted to critical care units after OHCA are at high risk for death, and neurologic deficits are common among those who survive. Targeted temperature management (also called therapeutic hypothermia), aiming for a constant temperature between 32 and 36 °C for at least 24 h, is indicated in patients who remain unconscious after resuscitation from cardiac arrest (of presumed cardiac cause) [14].

7 Cardiogenic Shock

Cardiogenic shock (CS) is one of the possible clinical presentations of acute MI and accounts for 81% of patients in cardiogenic shock.

This challenging and severe clinical condition must be promptly recognized in association to MI, because it complicates 5–10% of cases of acute MI and is the leading cause of death after ACS. ST-segment-elevation myocardial infarction (STEMI) is associated with a twofold increased risk for development of CS compared with non-ST-segment-elevation myocardial infarction (NSTEMI), but patients with NSTEMI-associated CS are less likely to undergo early cardiac catheterization, delaying coronary reperfusion, which is an essential therapeutic intervention, therefore increasing the risk of mortality compared with patients with STEMI-associated CS. Key elements for optimal treatment are rapid diagnosis, including other shock etiologies, differential integration of hemodynamic and metabolic data for diagnosis and risk stratification, and early evaluation and appropriate initiation of acute mechanical circulatory support devices with an organized algorithmic approach to decision-making together with well-defined hub and spoke strategies.

8 Cardiac Biomarkers

8.1 Serial Troponin Values

Although significant differences in the distribution of baseline or peak cTn levels are evident in several studies, overlapping ranges limit the use of cTn levels to accurately differentiate between etiologies of myocardial injury.

Nestelberger et al. found a statistically significant difference in the median baseline and 1-h change between patients with type 2 MI with or without the presence of CAD, patients with type 1 MI, and those with nonischemic myocardial injury; significant overlap in the interquartile ranges for both measures was evident [15]. Furthermore, although peak cTn values were higher in type 1 versus type 2 MI [1], both the absolute cTn level and the change over time provided poor discrimination for type 1 from type 2 MI (area under the receiver-operator characteristic curve, 0.51–0.62) [16]. Serial cTn testing to determine whether there is a rise or fall in cTn concentrations is required to differentiate between acute and chronic cTn elevation: a nonischemic ECG and stable pattern of cTn elevation are most consistent with chronic myocardial injury [4]. Dynamic cTn elevation is consistent with acute myocardial injury. The UDMI suggests using a 20% change in cTn4 to differentiate a stable versus a dynamic cTn pattern, but also recognizes that the optimal change criteria require individualization based on the timing of presentation, absolute cTn concentration, results of prior testing if available, cTn assay characteristics, and pretest probability of an acute versus chronic insult [17]. A relative change of 20% in an individual with low cTn concentrations shows poor specificity and positive predictive value for acute MI versus a similar change at higher concentrations. Thus, some experts have proposed using a 50% change near the 99th percentile and a 20% change when the baseline value is more substantially elevated to define a significant cTn change [18]. Furthermore, it may be more efficacious to use absolute changes as opposed to relative changes in cTn to delineate acute from chronic myocardial injury, in particular, with high-sensitivity cTn assays and when absolute cTn values are low [19].

9 Invasive Imaging

Coronary angiography is considered the gold standard for defining coronary anatomy and is widely used to identify patients with evidence of plaque rupture and coronary thrombosis among patients with suspected **type 1 MI.**

Although the last **Universal Definition of Myocardial Infarction** acknowledges that coronary angiography may aid in the distinction between type 1 MI, type 2 MI, and acute nonischemic myocardial injury, it is emphasized that coronary angiography is not always clinically indicated or required [4]. Rigorous diagnostic studies for differentiating thrombus from stable fibrotic plaque are few and reveal low sensitivity for identifying coronary thrombosis. As such, there are limited quantitative data on the efficacy of coronary angiography for the differentiation of type 1 from type 2 MI. Specificity for identifying highly probable thrombotic lesions was 99–100% for spherical, ovoid, or irregular filling defects and intraluminal staining, but sensitivity was very low for all tested angiographic characteristics (17–60%) [20]. Using postmortem angiography, Levin and Fallon [21] showed that 79% of lesions with complex morphology were associated with plaque rupture, plaque hemorrhage, superimposed partially occluding thrombus, or recanalized thrombus. However, postmortem, angiography on a non-beating heart is of questionable relevance to clinical angiography. Advanced invasive coronary imaging techniques, such as intravascular ultrasound and **optical coherence topography (OCT)**, have also been used to define plaque disruption and intracoronary thrombus. Among patients with acute MI and a culprit lesion identified by conventional angiography, imaging consistent with plaque disruption was found in 73% by OCT, 47% by angioscopy, and 40% by intravascular ultrasound [22].

Therefore, plaque disruption alone does not provide unequivocal evidence of type 1 MI, and thrombus formation and resolution as a consequence of endogenous fibrinolysis may add to diagnostic uncertainty. Although OCT and angioscopy have moderate sensitivity and excellent specificity for the identification of plaque disruption and coronary thrombosis, the expense, invasiveness required, and high level of expertise needed to perform these techniques currently preclude routine use [4].

10 Noninvasive Imaging

Noninvasive imaging may be helpful for differentiating type 1 MI from other causes of myocardial injury by 1. directly assessing the coronary arterial anatomy for evidence of atherosclerotic disease and thrombus; 2. evaluating the presence and pattern of myocardial edema, inflammation, or scar; and 3. identifying noncoronary cardiac pathologies associated with myocardial injury.

10.1 Computed Tomography Coronary Angiography

Because of its superior spatial resolution over other modalities such as magnetic resonance imaging (MRI), coronary computed tomography angiography (CTA) currently is best suited to noninvasively assess the coronary anatomy. CTA can detect small atherosclerotic plaques, and its assessment of the coronary anatomy correlates well with intravascular ultrasound. However, thrombus is difficult to differentiate from noncalcified atherosclerotic plaque by CTA. Plaque ruptures may be seen by CTA; however, sensitivity is modest in comparison with intravascular ultrasound [23]. Because atherosclerotic disease is a requisite for type 1 MI, absence of coronary atherosclerotic disease by CTA largely excludes this possibility and suggests type 2 MI or nonischemic myocardial injury in the setting of cTn elevation. Spontaneous coronary dissection is an increasingly recognized entity that is suspected to be the cause of acute MI in more than one-third of women <50 years of age. CTA may be useful to identify patients with spontaneous coronary dissection and thus differentiate type 1 versus type 2 MI attributable to spontaneous coronary dissection [24].

11 Structural and Functional Imaging

Echocardiography is widely available and relatively inexpensive. It can detect abnormalities in myocardial thickening and motion within minutes of the onset of ischemia, and its sensitivity is limited in individuals with small myocardial insults [25]. Detection of specific patterns of myocardial contractile abnormalities (i.e., regional wall motion abnormalities in a coronary territory or characteristics of stress cardiomyopathy) may support specific types of myocardial injury. Furthermore, type 2 MI (i.e., attributable to dissection, spasm, embolization, or supply/demand mismatch in the setting of fixed obstructive CAD) may result in regional wall motion abnormalities similar to type 1 MI, limiting the use of echocardiography to differentiate between some type 2 MIs and type 1 MIs. Echocardiography may be useful for detecting noncoronary pathologies of myocardial injury, such as severe aortic stenosis or cardiomyopathy. Regional perfusion abnormalities, in particular, within specific vascular distributions, increase the probability of type 1 MI or no atherothrombotic coronary abnormalities (i.e., coronary dissection, supply/demand mismatch in the setting of fixed obstructive CAD) resulting in type 2 MI, whereas diffuse myocardial perfusion abnormalities or normal perfusion may suggest more systemic insults from ischemic or nonischemic myocardial injury [4]. Myocardial perfusion imaging may be performed with **contrast echocardiography**, single photon emission computerized tomography, positron-emission tomography, computed tomography, or MRI.

Cardiac magnetic resonance (CMR) is a noninvasive imaging modality for assessing myocardial dysfunction and, in conjunction with delayed contrast enhancement, can differentiate between acute and chronic myocardial injury via the presence of tissue edema [26]. Ischemia-induced myocardial injury typically extends from the subendocardium to the epicardium, whereas nonischemic myocardial injury can be seen at the epicardium, mid-wall, or insertion points of the right ventricle. CMR is not well suited to assess the coronary arterial anatomy because of its limited spatial resolution with standard protocols. CMR is useful to identify condition associated with myocardial injury not related to MI. Among patients presenting with suspected acute MI in whom obstructive CAD was excluded, MRI found evidence of acute myocarditis with high accuracy. Cardiomyopathies and stress cardiomyopathy are well characterized by MRI [27].

11.1 Diagnostic Doubts

Clear diagnosis among type 1 MI, type 2 MI, or myocardial injury is not always easy. In the presence of signs and symptoms consistent with ischemia (e.g., typical chest pain) first diagnosis should be type 1 MI in order not to delay prompt reperfusion.

When subsequent evaluation fails to confirm coronary atherothrombosis, further consideration of alternative causes of acute ischemic (MINOCA; takotsubo syndrome (TTS)) or nonischemic myocardial injury (e.g., myocarditis, pulmonary embolism) is necessary.

Many patients with signs and symptoms of ACS present tachycardia, hypertension, and anemia, which lead to overdiagnosis or underdiagnosis of type 1 MI and therefore delay or withholding of appropriate treatments.

In the absence of clear evidence of ischemia and supply/demand mismatch, diagnosis of acute nonischemic myocardial injury should be the first diagnostic hypothesis.

11.2 Risk Assessment

Shortly after AMI diagnosis, all AMI patients should have an early assessment of evaluation of the extent of myocardial damage, evidence of successful reperfusion, and risk of further events.

Risk assessment should include several risk scores that have been developed. The Global Registry of Acute Coronary Events (GRACE) risk score [3] is recommended for risk assessment and adjustment. Besides information on CAD severity, quality of reperfusion, residual ischemia, occurrence of complications during hospitalization, and LV function (LVEF) should be carefully assessed before discharge because of its strong potential for risk stratification. Routine echocardiography after primary PCI is recommended to assess resting LV function as well as RV and valve function, to exclude postinfarction mechanical complications and LV thrombi. Left ventriculography should be considered during catheterization if echocardiography has not been performed yet. In limited cases in which echocardiography may be suboptimal or inconclusive, CMR can be a good alternative. In patients with multivessel disease, in which only the IRA lesion has been treated, assessment for residual ischemia is important for risk stratification. Timing and best imaging technique (echocardiography, SPECT, CMR, PET) to detect residual ischemia and myocardial viability have to be determined, and it also depends on local expertise and available.

12 Special New Conditions

12.1 Acute Myocardial Infarction in COVID-19 Pandemic Outbreak

COVID-19 has comparable cardiac manifestations to previous outbreaks of other coronaviruses, which are associated with worse outcomes of COVID-19. CVD comorbidity in COVID-19 may be either primary or secondary due to acute lung injury, leading to increased cardiac workload. Myocardial injury is often present during COVID-19 infection, especially if preexisting CVD risk factors are present [28, 29]. The potential mechanism underlying myocardial injury could be related to a type 1 and/or type 2 MI occurrence. Myocardial injury complicating COVID-19 infection is very often due to a mismatch between oxygen supply and oxygen needs due to hypoxia, tachycardia, and septic state (type 2 MI). In some cases, a typical type 1 MI may be linked to plaque disruption, epicardial coronary arteries, or microvessel thrombosis and occlusion. COVID-19-related abnormal platelet function and/or endothelial function have been postulated as the cause of increased thrombotic burden [30].

13 STEMI (STE-ACS)

The COVID-19 pandemic should not compromise timely reperfusion of ST-segment-elevation STEMI [31, 32]. Current guidelines recommend reperfusion therapy in patients with symptoms of ischemia of <12-h duration and persistent ST-segment elevation in at least two contiguous ECG leads [33].

In the absence of previous SARS-CoV-2 testing, all STEMI patients should be managed as they are COVID-19 positive. STEMI management in COVID-19 outbreak maximum delay between FMC/STEMI diagnosis and reperfusion should be <120 min (door-to-balloon time). Primary PCI within 120 min is treatment of choice in order to obtain adequate reperfusion safely also from the point of view of infection prevention.

Primary PCI pathways may be delayed due to implementation of protective measures.

STEMI patients should be considered potentially infected as long as SARS-CoV-2 test results are available and should undergo, as soon as possible, testing for SARS-CoV-2 following FMC, irrespective of reperfusion strategy, taking all precautionary measures. If optimal door-to-balloon time cannot be guaranteed and it is not contraindicated, fibrinolysis can be performed as an alternative to primary PCI [1].

In the presence of multiple-vessel disease, complete revascularization can be considered, if indicated, to avoid staged procedures and reduce hospital stay.

14 NSTEMI (NSTE-ACS)

In patients with NSTEMI-ACS, a careful risk stratification and proper management should be obtained, together with testing for SARS-CoV-2 as soon as possible [34]. In high-risk patients, the aim is clinical stabilization and early (<24 h) reperfusion. Time to invasive strategy may be longer than 24 h, according to testing results.

Patients at intermediate risk should be carefully evaluated considering alternative diagnoses, such a type 2 MI, myocarditis, myocardial injury due to respiratory distress, or takotsubo. In the event of any of plausible differential diagnosis, a noninvasive strategy should be considered and coronary computed tomography angiography (CCTA) should be favored. Patients with troponin rise and no acute clinical signs of instability (ECG changes, recurrence of chest pain) might be managed with a primarily conservative approach, speeding up risk stratification using CCTA if available [35–38].

14.1 Clinical Manifestations and Initial Diagnosis

- Profound hypoxemia, always present in moderate-to-severe COVID-19, together with tachycardia may result in chest pain, dyspnea, and electrocardiographic changes suggestive of myocardial ischemia. Chest pain or tightness is common in patients with active COVID-19. Chest pain on admission can be misdiagnosed due to the coexistence of other severe symptoms (i.e., acute dyspnea), making differential diagnosis more difficult. Real prevalence and characteristics of chest pain among COVID-19 patients are unknown. Biomarker elevation in conjunction with ECG changes suggests MI. The same ECG diagnostic criteria for ACS apply in patients with COVID-19. During COVID-19 outbreak, diagnostic workup of patients admitted to emergency department (ED) for dyspnea may often include computed tomography (CT) scan and therefore diagnosis of acute myocardial infarction may be occasional. As for patients with ACS with no COVID-19, echocardiography should not be performed routinely to rule out STEMI, in order not to delay time to reperfusion. Echocardiography can be used lately to stratify prognosis and confirm the efficacy of reperfusion as well as presence of possible mechanical complications. Left ventriculography can be performed if echocardiography was not yet performed.

Sometimes, initial presentation of MI in COVID-19 patients can be a clinical picture of acute heart failure, cardiogenic shock (CS), or out-of-hospital cardiac arrest (OHCA). Incidence of OHCA increased during first months of pandemic with an important reduction of people admitted alive at ED. In the first phase of outbreak, physicians reported a significant reduction of ACS patients' admission to ED due to fear of exposure to patients with COVID-19. These patients suffered unnecessary morbidity and mortality without proper ACS diagnosis and management.

15 Myocardial Infarction with Nonobstructive Coronary Arteries (MINOCA)

Myocardial infarction (MI) in the absence of obstructive coronary artery disease (MINOCA) can be found in 5–6% of MI, accounting for 5–25% of patients in large registries [3]. All traditional CV risk factors are less frequent in MINOCA with patients being younger and frequently female.

MINOCA is a heterogeneous entity comprising multiple causes and represents a conundrum for clinicians. The underlying pathogenesis ranges from functional alterations of epicardial coronary arteries (atherosclerosis, coronary thromboembolism, vasospasm, spontaneous dissection) to microvascular dysfunction, which accounts for about 70% of coronary resistance in the absence of obstructive CAD [3]. MINOCA patients suffer from a not benign condition despite not having epicardial coronary artery stenosis and are at higher risk of mortality, rehospitalization, disability, and angina burden at follow-up as compared to the general population without cardiovascular disease.

16 MINOCA Diagnostic Workup

MINOCA is a type 2 AMI that is myocardial cell necrosis due to supply/demand mismatch, with elevated cardiac biomarkers in addition to at least one of the other criteria for AMI in the presence of potential cardiac ischemic causes.

Noncardiac causes for troponin rise should be ruled out as sepsis, pulmonary embolism, cardiac contusion, and aortic dissection. Myocardial disorders, including myocarditis, takotsubo cardiomyopathy (TTS), and other cardiomyopathies, are excluded from MINOCA definition [39].

A systematic global approach is needed, including invasive and noninvasive techniques, in order to tailor the perfect management to the specific pathophysiological mechanism. Assessment of the clinical contest is the first step evaluation when MINOCA is suspected.

A suspicion of myocardial injury due to pulmonary embolism needs D-dimer testing, N-type natriuretic peptide (BNP), and or/or CT pulmonary angiography. Other causes of supply/demand mismatch of myocardial injury may be hypertensive crisis, sepsis, tachyarrhythmias, severe anemia, as well as noncardiac causes for troponin elevation. A history of atrial fibrillation, dilated cardiomyopathy, prothrombotic risk factors, recent deep vein thrombosis or pulmonary embolism, prosthetic heart valves, infective endocarditis, atrial myxoma, and patent foramen oval may suggest for a coronary embolism as the cause of MINOCA.

Coronary Angiography: Working diagnosis should exclude a significant coronary obstruction as well as small-vessel occlusions due to plaque rupture or distal embolization.

Echocardiography: Regional wall motion abnormalities corresponding to a clear coronary flow distribution suggest an ischemic mechanism of MINOCA.

Cardiac Magnetic Resonance: This can be helpful to elucidate underlying causes leading to MINOCA, being a powerful tool in differentiating other causes of myocardial injury. Transient wall motion abnormalities, typical myocardial edema, and absence of late gadolinium enhancement (LGE) indicate TTS, while nonischemic LGE together with myocardial edema suggests myocarditis.

Intravascular Imaging: Both IVUS and OCT may be helpful for identifying MINOCA mechanisms such as plaque disruption or coronary dissection, even if their diagnostic value depends strongly on time from FMC. Intracoronary acetylcholine or ergonovine testing may be associated when microvascular spasm is suspected.

References

1. Ibanez B, James S, Agewall S, Antunes MJ, Bucciarelli-Ducci C, Bueno H, ALP C, Crea F, Goudevenos JA, Halvorsen S, Hindricks G, Kastrati A, Lenzen MJ, Prescott E, Roffi M, Valgimigli M, Varenhorst C, Vranckx P, Widimský P. ESC Guidelines for the management of acute myocardial infarction in patients presenting with ST-segment elevation: The Task Force for the management of acute myocardial infarction in patients presenting with ST-T elevation of the European Society of Cardiology (ESC). Eur Heart J. 2018 Jan 7. 2017;39(2):119–77.
2. Thygesen K, Alpert JS, Jaffe AS, Chaitman BR, Bax JJ, Morrow DA, White HD, Executive Group on behalf of the Joint European Society of Cardiology (ESC)/American College of Cardiology (ACC)/American Heart Association (AHA)/World Heart Federation (WHF) Fourth Universal Definition of Myocardial Infarction. Task Force for the Universal Definition of Myocardial Infarction. J Am Coll Cardiol. 2018;72(18):2231–64.

3. Collet JP, Thiele H, Barbato E, Barthélémy O, Bauersachs J, Bhatt DL, Dendale P, Dorobantu M, Edvardsen T, Folliguet T, et al. ESC Guidelines for the management of acute coronary syndromes in patients presenting without persistent ST-segment elevation: The Task Force for the management of acute coronary syndromes in patients presenting without persistent ST-segment elevation of the European Society of Cardiology (ESC). European Heart Journal. 2020;42(14):1289–367.
4. De Filippis AP, Chapman AR, Mills NL, de Lemos JA, Arbab-Zadeh A, Newby LK, Morrow DA. Assessment and Treatment of Patients with Type 2 Myocardial Infarction and Acute non-Ischemic Myocardial Injury. Circulation. 2012;140(20):1661–78.
5. Canto JG, Shlipak MG, Rogers WJ, Malmgren JA, Frederick PD, Lambrew CT, Ornato JP, Barron HV, Kiefe CI. Prevalence, clinical characteristics, and mortality among patients with myocardial infarction presenting without chest pain. JAMA. 2000;283:3223–9.
6. Culić V, Eterović D, Mirić D, Silić N. Symptom presentation of acute myocardial infarction: influence of sex, age, and risk factors. Am Heart J. 2002;144:1012–7.
7. Tubaro M, Danchin N, Goldstein P, Filippatos G, Hasin Y, Heras M, Jansky P, Norekval TM, Swahn E, Thygesen K, Vrints C, Zahger D, Arntz HR, Bellou A, De La Coussaye JE, De Luca L, Huber K, Lambert Y, Lettino M, Lindahl B, McLean S, Nibbe L, Peacock WF, Price S, Quinn T, Spaulding C, Tatu-Chitoiu G, Van De Werf F. Pre-hospital treatment of STEMI patients. A scientific statement of the Working Group Acute Cardiac Care of the European Society of Cardiology. Acute Card Care. 2011;13(2):56–67.
8. Chan AW, Kornder J, Elliott H, Brown RI, Dorval JF, Charania J, Zhang R, Ding L, Lalani A, Kuritzky RA, Simkus GJ. Improved survival associated with pre-hospital triage strategy in a large regional ST-segment elevation myocardial infarction program. JACC Cardiovasc Interv. 2012;5(12):1239–46.
9. Dhruva VN, Abdelhadi SI, Anis A, Gluckman W, Hom D, Dougan W, Kaluski E, Haider B, Klapholz M. ST-Segment Analysis Using Wireless Technology in Acute Myocardial Infarction (STAT-MI) trial. J Am Coll Cardiol. 2007;50(6):509–13.
10. Lopes RD, Siha H, Fu Y, Mehta RH, Patel MR, Armstrong PW, Granger CB. Diagnosing acute myocardial infarction in patients with left bundle branch block. Am J Cardiol. 2011;108(6):782–8.
11. Madias JE. The non-specificity of ST-segment elevation > or = 5.0mm in V1-V3 in the diagnosis of acute myocardial infarction in the presence of ventricular paced rhythm. J Electrocardiol. 2004;37(2):135–9.
12. From AM, Best PJ, Lennon RJ, Rihal CS, Prasad A. Acute myocardial infarction due to left circumflex artery occlusion and significance of ST-segment elevation. Am J Cardiol. 2010;106(8):1081–5.
13. Yan AT, Yan RT, Kennelly BM, Anderson FA Jr, Budaj A, Lopez-Sendon J, Brieger D, Allegrone J, Steg G, Goodman SG. Relationship of ST elevation in lead aVR with angiographic findings and outcome in non-ST elevation acute coronary syndromes. Am Heart J. 2007;154(1):71–8.
14. Larsen JM, Ravkilde J. Acute coronary angiography in patients resuscitated from out-of-hospital cardiac arrest: a systematic review and meta-analysis. Resuscitation. 2012;83(12):1427–33.
15. Nikolaou NI, Welsford M, Beygui F, Bossaert L, Ghaemmaghami C, Nonogi H, O'Connor RE, Pichel DR, Scott T, Walters DL, Woolfrey KG. Part 5: Acute coronary syndromes: 2015 International Consensus on Cardiopulmonary Resuscitation and Emergency Cardiovascular Care Science with Treatment Recommendations. Resuscitation. 2015;95:e121–46.
16. Nestelberger T, Boeddinghaus J, Badertscher P, Twerenbold R, Wildi K, Breitenbücher D, Sabti Z, Puelacher C, Rubini Giménez M, Kozhuharov N, et al. APACE Investigators. Effect of definition on incidence and prognosis of type 2 myocardial infarction. J Am Coll Cardiol. 2017;70:1558–68.
17. Sandoval Y, Thordsen SE, Smith SW, Schulz KM, Murakami MM, Pearce LA, Apple FS. Cardiac troponin changes to distinguish type 1 and type 2 myocardial infarction and 180-day mortality risk. Eur Heart J Acute Cardiovasc Care. 2014;3:317–25.

18. Apple FS, Sandoval Y, Jaffe AS, Ordonez-Llanos J, IFCC Task Force on Clinical Applications of Cardiac Bio-Markers. Cardiac troponin assays: guide to understanding analytical characteristics and their impact on clinical care. Clin Chem. 2017;63:73–81.
19. Thygesen K, Mair J, Giannitsis E, Mueller C, Lindahl B, Blankenberg S, Huber K, Plebani M, Biasucci LM, Tubaro M, et al. Study Group on Bio-markers in Cardiology of ESC Working Group on Acute Cardiac Care. How to use high-sensitivity cardiac troponins in acute cardiac care. Eur Heart J. 2012;33:2252–7.
20. Reichlin T, Irfan A, Twerenbold R, Reiter M, Hochholzer W, Burkhalter H, Bassetti S, Steuer S, Winkler K, Peter F, et al. Utility of absolute and relative changes in cardiac troponin concentrations in the early diagnosis of acute myocardial infarction. Circulation. 2011;124:136–45.
21. Amraotkar AR, Ghafghazi S, Trainor PJ, Hargis CW, Irfan AB, Rai SN, Bhatnagar A, DeFilippis AP. Presence of multiple coronary angiographic characteristics for the diagnosis of acute coronary thrombus. Cardiol J. 2017;24:25–34.
22. Levin DC, Fallon JT. Significance of the angiographic morphology of localized coronary stenoses: histopathologic correlations. Circulation. 1982;66:316–20.
23. Kubo T, Imanishi T, Takarada S, Kuroi A, Ueno S, Yamano T, Tanimoto T, Matsuo Y, Masho T, Kitabata H, et al. Assessment of culprit lesion morphology in acute myocardial infarction: ability of optical coherence tomography compared with intravascular ultrasound and coronary angioscopy. J Am Coll Cardiol. 2007;
24. Obaid DR, Calvert PA, Brown A, Gopalan D, West NEJ, Rudd JHF, Bennett MR. Coronary CT angiography features of ruptured and high-risk atherosclerotic plaques: correlation with intravascular ultrasound. J Cardiovasc Comput Tomogr. 2017;11:455–61.
25. Tweet MS, Gulati R, Williamson EE, Vrtiska TJ, Hayes SN. Multimodality imaging for spontaneous coronary artery dissection in women. JACC Cardiovasc Imaging. 2016;9:436–50.
26. Neglia D, Rovai D, Caselli C, Pietila M, Teresinska A, Aguade-Bruix S, Pizzi MN, Todiere G, Gimelli A, Schroeder S, et al. Detection of significant coronary artery disease by noninvasive anatomical and functional imaging. Circ Cardiovasc Imaging. 2015;8:e002179.
27. Rajiah P, Desai MY, Kwon D, Flamm SD. MR imaging of myocardial infarction. Radiographics. 2013;33:1383–412.
28. Ferreira VM, Schulz-Menger J, Holmvang G, Kramer CM, Carbone I, Sechtem U, Kindermann I, Gutberlet M, Cooper LT, Liu P, et al. Cardiovascular magnetic resonance in nonischemic myocardial inflammation: expert recommendations. J Am Coll Cardiol. 2018;72:3158–76.
29. Pareek M, Singh A, Vadlamani L, et al. Relation of cardiovascular risk factors to mortality and cardiovascular events in hospitalized patients with coronavirus disease 2019 (from the Yale COVID-19 Cardiovascular Registry). Am J Cardiol. 2021;146:99–106.
30. Bavishi C, Bonow RO, Trivedi V, Abbott JD, Messerli FH, Bhatt DL. Special article-Acute myocardial injury in patients hospitalized with COVID-19 infection: a review. Prog Cardiovasc Dis. 2020;63:682–9.
31. Choudry FA, Hamshere SM, Rathod KS, et al. High thrombus burden in patients with COVID-19 presenting with ST-segment elevation myocardial infarction. JAm Coll Cardiol. 2020;76:1168–76.
32. De Rosa S, Spaccarotella C, Basso C, et al. Societa` Italiana di Cardiologia and the CCU Academy investigators group. Reduction of hospitalizations for myocardial infarction in Italy in the COVID-19 era. Eur Heart J. 2020;41:2083–8.
33. Rodriguez-Leor O, Cid Alvarez AB, de Prado AP, et al. In-hospital outcomes of patients with ST-segment elevation myocardial infarction and COVID-19. EuroIntervention. 2021;16:1426–33.
34. Ibanez B, James S, Agewall S, et al. ESC Scientific Document Group. 2017 ESC Guidelines for the management of acute myocardial infarction in patients presenting with ST-segment elevation: the Task Force for the management of acute myocardial infarction in patients pre-

senting with ST-segment elevation of the European Society of Cardiology (ESC). Eur Heart J. 2018;39:119–77.
35. Roffi M, Patrono C, Collet JP, et al. ESC Scientific Document Group. 2015 ESC Guidelines for the management of acute coronary syndromes in patients presenting without persistent ST-segment elevation: Task Force for the Management of Acute Coronary Syndromes in Patients Presenting without Persistent ST-Segment Elevation of the European Society of Cardiology (ESC). Eur Heart J. 2016;37:267–315.
36. Imazio M, Klingel K, Kindermann I, et al. COVID-19 pandemic and troponin: indirect myocardial injury, myocardial inflammation or myocarditis? Heart. 2020;106:1127–31.
37. Stefanini GG, Chiarito M, Ferrante G, et al. Humanitas COVID-19 Task Force. Early detection of elevated cardiac biomarkers to optimise risk stratification in patients with COVID-19. Heart. 2020;106:1512–8.
38. Pontone G, Baggiano A, Conte E, et al. "Quadruple rule-out" with computed tomography in a COVID-19 patient with equivocal acute coronary syndrome presentation. JACC Cardiovasc Imaging. 2020;13:1854–6.
39. Mele M, Casavecchia G, Ieva R, Brunetti ND. Diagnosis of acute myocardial infarction in the time of the COVID-19 pandemic. Eur Heart J. 2021;42(3):286.

Indications for Myocardial Revascularization

Francesca Chiaramonti

Abbreviations

BMS	Bare-metal stents
CABG	Coronary artery bypass grafting
CAD	Coronary artery disease
DES	Drug-eluting stents
LAD	Left anterior descending
LM	Left main
MACE	Major adverse cardiovascular event
NSTE-ACS	Non-ST-segment-elevation-acute coronary syndrome
PCI	Percutaneous coronary intervention
RCTs	Randomized clinical trials
STEMI	ST-segment-elevation myocardial infarction
SYNTAX	Synergy between PCI with Taxus and Cardiac Surgery

1 Introduction

In 1964, the first coronary artery bypass graft (CABG) procedure was performed [1], while the first percutaneous coronary revascularization procedure was performed only 13 years thereafter, in 1977 [2]. Since their first introduction, surgical revascularization techniques gained expertise and clinical relevance worldwide, becoming one of the most com-

F. Chiaramonti (✉)
Adult Cardiac Surgery Unit, Ospedale del Cuore "G. Pasquinucci", Fondazione Toscana G. Monasterio, Massa, Italy
e-mail: chiaramonti@ftgm.it

G. Concistrè (ed.), *Ischemic Heart Disease*,
https://doi.org/10.1007/978-3-031-25879-4_17

monly performed interventions in modern medicine. Sigwart et al. [3] introduced the first bare-metal stent (BMS) in 1986. In 2002, the first DES came to the markets in Europe [4] starting a new era in PCR. While both interventions have witnessed significant technological advances, their role in the treatment of patients presenting with stable CAD is being challenged by advances in medical treatment, referred to as optimal medical therapy (OMT), which include intensive lifestyle and pharmacological management. Furthermore, the differences between the two revascularization strategies should be recognized.

Since its introduction, PCI has been subjected to more randomized clinical trials (RCTs) than any other interventional procedure. Several trials have been made in order to compare treatments available and to choose the best revascularization modality for each single patient. The best known and probably the most important of these studies is the Synergy between PCI with Taxus and Cardiac Surgery (SYNTAX) trial. This was a non-inferiority trial that compared percutaneous coronary intervention (PCI) using first-generation paclitaxel-eluting stents with coronary artery bypass grafting (CABG) in patients with de novo three-vessel and left main coronary artery disease. Further information has been gained from its extension on 10-year follow-up. A great number of clinical practice guidelines have been issued in recent years both by the ESC and by other societies and organizations. Because of the impact on clinical practice, quality criteria for the development of guidelines have been established in order to make all decisions transparent to the user. Guidelines summarize and evaluate all available evidence, at the time of the writing process, on a particular issue with the aim of assisting health professionals in selecting the best management strategies for an individual patient with a given condition, taking into account the impact on outcome, as well as the risk–benefit ratio of particular diagnostic or therapeutic means. Latest ESC/EACTS Guidelines on myocardial revascularization [5] date back to 2018, while latest ACC/AHA Clinical Practice Guidelines were published in January 2022.

2 European Guidelines

At the European Society for Cardiology annual meeting in Stockholm on August 2010, the new joint European Society of Cardiology (ESC) and European Association for Cardio-Thoracic Surgery (EACTS) guidelines on myocardial revascularization were presented [6]. This is a completely new set of guidelines in which was recognized the need for cooperation between cardiologists and cardiac surgeons on the management of the entire spectrum of coronary artery disease.

These guidelines consisted of 14 sections dealing with all aspects of coronary artery disease starting from diagnosis, through treatment with lifestyle changes and medication and intervention by stents or surgery where appropriate, to secondary prevention. There were details of and recommendations for risk stratification, diagnosis, and imaging, and revascularization strategies in stable and unstable disease as well as in the setting of ST-segment-elevation myocardial infarction (STEMI). Specific chapters described the implications of coronary artery disease in the settings of diabetes, chronic renal disease, valvular heart disease, and chronic heart failure.

Evidences on which these guidelines are based showed how CABG still offers a survival benefit in the most severe and complex coronary artery disease; CABG and stents appear to offer similar survival outcome, at least over the short to medium term, in patients with lower tertile SYNTAX score severity coronary artery disease. It has been supposed that differences in cardiac outcome can be attributed in part to the different pathophysiological consequences of the two interventions, while in CABG, bypass grafts are placed to the mid-coronary vessel beyond the "culprit" lesion(s), providing extra sources of nutrient blood flow to the myocardium and offering protection against the consequences of further proximal obstructive disease. In PCI, coronary stents aim to restore the normal conductance of the native coronary vasculature without offering protection against new disease proximal to the stent [7].

The 2014 ESC/EACTS guidelines update and extend the effort started in 2010. Importantly, this latest edition provided a systematic review of all randomized clinical trials performed since 1980, comparing different strategies of myocardial revascularization, including CABG, balloon angioplasty, PCI with bare-metal stents (BMS), and first- and second-generation drug-eluting stents (DES), and retrieved 100 RCTs involving 93,553 patients with 262,090 patient-years of follow-up.

These guidelines further extended the importance of the heart team discussion, introduced in the 2010 edition, by inciting the development of shared institutional protocols, in order to better select the patients that deserve a multidisciplinary evaluation, saving time, resources, and delays of urgent procedures, especially in centers without on-site surgery. In the same setting, the 2014 ESC/EACTS revascularization guidelines deepened the risk score section. The Society of Thoracic Surgeons (STS) score has been recognized as the appropriate recommended tool to stratify surgical risk during CABG, whereas the role of the EuroSCORE has been reconsidered and its use is no longer indicated, based on the concern that it overestimates the surgical risk. However, the newly introduced EuroSCORE II overcomes this limitation, and its use should be preferred over the first iteration of this surgical risk score. The Synergy Between Percutaneous Coronary Intervention with Taxus and Cardiac Surgery (SYNTAX) score, introduced in the previous edition, was now recommended for the risk stratification of patients who undergo revascularization (CABG vs. PCI).

Another difference from the previous guidelines consisted of the indication on myocardial revascularization modality in patients with left main coronary artery stenosis (LMD). The results borrowed from the SYNTAX trial that evaluated a subgroup of patients with predominant distal left main disease showed that CABG and PCI had a comparable rate of the primary endpoint (a composite of death, myocardial infarction, stroke, and repeat revascularization) in the low and intermediate SYNTAX tertile (SYNTAX score ≤22 and SYNTAX score 23–32). In contrast, it observed a numerical increase of deaths and a significant increase of repeat revascularizations in the PCI group with the highest SYNTAX tertile (SYNTAX >32). Based on these data, the indication for PCI of LMD with low anatomical complexity (SYNTAX score ≤22) has been upgraded and now equated to CABG, whereas in anatomies with intermediate (SYNTAX score 23–32) complexity, PCI should be considered, but CABG remains the preferred revascularization modality. Similar to the 2010 edition, these guidelines reiterated the contraindication to the elective treatment of LMS with PCI, in case of high anatomical complexity (SYNTAX >32) in patients who have an acceptable surgical risk. Firstly, the indications for revascularization were simplified in patients with stable angina or silent ischemia.

An upgrade was performed also on the indications of revascularization of the proximal left anterior descending artery (LAD), where accordingly with the results of studies comparing PCI with DES and CABG in patients with isolated proximal LAD disease and two-vessel disease including proximal LAD, which demonstrated similar outcomes, PCI was equally recommended as CABG for the treatment of proximal LAD alone as well as in the context of a two-vessel disease.

Based on the results of 5-year follow-up of SYNTAX trial, at variance with previous guidelines, PCI was now equally recommended as CABG for the treatment of three-vessel disease with a low anatomical complexity (SYNTAX score ≤22).

Based on the results of FREEDOM trial [8], CABG was strongly recommended, with preference toward off-pump CABG over the on-pump approach, if possible, over PCI for patients with diabetes and multivessel disease, when surgical risk is acceptable. In cases where a percutaneous treatment is indicated, new-generation DES must be preferred over bare-metal stents.

In 2018, the latest ESC/EACTS Guidelines on myocardial revascularization were published. These Guidelines represent the third revision of preexisting guidelines made by the Task Force on myocardial revascularization of the European Society of Cardiology (ESC) and the European Association for Cardio-Thoracic Surgery (EACTS).

There is considerable overlap of this current document with other guidelines, specifically those on stable coronary artery disease, non-ST-elevation myocardial infarction, ST-elevation myocardial infarction, heart failure, and valvular heart disease, and the Focused Update on Dual Antiplatelet Therapy. Unless supported by new evidence, the recommendations of these guidelines were followed. Both percutaneous coronary intervention (PCI) and coronary artery bypass grafting (CABG) are demonstrated to be highly efficient in alleviating symptoms of myocardial ischemia, and both are capable of improving prognosis. There remains a gap between PCI and CABG, with PCI being associated with faster recovery and lower risk of early events, including stroke, and CABG being associated with improved survival and reduced risk of spontaneous myocardial infarction and repeat intervention in the long run. The difference in the risk of recurrent ischemic events, favoring CABG, mainly depends on the complexity of coronary artery disease and the presence of diabetes mellitus. Thus, the difference in long-term outcomes between CABG and PCI is negligible with low-complexity coronary artery disease, but substantial with high complexity, especially when combined with diabetes. To establish indications for myocardial revascularization by percutaneous coronary intervention (PCI) or coronary artery bypass grafting (CABG), it is highlighted how the evidence of the functional relevance of coronary artery stenoses is needed either by noninvasive imaging function tests or by intravascular hemodynamic measurements. The prognostic and symptomatic benefits of myocardial revascularization depend on whether complete revascularization can be achieved. This needs to be considered when choosing the most appropriate revascularization strategy.

The concept of heart team is further highlighted, and the choice of the revascularization method is a shared decision, involving the patient being informed by the heart team of the early and long-term benefits and risks of the recommended revascularization strategy and its alternative. These guidelines suggest evidence-based criteria that inform individual treatment decisions and facilitate a reasonable selection of the optimal revascularization strategy to be offered to the patient. Below are the tables with the updated indications for the treatment of possible scenarios of coronary artery disease.

At the end of the chapter are reported the key messages which we can extrapolate and keep in mind from these guidelines:

- Myocardial revascularization is performed for the relief of symptoms of myocardial ischemia and the improvement of prognosis. In SCAD, the prognostic benefit is dependent on the extent of myocardium subject to ischemia.
- The prognostic and symptomatic benefits of myocardial revascularization critically depend on the completeness of revascularization. Therefore, the ability to achieve complete revascularization is a key issue when choosing the appropriate treatment strategy.
- Apart from the issues of individual operative risk and technical feasibility, diabetes mellitus and anatomical complexity of CAD determine the relative benefits of PCI and CABG.
- The SYNTAX score is the recommended tool to gauge the anatomical complexity of coronary disease.
- In some instances, both PCI and CABG are equally reasonable, or sometimes even equally problematic, options. This calls for the heart team to be consulted to develop individualized treatment concepts, with respect for the preferences of the patient who has been informed about early and late outcomes.
- Timely PCI of the culprit lesion remains the mainstay of treatment of ACS.
- After PCI of the culprit lesion in ACS, the choice of further revascularization modality should follow the criteria applied to patients with SCAD.
- Radial access is preferred for any PCI irrespective of clinical presentation, unless there are overriding procedural considerations.
- DES is recommended for any PCI irrespective of clinical presentation, lesion type, anticipated duration of DAPT, or concomitant anticoagulant therapy.
- Even though 6 months of DAPT is generally recommended after PCI in SCAD and 12 months of DAPT after ACS, the type and duration of DAPT should be individualized according to the ischemic and bleeding risks and appropriately adapted during follow-up. Based on this judgement, treatment durations for DAPT after DES that are as short as 1 month or even as long as lifelong may be reasonable.

- Off-pump surgery with no-touch aorta for high-risk patients should be considered when expertise exists.
- Multiple arterial grafting should be considered using the radial artery for high-grade stenosis and/or BIMA grafting for patients who do not have an increased risk of sternal wound infection.

3 AHA/ACC Guidelines

In January 2022, the 2021 ACC/AHA/SCAI Guideline for Coronary Artery Revascularization was published. This guideline replaces the 2011 coronary artery bypass graft surgery and the 2011 and 2015 percutaneous coronary intervention guidelines, providing a patient-centric approach to guide clinicians in the treatment of patients with significant coronary artery disease undergoing coronary revascularization as well as the supporting documentation to encourage their use. The paper that reported these guidelines highlighted the "TOP 10 TAKE-HOME MESSAGES" from these.

1. Treatment decisions regarding coronary revascularization in patients with coronary artery disease should be based on clinical indications, regardless of sex, race, or ethnicity, because there is no evidence that some patients benefit less than others, and efforts to reduce disparities of care are warranted.
2. In patients being considered for coronary revascularization for whom the optimal treatment strategy is unclear, a multidisciplinary heart team approach is recommended. Treatment decisions should be patient centered, incorporate patient preferences and goals, and include shared decision-making.

For patients with significant left main disease, surgical revascularization is indicated to improve survival relative to that likely to be achieved with medical therapy. Percutaneous revascularization is a reasonable option to improve survival, compared with medical therapy, in selected patients with low to medium anatomic complexity of coronary artery disease and left main disease that is equally suitable for surgical or percutaneous revascularization.

1. Updated evidence from contemporary trials supplements older evidence with regard to mortality benefit of revascularization in patients with stable ischemic heart disease, normal left ventricular ejection fraction, and triple-vessel coronary artery disease. Surgical revascularization may be reasonable to improve survival. A survival benefit with percutaneous revascularization is uncertain. Revascularization decisions are based on the consideration of disease complexity, technical feasibility of treatment, and a heart team discussion.
2. The use of a radial artery as a surgical revascularization conduit is preferred versus the use of a saphenous vein conduit to bypass the second most important target vessel with

significant stenosis after the left anterior descending coronary artery. Benefits include superior patency, reduced adverse cardiac events, and improved survival.

3. Radial artery access is recommended in patients undergoing percutaneous intervention who have acute coronary syndromes or stable ischemic heart disease, to reduce bleeding and vascular complications compared with a femoral approach. Patients with acute coronary syndromes also benefit from a reduction in mortality rate with this approach.
4. A short duration of dual-antiplatelet therapy after percutaneous revascularization in patients with stable ischemic heart disease is reasonable to reduce the risk of bleeding events. After consideration of recurrent ischemia and bleeding risks, select patients may safely transition to P2Y12 inhibitor monotherapy and stop aspirin after 1–3 months of dual-antiplatelet therapy.
5. Staged percutaneous intervention (while in hospital or after discharge) of a significantly stenosed nonculprit artery in patients presenting with an ST-segment-elevation myocardial infarction is recommended in select patients to improve outcomes. Percutaneous intervention of the nonculprit artery at the time of primary percutaneous coronary intervention is less clear and may be considered in stable patients with uncomplicated revascularization of the culprit artery, low-complexity nonculprit artery disease, and normal renal function. In contrast, percutaneous intervention of the nonculprit artery can be harmful in patients in cardiogenic shock.
6. Revascularization decisions in patients with diabetes and multivessel coronary artery disease are optimized by the use of a heart team approach. Patients with diabetes who have triple-vessel disease should undergo surgical revascularization; percutaneous coronary intervention may be considered if they are poor candidates for surgery.
7. Treatment decisions for patients undergoing surgical revascularization of coronary artery disease should include the calculation of a patient's surgical risk with the Society of Thoracic Surgeons score. The usefulness of the SYNTAX score calculation in treatment decisions is less clear because of the interobserver variability in its calculation and its absence of clinical variables.

4 SYNTAX Trial and Its Extension

Discussing the indications to myocardial revascularization, it is mandatory to spend a paragraph on the Synergy between PCI with Taxus and Cardiac Surgery (SYNTAX) trial. To date, there are more than 20 randomized controlled trials testing the efficacy and safety of CABG versus PCI in approximately 15,000 patients. Nevertheless, the optimal revascularization strategy for individual patients with complex coronary artery disease is still debated. By contrast with previous randomized controlled trials, which enrolled highly selected populations, the Synergy between PCI with Taxus and Cardiac Surgery (SYNTAX) trial was a landmark study comparing CABG with PCI (using first-generation drug-eluting stents) in all-comer patients with de novo three-vessel disease or left main coronary artery disease, or both [9–11].

One thousand eight hundred patients with three-vessel or LMD were randomly assigned to undergo CABG or PCI (in a 1:1 ratio). For all these patients, the local cardiac surgeon and interventional cardiologist determined that equivalent anatomical revascularization could be achieved with either treatment. A non-inferiority comparison of the two groups was performed for the primary endpoint—a major adverse cardiac or cerebrovascular event (i.e., death from any cause, stroke, myocardial infarction, or repeat revascularization) during the 12-month period after randomization.

After the 12-month follow-up period, the non-inferiority of PCI as compared with CABG was not demonstrated; CABG proved to be superior. Rates of death and myocardial infarction at 1 year were similar between patients who underwent CABG and those who underwent PCI with DES, whereas the rate of stroke was increased in the CABG group and the rate of repeat revascularization was increased in the PCI group. The increase in the rate of repeat revascularization with PCI as compared with CABG did not appear to translate into a significant overall increase in the rate of death or myocardial infarction. The risk of repeat revascularization after PCI needs to be balanced against the invasiveness of CABG and the risk of stroke, as previously reported without a concomitant decrease in survival.

Following the publication of the primary results of the SYNTAX trial and subgroup analyses in 2009, the 2010 European Society of Cardiology and European Association for Cardio-Thoracic Surgery guidelines on myocardial revascularization introduced an algorithm based on the type (three-vessel disease or left main coronary artery disease), extent, and severity of coronary artery disease, as assessed by the anatomical SYNTAX score [12–14]. This stratification has been maintained in the 2018 version of the guidelines. Higher SYNTAX scores, indicative of more complex disease, are hypothesized to represent a bigger therapeutic challenge and to have potentially worse prognosis. To calculate the SYNTAX score, the arterial tree was divided into 16 segments and was made into an algorithm. Anatomical risk factors, including the number of lesions, lesion location, presence of bi/trifurcations, aorto-ostial stenosis, tortuosity, lesion length >20 mm, calcification, thrombus, and small-vessel/diffuse disease, are considered in the SYNTAX score. The SYNTAX score algorithm takes into account the location of a lesion (coronary tree segments are weighted depending on their location), if a lesion is occlusive or nonocclusive (multiplication factor of 5 or 2, respectively), and all other adverse lesion characteristics (assigned additive values). Importantly, it does not include other patient-related clinical risk factors. A computer program calculates the SYNTAX score after answering a set of interactive, self-guided questions. The online SYNTAX score calculator consists of 11 questions. They can be divided into two groups: The first three determine the dominance, the total number of lesions, and the vessel segments involved per lesion. The maximum number of lesions allowed is 12, and each lesion is characterized by a number, 1–12. Each lesion can involve one or more segments. In this case, each vessel segment involved contributes to the lesion scoring. There is no limit in the number of segments involved per lesion. The last nine questions refer to detailed adverse lesion characteristics and will be repeated for each lesion separately. The SYNTAX score calculates a point value for each lesion, which will be summed to generate the patient's overall SYNTAX score. A dedicated Web site (www.syntaxscore.com) was developed, allowing clinicians to calculate patients' SYNTAX scores anytime.

However, the SYNTAX score merely provides the heart team with an anatomical stratification of treatment recommendations and does not consider major clinical characteristics and comorbidities. When the SYNTAX randomized cohort was stratified by tertiles of the SYNTAX score, there were similar or nonsignificantly different MACE rates in those with low or intermediate scores; however, in the top tertile, the MACE rate was greater in those receiving PCI compared to CABG. The ultimate goal was to create an angiographic tool grading the complexity of coronary artery disease and obtain evidence-based guidelines for selecting the optimal technique of revascularization (CABG or PCI). In addition, it will allow comparison of coronary artery disease complexity in individual patients and entire patient cohorts, as well as assessment of adequacy and completeness of revascularization.

In 2019, the SYNTAX Extended Survival (SYNTAXES) study reported 10-year all-cause death in patients included in the original SYNTAX trial [15]. The SYNTAX Extended Survival (SYNTAXES) study [16] was an investigator-driven extension follow-up of a multicenter, randomized controlled trial done between March 2005 and April 2007. Using data from the SYNTAX trial and the extended follow-up SYNTAXES study, the SYNTAX score II (termed SYNTAX score II 2020) was redeveloped, with two prespecified effect modifiers selected on the basis of previous evidence for predicting the 10-year death risk and 5-year risk of having MACE. The SYNTAX score II 2020 provides individuals with a predicted treatment benefit of CABG over PCI, in terms of the 10-year death risk and 5-year risk of having a major adverse cardiovascular event, based on key angiographic and clinical variables obtained at the time of decision-making. An online calculator is available.

Takahashi [J] then assessed the ability of the models available to predict the risk of death or a major adverse cardiovascular event and their differences (i.e., the estimated benefit of CABG versus PCI by calculating the absolute risk difference between the two strategies) by cross-validation with the SYNTAX trial (n=1800 participants) and external validation in the pooled population (n=3380 participants) of the FREEDOM [16], BEST [17], and PRECOMBAT [18] trials. At cross-validation, the newly developed SYNTAX score II showed a helpful discriminative ability in both treatment groups for predicting 10-year all-cause deaths and 5-year major adverse cardiovascular events. At external validation, the SYNTAX score II 2020 showed helpful discrimination and good calibration for predicting 5-year major adverse cardiovascular events. Further adequately powered, randomized trials of PCI versus CABG, with 5–10-year follow-up, which employ contemporary revascularization techniques, devices, and adjunctive medical therapy, should be done to prospectively validate the SYNTAX score II 2020 model.

References

1. Head SJ, Kieser TM, Falk V, Huysmans HA, Kappetein AP. Coronary artery bypass grafting: part 1—the evolution over the first 50 years. Eur Heart J. 2013;34(37):2862–72. https://doi.org/10.1093/eurheartj/eht330.
2. Gruntzig A. Transluminal dilatation of coronary-artery stenosis. Lancet. 1978;1(8058):263. https://doi.org/10.1016/s0140-6736(78)90500-7.
3. Sigwart U, Puel J, Mirkovitch V, Joffre F, Kappenberger L. Intravascular stents to prevent occlusion and restenosis after transluminal angioplasty. N Engl J Med. 1987;316(12):701–6. https://doi.org/10.1056/NEJM198703193161201.
4. Stone GW, Ellis SG, Cox DA, Hermiller J, O'Shaughnessy C, Mann JT, Turco M, Caputo R, Bergin P, Greenberg J, Popma JJ, Russell ME, TAXUS-IV Investigators. One-year clinical results with the slow-release, polymer-based, paclitaxel-eluting TAXUS stent: the TAXUS-IV trial. Circulation. 2004;109(16):1942–7.
5. Neumann FJ, Sousa-Uva M, Ahlsson A, Alfonso F, Banning AP, Benedetto U, Byrne RA, Collet JP, Falk V, Head SJ, Jüni P, Kastrati A, Koller A, Kristensen SD, Niebauer J, Richter DJ, Seferovic PM, Sibbing D, Stefanini GG, Windecker S, Yadav R, Zembala MO, ESC Scientific Document Group. 2018 ESC/EACTS guidelines on myocardial revascularization. Eur Heart J. 2019;40(2):87–165. https://doi.org/10.1093/eurheartj/ehy394.
6. Wijns W, Kolh P, Danchin N, Di Mario C, Falk V, Folliguet T, Garg S, Huber K, James S, Knuuti J, Lopez-Sendon J, Marco J, Menicanti L, Ostojic M, Piepoli MF, Pirlet C, Pomar JL, Reifart N, Ribichini FL, Schalij MJ, Sergeant P, Serruys PW, Silber S, Sousa Uva M, Taggart D. Task Force on Myocardial Revascularization of the European Society of Cardiology (ESC) and the European Association for Cardio-Thoracic Surgery (EACTS); European Association for Percutaneous Cardiovascular Interventions (EAPCI), Guidelines on myocardial revascularization. Eur Heart J. 2010;31(20):2501–55. https://doi.org/10.1093/eurheartj/ehq277. Epub 2010 Aug 29
7. Taggart DP. Thomas B. Ferguson Lecture. Coronary artery bypass grafting is still the best treatment for multivessel and left main disease, but patients need to know. Ann Thorac Surg. 2006;82:1966–75.
8. Sajja LR, Mannam G, Chakravarthi RM, Sompalli S, Naidu SK, Somaraju B, Penumatsa RR. Coronary artery bypass grafting with or without cardiopulmonary bypass in patients with preoperative non-dialysis dependent renal insufficiency: a randomized study. J Thorac Cardiovasc Surg. 2007;133(2):378–88. https://doi.org/10.1016/j.jtcvs.2006.09.028.
9. Ong AT, Serruys PW, Mohr FW, et al. The SYNergy between percutaneous coronary intervention with TAXus and cardiac surgery (SYNTAX) study: design, rationale, and run-in phase. Am Heart J. 2006;151:1194–204.
10. Serruys PW, Morice MC, Kappetein AP, et al. Percutaneous coronary intervention versus coronary artery bypass grafting for severe coronary artery disease. N Engl J Med. 2009;360:961–72.
11. Kappetein AP, Feldman TE, Mack MJ, et al. Comparison of coronary bypass surgery with drug-eluting stenting for the treatment of left main and/or three-vessel disease: 3-year follow-up of the SYNTAX trial. Eur Heart J. 2011;32:2125–34.
12. Serruys PW, Chichareon P, Modolo R, et al. The SYNTAX score on its way out or... towards artificial intelligence: part I. EuroIntervention. 2019;16:44–59.
13. Serruys PW, Chichareon P, Modolo R, et al. The SYNTAX score on its way out or... towards artificial intelligence: part II. EuroIntervention. 2019;16:60–75.
14. Task Force on Myocardial Revascularization of the European Society of Cardiology and the European Association for Cardio-Thoracic Surgery, European Association for Percutaneous Cardiovascular Interventions, Wijns W, et al. Guidelines on myocardial revascularization. Eur Heart J. 2010;31:2501–55.

15. Thuijs D, Kappetein AP, Serruys PW, et al. Percutaneous coronary intervention versus coronary artery bypass grafting in patients with three-vessel or left main coronary artery disease: 10- year follow-up of the multicentre randomised controlled SYNTAX trial. Lancet. 2019;394:1325–34.
16. Takahashi K, Serruys PW, Fuster V, Farkouh ME, Spertus JA, Cohen DJ, Park SJ, Park DW, Ahn JM, Kappetein AP, Head SJ, Thuijs DJ, Onuma Y, Kent DM, Steyerberg EW, van Klaveren D, SYNTAXES, FREEDOM, BEST, and PRECOMBAT Trial Investigators. Redevelopment and validation of the SYNTAX score II to individualise decision making between percutaneous and surgical revascularisation in patients with complex coronary artery disease: secondary analysis of the multicentre randomised controlled SYNTAXES trial with external cohort validation. Lancet. 2020;396(10260):1399–412. https://doi.org/10.1016/S0140-6736(20)32114-0. Epub 2020 Oct 8
17. Park SJ, Ahn JM, Kim YH, Park DW, Yun SC, Lee JY, Kang SJ, Lee SW, Lee CW, Park SW, Choo SJ, Chung CH, Lee JW, Cohen DJ, Yeung AC, Hur SH, Seung KB, Ahn TH, Kwon HM, Lim DS, Rha SW, Jeong MH, Lee BK, Tresukosol D, Fu GS, Ong TK. BEST Trial Investigators. Trial of everolimus-eluting stents or bypass surgery for coronary disease. N Engl J Med. 2015;372(13):1204–12. https://doi.org/10.1056/NEJMoa1415447. Epub 2015 Mar 16
18. Park SJ, Kim YH, Park DW, Yun SC, Ahn JM, Song HG, Lee JY, Kim WJ, Kang SJ, Lee SW, Lee CW, Park SW, Chung CH, Lee JW, Lim DS, Rha SW, Lee SG, Gwon HC, Kim HS, Chae IH, Jang Y, Jeong MH, Tahk SJ, Seung KB. Randomized trial of stents versus bypass surgery for left main coronary artery disease. N Engl J Med. 2011;364(18):1718–27. https://doi.org/10.1056/NEJMoa1100452. Epub 2011 Apr 4

Multidisciplinary Approach to Treatment of Ischaemic Heart Disease: The Role of the Heart Team

Giovanni Concistrè

1 Introduction

With an increasing number of therapeutic options, MDM has become increasingly important for the evaluation of options in medicine, especially in patients with complex diseases. MDM has proven value in disciplines such as cancer treatment, where comprehensive decision-making in so-called tumour boards resulted in a change of diagnostic or therapeutic strategies and improved outcomes [1, 2].

Heart teams, as multidisciplinary teams in cardiovascular disease are usually named, have played a crucial role in decision-making. The European Society of Cardiology recommends the consultation of a heart team in the management of valvular heart disease [3], heart failure [4] and myocardial revascularization [5]. A heart team usually consists of cardiologists, cardiac surgeons, interventionists, imaging specialists, anaesthetists and midlevel providers. In some cases, the expert opinion of a general practitioner, geriatrician or intensive care specialist can be of additional value.

The evolution of the heart team concept started with a focus on CAD. Initially, the options for treatment of CAD were optimal medical therapy and CABG. The introduction of PCI revolutionized the treatment of CAD and became an alternative treatment option to CABG. Some studies showed, however, that patients who would benefit most of CABG actually received PCI treatment due to the less invasive nature of PCI [6]. This resulted in a call for standardized preoperative assessment of patients [7].

G. Concistrè (✉)
Adult Cardiac Surgery Unit, Ospedale del cuore "G. Pasquinucci", Fondazione Toscana G. Monasterio, Massa, Italy

G. Concistrè (ed.), *Ischemic Heart Disease*,
https://doi.org/10.1007/978-3-031-25879-4_18

The purpose of this chapter is to discuss the rationale for involvement of a heart team in decision-making. Furthermore, patient categories to be discussed with MDM, use of preoperative surgical risk scores, professionals to be involved in decision-making and limitations and other advantages of shared decision-making in ischaemic heart disease are discussed.

2 Advantages of a Multidisciplinary Approach

On the face of it, decision-making in a multidisciplinary team like a heart team has important advantages over solitary decision-making. Figure 1 represents the conceptual strengths and weaknesses of the heart team model. First, medicine is becoming increasingly complex with various therapeutic options to be considered in older patients with more comor-

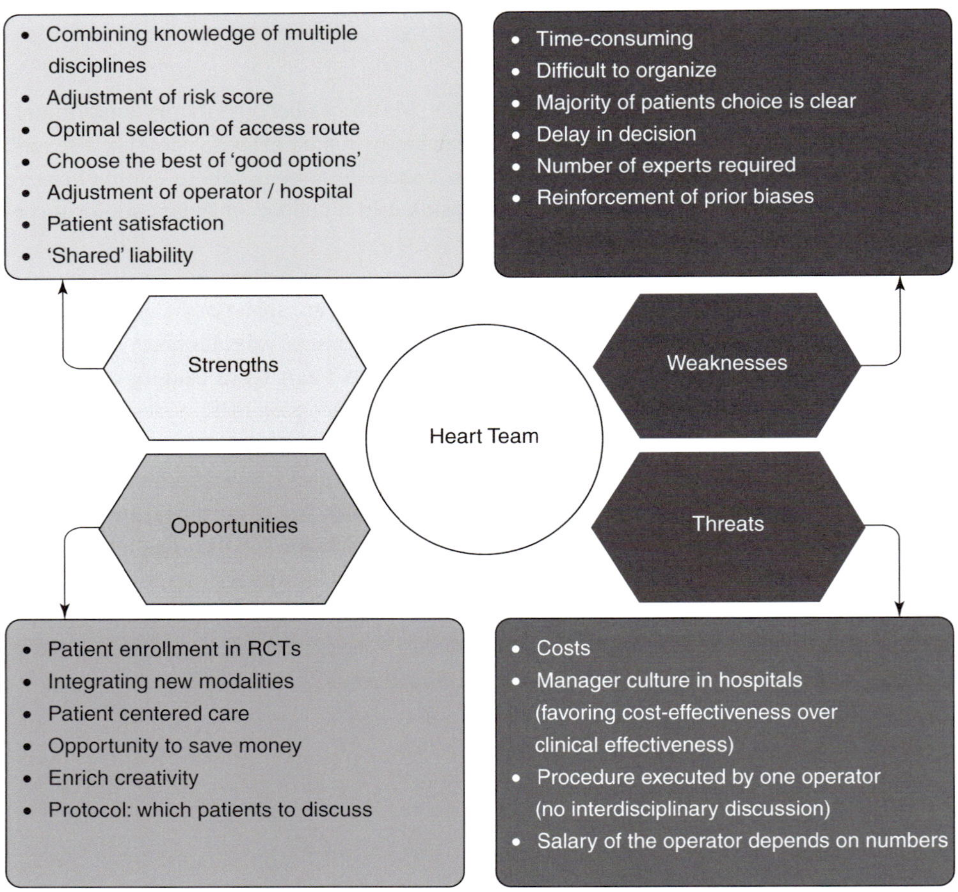

Fig. 1 The heart team illustrated according to the strengths, weaknesses, opportunities, and threats model (SWOT)

bidities. The combined expertise of a heart team provides the basis for a more balanced appraisal of a specific case. This is specifically important if the availability of clear supportive evidence (e.g. risk scores) is limited.

Secondly, use of expensive therapeutic options is likely to be restricted in patients where the benefits of treatment are questionable. Additionally, if an invasive treatment is deemed not to be beneficial for patients, extensive and detailed non-invasive care can be organized immediately. At the same time, underutilization of therapeutic options can be avoided. Furthermore, an open-minded, multidisciplinary approach minimizes disagreements between individual clinicians.

Another advantage of the heart team is that the preoperative diagnostic workup will become more standardized, since a protocolized and complete preoperative assessment is a requirement to have a successful multidisciplinary meeting. Finally, an open discussion about therapeutic options in complex patients creates an environment for clinicians to discuss and expand their knowledge ('Every day is a school day').

Moreover, complex cases sometimes require creative solutions which are not always supported by protocols and guidelines. The heart team offers a platform for 'creative solutions', and an opportunity to share responsibility for these treatments. Finally, these discussions can deliver an important contribution to the education of medical students and clinical residents in one of the most difficult and rapidly evolving subjects of medicine.

Although evidence of the benefit of heart teams is limited, one report has shown that in-hospital mortality and 1-year mortality in patients admitted to the hospital for heart failure were significantly lower if they were discussed in a heart team, compared to patients not discussed in a heart team [4].

3 Patient and Carer Involvement

The heart team should provide a consensus view as to which treatment strategy is superior based on the available evidence as well as the collective experience of individual specialists and their unit generally. By necessity, the meeting is a technical one, involving explicit discussions about risk and prognosis. Most would agree that it would be impracticable for the patient or their carer to be present during those discussions. Nevertheless, patients' wishes need to be accommodated in any decision-making process. Thus, mechanisms should be in place for the patient to be informed of the MDM recommendation in a manner that allows their wishes to be taken into account. It is, therefore, recommended that a clinician who is familiar with the patient and their wishes, and who can thereby act on their behalf, should present their case to be discussed in the MDM. Once the MDM decision has been reached, it should be that clinician's responsibility to ensure that the patient is informed. While a letter or telephone call might accomplish this, it is probably more expedient to make arrangements for the clinician to see the patient and their carer or family in an outpatient setting. That would not only allow the MDM decision to be summarized in a way that can be understood by all parties, but would also provide the fundamentals of the consenting process that will be required to precede any revascularization procedure.

Patients referred for CABG are usually seen in an outpatient clinic by the consultant surgeon who will perform the operation. Likewise, those referred for PCI should see the interventional cardiologist in a similar setting. There will inevitably be cases in which the MDM discussion condenses into a position of equipoise. In such situations, it is advised that the options be put to the patient and for the patient to choose his/her preferred management plan. Either the cardiac surgeon or the cardiologist could present these options to the patient. The paramount issue is that any perception of indecision should be avoided. Indeed, such a position should be—and expressed as—advantageous in that more than one treatment option is available. The use of patient information leaflets based on the locally available expertise and outcomes as well as lay description of the various treatment options may prove beneficial.

4 Clinical Composition, Attendance and Frequency

The overarching principles of an MDM meeting are that (1) it is quorate and (2) the frequency is sufficient to meet the demands of—but not so as to impede—the efficient running of a service. A robust MDM that seeks to discuss all the issues relevant to patients' management should comprise a minimum core group of individuals with the necessary range of expertise. Thus, in addition to cardiac surgeons and interventional cardiologists, there should also be a non-interventional cardiologist. The subspecialty interest of such individuals need not be specified, acknowledging that expertise in imaging, heart failure, device therapy or electrophysiology may all add value to discussion around individual patients. This varied expertise in attendance is in keeping with the results of a UK survey that indicated that the majority of current MDM meetings are attended predominantly by consultants in these disciplines. Although there may be some benefit in having members of other medical specialties (e.g. cardiac anaesthetists, geriatricians, diabetologists) and allied healthcare professionals (e.g. nurses) to be present at all the MDM meetings, it is recognized that this may not be practical. However, should the Chair identify such a need, then, in order to aid discussion of patients with complex disease, significant comorbidity or other medical conditions, a cardiac anaesthetist or a geriatrician may be asked to attend. Junior doctors should be encouraged to attend in order to become familiar with the process and derive benefit from its educational value. Other disciplines allied to medicine, e.g. nursing, pharmacy and audit staff, as well as research nurses, should be encouraged to attend given the multidisciplinary scope of the meeting and its potential educational value. Attendance by such colleagues would also enhance data collection for any proposed audit projects as well as recruitment into trials.

The meeting should be chaired by a consultant. The speciality of the Chair should be rotated between surgeons and interventional/non-interventional cardiologists. The function of the Chair is to ensure that sufficient time is allocated to discuss all cases presented, that all necessary data are available for each case and that discussion is directed towards producing a consensus view. The Chair should also ensure that the recommendations of the MDM are documented and that particular issues relevant to that decision are also recorded accurately (see below). It is not the function of the Chair to provide any form of 'casting vote' in situations of equipoise.

The frequency and duration of meetings will vary according to local needs and the number and type of cases discussed. Our survey and NCBC data suggest that, in most centres, this is one or two times per week and in each case lasting 1–2 h.

5 Facilities and Technical Considerations

A room dedicated to the MDM should be provided with adequate seating for all attendees and be sufficiently private in order to allow confidential discussion to take place. Seating should be such as to allow all members to be able to see clearly any data presented on a display screen. Facilities should be available to display and view all cardiac imaging modalities such as coronary angiograms, CT scan, MRI and nuclear scan results and echocardiograms in high quality and sufficient to meet diagnostic medical standards. In addition to the results of current investigations, easy and rapid access to archived images will also be required.

Acknowledging that patients from remote centres may also be discussed, the ability to transfer and display their images will also be required and access to any electronic reports should also be available. These requirements will depend greatly on existing local information technology facilities and support. Information technology and audiovisual support should be readily available during MDM meetings in order to address particular issues as they occur and thereby avoid delaying or postponing meetings.

6 Administration and Managerial Support

A dedicated MDM coordinator forms an essential component of these meetings and should be present to document the personnel attending, together with the outcome and recommendations reached after discussion for each patient. Issues resulting from detailed or complex discussion may require specific recording and more exact documentation, as directed by the Chair [8]. In order to cover periods of absence, leave or sickness, two dedicated coordinators will be required. The MDM coordinator should be notified prior to the meeting as to which patients are to be discussed. The coordinator will then ensure that all relevant investigations are available prior to the start of the meeting. Patient's information, including clinical details and results of relevant investigations and other data such as risk scores, should be documented on a dedicated MDM proforma made available to the MDM coordinator prior to the meeting. Once the proforma is completed to include the meeting's recommendation, it should then be signed by the Chair and incorporated into the patient's case notes. A copy should also be retained by the coordinator in order to enable later auditing of the MDM process. Documentation would be facilitated by the use of a computer database that would allow easier analysis of attendance, frequency, duration and outcome of meetings that would assist in audit, research and production of annual reports. An electronic version of the MDM proforma will also facilitate the subsequent circulation of the MDM discussion and its outcome to all relevant stakeholders such as the patient, the referring cardiologist, the patient's general practitioner and the cardiac surgeon.

7 The Type and Range of Cases to Be Discussed

Defining which cases should come to a formal MDM meeting is notoriously difficult. An ideal might be that all cases in which the possibility of any form of revascularization is considered should be discussed in an MDM forum. This policy might be seen as impractical and in some circumstances might even delay or jeopardize ideal patient care. Some centres are currently working with systems that routinely incorporate ad hoc or follow-on PCI in elective cases undergoing diagnostic angiography. Such an approach has both advantages (e.g. a single patient admission, one arterial puncture and one invasive radiographic procedure) and disadvantages (e.g. issues with the validity of the consenting process prior to the procedure when the exact nature of any intervention is unknown).

The ESC/EACTS guidelines for myocardial revascularization refer to cases that should undergo heart team discussion and provide a basis for any recommendations. When reviewing these criteria, it is clear that they highlight particularly the presence of obstruction of LMS or the proximal segment of its LAD branch, particularly if this is a component of triple-vessel disease.

Some patients undergoing investigation with coronary angiography may proceed directly to PCI without formal discussion, so-called ad hoc or follow-on cases. This applies particularly to urgent or emergency situations and is therefore recommended in haemodynamically unstable patients. Examples include addressing the culprit lesion in patients presenting with acute ST-segment-elevation myocardial infarction. An ad hoc approach may also be applied to elective cases with single- or double-vessel disease acknowledging the guidance above. A decision to proceed to PCI in such cases should take into account the validity of the consenting process and consideration as to whether CABG in such circumstances might confer prognostic—as well as symptomatic—advantage. An explanation for proceeding in such a situation should be documented in the case notes.

8 Minimum Data Discussed and Method of Presentation

In addition to basic patient demographics, other data should comprise the clinical presentation and severity of symptoms, together with the source of referral. The results of any stress investigations, the coronary anatomy and an assessment of left ventricular performance are also essential elements [9]. Associated medical conditions, particularly if they are known to confer additional risk for either PCI or CABG, should be itemized in order to calculate a formal score for either approach. While a number of risk scores are available, individual centres should decide upon which ones they feel should be used for both revascularization modalities and document them during the MDT meeting. The most commonly used system for CABG in Europe is EuroSCORE II [10].

The SYNTAX score is also being increasingly incorporated into MDM discussion [11]. While this does not quantify procedural risk for PCI, it nevertheless represents an individual's burden of disease and therefore a surrogate for the procedural time, contrast volume and number of stents that might be anticipated if PCI were to be recommended. Indeed, high SYNTAX scores are seen as a valuable discriminator in cases in which PCI and CABG are both feasible and may then sway the consensus view in favour of surgery [12].

9 Multidisciplinary Team Considerations and Functioning in Non-surgical Cardiology Centres

Multidisciplinary meetings should occur regularly in both the surgical centre and in each non-surgical cardiology centre within any region. The demand for a regular forum in a non-surgical cardiology centre not only requires a surgeon to travel to that unit, which is time consuming, but also has the disadvantage of involving and, therefore, relying upon a single surgeon. These constraints can be overcome by teleconferencing facilities, provided that the technology is robust, reliable and of high quality. In this way, the MDM can incorporate several members of the surgical centre team. It also allows for the heart team meeting to be 'attended' by high-volume PCI operators from other units, who will have experience in complex PCI cases, and thus make additional contributions to any case discussion.

Any teleconferencing facilities should support the viewing of multimodality imaging such as angiography, echocardiography and CT/MRI/nuclear scans, and it is preferable if those involved can have 'face-to-face' contact.

Documentation of the decisions made by the heart team should be consistent with those made in the surgical centre and be available electronically both locally and in the surgical centre. An effective Chair is important at each end to ensure open and democratic engagement. Core membership should be agreed upon, and attendance should be recorded. There should be a written policy of which cases should be discussed, and this could be guided by the guidelines.

10 Timing and Integration into Job Planning

The MDM forum is a pivotal requirement in the management pathway and is therefore a component of the planned activity that reflects direct patient care. Nevertheless, data from a UK survey and from NCBC comparisons suggested that although MDM meetings were held within ‘office hours’ in the majority of units sampled, they were only incorporated into consultant job plans in 60% of respondents. Dedicated time should be committed and agreed upon by managers and clinical directors in order for consultant staff to attend a sufficient proportion of MDT meetings and thereby ensure consistency of decision-making. It is not inconceivable that in the near future the reimbursement bodies (specialized commissioners, clinical commissioning groups or even private health insurers) for cardiac procedures would demand that the management plan for patients with CAD to have been discussed and validated by a heart team before payment is issued.

It is recognized that some cases may present urgently or as an emergency and require a more rapid discussion that may involve both interventional and surgical input. Most centres can work flexibly and be responsive enough to allow this important process to occur, the nature and results of which should be documented into the case notes.

11 Documentation, Feedback and Audit of Outcomes

It is a fundamental requirement that the recommendations reached by consensus are documented and signed off by the Chair. This ensures transparency. This record should be filed into the case notes. There will be cases in which the decision-making is not straightforward and in such circumstances the MDM documentation should attempt to capture the essential elements of that discussion in order to further justify any decision reached. The role of the Chair is also important here in guiding the MDM coordinator in documenting the outcome as accurately as is necessary.

In addition to making recommendations regarding the requirement and mode of revascularization, the MDM should also provide a view as to whether this should take place during the current hospital admission (if the patient has presented with an acute coronary syndrome), at an early juncture after discharge or as an elective case on a routine waiting list.

Feedback is important in order to demonstrate that the process is robust. Units should therefore ensure that a system is in place that follows up the cases discussed and correlates their eventual management with original MDM recommendation. Any aberration from the original outcome should be brought back to the MDM for discussion [13]. In addition, there should be a system in place that reviews those patients undergoing either PCI or CABG without MDM discussion in order to ensure that this was appropriate. Such processes can provide educational value as well as inform any future decisions in similar patients.

Some units have tested the reproducibility of the MDM using the representation of cases already discussed to examine whether the heart team outcome then differs from the original recommendations [9]. While this is an area of research interest, there are data to suggest that a proportion of outcomes are indeed different. This is to be expected given the dynamics of group discussion and the variability in attendance. This is usually in cases in which there is genuine equipoise and in which more than one management plan would be acceptable.

It is acknowledged that there may be instances where the clinician delivering the final decision of the MDM (e.g. PCI or CABG) may not have been part of the MDM discussion and does not share the MDM decision. In such instances, this should be documented in the patient's medical records and the patient rediscussed at the earliest convenient MDM meeting to avoid delays in treatment. Likewise, it may be that a patient may not wish to proceed with the MDM recommendation. In such cases, the reasons for aberration should be documented. Ideally, the MDM should be updated at the earliest appropriate opportunity of this change in decision.

It is acceptable that the MDM documentation processes (referral, MDM discussion, MDM decision and decision enactment) are done electronically if available at local Trust level.

References

1. Van Hagen P, Spaander MCW, Van Der Gaast A, et al. Impact of a multidisciplinary tumour board meeting for upper-GI malignancies on clinical decision making: a prospective cohort study. Int J Clin Oncol. 2013;18(2):214–9.
2. Kesson EM, Allardice GM, George WD, Burns HJG, Morrison DS. Effects of multidisciplinary team working on breast cancer survival: retrospective, comparative, interventional cohort study of 13 722 women. BMJ. 2012;344(e2718):1–9.
3. Vahanian A, Alfieri O, Andreotti F, et al. Guidelines on the management of valvular heart disease (version 2012). The joint task force on the management of valvular heart disease of the European Society of Cardiology (ESC) and the European Association for Cardio-Thoracic Surgery (EACTS). Eur Heart J. 2012;33(19):2451–96.
4. Ponikowski P, Voors AA, Anker SD, et al. ESC guidelines for the diagnosis and treatment of acute and chronic heart failure. The task force for the diagnosis and treatment of acute and chronic heart failure of the European Society of Cardiology (ESC) developed with the special contribution of the Heart Failure Association (HFA) of the ESC. Eur Heart J. 2016;37(27):2129–200.
5. Windecker S, Kolh P, Alfonso F, et al. ESC/EACTS guidelines on myocardial revascularization. The task force on myocardial revascularization of the European Society of Cardiology (ESC) and the European Association for Cardio-Thoracic Surgery (EACTS) developed with the special contribution of the European Association of Percutaneous Cardiovascular Interventions (EAPCI). Eur Heart J. 2014;35(37):2541–619.
6. Hannan EL, Racz MJ, Gold J, et al. Adherence of catheterization laboratory cardiologists to American College of Cardiology/American Heart Association guidelines for percutaneous coronary interventions and coronary artery bypass graft surgery. What happens in actual practice? Circulation. 2010;121(2):267–75.
7. Head SJ, Kaul S, Mack MJ, et al. The rationale for heart team decision-making for patients with stable, complex coronary artery disease. Eur Heart J. 2013;34(32):2510–8.
8. Jalil R, Lamb B, Russ S, Sevdalis N, Green JS. The cancer multi-disciplinary team from the coordinators' perspective: results from a national survey in the UK. BMC Health Serv Res. 2012;12:457.

9. Long J, Luckraz H, Thekkudan J, Maher A, Norell M. Heart team discussion in managing patients with coronary artery disease: outcome and reproducibility. Interact Cardiovasc Thorac Surg. 2012;14:594–8.
10. Nashef SA, Roques F, Sharples LD, Nilsson J, Smith C, Goldstone AR, et al. EuroSCORE II. Eur J Cardiothorac Surg. 2012;41:734–45.
11. Sianos G, Morel MA, Kappetein AP, Morice MC, Colombo A, Dawkis K, et al. The SYNTAX Score: an angiographic tool grading the complexity of coronary artery disease. EuroInterv. 2005;1:219–27.
12. Mohr FW, Morice MC, Kappetein AP, Feldman TE, Stahle E, Colombo A, et al. Coronary artery bypass graft surgery versus percutaneous coronary intervention in patients with three-vessel disease and left main coronary disease: 5-year follow-up of the randomised, clinical SYNTAX trial. Lancet. 2013;381:629–38.
13. Mishra P, Luckraz H, Dincer A, Thekkudan J, Mahboob S, Norell M. How does MDT decision get enacted for patients with coronary artery disease? Heart Asia. 2014;0:30–3.

Pharmacological Treatment of Ischemic Heart Disease

Alberto Giannoni, Francesco Gentile, and Chiara Borrelli

Few things are more distressing to a physician than to stand beside a suffering patient who is anxiously looking to him for that relief from pain which he feels himself utterly unable to afford. His sympathy for the sufferer, and the regret he feels for the impotence of his art, engrave the picture indelibly on his mind, and serve as a constant and urgent stimulus in his search after the causes of the pain, and the means by which it may be alleviated.

—T. Lauder Brunton, July 27, 1867.

1 Introduction

Chronic myocardial ischemia may be a consequence of obstructive coronary artery disease (CAD), secondary to luminal stenosis and reduced coronary flow reserve, and/or of other conditions, such as vasospasm, microvascular dysfunction, and energetic mismatch [1–3]. According to the latest European guidelines, whenever a macro- or microvascular coronary disorder is documented, the clinical condition could be denoted as chronic coronary syndrome (CCS) [1].

A. Giannoni (✉)
Institute of Life Sciences, Scuola Superiore Sant'Anna, Pisa, Italy

Cardiology and Cardiovascular Medicine Department, Fondazione Toscana G. Monasterio, Pisa, Italy
e-mail: a.giannoni@santannapisa.it; agiannon@ftgm.it

F. Gentile · C. Borrelli
Cardiology and Cardiovascular Medicine Department, Fondazione Toscana G. Monasterio, Pisa, Italy

Pisa University Hospital, Pisa, Italy
e-mail: fgentile@monasterio.it; cborrelli@ftgm.it

G. Concistrè (ed.), *Ischemic Heart Disease*,
https://doi.org/10.1007/978-3-031-25879-4_19

Of note, myocardial ischemia is often but not always accompanied by chest pain or angina. Indeed, angina is only the final clinical manifestation of a series of pathophysiological changes induced by myocardial energetic unbalance and named the "*ischemic cascade*," including diminished left ventricular compliance, decreased contractility, increased left ventricular end-diastolic pressure, and electrocardiographic changes [4]. The threshold of ischemia associated with symptoms may vary among patients and within the same patient, or may also be absent in conditions of neuropathic functional denervation (i.e., diabetes) [5, 6]: therefore, episodes of silent ischemia may occur.

Although observational studies suggested that silent myocardial ischemia could compromise contractile function and electrical stability, with negative hemodynamic consequences [7], and life-threatening arrhythmias [8–11], there is currently no evidence showing a prognostic benefit of anti-ischemic therapies in this context. Therefore, current guidelines discourage functional testing in asymptomatic individuals [1] and highlight that the main aim of medical therapy in CCS is to target angina rather than ischemia [1].

As for symptomatic patients, while meta-analyses show that all antianginal drugs are similarly efficacious in alleviating angina and increasing exercise tolerance, evidence for improvement in event-free survival is generally missing, apart from beta-blockers (BBs) in patients with heart failure and reduced ejection fraction, and nicorandil for angina-related hospitalization [12, 13].

Nonetheless, treating ischemia may prove value in specific subsets (e.g., in the presence of an extensive ischemic burden and/or of left ventricular systolic dysfunction) [1], and this topic still remains a matter of debate [14, 15].

2 Pathophysiological Mechanisms of Ischemia and Potential Targets

As detailed in the chapter "Pathophysiology of Ischemic Syndromes in Coronary Artery Disease", in the last century, a plethora of elegant physiological and pharmacological studies have outlined the heterogenous pathophysiological determinants of myocardial ischemia [16]. Whereas an impaired oxygen/nutrients' supply due to either coronary (e.g., epicardial artery stenosis, vasospasm, microvascular dysfunction) or noncoronary causes (e.g., anemia, hypoxia, toxic and metabolic disorders) and an unbalanced increase in energetic demand (secondary to increased myocardial contractility, wall stress, or heart rate) are key determinants of myocardial ischemia, more subtle abnormalities in cardiomyocyte metabolism have been observed as well [16–19]. Importantly, these mechanisms are not exclusive but could be variously intertwined and declined in the single patient, fostering the research for a tailored and integrated therapeutic approach (Fig. 1) [20, 21].

Beyond its conduit function, coronary circulation is responsible for modulating myocardial blood flow to match energetic demand across a wide spectrum of physiological conditions, through the mechanisms of autoregulation and autonomic control [22, 23]. Accordingly, in conditions of increased myocardial requests (e.g., physical exercise, emo-

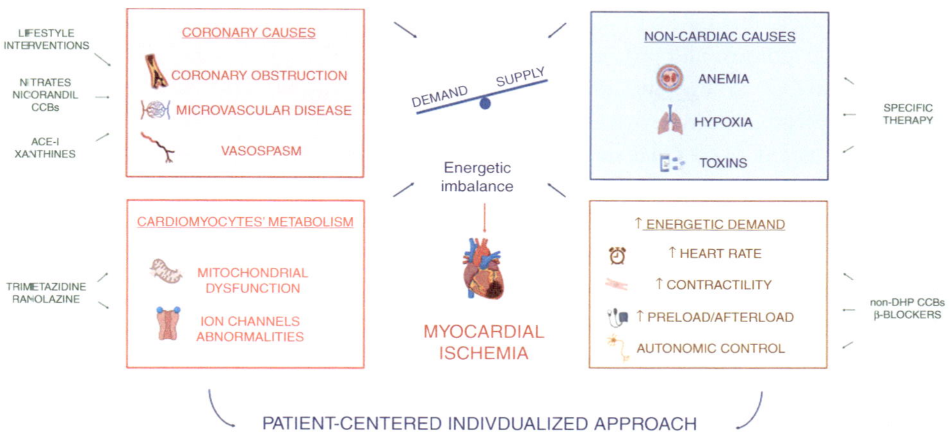

Fig. 1 Pathophysiology-driven pharmacological management of myocardial ischemia. *ACE-i* angiotensin-converting enzyme inhibitors; *CCBs* calcium channel blockers; *DHP* dihydropyridines

tional stress), coronary flow increases proportionally [24]. On the other hand, in the presence of a significant luminal obstruction in an epicardial artery, the downstream flow is usually maintained at rest at the price of exhausting the vasodilatory reserve, so that myocardial ischemia may emerge when a further increase in energetic demand is not adequately counterbalanced [25]. Nevertheless, a certain degree of vasodilation may be obtained through some drugs (e.g., nitric oxide (NO) donors, nicorandil, and calcium channel blockers (CCBs)), which are therefore effective anti-ischemic agents in this setting [26–28].

Although such a hydraulic mechanism has long been considered the fundament of chronic myocardial ischemia and angina, it is nowadays established that this may occur also in the absence of obstructive CAD and persist also after successful revascularization [29–31]. In this regard, vasospasm has been identified as a potential contributor. Although the so-called resting vasospastic or Prinzmetal angina, as originally described [32], represents a rare condition, macro- and/or microvascular spasm may be frequently observed independently of the concomitant atherosclerotic burden [33, 34]. A paradoxical vasoconstrictive response to acetylcholine, which is normally associated with a NO-mediated vasodilation, characterizes coronary vasospasm, implying a pivotal role of endothelial dysfunction [35, 36]. In this context, CCBs (both dihydropyridines—DHP and non-DHP) are a well-established first-line therapy [37, 38], while other vasodilators such as nitrates and nicorandil represent possible alternatives or add-on therapies in refractory cases [39, 40]. On the contrary, BBs are usually not recommended since vasospasm could be exacerbated by the blockage of the "vasodilative" β_2-adrenergic receptors and a paradoxical overstimulation of the "vasoconstrictive" α_1-adrenergic receptors on coronaries' walls [41].

Microvascular disease may underlie myocardial ischemia and angina, also in the absence of detectable epicardial coronary stenosis and vasospasm or other cardiac conditions, due to endothelial and autonomic dysfunction, exaggerated vasoconstrictive and nociceptive responses, and pro-inflammatory signals [3, 42, 43]. Although NO-mediated pathways and Ca^{2+} inflow modulate microvascular tone, too [44], both nitrates and CCBs are poorly effective on microvascular angina [45, 46], particularly when no vasospasm could be detected [47]. Conversely, more promising findings have been obtained for angiotensin-converting enzyme inhibitors, since angiotensin II is a direct modulator of microvascular tone [48] and for xanthines, which may favor flow redistribution toward ischemic areas (by inhibiting the arteriolar vasodilator effects of adenosine) and antagonize adenosine-mediated pain afferents, relieving angina [49].

As anticipated, also the reduction of myocardial energetic demand is an effective strategy to alleviate ischemia and angina and may be achieved by lowering blood pressure and, most importantly, heart rate [50]. Beyond reducing oxygen consumption, a lower heart rate prolongs coronary diastolic perfusion, so that the net effect of negative chronotropic drugs may be an improved contractility of ischemic regions, despite their possible negative inotropic action [51]. Therefore, BBs and non-DHP CCBs play a central role among antianginal therapies [52], while their anti-ischemic efficacy in asymptomatic patients is still controversial [50, 53]. Alternatively, a lower heart rate may be achieved by inhibiting the I_f current with ivabradine, considered a second-line antianginal drug, with no negative inotropic or lusitropic effect [52, 54].

Finally, further targets for anti-ischemic therapies have been identified by shifting the focus on the cardiomyocyte. Indeed, whereas its energetic metabolism is primarily based on mitochondrial oxidation of fatty acids and other substrates (e.g., glucose, ketones) are less utilized in physiological condition [55], in the presence of ischemia, such pathways may be corrupted and anaerobic glycolysis favored, resulting in acidosis, Na^+ and Ca^{2+} overload, and decreased cardiac function [19, 55]. Promoting the shift toward a more efficient energetic asset has therefore emerged as an intriguing strategy and may be achieved by favoring glucose instead of fatty acid utilization. As detailed below in this chapter, two anti-ischemic drugs, i.e., trimetazidine and ranolazine, act in modulating these pathways [56, 57].

3 Medical Therapy of Ischemic Heart Disease

Historically, the first class of drugs that have been used as antianginal were nitrates, followed almost a century after by BBs, then CCBs, trimetazidine, nicorandil, ivabradine, and, finally, ranolazine [58–64] (Fig. 2).

Considering the number of antianginal drugs now available for clinical use, it may be difficult to identify the optimal treatment. Ideally, the best option should control symptoms, improve quality of life, maximize patient's adherence, and minimize drug-related side effects. Furthermore, as suggested by the current guidelines, the therapeutic choice should also be adapted to the patient's characteristics, such as cardiac and noncardiac

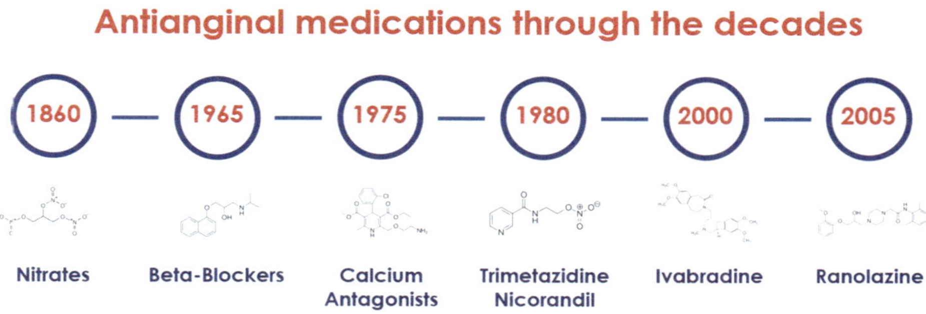

Fig. 2 Antianginal medications through the decades

comorbidities, to improve (soft) outcomes and avoid undesirable side effects [1, 18, 19]. Furthermore, targeting the pathophysiological substrate of myocardial ischemia may further improve therapeutic efficacy [65].

Antianginal drugs are classified as being first-line (BBs, CCBs, and short-acting nitrates on request) or second-line (long-acting nitrates, nicorandil, ivabradine, trimetazidine, and ranolazine) [1]. Second-line medications are usually destinated to patients who have contraindications, do not tolerate, or remain symptomatic despite first-line agents. However, no randomized clinical trial (RCT) has shown superiority of first-line over second-line treatments [1, 21]. A recent systematic review and meta-analysis has also showed that no one antianginal drug is superior to another and that equivalence has only been demonstrated for the use of BBs (atenolol), DHP CCBs (amlodipine, nifedipine), and I_f current inhibitors (ivabradine) [21].

Another meta-analysis supports the combination of DHP CCBs with BBs over monotherapy and to ranolazine added to either BBs or CCBs [66]. According to the same meta-analysis, adding long-acting nitrates and trimetazidine may be effective as well, although the evidence seems more scattered [66]. Similarly, ivabradine was shown to increase exercise time, angina attacks, and use on nitrates when added to BBs in the ASSOCIATE [67] and ADDITIONS [68] trials. There are no significant data for nicorandil as far as combination therapy is concerned [69].

Some authors have also highlighted that each drug/combination may have beneficial or detrimental effects on patients' specific characteristics, and thus a "*diamond*" approach similar to that employed in hypertension (i.e., leaving physician free to choose the most appropriate drug/combination according to patient-specific needs) has been proposed [18]. Considering the mechanisms of action, association of BBs or ivabradine with non-DHP CCBs is not recommended, whereas other combinations (i.e., nitrates/nicorandil with CCBs or ranolazine with trimetazidine) might be partially redundant, unless specific pathophysiology is considered (e.g., vasospastic angina) [18].

3.1 Vasodilators

3.1.1 Nitrates

Short- and long-acting nitrates represent an established class of antianginal drugs, whose effects depend on the release of NO through an enzymatic process (i.e., denitrification) taking place in the vessel walls [70]. By stimulating the soluble guanylyl cyclase of smooth muscle cells, NO promotes the production of cyclic guanosine monophosphate, leading to membrane hyperpolarization and reduction of Ca^{2+} inflow, with consequent vasodilation [70]. Whereas at low doses nitrates act mostly on the venous system (hence reducing pre-load), arterial vasodilation occurs at higher doses, favoring epicardial coronaries and collateral blood flow perfusion (even in the presence of luminal obstruction) and reducing post-load [71]. Although the potential reduction of myocardial oxygen consumption secondary to reduced pre- and post-load may be partially counterbalanced by an autonomic mediated increase in heart rate, the concomitant use of negative chronotropic drugs (e.g., BBs) may result in synergetic anti-ischemic effect [72]. Furthermore, thanks to their NO-dependent action, nitrates are also effective in relieving vasospastic [73] but not microvascular angina, probably because of the lower sensitivity of resistance arterioles to such signals at clinically used dosages [74].

As recommended by the current guidelines, short-acting nitrates are the first-line therapy to relieve effort angina (class of recommendation (CoR) I, level of evidence (LoE) B), while long-acting nitrates are second-line choices in the long term compared to BBs and non-DHP CCBs (CoR IIa, LoE B) [52]. Indeed, several RCTs have examined the efficacy of nitrates, and in a meta-analysis of 51 studies including a total of 3595 patients with stable angina, their long-term administration was found to be beneficial in preventing angina and improving exercise tolerance but not the overall quality of life [75]. On the other hand, only a few studies have evaluated the survival benefits of chronic nitrate administration in different subsets, yielding substantially neutral results [76–78].

Finally, because of their intense systemic vasodilator action, the use of nitrates may exacerbate various adverse effects, including headache, flushing, and hypotension, while they are not indicated in patients with intraventricular obstruction, severe aortic or mitral stenosis, and constrictive pericarditis, and they should be used with caution in concomitance with other vasodilators [71]. Another limitation for the use of nitrates is the risk of tolerance, with a reduction in their anti-ischemic efficacy [79], so that nitrate-free or low-nitrate intervals are suggested in patients on chronic therapy (CoR IIa, LoE B) [52]. Although the underlying mechanisms are still to be completely clarified, oxidative stress may contribute [79], while the use of alternative molecules may overcome such problem [80].

3.1.2 Nicorandil

Nicorandil is a nicotinamide-nitrate ester holding anti-ischemic properties related to its NO-donor capacity and to a direct stimulation of adenosine triphosphate-sensitive K^+ channels on arterial walls, together leading to vasodilatation, but also to possible metabolic effects [81–83]. Moreover, nicorandil may be effective in alleviating vasospasm [84], and growing evidence sustains a possible role also in the context of microvascular dysfunction, even though further research seems necessary to confirm such assumption and to clarify the biological mechanisms involved [85, 86].

The use of nicorandil in patients with stable angina has been evaluated in various RCTs, demonstrating good efficacy [20, 52]. Most notably, among 5126 patients with stable angina, nicorandil, compared to placebo, significantly reduced a composite endpoint of cardiovascular events, but not cardiac death or nonfatal myocardial infarction [87]. Therefore, it is considered a second-line treatment to reduce angina frequency and improve exercise tolerance (CoR IIa, LoE B) [52].

Despite the similar mechanisms of action, the use of nicorandil is associated with a lower risk of tolerance than nitrates, whereas nausea, vomiting, mucosal ulcerations, and, most importantly, headache are potential adverse effects, which could affect therapeutic adherence [52, 87].

3.1.3 Dihydropyridine Calcium Channel Blockers

CCBs are a heterogenous class of drugs, characterized by the inhibition of high-voltage-activated L-type Ca^{2+} channels on vascular smooth muscle cells and cardiomyocytes [88]. DHP CCBs (e.g., amlodipine, nicardipine, nifedipine) act more specifically on vascular channels, causing an intense coronary and systemic vasodilation, while they do not act on cardiomyocytes [89].

Beyond vasodilatation, DHP CCBs reduce myocardial oxygen demand by lowering systemic blood pressure (i.e., cardiac post-load) [88, 90] and are effective also in the case of vasospastic [91] and microvascular angina [92, 93], whereas the reflex increase in heart rate could be blunted by the use of BBs, further improving their anti-ischemic efficacy (CoR IIa, LoE B) [52, 94, 95]. In patients with stable angina, the use of nifedipine was associated with a reduced need for coronary angiography and intervention, despite no difference in cardiac death or myocardial infarction [96], while the use of amlodipine reduced the risk of adverse cardiovascular events and of atherosclerosis progression [97].

Although headache, ankle swelling, and hypotension represent possible side effects [89], DHP CCBs are usually well tolerated and represent first-line antianginal therapies (CoR I, LoE A) [52].

3.2 Drugs Reducing Myocardial Oxygen Consumption

3.2.1 Non-dihydropyridine Calcium Channel Blockers

Differently from DHP CCB, diltiazem and verapamil (i.e., non-DHP CCB) show a higher selectivity for myocardial than for vascular Ca^{2+} channels, and their anti-ischemic efficacy mostly relies upon the reduction of myocardial oxygen demand secondary to a negative inotropic and heart rate-dependent chronotropic effects [88, 89, 98]. The use of these drugs is therefore recommended to control heart rate and symptoms in patients with stable effort angina (CoR I, LoE A) [1], while they are routinely used also in patients with vasospastic angina [99] and may be effective in the case of microvascular dysfunction [100], where ongoing studies (e.g., NCT04777045) are expected to confirm such findings.

Although generally safe, RCTs failed to show any survival benefit with the use of diltiazem [101], while verapamil was shown to reduce adverse events only in patients after myocardial infarction and without heart failure [102]. Moreover, they share similar side effects with DHP CCBs, and they should be used with caution in patients at risk of sinus bradycardia or atrioventricular blocks and in those with systolic dysfunction [52, 88, 89].

3.2.2 Beta-Blockers

BBs are very effective antianginal therapies, as demonstrated by the high rate of patients free from anginal events after optimization of medical therapy in both the COURAGE (87% receiving BBs) [103] and the ORBITA (77% receiving BBs) [104] trials, and thus represent a first-line treatment to control heart rate and symptoms in patients with stable effort angina (CoR I, LoE A) [1].

Similarly to non-DHP CCBs, BBs' antianginal action mainly relies on the reduction of myocardial oxygen demand [19]. Their primary action is to decrease heart rate and thus to increase diastolic duration and coronary perfusion, in particular blood flow per heartbeat [105]. Although BBs have negative inotropic effects (less than non-DHP CCBs), by decreasing oxygen consumption in the healthy myocardium, they may increase perfusion to the post-stenotic myocardium and also its regional contractility [106, 107], but only if heart rate reduction is achieved [51]. However, they may also favor coronary vasoconstriction by blocking $\beta 2$-adrenergic receptors, so $\beta 1$-selective compounds, or BBs with vasodilatation capability, such as carvedilol—an α-β-blocker [108] [109]—or nebivolol, through NO release [110], are usually preferred in the treatment of CCS, unless a vasospastic component is hypothesized. In that case, BBs should be used with caution (i.e., low dose or adding a vasodilator) or avoided, similarly to other conditions such as asthma, baseline bradycardia, or evidence of atrioventricular conduction abnormalities.

Although several studies have investigated the prognostic effects of BBs, according to the main RCTs and meta-analyses [111], this seems limited to patients receiving BBs early after myocardial infarction [112] or with left ventricular systolic dysfunction [113].

3.2.3 Ivabradine

As non-DHP CCBs and BBs, also ivabradine's antianginal capacity derives from a reduction of heart rate. This is obtained through a selective inhibition of the I_f (or "funny," inward Na^+-K^+) current of the sinoatrial node [114, 115], which has a key role in the generation of spontaneous depolarization of pacemaker cells and in mediating the autonomic control of heart rate [116]. By inhibiting I_f current, ivabradine causes a decrease in the slope of depolarization, lowering heart rate [105] and promoting a proportionate improvement in ischemic regional blood flow and contractile function [117].

The risk of bradycardia with ivabradine is low, since its effect is heart rate dependent by acting on open channels [118]. Furthermore, ivabradine does not affect myocardial work or vascular tone, favoring its use when such effects would be undesirable (i.e., patients with hypotension) [119].

Despite those premises, the increased risk of cardiovascular death and nonfatal myocardial infarction observed in patients with CCS treated with ivabradine in the SIGNIFY trial [120] raised some concerns, which could have been at least partially explained by the concomitant use of non-DHP CCBs (which may inhibit the ivabradine-metabolizing cytochrome p450, i.e., CYP3A4) causing bradycardia in a relevant proportion of patients. Hence, this association should be avoided. On the contrary, no safety concerns were observed when administering ivabradine with BBs, in the BEAUTIFUL trial, in which ivabradine was however shown not to improve outcome in patients with CCS and left ventricular systolic dysfunction [121], apart from decreasing the risk of hospitalization for myocardial infarction or coronary revascularization in patients with a heart rate ≥70 bpm.

Of note, ivabradine may also be useful in improving symptoms in patients with microvascular dysfunction [122], even though future studies should confirm such findings. Finally, outside the CCS scenario, ivabradine was found to decrease the combined outcome of cardiovascular mortality and hospitalization (mainly driven by reduced hospitalizations for worsening heart failure) in patients with heart failure and reduced ejection fraction (89% on BBs) [123].

3.3 Myocyte Metabolism Modulators

3.3.1 Trimetazidine

Trimetazidine increases cellular tolerance to ischemia by decreasing fatty acid metabolism through the inhibition of 3-ketoacyl CoA thiolase, shifting myocardial metabolism toward pyruvate oxidation [56, 61]. Trimetazidine also stimulates glucose metabolism and insulin sensitivity [124].

The antianginal/anti-ischemic effects of trimetazidine are similar to those obtained with BBs or CCBs [125]. Of note, the absence of relevant hemodynamic consequences [126] prompts the use of this molecule as a second-line treatment in patients that do not tolerate, have contraindications to, or whose symptoms are not adequately controlled by BBs, CCBs, and long-acting nitrates (CoR IIa, LoE B) [1]. When used in combination with metoprolol, trimetazidine was shown to decrease angina and increase exercise duration and time to ST-segment depression compared to metoprolol alone in 426 patients with stable, effort-induced angina and documented CAD (TRIMPOL II trial) [127]. Similar findings were obtained adding trimetazidine to atenolol in the VASCO trial [128] or to diltiazem [129]. The overall beneficial effect of trimetazidine on anginal attacks, daily use of nitrates, exercise duration, and time to ST-segment depression has been confirmed also in three meta-analyses [130–132]. Trimetazidine prolonged exercise time and time to ST depression also in patients with microvascular angina in a small placebo-controlled RCT [133]. On the contrary, ranolazine seems ineffective on major cardiovascular adverse events or angina recurrence in patients who have undergone successful percutaneous coronary intervention from the ATPCI trial (n = 6007) [134]. Trimetazidine remains contraindicated in Parkinson's disease and motion disorders, such as tremor (shaking), muscle rigidity, walking disorders, and restless leg syndrome [1].

3.3.2 Ranolazine

Ranolazine, similarly to trimetazidine, is a metabolic antianginal agent, which inhibits fatty acid oxidation in the mitochondria and favors glucose metabolism [135]. Its main mechanism of action is however to increase myocardial relaxation by reducing Ca^{2+} overload caused by inhibition of late Na^{+} currents [136]. Like trimetazidine, also ranolazine does not affect heart rate or blood pressure and therefore may be used in patients with hypotension or bradycardia [137, 138].

The antianginal properties of ranolazine have been evaluated in several RCTs. In patients with CCS, the use of ranolazine was associated with fewer angina episodes and longer exercise duration compared to placebo [138], in both patients without other antianginal therapies or already on standard treatment [139–141]. Ranolazine was shown to improve angina and use of nitrate in patients with diabetes compared to placebo [142], but did not reduce angina, need for repeated revascularization, or angina-related hospitalizations in patients with incomplete revascularization: a high nonadherence to the drug may partly explain such findings [143]. Likewise, ranolazine seems ineffective in patients with microvascular disease [144]. An exception seems to be represented by women with microvascular angina, in whom ranolazine was shown to improve angina and myocardial ischemia, albeit only in those with reduced coronary flow reserve [145]. Ranolazine seems to be also not beneficial in patients with acute coronary syndrome as shown in the MERLIN-TIMI trial [146], even though a possible antiarrhythmic effect has been observed in this scenario [147].

In 2017, a Cochrane systematic review and meta-analysis on the use of ranolazine in patients with CCS has been published, highlighting the positive effect of ranolazine on angina (moderate quality of data), some evidence of increased risk of nonserious side effects (low quality of data), and an uncertain effect on both overall and cardiovascular mortality (low quality of data) [148].

Side effects of ranolazine, such as dizziness, nausea, and constipation, are dose dependent [149]. The inhibition of late sodium currents, together with its effect on delayed rectifier potassium currents, also causes prolongation of QT interval [149], and thus ranolazine should be avoided in patients with long QT interval or already taking QT-prolonging drugs. However, no significant increase in life-threatening arrythmias has been noticed in multiple safety studies [150].

4 Novel Perspectives from Animal Models and Human Studies

Therapeutic efficacy, safety profile, and cost-effectiveness are essential factors to be considered when designing a novel drug [151]. Standing this premise, several anti-ischemic compounds are on the pipeline. Novel vasodilators, metabolic modulators, as well as angiogenetic factors and cell therapies represent possible opportunities, especially for patients with refractory angina (Fig. 3).

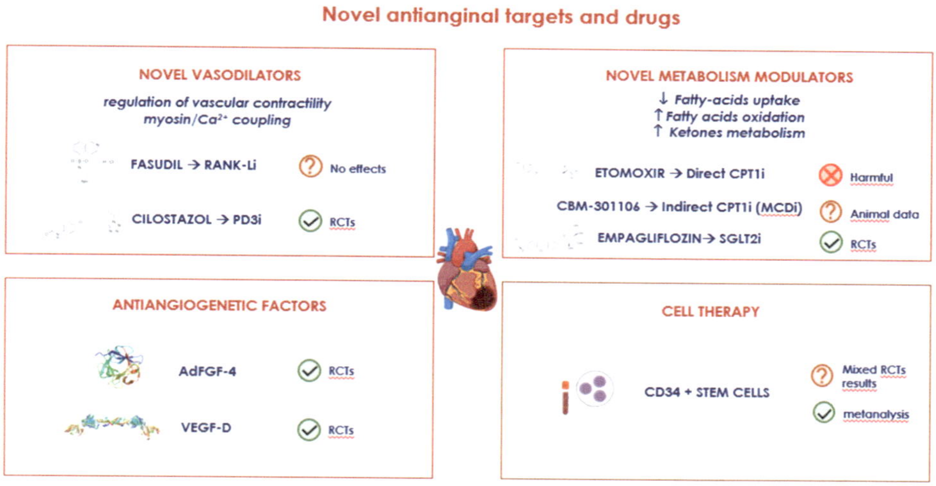

Fig. 3 Novel antianginal targets and drugs. *CPT1i* inhibitor of carnitine palmitoyltransferase I; *FGF* fibroblast growth factor; *MCDi* inhibitor of malonyl-CoA decarboxylase; *PDE3i* inhibitor of phosphodiesterase 3; *RANKL-i* inhibitor of the receptor activator of nuclear factor kappa-B ligand; *RCTs* randomized controlled trials; *SGLT2i* inhibitor of sodium glucose transporter 2; *VEGF* vascular endothelial growth factor

4.1 Novel Compounds with Vasodilatory Effects

The small guanosine triphosphatase RhoA and its downstream effector Rho-kinase are involved in the regulation of vascular contractility, leading through inhibition myosin light-chain phosphatase to Ca^{2+} sensitization in response to vasoconstrictor stimuli [152]. Fasudil, a Rho-kinase inhibitor approved in Japan for the prevention of cerebral artery vasospasm in the setting of subarachnoid hemorrhage [153], has been tested in animal studies and in small trials in patients with microvascular spasm [154] and in patients with stable angina [155]. While fasudil intracoronary infusion was shown to prevent Ach-mediated vasoconstriction [153], fasudil oral administration only increased time to ST depression and had no effect on symptoms in humans [155]. To date, no Rho-kinase inhibitor has been approved for the treatment of vasospastic angina, and more clinical evidence is needed.

A selective phosphodiesterase-3-inhibitor, cilostazol, has also been shown to be efficacious in vasospastic angina in small clinical trials [156, 157], although its mechanism of action remains to be elucidated. In 49 patients with vasospastic angina, cilostazol decreased weakly angina episodes, proportion of angina-free period of angina severity compared to placebo, at the cost of increased rate of headache [157]. Still, its efficacy, dosage, and safety should be confirmed in larger RCTs.

4.2 Novel Modulators of Myocardial Metabolism

Since alterations in myocardial substrate preference contribute to energetic inefficiency, contractile dysfunction, and severity of ischemia, novel drugs inhibiting fatty acid oxidation or increasing the coupling of glycolysis to glucose oxidation represent promising approaches in CCS [158].

Decreasing myocardial fatty acid uptake may be obtained by acting on CD-36 (a sarcolemmal transporter responsible for up to 50% of cardiac fatty acid uptake) [159], and sulfo-N-succinimidyl-oleate was shown to inhibit fatty acid uptake in vitro in various cell lines including cardiomyocytes [160]. Interestingly, its infusion increased the glycolytic rate by 46% and pyruvate-dehydrogenase activity by 53%, while it decreased lactate efflux rate by 56% in the hearts of diabetic rats during hypoxia, compared with untreated rats, preventing cardiac dysfunction in hypoxic conditions. Although promising, whether this compound might be beneficial in CCS is still to be demonstrated.

The rate of cardiac fatty acid oxidation is regulated by the activity of carnitine palmitoyltransferase-I. While the use of direct inhibitors (e.g., etomoxir, perhexiline, oxfenicine, teglicar) may be burdened by hepatotoxic and cardiotoxic effects due to unspecific mitochondrial effects [161], an indirect inhibition of this pathway by malonyl-CoA may be a promising approach. CBM-301106 inhibits malonyl-CoA decarboxylase, which catalyzes degradation of malonyl-CoA converting it to acetyl-CoA and thus decreases long-chain fatty acid metabolism [161]. This molecule reduced fatty acid oxidation and lactate production during demand-induced ischemia in various rat and pig models of ischemic heart disease [162–164], but it has to be tested in humans.

The role of ketones in cardiac energetics may be important in the condition of limited energy supply, as in the case of the failing heart [165]. Whether ketone metabolism may be a "super-fuel," increasing cardiac efficiency or changing fatty acid oxidation or glucose metabolism, is still debated [166, 167]. In this respect, the positive effects of Na^+-glucose-cotransporter-2-inhibitors (SGLT2-i) on cardiovascular outcomes in diabetic patients and in those with heart failure could be partially ascribed to an increased cardiac consumption of ketone bodies [168, 169]. However, the increase in ketone bodies following administration of SGLT2-i is usually mild and higher during fasting (i.e., at night) [169]. Therefore, it is currently unknown whether this may be sufficient to change myocardial metabolism (especially during daily activity), so as to have favorable effects on patients with CCS. Of note, empagliflozin has been recently shown to decrease contractile dysfunction and arrhythmias following ischemia in Langendorff-perfused rabbit heart [170], but the effects on ketone bodies were not assessed. This topic should be then addressed by dedicated studies.

4.3 Angiogenetic Factors

Vascular endothelial growth factors (VEGF) and fibroblast growth factors (FGF) have been tested in a few studies mainly in the setting of refractory angina [171], starting from the pioneering works in rabbit with hindlimb ischemia by Takeshita [172] and in humans by the group of Isner [173]. However, in the setting of RCTs, the percutaneous intracoronary administration or epicardial injection of VEGF (during bypass surgery) via naked plasmid or adenoviral vectors failed to deliver significant clinical effects, although no significant long-term side effect was observed [174].

On the other hand, intracoronary adenoviral mediated FGF-4 delivery improved exercise time in postmenopausal women as shown in a pooled analysis of the AGENT-3 and AGENT-4 trials [171]. The results of two similar trials, the Russian ASPIRE trial (NCT01550614) [174] based on intracoronary administration of Ad5FGF-4 (open-label design, no placebo, completed in 2016) and the AWARE trial [174] based on intracoronary administration of AdFGF-4 only in women with stable angina, have never been published.

Finally, intramyocardial adenoviral delivery of VEGF-D showed promising results in the KAT301 (phase I–IIa, $n = 60$) trial [175], where VEGF-D administration was associated with a significant improvement of myocardial perfusion reserve, reduction of angina, and improvement of quality of life, differently from placebo, especially in patients with high lipoprotein (a) levels. A larger phase IIb multicentric trial on VEFG-D is currently ongoing [171].

4.4 Cell Therapy

Similarly to angiogenetic factors, cell therapy has also been tested in refractory angina [171], but also in myocardial infarction and heart failure [176]. Although bone marrow-derived progenitors do not transform into myocytes, they may exert paracrine effects. Different pro-angiogenic cells were administered in an autologous setting, including unfractionated bone marrow-derived mononuclear cells, selected endothelial progenitors (i.e., CD34+ and CD133+ cells), or mesenchymal stem [177].

In the ACT34-CMI placebo-controlled trial ($n = 167$), patients with refractory angina receiving intramyocardial injection of CD34+ stem cells showed improved exercise tolerance ($p = 0.01$) and angina frequency ($p = 0.02$), also after a 2-year follow-up, where a trend of reduction in major events was observed as well [178]. Conversely, the RENEW trial was prematurely terminated by the sponsor for strategic consideration after enrolling only 112 of the 444 patients originally planned, showing a borderline reduction ($p = 0.05$) in angina frequency and only a trend toward an increase in exercise time at 3 months ($p = 0.06$), lost at 6 and 12 months. In a meta-analysis [179] including 3 phase II trials and 269 patients, intramyocardial therapy with CD34+ stem cells was superior to placebo in improving angina frequency, increasing exercise time, and decreasing mortality, without significant adverse events, thus supporting future larger trials in refractory angina patients.

5 Conclusions

Various anti-ischemic medications are currently available and extensively used in the routine clinical practice. Although their prognostic benefits are poor or scarcely investigated, they seem to be equally effective in relieving angina and improving quality of life. However, considering the multifactorial pathophysiology of myocardial ischemia and the heterogeneity of patients with CCS, a more rational patient-tailored use of anti-ischemic drugs may yield further benefits. Finally, various promising molecules are emerging from exploratory animal and preliminary clinical studies and may prove their value in the next future.

References

1. Knuuti J, Wijns W, Saraste A, Capodanno D, Barbato E, Funck-Brentano C, et al. 2019 ESC Guidelines for the diagnosis and management of chronic coronary syndromes: the Task Force for the Diagnosis and Management of Chronic Coronary Syndromes of the European Society of Cardiology (ESC). Eur Heart J. 2020;41(3):407–77.
2. Kaski J-C, Crea F, Gersh BJ, Camici PG. Reappraisal of ischemic heart disease. Circulation. 2018;138(14):1463–80.
3. Crea F, Camici PG, Bairey Merz CN. Coronary microvascular dysfunction: an update. Eur Heart J. 2014;35(17):1101–11.
4. Nesto RW, Kowalchuk GJ. The ischemic cascade: temporal sequence of hemodynamic, electrocardiographic and symptomatic expressions of ischemia. Am J Cardiol. 1987;59(7):C23–30.
5. O'Sullivan JJ, Conroy RM, MacDonald K, McKenna TJ, Maurer BJ. Silent ischaemia in diabetic men with autonomic neuropathy. Br Heart J. 1991;66(4):313–5.
6. Marchant B, Umachandran V, Stevenson R, Kopelman PG, Timmis AD. Silent myocardial ischemia: role of subclinical neuropathy in patients with and without diabetes. J Am Coll Cardiol. 1993;22(5):1433–7.
7. Deedwania PC, Carbajal EV. Silent myocardial ischemia: a clinical perspective. Arch Intern Med. 1991;151(12):2373–82.
8. Group MRFITR. Exercise electrocardiogram and coronary heart disease mortality in the Multiple Risk Factor Intervention Trial. Am J Cardiol. 1985 Jan;1(55):16–24.
9. Yeung AC, Barry J, Orav J, Bonassin E, Raby KE, Selwyn AP. Effects of asymptomatic ischemia on long-term prognosis in chronic stable coronary disease. Circulation. 1991;83(5):1598–604.
10. Laukkanen JA, Kurl S, Lakka TA, Tuomainen T-P, Rauramaa R, Salonen R, et al. Exercise-induced silent myocardial ischemia and coronary morbidity and mortality in middle-aged men. J Am Coll Cardiol. 2001;38:72–9.

11. Sajadieh A, Nielsen OW, Rasmussen V, Hein HO, Hansen JF. Prevalence and prognostic significance of daily-life silent myocardial ischaemia in middle-aged and elderly subjects with no apparent heart disease. Eur Heart J. 2005;26(14):1402–9.
12. Ferrari R, Camici PG, Crea F, Danchin N, Fox K, Maggioni AP, et al. A "diamond" approach to personalized treatment of angina. Nat Rev Cardiol. 2018;15:120–32.
13. Group TIS. Effect of nicorandil on coronary events in patients with stable angina: the Impact Of Nicorandil in Angina (IONA) randomised trial. Lancet. 2002;359(9314):1269–75.
14. Newby DE, Williams MC. Dweck MR. Forget ischemia: it's all about the plaque: Circulation; 2021. p. 1039–41.
15. Ryan M, Morgan H, Chiribiri A, Nagel E, Cleland J, Perera D. Myocardial viability testing: all STICHed up, or about to be REVIVED? Eur Heart J. 2021:ehab729.
16. Crossman DC. The pathophysiology of myocardial ischaemia. Heart. 2004;90(5):576.
17. Marzilli M, Merz CNB, Boden WE, Bonow RO, Capozza PG, Chilian WM, et al. Obstructive coronary atherosclerosis and ischemic heart disease: an elusive link! J Am Coll Cardiol. 2012;60(11):951–6.
18. Ferrari R, Camici PG, Crea F, Danchin N, Fox K, Maggioni AP, et al. Expert consensus document: a "diamond" approach to personalized treatment of angina. Nat Rev Cardiol. 2018;15(2):120–32.
19. Bertero E, Heusch G, Münzel T, Maack C. A pathophysiological compass to personalize antianginal drug treatment. Nat Rev Cardiol. 2021;18(12):838–52.
20. Husted SE, Ohman EM. Pharmacological and emerging therapies in the treatment of chronic angina. Lancet (London, England). 2015;386(9994):691–701.
21. Ferrari R, Pavasini R, Camici PG, Crea F, Danchin N, Pinto F, et al. Anti-anginal drugs–beliefs and evidence: systematic review covering 50 years of medical treatment. Eur Heart J. 2019;40(2):190–4.
22. Mosher P, Ross J, Mcfate P, Shaw R. Control of coronary blood flow by an autoregulatory mechanism. Circ Res. 1964;14:250–9.
23. Heusch G. The paradox of α-adrenergic coronary vasoconstriction revisited. J Mol Cell Cardiol. 2011;51(1):16–23.
24. Deussen A, Ohanyan V, Jannasch A, Yin L, Chilian W. Mechanisms of metabolic coronary flow regulation. J Mol Cell Cardiol. 2012;52(4):794–801.
25. Gould KL, Lipscomb K. Effects of coronary stenoses on coronary flow reserve and resistance. Am J Cardiol. 1974;34(1):48–55.
26. Aversano T, Becker LC. Persistence of coronary vasodilator reserve despite functionally significant flow reduction. Am J Phys 1985;248(3 Pt 2).
27. Canty JM, Klocke FJ. Reduced regional myocardial perfusion in the presence of pharmacologic vasodilator reserve. Circulation. 1985;71(2):370–7.
28. Heusch G, Guth BD, Seitelberger R, Ross J. Attenuation of exercise-induced myocardial ischemia in dogs with recruitment of coronary vasodilator reserve by nifedipine. Circulation. 1987;75(2):482–90.
29. Patel MR, Peterson ED, Dai D, Brennan JM, Redberg RF, Anderson HV, et al. Low diagnostic yield of elective coronary angiography. N Engl J Med. 2010;362(10):886–95.
30. Douglas PS, Patel MR, Bailey SR, Dai D, Kaltenbach L, Brindis RG, et al. Hospital variability in the rate of finding obstructive coronary artery disease at elective, diagnostic coronary angiography. J Am Coll Cardiol. 2011;58(8):801–9.
31. Arnold JR, Karamitsos TD, Van Gaal WJ, Testa L, Francis JM, Bhamra-Ariza P, et al. Residual ischemia after revascularization in multivessel coronary artery disease: insights from measurement of absolute myocardial blood flow using magnetic resonance imaging compared with angiographic assessment. Circ Cardiovasc Interv. 2013;6(3):237–45.

32. Prinzmetal M, Kennamer R, Merliss R, Wada T, Bor N. Angina pectoris I. A variant form of angina pectoris: preliminary report. Am J Med. 1959;27(3):375–88.
33. Sun H, Mohri M, Shimokawa H, Usui M, Urakami L, Takeshita A. Coronary microvascular spasm causes myocardial ischemia in patients with vasospastic angina. J Am Coll Cardiol. 2002;39(5):847–51.
34. Ong P, Athanasiadis A, Borgulya G, Mahrholdt H, Kaski JC, Sechtem U. High prevalence of a pathological response to acetylcholine testing in patients with stable angina pectoris and unobstructed coronary arteries: the ACOVA study (Abnormal COronary VAsomotion in patients with stable angina and unobstructed coronary arteries). J Am Coll Cardiol. 2012;59(7):655–62.
35. Furchgott RF, Zawadzki JV. The obligatory role of endothelial cells in the relaxation of arterial smooth muscle by acetylcholine. Nature. 1980;288(5789):373–6.
36. Yasue H, Horio Y, Nakamura N, Fujii H, Imoto N, Sonoda R, et al. Induction of coronary artery spasm by acetylcholine in patients with variant angina: possible role of the parasympathetic nervous system in the pathogenesis of coronary artery spasm. Circulation. 1986;74(5):955–63.
37. Rosenthal SJ, Ginsburg R, Lamb IH, Baim DS, Schroeder JS. Efficacy of diltiazem for control of symptoms of coronary arterial spasm. Am J Cardiol. 1980 Dec;46(6):1027–32.
38. Antman E, Muller J, Goldberg S, MacAlpin R, Rubenfire M, Tabatznik B, et al. Nifedipine therapy for coronary-artery spasm. Experience in 127 patients. N Engl J Med. 1980;302(23):1269–73.
39. Conti CR. Large vessel coronary vasospasm: diagnosis, natural history and treatment. Am J Cardiol. 1985;55(3).
40. Aizawa T, Ogasawara K, Nakamura F, Hirosaka A, Sakuma T, Nagashima K, et al. Effect of nicorandil on coronary spasm. Am J Cardiol. 1989;63(21).
41. Marie Robertson R, Wood AJ, Vaughn WK, Robertson D. Exacerbation of vasotonic angina pectoris by propranolol. Circulation. 1982;65:281–5.
42. Crea F, Lanza GA. Angina pectoris and normal coronary arteries: cardiac syndrome X. Heart. 2004;90(4):457–63.
43. Camici PG, Crea F. Coronary microvascular dysfunction. N Engl J Med. 2009;356(8):830–40.
44. Lundberg JO, Weitzberg E, Gladwin MT. The nitrate–nitrite–nitric oxide pathway in physiology and therapeutics. Nat Rev Drug Discov. 2008;7(2):156–67.
45. Kaski JC, Rosano GMC, Collins P, Nihoyannopoulos P, Maseri A, Poole-Wilson PA. Cardiac syndrome X: clinical characteristics and left ventricular function. Long-term follow-up study. J Am Coll Cardiol. 1995;25(4):807–14.
46. Sütsch G, Oechslin E, Mayer I, Hess OM. Effect of diltiazem on coronary flow reserve in patients with microvascular angina. Int J Cardiol. 1995;52(2):135–43.
47. Ohba K, Sugiyama S, Sumida H, Nozaki T, Matsubara J, Matsuzawa Y, et al. Microvascular coronary artery spasm presents distinctive clinical features with endothelial dysfunction as nonobstructive coronary artery disease. J Am Heart Assoc. 2012;1(5).
48. Pauly DF, Johnson BD, Anderson RD, Handberg EM, Smith KM, Cooper-Dehoff RM, et al. In women with symptoms of cardiac ischemia, nonobstructive coronary arteries, and microvascular dysfunction, angiotensin-converting enzyme inhibition is associated with improved microvascular function: a double-blind randomized study from the National Hea. Am Heart J. 2011;162(4):678–84.
49. Crea F, Pupita G, Galassi AR, El-Tamimi H, Kaski JC, Davies G, et al. Role of adenosine in pathogenesis of anginal pain. Circulation. 1990;81(1):164–72.
50. Ferrari R, Fox K. Heart rate reduction in coronary artery disease and heart failure. Nat Rev Cardiol. 2016;13(8):493–501.
51. Guth BD, Heusch G, Seitelberger R, Ross J. Mechanism of beneficial effect of beta-adrenergic blockade on exercise-induced myocardial ischemia in conscious dogs. Circ Res. 1987;60(5):738–46.

52. Neumann FJ, Sechtem U, Banning AP, Bonaros N, Bueno H, Bugiardini R, et al. 2019 ESC Guidelines for the diagnosis and management of chronic coronary syndromes. The Task Force for the diagnosis and management of chronic coronary syndromes of the European Society of Cardiology (ESC). Eur Heart J. 2020;41(3):407–77.
53. Steg PG, De Silva R. Beta-blockers in asymptomatic coronary artery disease no benefit or no evidence? J Am Coll Cardiol. 2014;64(3):253–5.
54. Borer JS, Le Heuzey JY. Characterization of the heart rate-lowering action of ivabradine, a selective I(f) current inhibitor. Am J Ther. 2008;15(5):461–73.
55. Stanley WC, Recchia FA, Lopaschuk GD. Myocardial substrate metabolism in the normal and failing heart. Physiol Rev. 2005;85(3):1093–129.
56. Kantor PF, Lucien A, Kozak R, Lopaschuk GD. The antianginal drug trimetazidine shifts cardiac energy metabolism from fatty acid oxidation to glucose oxidation by inhibiting mitochondrial long-chain 3-ketoacyl coenzyme A thiolase. Circ Res. 2000;86(5):580–8.
57. Hasenfuss G, Maier LS. Mechanism of action of the new anti-ischemia drug ranolazine. Clin Res Cardiol. 2008;97(4):222.
58. Lauder Brunton T. ON THE USE OF NITRITE OF AMYL IN ANGINA PECTORIS. Lancet. 1867;90(2291):97–8.
59. Srivastava SC, Dewar HA, Newell DJ. Double-blind Trial of Propranolol (Inderal) in Angina of Effort. Br Med J. 1964;2(5411):724 LP–725.
60. Melville KI, Shister HE, Huq S. Iproveratril: experimental data on coronary dilatation and antiarrhythmic action. Can Med Assoc J. 1964;90(13):761–70.
61. Mehrotra TN, Bassadone ET. Trimetazidine in the treatment of angina pectoris. Br J Clin Pr. 1967;21(11):553–4.
62. Sakai K, Shiraki Y, Nabata H. Cardiovascular effects of a new coronary vasodilator N-(2-hydroxyethyl)nicotinamide nitrate (SG-75): comparison with nitroglycerin and diltiazem. J Cardiovasc Pharmacol. 1981;3(1).
63. Vilaine JP. The discovery of the selective if current inhibitor ivabradine: a new therapeutic approach to ischemic heart disease. Pharmacol Res. 2006;53(5):424–34.
64. Jain D, Dasgupta P, Hughes LO, Lahiri A, Raftery EB. Ranolazine (RS-43285): a preliminary study of a new anti-anginal agent with selective effect on ischaemic myocardium. Eur J Clin Pharmacol. 1990;38(2):111–4.
65. Ford TJ, Stanley B, Good R, Rocchiccioli P, McEntegart M, Watkins S, et al. Stratified medical therapy using invasive coronary function testing in angina: the CorMicA trial. J Am Coll Cardiol. 2018;72(23):2841–55.
66. Klein WW, Jackson G, Tavazzi L. Efficacy of monotherapy compared with combined antianginal drugs in the treatment of chronic stable angina pectoris: a meta-analysis. Coron Artery Dis. 2002;13(8):427–36.
67. Tardif J-C, Ponikowski P, Kahan T, Investigators AS. Efficacy of the I(f) current inhibitor ivabradine in patients with chronic stable angina receiving beta-blocker therapy: a 4-month, randomized, placebo-controlled trial. Eur Heart J. 2009;30(5):540–8.
68. Werdan K, Ebelt H, Nuding S, Höpfner F, Hack G, Müller-Werdan U. Ivabradine in combination with beta-blocker improves symptoms and quality of life in patients with stable angina pectoris: results from the ADDITIONS study. Clin Res Cardiol. 2012;101(5):365–73.
69. Belsey J, Savelieva I, Mugelli A, Camm AJ. Relative efficacy of antianginal drugs used as add-on therapy in patients with stable angina: a systematic review and meta-analysis. Eur J Prev Cardiol. 2015;22(7):837–48.
70. Torfgård KE, Ahlner J. Mechanisms of action of nitrates. Cardiovasc Drugs Ther. 1994;8(5):701–17.
71. Parker JD, Parker JO. Nitrate therapy for stable angina pectoris. NEJM. 2009;338(8):520–31.

72. Andersson KE, Hoglund P. Combination of nitrates with other antianginal drugs. Drugs. 1987;33 Suppl 4(4):43–8.
73. Harris JR, Hale GM, Dasari TW, Schwier NC. Pharmacotherapy of vasospastic angina. J Cardiovasc Pharmacol Ther. 2016;21(5):439–51.
74. Lanza GA, Manzoli A, Bia E, Crea F, Maseri A. Acute effects of nitrates on exercise testing in patients with syndrome X. Clinical and pathophysiological implications. Circulation. 1994;90(6):2695–700.
75. Wei J, Wu T, Yang Q, Chen M, Ni J, Huang D. Nitrates for stable angina: a systematic review and meta-analysis of randomized clinical trials. Int J Cardiol. 2011;146(1):4–12.
76. Kojima S, Matsui K, Sakamoto T, Ishihara M, Kimura K, Miyazaki S, et al. Long-term nitrate therapy after acute myocardial infarction does not improve or aggravate prognosis. Circ J. 2007;71(3):301–7.
77. Takahashi J, Nihei T, Takagi Y, et al. Prognostic impact of chronic nitrate therapy in patients with vasospastic angina: multicentre registry study of the Japanese coronary spasm association. Eur Heart J. 2015;36(4):228–37.
78. Ural D, Kandemir AŞ, Karaüzüm K, Baydemir C, Karaüzüm İY, Bozyel S, et al. Effect of oral nitrates on all-cause mortality and hospitalization in heart failure patients with reduced ejection fraction: a propensity-matched analysis. J Card Fail. 2017;23(4):286–92.
79. Münzel T, Daiber A, Mülsch A. Explaining the phenomenon of nitrate tolerance. Circ Res. 2005;97(7):618–28.
80. Sekiya M, Sato M, Funada J, Ohtani T, Akutsu H, Watanabe K. Effects of the long-term administration of nicorandil on vascular endothelial function and the progression of arteriosclerosis. J Cardiovasc Pharmacol. 2005;46(1):63–7.
81. Suryapranata H, Serruys PW, De Feyter PJ, Verdouw PD, Hugenholtz PG. Coronary vasodilatory action after a single dose of nicorandil. Am J Cardiol. 1988;61(4):292–7.
82. Ogino K, Osaki S, Noguchi N, Kitamura H, Omodani H, Kato M, et al. Nicorandil suppressed myocardial purine metabolism during exercise in patients with angina pectoris. Eur J Clin Pharmacol. 1995;48(3–4):189–94.
83. Cheng K, Alhumood K, El Shaer F, De Silva R. The role of nicorandil in the management of chronic coronary syndromes in the gulf region. Adv Ther. 2021;38(2):925–48.
84. Kaski JC. Management of vasospastic angina--role of nicorandil. Cardiovasc Drugs Ther. 1995;9(2 Supplement):221–7.
85. Jia Q, Shi S, Yuan G, Shi J, Shi S, Wei Y, et al. The effect of nicorandil in patients with cardiac syndrome X: a meta-analysis of randomized controlled trials. Medicine (Baltimore). 2020;99(37):e22167.
86. Hirohata A, Yamamoto K, Hirose E, Kobayashi Y, Takafuji H, Sano F, et al. Nicorandil prevents microvascular dysfunction resulting from PCI in patients with stable angina pectoris: a randomised study. EuroIntervention. 2014;9(9):1050–8.
87. Dargie HJ. Effect of nicorandil on coronary events in patients with stable angina: the Impact Of Nicorandil in Angina (IONA) randomised trial. Lancet (London, England). 2002;359(9314):1269–75.
88. Abernethy DR, Schwartz JB. Calcium-antagonist drugs. NEJM. 2008;341(19):1447–57.
89. Godfraind T. Discovery and development of calcium channel blockers. Front Pharmacol. 2017;8:286.
90. Ezekowitz MD, Hossack K, Mehta JL, Thadani U, Weidler DJ, Kostuk W, et al. Amlodipine in chronic stable angina: results of a multicenter double-blind crossover trial. Am Heart J. 1995;129(3):527–35.
91. Chahine RA, Feldman RL, Giles TD, Nicod P, Raizner AE, Weiss RJ, et al. Randomized placebo-controlled trial of amlodipine in vasospastic angina. Amlodipine Study 160 Group. J Am Coll Cardiol. 1993;21(6):1365–70.

92. Cannon RO, Watson RM, Rosing DR, Epstein SE. Efficacy of calcium channel blocker therapy for angina pectoris resulting from small-vessel coronary artery disease and abnormal vasodilator reserve. Am J Cardiol. 1985;56(4):242–6.
93. Ong P, Athanasiadis A, Sechtem U. Pharmacotherapy for coronary microvascular dysfunction. Eur Hear J Cardiovasc Pharmacother. 2015;1(1):65–71.
94. Leon MB, Rosing DR, Bonow RO, Epstein SE. Combination therapy with calcium-channel blockers and beta blockers for chronic stable angina pectoris. Am J Cardiol. 1985;55(3):69B–80B.
95. Frishman WH, Glasser S, Stone P, Deedwania PC, Johnson M, Fakouhi TD. Comparison of controlled-onset, extended-release verapamil with amlodipine and amlodipine plus atenolol on exercise performance and ambulatory ischemia in patients with chronic stable angina pectoris. Am J Cardiol. 1999;83(4):507–14.
95. Poole-Wilson PPA, Lubsen PJ, Kirwan BA, Van Dalen FJ, Wagener G, Danchin PN, et al. Effect of long-acting nifedipine on mortality and cardiovascular morbidity in patients with stable angina requiring treatment (ACTION trial): randomised controlled trial. Lancet (London, England). 2004;364(9437):849–57.
97. Nissen SE, Tuzcu EM, Libby P, Thompson PD, Ghali M, Garza D, et al. Effect of antihypertensive agents on cardiovascular events in patients with coronary disease and normal blood pressure: the CAMELOT study: a randomized controlled trial. JAMA. 2004;292(18):2217–26.
98. Talajic M, Nattel S. Frequency-dependent effects of calcium antagonists on atrioventricular conduction and refractoriness: demonstration and characterization in anesthetized dogs. Circulation. 1986;74(5):1156–67.
99. Schroeder JS, Feldman RL, Giles TD, Friedman MJ, DeMaria AN, Kinney EL, et al. Multiclinic controlled trial of diltiazem for Prinzmetal's angina. Am J Med. 1982;72(2):227–32.
100. Zhang X, Li Q, Zhao J, Li X, Sun X, Yang H, et al. Effects of combination of statin and calcium channel blocker in patients with cardiac syndrome X. Coron Artery Dis. 2014;25(1):40–4.
101. The effect of diltiazem on mortality and reinfarction after myocardial infarction. N Engl J Med. 1988;319(7):385–92.
102. Hansen JF, Mellemgaard K, Pedersen-Bjergaard O, Rasmussen B, Launbjerg J, Fruergaard P, et al. Effect of verapamil on mortality and major events after acute myocardial infarction (the Danish Verapamil Infarction Trial II--DAVIT II). Am J Cardiol. 1990;66(10):779–85.
103. Weintraub WS, Spertus JA, Kolm P, Maron DJ, Zhang Z, Jurkovitz C, et al. Effect of PCI on quality of life in patients with stable coronary disease. NEJM. 2008;359(7):677–87.
104. Al-Lamee R, Thompson D, Dehbi H-M, Sen S, Tang K, Davies J, et al. Percutaneous coronary intervention in stable angina (ORBITA): a double-blind, randomised controlled trial. Lancet. 2018;391(10115):31–40.
105. Heusch G. Heart rate in the pathophysiology of coronary blood flow and myocardial ischaemia: benefit from selective bradycardic agents. Br J Pharmacol. 2008;153(8):1589–601.
106. Buck JD, Hardman HF, Warltier DC, Gross GJ. Changes in ischemic blood flow distribution and dynamic severity of a coronary stenosis induced by beta blockade in the canine heart. Circulation. 1981;64(4):708–15.
107. Matsuzaki M, Patritti J, Tajimi T, Miller M, Kemper WS, Ross J. Effects of beta-blockade on regional myocardial flow and function during exercise. Am J Physiol Circ Physiol. 1984;247(1):H52–60.
108. Tham TC, Guy S, McDermott BJ, Shanks RG, Riddell JG. The dose dependency of the alpha- and beta-adrenoceptor antagonist activity of carvedilol in man. Br J Clin Pharmacol. 1995;40(1):19–23.
109. Seitelberger R, Guth BD, Heusch G, Lee JD, Katayama K, Ross J. Intracoronary alpha 2-adrenergic receptor blockade attenuates ischemia in conscious dogs during exercise. Circ Res. 1988;62(3):436–42.

110. Bowman AJ, Chen CP, Ford GA. Nitric oxide mediated venodilator effects of nebivolol. Br J Clin Pharmacol. 1994;38(3):199–204.
111. Safi S, Sethi NJ, Nielsen EE, Feinberg J, Jakobsen JC, Gluud C. Beta-blockers for suspected or diagnosed acute myocardial infarction. Cochrane Database Syst Rev. 2019;12(12):CD012484.
112. COMMIT (ClOpidogrel and Metoprolol in Myocardial Infarction Trial) collaborative group. Early intravenous then oral metoprolol in 45852 patients with acute myocardial infarction: randomised placebo-controlled trial. Lancet. 2005;366(9497):1622–32.
113. Dondo TB, Hall M, West RM, Jernberg T, Lindahl B, Bueno H, et al. β-blockers and mortality after acute myocardial infarction in patients without heart failure or ventricular dysfunction. J Am Coll Cardiol. 2017;69(22):2710–20.
114. Thollon C, Cambarrat C, Vian J, Prost JF, Peglion JL, Vilaine JP. Electrophysiological effects of S 16257, a novel sino-atrial node modulator, on rabbit and guinea-pig cardiac preparations: comparison with UL-FS 49. Br J Pharmacol. 1994;112(1):37–42.
115. DiFrancesco D, Ferroni A, Mazzanti M, Tromba C. Properties of the hyperpolarizing-activated current (if) in cells isolated from the rabbit sino-atrial node. J Physiol. 1986;377:61–88.
116. Brown H, Difrancesco D. Voltage-clamp investigations of membrane currents underlying pacemaker activity in rabbit sino-atrial node. J Physiol. 1980;308:331–51.
117. Heusch G, Skyschally A, Gres P, van Caster P, Schilawa D, Schulz R. Improvement of regional myocardial blood flow and function and reduction of infarct size with ivabradine: protection beyond heart rate reduction. Eur Heart J. 2008;29(18):2265–75.
118. Bucchi A, Baruscotti M, DiFrancesco D. Current-dependent block of rabbit sino-atrial node I(f) channels by ivabradine. J Gen Physiol. 2002;120(1):1–13.
119. Savelieva I, Camm A. Novel I_f current inhibitor ivabradine: safety considerations. In: Advances in cardiology. 2006. p. 79–96.
120. Fox K, Ford I, Steg PG, Tardif J-C, Tendera M, Ferrari R. Ivabradine in stable coronary artery disease without clinical heart failure. N Engl J Med. 2014;371(12):1091–9.
121. Fox K, Ford I, Steg PG, Tendera M, Robertson M, Ferrari R, et al. Relationship between ivabradine treatment and cardiovascular outcomes in patients with stable coronary artery disease and left ventricular systolic dysfunction with limiting angina: a subgroup analysis of the randomized, controlled BEAUTIFUL trial. Eur Heart J. 2009;30(19):2337–45.
122. Villano A, Di Franco A, Nerla R, Sestito A, Tarzia P, Lamendola P, et al. Effects of ivabradine and ranolazine in patients with microvascular angina pectoris. Am J Cardiol. 2013;112(1):8–13.
123. Swedberg K, Komajda M, Böhm M, Borer JS, Ford I, Dubost-Brama A, et al. Ivabradine and outcomes in chronic heart failure (SHIFT): a randomised placebo-controlled study. Lancet. 2010;376(9744):875–85.
124. Tuunanen H, Engblom E, Naum A, Någren K, Scheinin M, Hesse B, et al. Trimetazidine, a metabolic modulator, has cardiac and extracardiac benefits in idiopathic dilated cardiomyopathy. Circulation. 2008;118(12):1250–8.
125. Koylan N, Bilge AK, Adalet K, Mercanoglu F, Buyukozturk K. Comparison of the effects of trimetazidine and diltiazem on exercise performance in patients with coronary heart disease. The Turkish trimetazidine study (TTS). Acta Cardiol. 2004;59(6):644–50.
126. Lopaschuk GD, Barr R, Thomas PD, Dyck JRB. Beneficial effects of trimetazidine in ex vivo working ischemic hearts are due to a stimulation of glucose oxidation secondary to inhibition of long-chain 3-ketoacyl coenzyme A thiolase. Circ Res. 2003;93(3):e33–7.
127. Szwed H, Sadowski Z, Elikowski W, Koronkiewicz A, Mamcarz A, Orszulak W, et al. Combination treatment in stable effort angina using trimetazidine and metoprolol. Results of a randomized, double-blind, multicentre study (TRIMPOL II). Eur Heart J. 2001;22(24):2267–74.
128. Vitale C, Spoletini I, Malorni W, Perrone-Filardi P, Volterrani M, Rosano GMC. Efficacy of trimetazidine on functional capacity in symptomatic patients with stable exertional angina; The VASCO-angina study. Int J Cardiol. 2013;168(2):1078–81.

129. Manchanda SC, Krishnaswami S. Combination treatment with trimetazidine and diltiazem in stable angina pectoris. Heart. 1997;78(4):353–7.
130. Ciapponi A, Pizarro R, Harrison J. WITHDRAWN: trimetazidine for stable angina. Cochrane Database Syst Rev. 2017;3(3):CD003614.
131. Danchin N, Marzilli M, Parkhomenko A, Ribeiro JP. Efficacy comparison of trimetazidine with therapeutic alternatives in stable angina pectoris: a network meta-analysis. Cardiology. 2011;120(2):59–72.
132. Peng S, Zhao M, Wan J, Fang Q, Fang D, Li K. The efficacy of trimetazidine on stable angina pectoris: a meta-analysis of randomized clinical trials. Int J Cardiol. 2014;177(3):780–5.
133. Nalbantgil S, Altintiğ A, Yilmaz H, Nalbantgil I, Önder R. The effect of trimetazidine in the treatment of microvascular angina. Int J Angiol. 1999;8(1):40–3.
134. Ferrari R, Ford I, Fox K, Challeton JP, Correges A, Tendera M, et al. Efficacy and safety of trimetazidine after percutaneous coronary intervention (ATPCI): a randomised, double-blind, placebo-controlled trial. Lancet. 2020;396(10254):830–8.
135. McCormack JG, Barr RL, Wolff AA, Lopaschuk GD. Ranolazine stimulates glucose oxidation in normoxic, ischemic, and reperfused ischemic rat hearts. Circulation. 1996;93(1):135–42.
136. Chaitman BR. Ranolazine for the treatment of chronic angina and potential use in other cardiovascular conditions. Circulation. 2006;113(20):2462–72.
137. Ohman EM. Chronic stable angina. N Engl J Med. 2016;374:1167–76.
138. Chaitman BR, Skettino SL, Parker JO, Hanley P, Meluzin J, Kuch J, et al. Anti-ischemic effects and long-term survival during ranolazine monotherapy in patients with chronic severe angina. J Am Coll Cardiol. 2004;43(8):1375–82.
139. Stone PH, Gratsiansky NA, Blokhin A, Huang I-Z, Meng L. Antianginal efficacy of ranolazine when added to treatment with amlodipine: the ERICA (Efficacy of Ranolazine in Chronic Angina) trial. J Am Coll Cardiol. 2006;48(3):566–75.
140. Chaitman BR, Pepine CJ, Parker JO, Skopal J, Chumakova G, Kuch J, et al. Effects of ranolazine with atenolol, amlodipine, or diltiazem on exercise tolerance and angina frequency in patients with severe chronic angina: a randomized controlled trial. JAMA. 2004;291(3):309–16.
141. Salazar CA, Basilio Flores JE, Veramendi Espinoza LE, Mejia Dolores JW, Rey Rodriguez DE, Loza Munárriz C. Ranolazine for stable angina pectoris. Cochrane Database Syst Rev. 2017;2017(2).
142. Kosiborod M, Arnold SV, Spertus JA, McGuire DK, Li Y, Yue P, et al. Evaluation of ranolazine in patients with type 2 diabetes mellitus and chronic stable angina: results from the terisa randomized clinical trial (Type 2 Diabetes Evaluation of Ranolazine in Subjects With Chronic Stable Angina). J Am Coll Cardiol. 2013;61(20):2038–45.
143. Weisz G, Généreux P, Iñiguez A, Zurakowski A, Shechter M, Alexander KP, et al. Ranolazine in patients with incomplete revascularisation after percutaneous coronary intervention (RIVER-PCI): a multicentre, randomised, double-blind, placebo-controlled trial. Lancet. 2016;387(10014):136–45.
144. Bairey Merz CN, Handberg EM, Shufelt CL, Mehta PK, Minissian MB, Wei J, et al. A randomized, placebo-controlled trial of late Na current inhibition (ranolazine) in coronary microvascular dysfunction (CMD): impact on angina and myocardial perfusion reserve. Eur Heart J. 2015;37(19):1504–13.
145. Mehta S, Liu PP, Fitzgerald FS, Allidina YK, Douglas Bradley T. Effects of continuous positive airway pressure on cardiac volumes in patients with ischemic and dilated cardiomyopathy. AJRCCM. 2012:13–5.
146. Morrow DA, Scirica BM, Karwatowska-Prokopczuk E, Murphy SA, Budaj A, Varshavsky S, et al. Effects of ranolazine on recurrent cardiovascular events in patients with non-ST-elevation acute coronary syndromes: the MERLIN-TIMI 36 randomized trial. JAMA. 2007;297(16):1775–83.

147. Scirica BM, Morrow DA, Hod H, Murphy SA, Belardinelli L, Hedgepeth CM, et al. Effect of ranolazine, an antianginal agent with novel electrophysiological properties, on the incidence of arrhythmias in patients with non-ST-segment–elevation acute coronary syndrome. Circulation. 2007;116(15):1647–52.
148. Salazar CA, Basilio Flores JE, Veramendi Espinoza LE, Mejia Dolores JW, Rey Rodriguez DE, Loza Munárriz C. Ranolazine for stable angina pectoris. Cochrane Database Syst Rev. 2017;2(2):CD011747.
149. Rayner-Hartley E, Sedlak T. Ranolazine: a contemporary review. J Am Heart Assoc. 2016;5(3):e003196.
150. Kumar K, Nearing BD, Bartoli CR, Kwaku KF, Belardinelli L, Verrier RL. Effect of ranolazine on ventricular vulnerability and defibrillation threshold in the intact porcine heart. J Cardiovasc Electrophysiol. 2008;19(10):1073–9.
151. Chong C-R, Ong GJ, Horowitz JD. Emerging drugs for the treatment of angina pectoris. Expert Opin Emerg Drugs. 2016;21(4):365–76.
152. Shimokawa H, Sunamura S, Satoh K. RhoA/Rho-kinase in the cardiovascular system. Circ Res. 2016;118(2):352–66.
153. Liu GJ, Wang ZJ, Wang YF, Xu LL, Wang XL, Liu Y, et al. Systematic assessment and meta-analysis of the efficacy and safety of fasudil in the treatment of cerebral vasospasm in patients with subarachnoid hemorrhage. Eur J Clin Pharmacol. 2012;68(2):131–9.
154. Mohri M, Shimokawa H, Hirakawa Y, Masumoto A, Takeshita A. Rho-kinase inhibition with intracoronary fasudil prevents myocardial ischemia in patients with coronary microvascular spasm. J Am Coll Cardiol. 2003;41(1):15–9.
155. Vicari RM, Chaitman B, Keefe D, Smith WB, Chrysant SG, Tonkon MJ, et al. Efficacy and safety of fasudil in patients with stable angina: a double-blind, placebo-controlled, phase 2 trial. J Am Coll Cardiol. 2005;46(10):1803–11.
156. Yoo SY, Song SG, Lee JH, Shin ES, Kim J-S, Park YH, et al. Efficacy of cilostazol on uncontrolled coronary vasospastic angina: a pilot study. Cardiovasc Ther. 2013;31:179–85.
157. Kim JH, Shin ES, Lee JH, Yoo SY, Park YW, Hong YJ, et al. A randomized multicenter double-blind placebo-controlled trial to evaluate the efficacy and safety of cilostazol in patients with vasospastic angina (STELLA trial). Eur Heart J. 2013;34(suppl_1).
158. Lopaschuk GD. Metabolic modulators in heart disease: past, present, and future. Can J Cardiol. 2017;33(7):838–49.
159. Goldberg IJ, Eckel RH, Abumrad NA. Regulation of fatty acid uptake into tissues: lipoprotein lipase and CD36-mediated pathways. J Lipid Res. 2009;50(Suppl):S86–90.
160. Coort S, Willems J, Coumans W, van der Vusse G, Bonen A, Glatz J, et al. Sulfo-N-succinimidyl esters of long chain fatty acids specifically inhibit fatty acid translocase (FAT/CD36)-mediated cellular fatty acid uptake. In: Glatz JFC, editor. Cellular lipid binding proteins. Developments in molecular and cellular biochemistry. Springer; 2002. p. 213–9.
161. Makrecka-Kuka M, Liepinsh E, Murray AJ, Lemieux H, Dambrova M, Tepp K, Puurand M, Käämbre T, Han WH, de Goede P, O'Brien KA, Turan B, Tuncay E, Olgar Y, Rolo AP, Palmeira CM, Boardman NT, Wüst RCI, Larsen T. Altered mitochondrial metabolism in the insulin-resistant heart. Acta Physiol (Oxf). 2020;228(3):e13430.
162. Stanley WC, Morgan EE, Huang H, McElfresh TA, Sterk JP, Okere IC, et al. Malonyl-CoA decarboxylase inhibition suppresses fatty acid oxidation and reduces lactate production during demand-induced ischemia. Am J Physiol Circ Physiol. 2005;289(6):H2304–9.
163. Ussher JR, Lopaschuk GD. Targeting malonyl CoA inhibition of mitochondrial fatty acid uptake as an approach to treat cardiac ischemia/reperfusion. Basic Res Cardiol. 2009;104(2):203–10.
164. Dyck JRB, Cheng J-F, Stanley WC, Barr R, Chandler MP, Brown S, et al. Malonyl coenzyme A decarboxylase inhibition protects the ischemic heart by inhibiting fatty acid oxidation and stimulating glucose oxidation. Circ Res. 2004;94(9):e78–84.

165. Lopaschuk GD, Karwi QG, Ho KL, Pherwani S, Ketema EB. Ketone metabolism in the failing heart. Biochim Biophys Acta Mol Cell Biol Lipids. 2020;1865(12):158813. https://www.sciencedirect.com/science/article/pii/S1388198120302055.
166. Kolwicz SC Jr, Airhart S, Tian R. Ketones step to the plate: a game changer for metabolic remodeling in heart failure? Circulation. 2016;133(8):689–91.
167. Ho KL, Zhang L, Wagg C, Al Batran R, Gopal K, Levasseur J, et al. Increased ketone body oxidation provides additional energy for the failing heart without improving cardiac efficiency. Cardiovasc Res. 2019;115(11):1606–16.
168. Cowie MR, Fisher M. SGLT2 inhibitors: mechanisms of cardiovascular benefit beyond glycaemic control. Nat Rev Cardiol. 2020;17(12):761–72.
169. Ferrannini E, Mark M, Mayoux E. CV protection in the EMPA-REG OUTCOME trial: a "thrifty substrate" hypothesis. Diabetes Care. 2016;39(7):1108 LP–1114.
170. Azam MA, Chakraborty P, Si D, Du B, Massé S, Lai PFH, et al. Anti-arrhythmic and inotropic effects of empagliflozin following myocardial ischemia. Life Sci. 2021;276:119440.
171. Davies A, Fox K, Galassi AR, Banai S, Ylä-Herttuala S, Lüscher TF. Management of refractory angina: an update. Eur Heart J. 2021;42(3):269–83.
172. Takeshita S, Zheng LP, Brogi E, Kearney M, Pu LQ, Bunting S, et al. Therapeutic angiogenesis. A single intraarterial bolus of vascular endothelial growth factor augments revascularization in a rabbit ischemic hind limb model. J Clin Invest. 1994;93(2):662–70.
173. Losordo DW, Vale PR, Symes JF, Dunnington CH, Esakof DD, Maysky M, et al. Gene therapy for myocardial angiogenesis. Circulation. 1998;98(25):2800–4.
174. Ylä-Herttuala S, Bridges C, Katz MG, Korpisalo P. Angiogenic gene therapy in cardiovascular diseases: dream or vision? Eur Heart J. 2017;38(18):1365–71.
175. Hartikainen J, Hassinen I, Hedman A, Kivelä A, Saraste A, Knuuti J, et al. Adenoviral intramyocardial VEGF-DΔNΔC gene transfer increases myocardial perfusion reserve in refractory angina patients: a phase I/IIa study with 1-year follow-up. Eur Heart J. 2017;38(33):2547–55.
176. Mathur A, Fernández-Avilés F, Dimmeler S, Hauskeller C, Janssens S, Menasche P, et al. The consensus of the Task Force of the European Society of Cardiology concerning the clinical investigation of the use of autologous adult stem cells for the treatment of acute myocardial infarction and heart failure: update 2016. Eur Heart J. 2017;38(39):2930–5.
177. Bassetti B, Rurali E, Gambini E, Pompilio G. Son of a lesser god: the case of cell therapy for refractory angina. Front Cardiov Med. 2021;8:818.
178. Henry TD, Schaer GL, Traverse JH, Povsic TJ, Davidson C, Lee JS, et al. Autologous CD34+ cell therapy for refractory angina: 2-year outcomes from the ACT34-CMI study. Cell Transplant. 2016;25(9):1701–11.
179. Velagapudi P, Turagam M, Kolte D, Khera S, Hyder O, Gordon P, et al. Intramyocardial autologous CD34+ cell therapy for refractory angina: a meta-analysis of randomized controlled trials. Cardiovasc Revasc Med. 2019;20(3):215–9.

Percutaneous Myocardial Revascularization

Luigi Ferrarotto, Alessio La Manna, and Corrado Tamburino

1 Historical Notes

The first PTCA was performed by Andreas Grüntzig on September 16th, 1977, in Zurich, with handmade balloon catheter. Jacques Puel implanted the world's first human coronary artery endoprosthesis, a BMS, in 1986, and over the next decades, balloon-expandable and self-expanding stents struggled to overcome various technical and clinical problems, including poor crimping of the stent on the balloon, incomplete and inaccurate deployment of the self-expanding "endoprosthesis," bulkiness, stiffness, and thrombogenic nature of these devices in coronary arteries [1]. The STRESS [2] and BENESTENT [3] trials demonstrated the efficacy of this new technique, but in-stent restenosis became the emerging problem and dual-antiplatelet therapy became a must [4, 5].

In 2002, the results of RAVEL [6] trial opened the era of DES, which changed the history of myocardial revascularization.

L. Ferrarotto · C. Tamburino (✉)
Division of Cardiology, Centro Alte Specialità e Trapianti (CAST), Azienda Ospedaliero-Universitaria Policlinico-San Marco, University of Catania, Catania, Italy
e-mail: Luigi.ferrarotto@studium.unict.it; Tambucor@unict.it

A. La Manna
Division of Cardiology, San Marco Hospital, Azienda Ospedaliero-Universitaria Policlinico-San Marco, University of Catania, Catania, Italy
e-mail: a.lamanna@policlinico.unict.it

G. Concistrè (ed.), *Ischemic Heart Disease*,
https://doi.org/10.1007/978-3-031-25879-4_20

2 Vascular Access

The femoral approach was historically the most used vascular access site; it provides the advantages of large vessel, which permits to accommodate larger (>6-French) sheath sizes, and excellent guide catheter support and manipulability, due to the typically straight path from the femoral artery to the ascending aorta. Severe peripheral arterial disease or peripheral vascular bypass grafts and requirement for immobilization after the procedure limit the use of the femoral approach in some patients. Performing ultrasound-guided puncture of femoral artery can reduce vascular complications compared with fluoroscopic guided puncture [7].

The brachial approach was used as an alternative to femoral access, but as the brachial artery provides the only circulation to the forearm and hand, any compromise of this artery can lead to severe ischemic complications.

The radial approach is nowadays the most used since it provides direct access to the ascending aorta, allows immediate mobilization following PCI, and reduces bleeding compared to the femoral access [8, 9]. Tortuosity of the brachiocephalic trunk may limit the use of the radial approach in 2–3% of patients. The small size of the radial artery could limit the size of guiding catheters that can be used, but sheathless catheters allow to use sheaths large up to 7.5-French using the radial approach. One of the benefits of transradial approach is the lower rates of vascular complications [10, 11]. The RIVAL (Radial vs. Femoral Access for Coronary Intervention) [12] trial showed no significant difference in the primary endpoint of major ischemic events or bleeding in patients undergoing PCI through transradial or femoral approach, but the rate of vascular complications was significantly lower in patients in whom the radial approach was performed. In the MATRIX [13] trial, radial access was associated with lower rates of net adverse clinical events compared with femoral access, and no significative difference in major adverse cardiovascular events was found at 1 year.

3 Coronary Devices

3.1 Balloon Catheters

Stand-alone balloon angioplasty is nowadays rarely used other than for very small vessels; it remains part of the PCI procedure for predilating and preparing the lesion before stent placement and optimizing stent expansion after its deployment.

Along with other coronary devices, balloon catheters developed over the years achieving lower profile and better support, providing more trackability and pushability.

There are several types of balloons used during PCIs: semi-compliant balloons, noncompliant balloons, and specialty balloons as OPN NC super high-pressure balloon (SIS Medical AG, Winterthur, Switzerland), AngioSculpt (Philips, Amsterdam, Netherlands),

Wolverine (Boston Scientific Corporation, MA, USA), and Chocolate balloon (Teleflex, PA, USA).

Lesion preparation with balloon dilatation is not always necessary before stenting, but it allows to expand the coronary lumen by stretching the atherosclerotic plaque and vessel wall and redistributing atherosclerotic plaque along its longitudinal axis. Vessel wall elastic recoil generally leaves a residual stenosis, and vessel dilatation can lead to coronary dissections, requiring stent implantation to achieve a better result.

Together with DES, DCB evolved during last decades, from passive vessel wall transmission of biophilic cytotoxic drugs to active penetration with electrostatic attachment and long-term residency of microspheres or even nanospheres containing hydrophilic cytostatic drugs. Initially used for small-vessel PCIs and in-stent restenosis with very good results [14], DCBs are being compared with DES in several ongoing studies including patients with large de novo coronary arteries.

3.2 Coronary Stents

First-generation DES showed less late luminal loss and major cardiac events than BMS. Sirolimus-eluting stent Cypher (Cordis, Warren, USA) and paclitaxel-eluting stent Taxus (Boston Scientific, MA, USA) were the most frequently used DES in the first decade of the new century and significantly reduced the rate of target-vessel revascularization [15, 16].

Second- and third-generation DESs were designed to overcome the issues of late and very late thrombosis, using different scaffolds, polymers, and cytostatic drugs. Various trials confirmed that a step forward was made in terms of DES manufacturing [17–22].

Nowadays, the stents have thinner struts made from different alloys that are less bulky than the initial stainless steel, with sophisticated platform designs and biocompatible, bioresorbable, or biostable coatings that reduced restenosis, thrombosis, and need for a long-lasting dual-antiplatelet therapy [23–26].

BRSs were designed aiming to avoid leaving "foreign bodies" in the coronary arteries, but they did not achieve the target rate of MACE compared with current DES [27–29].

3.3 Intracoronary Imaging

Intracoronary imaging was developed to acquire information about vessel wall and plaque morphology that are not showed by conventional coronary angiography (plaque composition, real lumen diameter, vessel diameter, endothelium injury, intravascular formations, etc.) [30].

IVUS devices are characterized by rapid-exchange catheters with a transducer on their tip and represent one of the most common tools used in daily interventional practice since they clearly provide information about plaque characteristics and composition and pres-

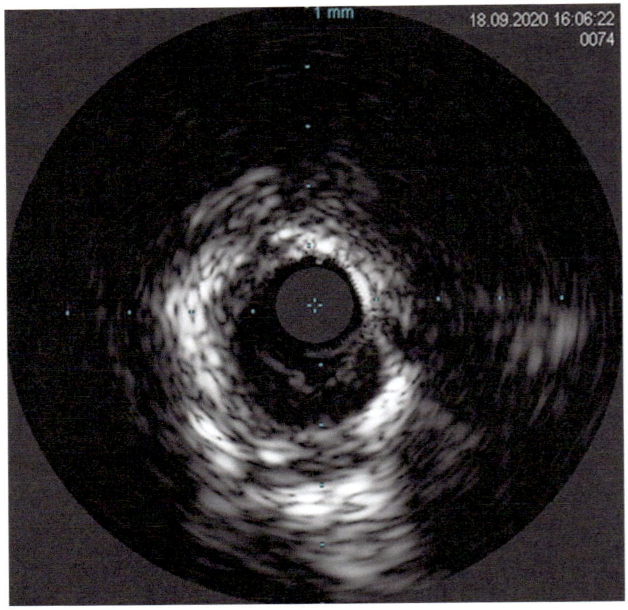

Fig. 1 Intravascular ultrasound (IVUS) evaluation showing calcific coronary plaque

ence of superficial or deep calcium (Fig. 1) [31, 32]. Moreover, IVUS provides information about lumen area and diameters and stent apposition, guiding the physicians during complex PCIs [33, 34]. As other coronary devices, IVUS developed over the years, and manufacturers developed catheter with smaller traducer dimensions and sharper images [35]. The importance of IVUS to obtain better procedural and clinical results has been confirmed in several trials and meta-analyses [36–40].

Similarly to IVUS, OCT is an intravascular imaging modality that provides cross-sectional images of the coronary artery, but it uses near-infrared light instead of ultrasounds, obtaining images of translucent or opaque material at a resolution equivalent to a microscope.

The images acquired with OCT have a higher resolution compared to IVUS, at the cost of a decrease in the depth of imaging. Performing OCT analysis requires contrast media injection to remove blood cells and reduce artifacts [41]; this characteristic potentially represents a limitation in its use in some scenarios (i.e., chronic kidney disease). Zero-contrast PCIs using dextran-based OCT have been proven to be feasible, overcoming the problem of contrast media injection in patients with renal insufficiency [42], but its application requires further evidence.

The OCT analysis generates a volumetric lumen profiling and three-dimensional rendering that includes the lesion and its adjacent reference segments. The information derived from these assessments can be very useful for the operators, helping them to interpret ambiguous angiographic findings (i.e., dissection, plaque erosion) and to optimize PCI result (Fig. 2).

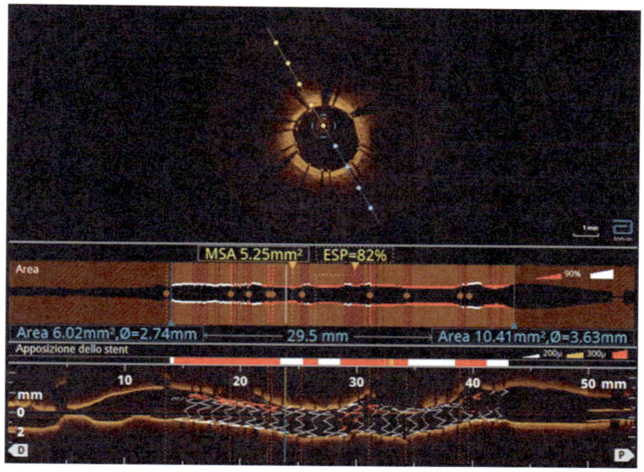

Fig. 2 Optical coherence tomography (OCT) analysis showing stent apposition (malapposed stent struts in *red*)

4 Calcific Coronary Lesions

Severe calcified coronary lesions represent a challenge for interventional cardiologists due to the higher likelihood of suboptimal PCI result with consequent poor clinical outcomes. They are found in 6–20% of patients undergoing percutaneous coronary intervention [43].

The presence of severe coronary calcification increases procedural complexity and fluoroscopic time, is associated with higher rates of procedural failure, and remains an important cause of stent under-expansion, which is a possible trigger for stent thrombosis, ISR, and target lesion revascularization [43].

Several devices, ranging from specialty balloon catheters to atherectomy systems, have been designed to tackle calcific lesions. These devices include super-high-pressure NC balloons, CB, SB, and IVL coronary system [44].

Rotablator (Boston Scientific, MA, USA) was the first atherectomy technology available on the market. It is based on "the differential cutting principle" provided by a diamond-tipped burr advanced over a dedicated guidewire. The differential cutting is the ability of selectively removing inelastic tissue (calcific or fibrotic) while not involving and maintaining the integrity of the surroundings. Recently, Boston Scientific launched the Rotapro system, which, compared with the previous Rotablator technology, represents a valuable technical improvement by the side of interventionalists, making the system more "user-friendly." The main scenarios that justify the use of RA are the preparation of severe calcified or fibrotic de novo lesions that cannot be adequately prepared by conventional balloon inflation, uncrossable de novo lesions, and ostial lesions. Complications associated with the use of RA include burr entrapment, slow/no-flow phenomenon, vessel dissection, or perforation [45, 46].

Diamondback 360 Coronary system (Cardiovascular Systems Inc., MN, USA) performs OA and consists of an eccentric diamond-coated crown mounted on the end of a drive shaft powered by a pneumatic drive console and advanced over a dedicated guidewire. OA system uses a 1.25 mm crown that ablates the calcium with an orbital and bidirectional movement, which should reduce the risk of distal embolization and burr entrapment as compared to Rotablator. Since the crown is in contact with only one side of the vessel wall, continuous blood flow during ablation is maintained and debulking particle size is constantly flushed away reducing thermal injury, temporary heart block, and slow/no-flow phenomenon. OA use is recommended in case of heavily calcified de novo lesion preparation [45]. The safety and the effectiveness of this technology have been proved by single-arm studies, showing adequate plaque modification and infrequent complication [47, 48].

RA and OA have not yet been compared in randomized trials.

Excimer laser atherectomy exerts photochemical, photothermal, and photomechanical effects. The CVX-300 (Philips) excimer laser system emits high-power ultraviolet pulses (wavelength 308 nm), which penetrate up to 30–50 μm and vaporize thin sections of tissue without causing significant surrounding damage. It represents a valid tool in case of ISR caused by incomplete stent expansion.

Intravascular lithotripsy creates fracture into calcific plaques with the aim of facilitating DES expansion and apposition [49]. The lithoplasty technology consists of transforming electric energy in mechanical energy. Electricity creates sparks that vaporize fluid and produce powerful pressure mechanical waves, which, travelling at the speed of sound, break the calcium leaving the soft tissue unharmed.

The sonic waves emitted from the transducers can penetrate even the deeper vascular layers. Therefore, IVL can disrupt both superficial and deeper calcium deposits with no significant surrounding damages and leaving calcium fragments in situ, avoiding distal embolization and microvascular impairment [49]. Several trials showed that coronary IVL safely and effectively facilitated stent implantation in severely calcified lesions [50, 51].

5 PCI of Bifurcations

A bifurcation coronary lesion is a lesion involving a significant division of a major epicardial coronary artery [52]. A "significant" SB is often defined as a SB >2.25 mm that the operator does not want to compromise.

Coronary bifurcations account for 15–20% of all percutaneous coronary interventions and remain one of the most challenging lesions in interventional cardiology in terms of procedural success rate as well as long-term cardiac events.

The most used classification for coronary bifurcations is the Medina one, which evaluates the MV, the MB, and the SB and attributes a 0 or a 1 to each segment if it is healthy or diseased, respectively (Fig. 3) [53].

The optimal management of bifurcation lesions is still the subject of considerable debate regarding the use of an initial one-stent technique, mainly represented by PS, or two-stent techniques, mainly represented by double kissing crush technique (DK crush).

The provisional stenting technique is one of the most used; it is chosen when a one-stent technique is preferred, leaving two-stent technique as a bailout option. In this tech-

Fig. 3 Medina classification. *MV* main vessel, *MB* main branch, *SB* side branch

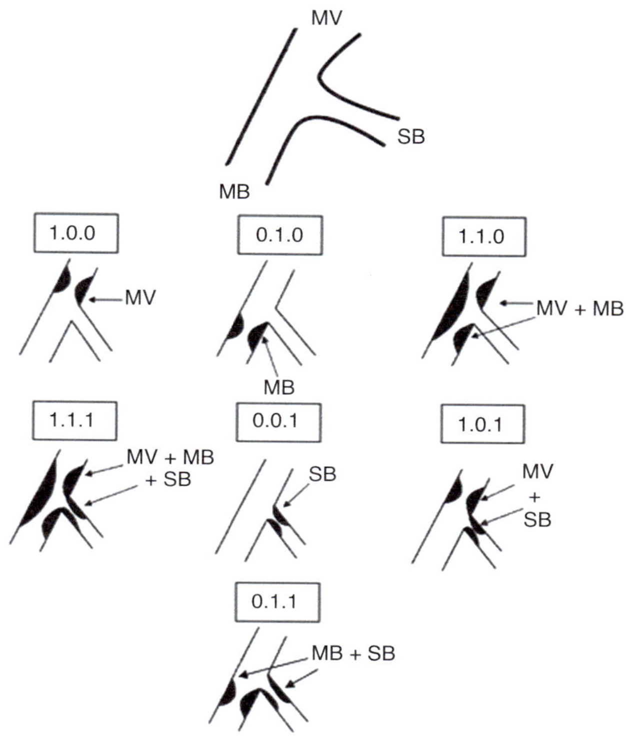

nique, the main vessel is stented first and the side branch is stented only in case of severe narrowing or flow limitation after MV stenting, ending with T, T and protruding (TAP), or culotte stenting technique.

DK crush technique consists of stenting the SB first, with a small protrusion into the MV; the protruding stent's struts are crushed into the lateral wall of MV with balloon inflation, the struts are opened towards the SB with KBI, MV is then stented, and POT, KBI, and final POT are performed.

Several trials comparing one-stent technique with two-stent techniques have been performed. Provisional stenting has been proved to be effective and superior to a planned two-stent approach in most randomized trials of non-LM bifurcation lesions [54–57]. However, the DK crush planned two-stent technique resulted in lower rates of TLR compared with PS in non-left main coronary bifurcation lesions [58], and lower rates of target vessel revascularization, ST, and composite major adverse cardiac events compared with provisional or culotte stenting in unprotected LM distal bifurcation lesions [59–61]. The recent EBC MAIN [62] trial showed nonsignificant difference between stepwise provisional approach and systematic dual-stent approach in terms of primary endpoint rate (a composite of death, myocardial infarction, and target lesion revascularization at 12 months) in patients undergoing unprotected LM bifurcation PCI. The discordance of the results of DK-CRUSH V and EBC MAIN trials may be explained by the difference in lesion complexity between the two populations and by the fact that systematic dual-stent techniques used in these two trials were different; in the DK-CRUSH V trial, the DK crush approach was used throughout, while in the EBC MAIN trial, most of the dual-stent procedures were culotte (53%) or T/TAP (33%).

6 Left Main PCI

The treatment of patients with left main disease has always been the object of contention between surgeons and interventional cardiologists, but recent studies questioned the supremacy of the formers.

PCI and CABG in the setting of LM coronary artery disease have been compared in several randomized clinical trials, but only two of them were conducted in the era of second-generation drug-eluting stents (DES) [63–69].

Capodanno et al. [70] conducted a meta-analysis of trials implementing first-generation DES with a total of 1611 patients, 809 assigned to PCI and 802 assigned to CABG.

PCI was associated with a higher 1-year rate of target vessel revascularization (TVR) compared to CABG (11.4 vs. 5.4%; OR: 2.25; 95% CI: 1.54–3.29; $p = 0.001$). Death (3.0 vs. 4.1%; OR: 0.74; 95% CI: 0.43–1.29; $p = 0.29$) and myocardial infarction (MI) (2.8 vs. 2.9%; OR: 0.98; 95% CI: 0.54–1.78; $p = 0.95$) were similar in the two groups at 1 year. CVA at 1 year was significantly less frequent with PCI compared with CABG (0.1 vs. 1.7%; OR: 0.15; 95% CI: 0.03–0.67; $p = 0.013$).

The EXCEL [67] trial, in which 1905 patients with LM coronary artery disease underwent randomization to PCI or CABG, showed non-inferiority of the former at 1 month and at 5 years.

In the NOBLE [68, 69] trial, the difference in favor of CABG was statistically significant, driven by significantly higher rates of non-procedural MI and repeat revascularization in the PCI arm.

The conclusions of the EXCEL and NOBLE trials appear discordant, but these findings could be explained by the differences in the type of DES used, MI definitions, and adverse events included in the primary endpoint [71].

To summarize, according to randomized controlled trials and meta-analyses, PCI represents a valuable option for myocardial revascularization in selected patients with unprotected LM coronary artery disease.

According to the European Society of Cardiology (ESC) practice guidelines, PCI is indicated (I A) in patients with a low SYNTAX (0–22). In patients with an intermediate SYNTAX score (22–32), PCI has a class IIa (level of evidence A) indication. In those with a SYNTAX score of ≥32, PCI has a class III recommendation (level of evidence B). In the setting of STEMI with the involvement of LM coronary artery, primary PCI is the preferred reperfusion strategy [72].

With regard to the American Heart Association/American College of Cardiology/Society for Cardiovascular and Angiographic Interventions (AHA/ACC/SCAI) guidelines, PCI has a class Ia recommendation (level of evidence B) in patients with a SYNTAX score <22 and clinical conditions that present a greater risk of adverse events with CABG. In patients presenting with acute coronary syndromes and ST-elevation myocardial infarction, unprotected LM coronary artery PCI has a class IIa (level of evidence B) recommendation [73].

7 Chronic Total Occlusions

CTO can be considered the final stage of obstructive CAD. It is defined as a complete occlusive lesion of a coronary artery with a Thrombolysis in Myocardial Infarction (TIMI) grade "0" flow since at least 3 months. CTOs are observed in approximatively 15–25% of patients undergoing coronary angiography.

A CTO is composed of a central body, a proximal and a distal cap that delimitates the occlusion, and collateral circulation. Proximal and distal caps are mostly tapered or blunt, although sometimes cap shape may not be clearly distinguished at the angiogram. CTO tapered caps are often characterized by the presence of luminal microchannels and loose connective fibrous tissue, which make these lesions easier to cross if compared to blunt stump CTOs.

A meticulous preparation and a detailed procedural planning are pivotal contributors for a successful CTO PCI. Pre-procedural planning is crucial to establish the strategy for successful CTO crossing and be prepared for any occurring scenarios, including complications. For these reasons, ad hoc CTO PCI is not recommended. Dual injection should always be performed in order to understand better CTO anatomy and collateral circulation.

Various scoring systems have been made to estimate the likelihood of CTO PCI success; the most used is the Japan-CTO score. It was developed to estimate the likelihood of successful guidewire crossing within 30 min, and it is based on five criteria (bend over 45 degrees within the CTO body, length >20 mm, blunt stump, calcification degree, and previously failed attempt) [74]. While historically CTOs of LCx coronary artery were associated with lower success rates and more complications [75], the development of CTO equipment and techniques during recent years has led to substantial improvement in success rates and new studies have showed no difference in success rates of CTO PCI in LCx compared to other coronary arteries [76].

Many devices, as dedicated guidewires and microcatheters, have been designed for CTO PCIs, and several techniques have been proposed. CTO recanalization can be finalized by either antegrade or retrograde approach, using several strategies that can be classified into TTT wire crossing techniques and DR techniques. Almost a decade ago, the North American operators proposed the "Hybrid Algorithm" that is based on the tendency of switching from a technique to another in order to increase the likelihood of success and proved to be safe and effective [77]. Nowadays, the hybrid approach is globally acknowledged and used. Recently, the Global Chronic Total Occlusion Crossing Algorithm has been published, including all the main contemporary techniques [78].

CTO PCIs' success rates have been continuously improving due to the continuous development of devices and techniques; furthermore, the rate of major complications has decreased to less than 2% and appears close to that of PCI of non-occluded coronary arteries [79].

References

1. Serruys PW, Ono M, Garg S, et al. Percutaneous coronary revascularization: JACC Historical breakthroughs in perspective. J Am Coll Cardiol. 2021;78:384–407.
2. George CJ, Baim DS, Brinker JA, et al. One-year follow-up of the stent restenosis (STRESS I) study. Am J Cardiol. 1998;81:860–5.
3. Serruys PW, de Jaegere P, Kiemeneij F, Macaya C, Rutsch W, Heyndrickx G, Emanuelsson H, Marco J, Legrand V, Materne P, et al. A comparison of balloon-expandable-stent implantation with balloon angioplasty in patients with coronary artery disease. Benestent study group. N Engl J Med. 1994;331:389–94.
4. Mehta SR, Yusuf S, Peters RJG, et al. Effects of pretreatment with clopidogrel and aspirin followed by long-term therapy in patients undergoing percutaneous coronary intervention: the PCI-CURE study. Lancet. 2001;358:527–33.
5. Steinhubl SR, Berger PB, Tift Mann J, Fry ETA, DeLago A, Wilmer C, Topol EJ, CInvestigators. Early and sustained dual Oral antiplatelet therapy following percutaneous coronary intervention: a randomized controlled trial. Journal of American Medical Association. 2002;288:2411–20.
6. Morice M-C, Serruys PW, Sousa JE, Fajadet J, Hayashi EB, Perin M, Colombo A, Schuler G, Barragan P, Guagliumi G, Molnàr F, Robert Falotico RSGroup. A randomized comparison of a sirolimus-eluting stent with a standard stent for coronary Revascularization. N Engl J Med. 2002;346:1773–80.
7. Piedimonte G, Bertagnin E, Castellana C, et al. Ultrasound versus fluoroscopy-guided femoral access for percutaneous coronary intervention of chronic total occlusions: insights from FOUND BLOOD CTO registry. Cardiovasc Revasc Med. 2021; https://doi.org/10.1016/j.carrev.2021.08.024.
8. Vavalle JP, Rao S, v. The association between the transradial approach for percutaneous coronary interventions and bleeding. J Invasive Cardiol. 2009:21.
9. Kern MJ. Cardiac catheterization on the road less traveled: navigating the radial versus femoral debate. JACC Cardiovasc Interv. 2009:2. https://doi.org/10.1016/j.jcin.2009.08.017.
10. Andò G, Porto I, Montalescot G, et al. Radial access in patients with acute coronary syndrome without persistent ST-segment elevation: systematic review, collaborative meta-analysis, and meta-regression. Int J Cardiol. 2016:222. https://doi.org/10.1016/j.ijcard.2016.07.228.
11. Jolly SS, Amlani S, Hamon M, Yusuf S, Mehta SR. Radial versus femoral access for coronary angiography or intervention and the impact on major bleeding and ischemic events: a systematic review and meta-analysis of randomized trials. Am Heart J. 2009:157. https://doi.org/10.1016/j.ahj.2008.08.023.
12. Jolly SS, Yusuf S, Cairns J, et al. Radial versus femoral access for coronary angiography and intervention in patients with acute coronary syndromes (RIVAL): a randomised, parallel group, multicentre trial. Lancet (London, England). 2011:377. https://doi.org/10.1016/S0140-6736(11)60404-2.
13. Valgimigli M, Frigoli E, Leonardi S, et al. Radial versus femoral access and bivalirudin versus unfractionated heparin in invasively managed patients with acute coronary syndrome (MATRIX): final 1-year results of a multicentre, randomised controlled trial. Lancet. 2018;392:835–48.

14. Cortese B, di Palma G, Guimaraes MG, et al. Drug-coated balloon versus drug-eluting stent for small coronary vessel disease: PICCOLETO II randomized clinical trial. JACC Cardiovasc Interv. 2020:13. https://doi.org/10.1016/j.jcin.2020.08.035.
15. Holmes DR, Leon MB, Moses JW, et al. Analysis of 1-year clinical outcomes in the SIRIUS trial. Circulation. 2004:109. https://doi.org/10.1161/01.CIR.0000112572.57794.22.
16. Stone GW, Ellis SG, Cox DA, et al. One-year clinical results with the slow-release, polymer-based, paclitaxel-eluting TAXUS stent: the TAXUS-IV trial. Circulation. 2004:109. https://doi.org/10.1161/01.CIR.0000127110.49192.72.
17. Kirtane AJ, Leon MB, Ball MW, et al. The "final" 5-year follow-up from the ENDEAVOR IV trial comparing a Zotarolimus-eluting stent with a paclitaxel-eluting stent. 2013.
18. Iqbal J, Serruys PW, Silber S, et al. Comparison of zotarolimus-and everolimus-eluting coronary stents: final 5-year report of the RESOLUTE all-comers trial. Circ Cardiovasc Interv. 2015:8. https://doi.org/10.1161/CIRCINTERVENTIONS.114.002230.
19. Onuma Y, Miquel-Hebert K, Serruys PW. Five-year long-term clinical follow-up of the XIENCE V everolimus-eluting coronary stent system in the treatment of patients with de novo coronary artery disease: the SPIRIT II trial. EuroIntervention. 2013:8. https://doi.org/10.4244/EIJV8I9A161.
20. Stone GW, Midei M, Newman W, et al. Randomized comparison of everolimus-eluting and paclitaxel-eluting stents: two-year clinical follow-up from the clinical evaluation of the Xience V Everolimus eluting coronary stent system in the treatment of patients with de novo native coronary artery lesions (SPIRIT) III trial. Circulation. 2009:119. https://doi.org/10.1161/CIRCULATIONAHA.108.803528.
21. Stone GW, Rizvi A, Newman W, et al. Everolimus-eluting versus paclitaxel-eluting stents in coronary artery disease. N Engl J Med. 2010:362. https://doi.org/10.1056/NEJMoa0910496.
22. Kereiakes DJ, Meredith IT, Windecker S, et al. Efficacy and safety of a novel bioabsorbable polymer-coated, everolimus-eluting coronary stent: the EVOLVE II randomized trial. Circ Cardiovasc Interv. 2015:8. https://doi.org/10.1161/CIRCINTERVENTIONS.114.002372.
23. Valgimigli M, Frigoli E, Heg D, et al. Dual antiplatelet therapy after PCI in patients at high bleeding risk. N Engl J Med. 2021;385:1643–55.
24. Hong S-J, Kim J-S, Hong SJ, et al. 1-month dual-antiplatelet therapy followed by aspirin monotherapy after polymer-free drug-coated stent implantation. J Am Coll Cardiol Intv. 2021;14:1801–11.
25. Mehran R, Cao D, Angiolillo DJ, et al. 3- or 1-month DAPT in patients at high bleeding risk undergoing Everolimus-eluting stent implantation. J Am Coll Cardiol Intv. 2021;14:1870–83.
26. Windecker S, Latib A, Kedhi E, et al. Polymer-based or polymer-free stents in patients at high bleeding risk. N Engl J Med. 2020;382:1208–18.
27. Stone GW, Kimura T, Gao R, et al. Time-varying outcomes with the absorb bioresorbable vascular scaffold during 5-year follow-up. JAMA Cardiol. 2019:4. https://doi.org/10.1001/jamacardio.2019.4101.
28. Wykrzykowska JJ, Kraak RP, Hofma SH, et al. Bioresorbable scaffolds versus metallic stents in routine PCI. N Engl J Med. 2017:376. https://doi.org/10.1056/NEJMoa1614954.
29. Sorrentino S, Giustino G, Mehran R, et al. Everolimus-eluting bioresorbable scaffolds versus Everolimus-eluting metallic stents. J Am Coll Cardiol. 2017:69. https://doi.org/10.1016/j.jacc.2017.04.011.
30. Bourassa MG. The history of cardiac catheterization. Can J Cardiol. 2005;21
31. Tobis JM, Mallery J, Mahon D, et al. Intravascular ultrasound imaging of human coronary arteries in vivo. Analysis of tissue characterizations with comparison to in vitro histological specimens. Circulation. 1991:83. https://doi.org/10.1161/01.cir.83.3.913.

32. St Goar FG, Pinto FJ, Alderman EL, Fitzgerald PJ, Stadius ML, Popp RL. Intravascular ultrasound imaging of angiographically normal coronary arteries: an in vivo comparison with quantitative angiography. J Am Coll Cardiol. 1991:18. https://doi.org/10.1016/0735-1097(91)90753-v.
33. di Mario C, Görge G, Peters R, et al. Clinical application and image interpretation in intracoronary ultrasound. Study group on intracoronary imaging of the working Group of Coronary Circulation and of the subgroup on intravascular ultrasound of the working Group of Echocardiography of the European Society of Cardiology. Eur Heart J. 1998:19. https://doi.org/10.1053/euhj.1996.0433.
34. Mintz GS, Nissen SE, Anderson WD, et al. American College of Cardiology Clinical Expert Consensus Document on standards for acquisition, measurement and reporting of intravascular ultrasound studies (IVUS). A report of the American College of Cardiology Task Force on clinical expert consensus documents. J Am Coll Cardiol. 2001:37. https://doi.org/10.1016/s0735-1097(01)01175-5.
35. Nissen SE, Yock P. Intravascular ultrasound: novel pathophysiological insights and current clinical applications. Circulation. 2001:103. https://doi.org/10.1161/01.cir.103.4.604.
36. Jang J-S, Song Y-J, Kang W, et al. Intravascular ultrasound-guided implantation of drug-eluting stents to improve outcome. J Am Coll Cardiol Intv. 2014:7. https://doi.org/10.1016/j.jcin.2013.09.013.
37. Ahn J-M, Kang S-J, Yoon S-H, et al. Meta-analysis of outcomes after intravascular ultrasound–guided versus angiography-guided drug-eluting stent implantation in 26,503 patients enrolled in three randomized trials and 14 observational studies. Am J Cardiol. 2014:113. https://doi.org/10.1016/j.amjcard.2013.12.043.
38. Nerlekar N, Cheshire C, Verma K, et al. Intravascular ultrasound guidance improves clinical outcomes during implantation of both first- and second-generation drug-eluting stents: a meta-analysis. EuroIntervention. 2017:12. https://doi.org/10.4244/EIJ-D-16-00769.
39. Bavishi C, Sardar P, Chatterjee S, et al. Intravascular ultrasound–guided vs angiography-guided drug-eluting stent implantation in complex coronary lesions: meta-analysis of randomized trials. Am Heart J. 2017:185. https://doi.org/10.1016/j.ahj.2016.10.008.
40. Buccheri S, Franchina G, Romano S, et al. Clinical outcomes following intravascular imaging-guided versus coronary angiography–guided percutaneous coronary intervention with stent implantation. J Am Coll Cardiol Intv. 2017:10. https://doi.org/10.1016/j.jcin.2017.08.051.
41. Yamaguchi T, Terashima M, Akasaka T, et al. Safety and feasibility of an intravascular optical coherence tomography image wire system in the clinical setting. Am J Cardiol. 2008:101. https://doi.org/10.1016/j.amjcard.2007.09.116.
42. Azzalini L, Mitomo S, Hachinohe D, Regazzoli D, Colombo A. Zero-contrast percutaneous coronary intervention guided by dextran-based optical coherence tomography. Can J Cardiol. 2018:34. https://doi.org/10.1016/j.cjca.2017.11.008.
43. Généreux P, Madhavan MV, Mintz GS, et al. Ischemic outcomes after coronary intervention of calcified vessels in acute coronary syndromes. J Am Coll Cardiol. 2014:63. https://doi.org/10.1016/j.jacc.2014.01.034.
44. Venuti G, Piedimonte G, Castellana C, et al. Using the coronary lithotripsy system for coronary artery disease. Futur Cardiol. 2021;17:59–71.
45. Barbato E, Shlofmitz E, Milkas A, Shlofmitz R, Azzalini L, Colombo A. State of the art: evolving concepts in the treatment of heavily calcified and undilatable coronary stenoses—From debulking to plaque modification, a 40-year-long journey. EuroIntervention. 2017;13 https://doi.org/10.4244/EIJ-D-17-00473.
46. Gupta T, Weinreich M, Greenberg M, Colombo A, Latib A. Rotational atherectomy: a contemporary appraisal. Interventional cardiology (London, England). 2019:14. https://doi.org/10.15420/icr.2019.17.R1.

47. Kini AS, Vengrenyuk Y, Pena J, et al. Optical coherence tomography assessment of the mechanistic effects of rotational and orbital atherectomy in severely calcified coronary lesions. Catheter Cardiovasc Interv. 2015:86. https://doi.org/10.1002/ccd.26000.
48. Shlofmitz E, Jeremias A, Shlofmitz R, Ali ZA. Lesion preparation with orbital atherectomy. Interventional cardiology (London, England). 2019:14. https://doi.org/10.15420/icr.2019.20.R1.
49. Ali ZA, Brinton TJ, Hill JM, et al. Optical coherence tomography characterization of coronary Lithoplasty for treatment of calcified lesions: first description. J Am Coll Cardiol Img. 2017:10. https://doi.org/10.1016/j.jcmg.2017.05.012.
50. Hill JM, Kereiakes DJ, Shlofmitz RA, et al. Intravascular lithotripsy for treatment of severely calcified coronary artery disease. J Am Coll Cardiol. 2020:76. https://doi.org/10.1016/j.jacc.2020.09.603.
51. Saito S, Yamazaki S, Takahashi A, et al. Intravascular lithotripsy for vessel preparation in severely calcified coronary arteries prior to stent placement—primary outcomes from the Japanese disrupt CAD IV study. Circ J. 2021;85:826–33.
52. Thomas M, Hildick-Smith D, Louvard Y, et al. Percutaneous coronary intervention for bifurcation disease. A consensus view from the first meeting of the European bifurcation Club. EuroIntervention. 2006;2
53. Medina A, Suárez de Lezo J, Pan M. A new classification of coronary bifurcation lesions. Revista Española de Cardiología (English Edition). 2006:59. https://doi.org/10.1016/S1885-5857(06)60130-8.
54. Steigen TK, Maeng M, Wiseth R, et al. Randomized study on simple versus complex stenting of coronary artery bifurcation lesions: the Nordic bifurcation study. Circulation. 2006:114. https://doi.org/10.1161/CIRCULATIONAHA.106.664920.
55. Colombo A, Bramucci E, Saccà S, et al. Randomized study of the crush technique versus provisional side-branch stenting in true coronary bifurcations: the CACTUS (coronary bifurcations: application of the crushing technique using sirolimus-eluting stents) study. Circulation. 2009:119. https://doi.org/10.1161/CIRCULATIONAHA.108.808402.
56. Hildick-Smith D, de Belder AJ, Cooter N, et al. Randomized trial of simple versus complex drug-eluting stenting for bifurcation lesions. Circulation. 2010:121. https://doi.org/10.1161/CIRCULATIONAHA.109.888297.
57. Ferenc M, Gick M, Kienzle R-P, et al. Randomized trial on routine vs. provisional T-stenting in the treatment of de novo coronary bifurcation lesions. Eur Heart J. 2008:29. https://doi.org/10.1093/eurheartj/ehn455.
58. Chen S-L, Santoso T, Zhang J-J, et al. A randomized clinical study comparing double kissing crush with provisional stenting for treatment of coronary bifurcation lesions: results from the DKCRUSH-II (double kissing crush versus provisional stenting technique for treatment of coronary bifurcation lesions) trial. J Am Coll Cardiol. 2011:57. https://doi.org/10.1016/j.jacc.2010.10.023.
59. Chen S-L, Xu B, Han Y-L, et al. Comparison of double kissing crush versus culotte stenting for unprotected distal left main bifurcation lesions: results from a multicenter, randomized, prospective DKCRUSH-III study. J Am Coll Cardiol. 2013:61. https://doi.org/10.1016/j.jacc.2013.01.023.
60. Chen S-L, Xu B, Han Y-L, et al. Clinical outcome after DK crush versus culotte stenting of distal left Main bifurcation lesions: the 3-year follow-up results of the DKCRUSH-III study. JACC Cardiovasc Interv. 2015:8. https://doi.org/10.1016/j.jcin.2015.05.017.
61. Chen X, Li X, Zhang JJ, et al. 3-year outcomes of the DKCRUSH-V trial comparing DK crush with provisional stenting for left Main bifurcation lesions. J Am Coll Cardiol Intv. 2019;12:1927–37.

62. Hildick-Smith D, Egred M, Banning A, et al. The European bifurcation club left Main coronary stent study: a randomized comparison of stepwise provisional vs. systematic dual stenting strategies (EBC MAIN). Eur Heart J. 2021;42:3829–39.
63. Buszman PE, Buszman PP, Banasiewicz-Szkróbka I, et al. Left Main stenting in comparison with surgical revascularization. J Am Coll Cardiol Intv. 2016;9:318–27.
64. Thuijs DJFM, Kappetein AP, Serruys PW, et al. Percutaneous coronary intervention versus coronary artery bypass grafting in patients with three-vessel or left main coronary artery disease: 10-year follow-up of the multicentre randomised controlled SYNTAX trial. Lancet. 2019;394:1325–34.
65. Morice M-C, Serruys PW, Kappetein AP, et al. Five-year outcomes in patients with left Main disease treated with either percutaneous coronary intervention or coronary artery bypass grafting in the synergy between percutaneous coronary intervention with Taxus and cardiac surgery trial. Circulation. 2014;129:2388–94.
66. Park D-W, Ahn J-M, Park H, et al. Ten-year outcomes after drug-eluting stents versus coronary artery bypass grafting for left Main coronary disease. Circulation. 2020;141:1437–46.
67. Stone GW, Kappetein AP, Sabik JF, et al. Five-year outcomes after PCI or CABG for left Main coronary disease. N Engl J Med. 2019;381:1820–30.
68. Mäkikallio T, Holm NR, Lindsay M, et al. Percutaneous coronary angioplasty versus coronary artery bypass grafting in treatment of unprotected left main stenosis (NOBLE): a prospective, randomised, open-label, non-inferiority trial. Lancet. 2016;388:2743–52.
69. Holm NR, Mäkikallio T, Lindsay MM, et al. Percutaneous coronary angioplasty versus coronary artery bypass grafting in the treatment of unprotected left main stenosis: updated 5-year outcomes from the randomised, non-inferiority NOBLE trial. Lancet. 2020;395:191–9.
70. Capodanno D, Stone GW, Morice MC, Bass TA, Tamburino C. Percutaneous coronary intervention versus coronary artery bypass graft surgery in left main coronary artery disease: a meta-analysis of randomized clinical data. J Am Coll Cardiol. 2011;58:1426–32.
71. Fajadet J, Capodanno D, Stone GW. Management of left main disease: an update. Eur Heart J. 2019;40:1454–65.
72. Neumann F-J, Sousa-Uva M, Ahlsson A, et al. 2018 ESC/EACTS Guidelines on myocardial revascularization. Eur Heart J. 2019;40:87–165.
73. Levine GN, Bates ER, Blankenship JC, et al. 2011 ACCF/AHA/SCAI guideline for percutaneous coronary intervention: executive summary: a report of the American College of Cardiology Foundation/American Heart Association task force on practice guidelines and the Society for Cardiovascular Angiography and Interventions. Catheter Cardiovasc Interv. 2012;79:453–95.
74. Morino Y, Abe M, Morimoto T, et al. Predicting successful guidewire crossing through chronic Total occlusion of native coronary lesions within 30 minutes. J Am Coll Cardiol Intv. 2011;4:213–21.
75. Christopoulos G, Karmpaliotis D, Wyman MR, et al. Percutaneous intervention of circumflex chronic total occlusions is associated with worse procedural outcomes: insights from a multicentre US registry. Can J Cardiol. 2014;30:1588–94.
76. Hagnäs MJ, Venuti G, Castellana C, et al. Does the left circumflex coronary artery location impact on the success of chronic total occlusion recanalization? A single-center cohort study. Scandinavian cardiovascular journal: SCJ. 2021;55:106–8.
77. Brilakis ES, Grantham JA, Rinfret S, et al. A percutaneous treatment algorithm for crossing coronary chronic total occlusions. JACC Cardiovasc Interv. 2012;5:367–79.
78. Wu EB, Brilakis ES, Mashayekhi K, et al. Global chronic Total occlusion crossing algorithm. J Am Coll Cardiol. 2021;78:840–53.
79. Galassi AR, Werner GS, Boukhris M, et al. Percutaneous recanalisation of chronic total occlusions: 2019 consensus document from the EuroCTO Club. EuroIntervention. 2019;15:198–208.

Anomalous Aortic Origin of a Coronary Artery: Clinical and Surgical Perspective

Chiara Marrone and Duccio Federici

Abbreviations

AAOCA	Anomalous aortic origin of a coronary artery
CA	Coronary artery
SCD	Sudden cardiac death
ALCA	Anomalous left coronary artery
ARCA	Anomalous right coronary artery
LM	Left main
TTE	Transthoracic echocardiography
CTA	Computed tomography angiography
cMRI	Cardiac magnetic resonance imaging
sNPI	Stress nuclear perfusion imaging
FFR	Fractional flow reserve
sCMR	Stress cardiac magnetic resonance
IVUS	Intravascular ultrasound
EST	Exercise stress test
TAR	Transection and reimplantation

C. Marrone · D. Federici (✉)
Ospedale del cuore "G. Pasquinucci", Massa, Italy
e-mail: marrone@ftgm.it; federici@ftgm.it

G. Concistrè (ed.), *Ischemic Heart Disease*,
https://doi.org/10.1007/978-3-031-25879-4_21

1 Clinical Management

AAOCA is a rare congenital abnormality of the origin or course of a CA that arises from the aorta at or above the inappropriate sinus of Valsalva by a separate ostium, by a shared or common ostium, or as a branch vessel. It can be characterized by different course subtypes: interarterial, subpulmonic (intraconal or intraseptal), pre-pulmonic, retroaortic, or retrocardiac [1].

Despite its rarity, CA anomalies have important public health implications, particularly AOOCA with interarterial course, representing the second leading cause of SCD in young athletes: about 14–17% of all cardiovascular deaths identified in this population [2–4].

In this review, we will focus on AOOCA with interarterial course: ALCA arising at or above the right sinus of Valsalva, ARCA arising at or above the left sinus of Valsalva, and the left main (LM) coronary artery with intraseptal or intraconal course.

The true prevalence of AAOCA in the general population is unknown, estimated to be 0.06–0.9% for ARCA, 0.02–0.1% for ALCA, and 0.004–0.04% for LMCA with intraseptal course [1, 5–7]. The wide variability in the prevalence data found in literature results from differences in age groups and presentation of various cohorts, variable inclusion criteria and AAOCA course descriptions, and limitations in the ability of each imaging modality used for the diagnosis.

1.1 Clinical Presentation

The clinical presentation of AAOCA is variable, symptoms may not be present in a large number of patients, and SCD might be the initial event in a few. About half of the patients with AAOCA are asymptomatic and the other half may present with symptoms highly suggestive for ischemia, on or following exertion, less frequently at rest: chest pain, palpitations, shortness of breath, dizziness, or syncope on exertion. However, it remains unknown why an athlete can participate vigorously in sports/exercise activities for many years until a cardiac event occurs [8, 9].

Basso et al. reported that only 10 (36%) of 27 cases presenting with SCD (23 ALCA and 4 ARCA) had symptoms prior to the event including syncope, chest pain, and palpitations. All cases had an acute angle takeoff and a slit-like ostium [9]. Eckart et al. reported that 11 (52%) of 21 military recruits with AAOCA suffering from SCD had previous symptoms of syncope, chest pain, and dyspnea [10]. Molossi et al. reported 163 patients with AOOCA (25 ALCA, 116 ARCA, 17 single CA, 5 anomalous circumflex CA), where the diagnosis was incidental in half ($n = 80$, 49%), while others presented with exertional symptoms ($n = 35$, 21%), non-exertional symptoms ($n = 32$, 20%), family history of cardiovascular disease ($n = 8$, 5%), sudden cardiac arrest or shock ($n = 5$, 3%), and arrhythmia/bradycardia ($n = 3$, 2%) [11]. Several autopsy studies demonstrated that ALCA and ARCA patients are associated with an increased risk of SCD, which is highest in young individuals <35 years of age and particularly in interarterial ALCA, during or following a strenuous exertion [12–14].

LMCA with intraconal course has been considered a benign entity for many years. However, some recent case report and series demonstrated that patients with this anatomy can develop symptoms of ischemia, such as exertional chest pain or syncope in association with documentable evidence of myocardial ischemia, although they seem to be at low risk for sudden death [15–17].

1.2 Anatomy and Mechanisms of Ischemia

ALCA and ARCA arise from the opposite sinus, generally just beyond the commissure between the anterior sinuses; have different ostial morphology and position, with often a slit-like ostium and high takeoff; and have an interarterial course with or without an intramural segment to reach the normal epicardial course, opposite the sinus [8]. LM coronary artery with intraseptal course has a different anatomy: a single coronary ostium from which both the right and left CA arise, with their origins being well away from the aorta and thus never being intramural; has wide-open ostia and does not have any acute angulation at their takeoff; and has an interarterial course through the conal muscle to reach the normal position behind the pulmonary artery. This intraconal course results in the LM coronary artery being at the very bottom of the "V" created by the aorta and pulmonary artery [18]. As a result of the different anatomies, the mechanisms of ischemia are also different. The pathophysiology of myocardial ischemia in ALCA and ARCA is not completely elucidated; however, the main mechanism is external compression of the abnormal coronary artery between the great arteries, as the arteries expand during strenuous exercise. The risk of ischemia is probably exacerbated in these cases by potential associated anatomical factors: flap closure of the slit-like deformation of the coronary ostium, acute (non-orthogonal) angle of takeoff, and kinking of the coronary artery as it exits from the aorta and hypoplasia and/or stenosis of the intramural segment, particularly at the level of the vulvar commissure. In addition, cumulative episodes of myocardial ischemia may lead to myocardial necrosis and fibrosis that can create the substrate for ventricular arrhythmias [19, 20].

The mechanism of ischemia in anomalous LMCA with an intraconal course is different, because generally there is a wide-open ostium without angulation or intramural segment and probably would be related to the long myocardial bridge (MB) or the coronary coursing at the bottom of the "V" between the aorta and pulmonary artery, where it is pinched between these structures. Therefore, there is a dynamic compression of the intramyocardial segment of the CA, which can cause delayed recovery of the luminal dimension in early diastole impairing diastolic blood flow, especially during exercise [21]. This can mediate multiple effects including endothelial dysfunction, venturi effect with increasing velocity and septal steal, impaired coronary flow reserve, and plaque fissure/rupture proximal to the MB, which can be potential mechanisms of ischemia [22, 23].

1.3 Diagnosis

(A) **Anatomy definition**

TTE is the first-line imaging modality for diagnosis of anomalous coronary origin, due to the low cost and wide availability [24, 25]. Although dependent on body habitus and operator technique, it can be helpful in the identification of critical anatomical features like interarterial course; however, it has limited accuracy in the assessment of anatomy of the coronary ostium, as well as the presence and the length of intramyocardial and intramural course [1]. Moreover, a variable agreement between TTE and surgical findings has been found in different reports [24–26].

Advanced noninvasive and invasive imaging modalities, such as CTA or cMRI and cardiac catheterization, are recommended for the evaluation of anomalous CA [27–34].

Retrospectively, ECG-gated coronary CTA is generally preferred because it has superior spatial and temporal resolution and provides an accurate noninvasive assessment of the coronary anatomy and detailed research of the anatomical "high-risk factors": high orifice, ostial stenosis, slit-like/fish mouth-shaped orifice, acute-angle takeoff, intramural course and its length, or interarterial course and hypoplasia of the proximal coronary artery [35–38]. It does not require sedation in younger children because of short scan time, but needs ionizing radiation, although the amount has significantly decreased with new-generation scanners.

Cardiac MRI provides a coronary artery noninvasive imaging without the use of radiation and iodinated contrast. Compared to cardiac CTA, it has lower spatial resolution and higher scan times, usually requiring general anesthesia in infants and small children. However, it provides a cardiac morphological and functional imaging, which complements the anatomic information. In small children, the fast and irregular heart rates, need for higher spatial resolution owing to small vessel size, and compensation of respiratory motion may limit the quality of the exam, although in experienced centers free-breathing cMRI visualizes the coronary takeoff and course in nearly all patients [39, 40], with sedation in the majority of young children (e.g., <7 years of age) [40].

Cardiac catheterization in combination with IVUS is generally a low-risk technique, offering high spatial resolution and excellent dynamic imaging to assess the degree of coronary stenosis in the intramural and intramyocardial segment, as demonstrated by Angelini et al. [41–45]. Although IVUS is low risk, engaging AAOCA vessels may be difficult in cases with ostial narrowing, an ostial ridge, or an acute angle takeoff [42]; moreover, additional care is needed during IVUS to distinguish vessel spasm from true narrowing [46]. Therefore, invasive imaging is not routinary recommended, but it can be helpful when there is concern about stenosis in the coronary artery or when concomitant delineation of potential mechanisms of flow restriction is needed (class IIa, level of evidence C) [34, 45].

(B) **Functional assessment of ischemia**

Assessment of physical stress-induced ischemia using advanced imaging modalities is the key to decision-making, and exercise stress is preferable when considering that a majority of SCD cases attributed to AAOCA occur with strenuous exercise [47]. However, the validity is yet to be clearly defined given reports of both false-positive and false-negative results [47]. As a consequence, the absence of ischemia during stress testing cannot completely exclude the risk of SCD, particularly when potentially high-risk anatomic features are present [45, 48].

Current guidelines recommend non-pharmacological functional imaging (e.g., nuclear study, echocardiography, or CMR with physical stress) for all symptomatic and asymptomatic patients with AOOCA (class I, level of evidence C) [47].

It is now clearly established from previous reports that ECG and EST have low sensitivity in identifying those patients at risk for myocardial ischemia and SCD, since a normal EST has been reported in patients with AAOCA presenting with concerning symptoms for myocardial ischemia and also experiencing sudden cardiac arrest or death [9, 13, 33, 49, 50].

Some centers use stress echocardiography to study myocardial ischemia by identification of wall motion abnormalities; however, techniques which can evaluate both myocardial perfusion and wall motion abnormalities at rest and stress, such as sNPI and stress cMRI, are preferred in anomalous CA. Exercise-stress NPI needs exposure to ionizing radiations and is often used although both false positive and false negative, decreased spatial resolution, and attenuation artifacts related to the body wall and diaphragm movement results question its reliability to identify true myocardial ischemia [11]. Uebleis et al. used 3-dimensional CTA and sNPI image fusion in adults with AAOCA showing poor correlation between the anomalous CA and the territory of stress-induced perfusion defect [50]. Molossi et al. also reported 14 patients (8.6%) with abnormal perfusion defects, 5 of those deemed false positive [11].

1.4 Cardiac MR

Cardiac MR (CMR) perfusion at rest and stress is a noninvasive imaging approach, which allows assessment of functional significance of CAD [3–8]. Both pharmacologic stress (vasodilators and beta-agonists) and physiologic stress testing (treadmill and bicycle ergometer) have been used in CMR perfusion [9–14]. Although pharmacologic stress has the advantage of providing uniformity in testing and a uniform vasodilator response, it cannot provide information regarding the patient's exercise capacity, hemodynamic response to exercise, and extent of physical activity that can reproduce the patient's symptoms during imaging. To address these limitations, the feasibility of CMR imaging after physical exercise using a supine ergometer or treadmill has been demonstrated previously. Both pharmacologic stress (vasodilators and beta-agonists) and physiologic stress testing (treadmill and bicycle ergometer) have been used in CMR perfusion [9–14]. Although pharmacologic stress has the advantage of providing uniformity in testing and a uniform vasodilator response, it cannot provide information regarding the patient's exercise capacity, hemodynamic response to exercise, and extent of physical activity that can reproduce the patient's symptoms during imaging. To address these limitations, the feasibility of CMR imaging after physical exercise using a supine ergometer or treadmill has been demonstrated previously [12, 13, 15–19, 51]. However, exercise perfusion in CMR still has several notable challenges, which have limited its clinical use. Specifically, imaging after physical exercise must be performed as close as possible to the peak heart rate, which requires minimal transition time between the end of exercise and imaging. Furthermore, subjects are unable to hold their breath immediately after exercise, and imaging must be performed under free-breathing conditions. The acquisition of multiple slices using single-shot imaging with sufficient spatial and temporal resolution necessitates the use of accelerated imaging techniques, especially for stress CMR perfusion.

sCMR imaging has been shown to have better sensitivity and specificity to nuclear techniques in assessing myocardial perfusion and wall motion abnormalities in the adult population [52, 53]. sCMR perfusion is based on the principle of altered coronary blood-flow derived coronary flow reserve and accounts for the entire coronary microvasculature. This technique provides high-quality cardiac imaging with excellent spatial resolution; it is feasible and well tolerated in children and does not utilize ionizing radiation [54]. Both pharmacologic and physiologic exercise stress testing have been used in CMR perfusion. Pharmacologic stress has the advantage of providing a uniform vasodilator response, although it cannot provide information regarding hemodynamic response to exercise and extent of physical activity that can reproduce the patient's symptoms during imaging [55]. However, exercise perfusion in CMR still has several changes, which have limited its clinical use; therefore, generally pharmacologic perfusion testing is most often used [54] and dobutamine is preferred as a provocative agent as it increases cardiac inotropy and chronotropy and simulates physiologic exercise condition [21, 54]. Atropine may also be used to achieve the desired increase to 85% predicted peak heart rate. Molossi et al. evaluated a total of 41 patients (25%) with pharmacologic sCMR and found abnormal results with perfusion defects in 9 (21%) patients, all in the high-risk group [11], thus concluding that sCMR seems to be a promising technique that may help in the future to identify myocardial perfusion defects in select patients and contribute to risk stratification.

Invasive assessment of coronary flow is performed with measurement of FFR during cardiac catheterization upon administration of adenosine and/or dobutamine, representing a reference standard given its inability to be affected by heart rate, myocardial contractility, and blood pressure [56–58]. Measurement of FFR proved to be very useful in risk stratification of patients with intramyocardial course or MB; thus, it has been described in some specialized centers as an emerging invasive technique to confirm myocardial ischemia in patients with LMNA with intraseptal course with specific clinical concerns such as symptoms ascribed to ischemia or myocardial perfusion abnormalities. Although the feasibility and safety have been demonstrated, the potential risks involved with coronary dissection, especially in children, must always be considered.

1.5 Decision-Making

Management of patients with AOOCA is even more challenging, as there is lack of long-term data on outcomes of both repaired and unrepaired populations. Moreover, the assessment of the risk of SCD and of the role of AAOCA in causing ischemia or symptoms is still difficult and principally based on data coming from autoptic studies. Autopsy series describe the anomalies found in patients who suffered from SCD in contrast to other causes of death [9, 10, 59–61]. Surgical case series describe findings before operation, operative anatomy, and postoperative course [9, 37, 60–63]. There are imaging studies describing the anatomy and potential pathophysiological abnormalities associated with AAOCA [6, 9–11]. There are surgical series describing improvement in symptoms after operation [37, 62, 63]. However, data proving that any particular management strategy prevents SCD are still lacking. As a consequence, decisions regarding whether surgery is necessary or exercise restriction or medical therapy might be beneficial are all tailored to an individual patient, on the basis of the age and the expected quality of life. Therefore, discussion with the patient and family is undertaken upon completing the evaluation and care should always be individualized.

Currently, in ALCA, surgery is recommended in symptomatic patients with typical symptoms who present with evidence of stress-induced myocardial ischemia in a matching territory or high-risk anatomy (class I, level of evidence C) and should be considered in asymptomatic patients in the presence of either evidence of myocardial ischemia or a high-risk anatomy, even without myocardial ischemia (class IIa, level of evidence C) [47].

In ARCA, surgery is recommended in symptomatic patients with typical symptoms who present with evidence of stress-induced myocardial ischemia in a matching territory or high-risk anatomy (class I, level of evidence C) and should be considered in asymptomatic patients with evidence of myocardial ischemia (class IIa, level of evidence C) [47]. Management of asymptomatic ARCA patients with high-risk anatomy and no evidence of myocardial ischemia is still debated. Due to the emerging accurate data on myocardial perfusion and wall motion assessment derived from advanced imaging techniques, such as cMRI, some high-specialized centers started to offer surgical intervention to ARCA patients with high-risk anatomy in the presence of myocardial perfusion abnormalities regardless of symptomatology, upon shared decision-making with the family and the patient [64].

Management of LMCA with intraseptal course is also debated, and there are no specific indications for surgery in the current guidelines, due to the recent challenging opinion regarding its benignity. However, some centers suggest surgery in symptomatic patients with myocardial ischemia, documented with noninvasive imaging and confirmed by invasive imaging with coronary angiography, IVUS, and FFR [64]. As an alternative strategy, exercise restriction and b-blocker therapy are recommended, again following extensive discussion with the family and shared decision-making [8].

2 Surgical Management

The surgical treatment of AAOCA relies on various techniques that currently find their specific indication on the base of the anatomical type of anomaly.

Nowadays, four types of surgical strategy are identifiable, each of which aims at the treatment of one or more pathological features of the coronary anomaly.

The four groups of surgical strategies are represented by:

1. Unroofing technique
2. Pulmonary translocation
3. Reimplantation (with or without aortic button)
4. Neo-ostioplasty (Vouhè technique)

The objectives of the aforementioned strategies, more or less achievable depending on the type of technique, are:

1. Correction of the intramural or intramuscular course
2. Correction of the slit-like coronary ostium
3. Correction of the interarterial tract
4. Restoration of a normal coronary takeoff angle

2.1 Unroofing Technique

Unroofing surgical techniques currently represent the first-choice strategy and undoubtedly the most widespread for the treatment of AAOCA. For the surgical treatment of ALCA and ARCA, the unroofing procedure consists of the correction, achievable with different techniques, of the entire intramural aortic tract of the anomalous coronary artery. In this way, the area of greatest restriction to coronary flow is eliminated and the native ostium is enlarged. The wall of intramural tract is therefore resected or electrically fulgurated depending on the technique adopted. The limitation of unroofing procedure consists of the fact that neither the interarterial course, susceptible to dynamic compressions by pulmonary trunk, nor the acute angle of coronary takeoff is treated.

In 2018, Sachdeva et al. [65] reported their experience of unroofing procedure performed by sharp excision for AAOCA in 63 patients with a median age of 13 years. The majority underwent unroofing for an intramural right coronary artery (79%). There was no surgical mortality, and no additional coronary reintervention was performed. The median duration of postoperative follow-up was 3.1 years. Despite a good immediate surgical outcome, symptoms either persisted or developed in 46% of patients at follow-up. This probably suggests an incomplete efficacy of unroofing procedure in treating all the pathophysiological features of the disease.

Vinnakota et al. [66] in 2019 reported their experience of unroofing procedure, performed by electrical fulguration or traditional sharp excision, in 40 adult patients with a mean age of 41 years. The majority of patients were ARCA (35/40). The authors reported no 30-day mortality or complications and no reintervention. The two techniques, sharp excision and electrical fulguration, were equally safe in the short term.

In 2020, Mostefa Kara et al. [67], from Marie Lannelongue Hospital Paris, reported their experience in 39 patients with a median age of 14 years. The patients underwent surgical correction of AAOCA (72% ARCA and 28% ALCA) by means of unroofing procedure (sharp excision) in the majority of cases. In two cases, direct right coronary reimplantation was performed, three had coronary artery bypass grafting and three had isolated pulmonary translocation. There were no early or late deaths, and all patients were free from symptoms at last follow-up. The authors pointed out the contraindications to unroofing procedure: In cases with a short intramural segment and juxta-commissural coronary takeoff (in particular in ARCA), unroofing could not be ideal to create a wide ostium and to prevent pulmonary compression of the interarterial segment. In these cases, direct reimplantation, although challenging in small children, could be preferable.

2.2 Unroofing Procedure for Intraseptal Left Coronary Artery

A particular type of unroofing technique is used for the treatment of the intraseptal subpulmonic LAD. In this condition, the goal is to release the common "intraconal" trunk of the left coronary artery from the muscle fibers of the conal septum, thus preventing it from undergoing dynamic compression phenomena. In its classical form, the unroofing operation for intraseptal LAD is very similar to the first part of Ross procedure: The pulmonary infundibulum is completely harvested with the aim of unroofing the intraconal coronary tract. Subsequently, the pulmonary infundibulum is reimplanted in the RVOT at a lower level than that of the released coronary artery [68].

Recently, variants have been proposed to the aforementioned technique in which access to the conal septum is obtained by means of a limited anterior infundibulotomy [69]. or by means of an upper retro-pulmonary approach that does not include any infundibulotomy [70].

2.3 Pulmonary Trunk Translocation

Pulmonary translocation surgery has the sole objective of preventing the interarterial coronary segment from undergoing dynamic compressions by the pulmonary artery. With this technique, neither the intramural segment nor the slit-like ostium and the takeoff angle are corrected. The technique involves transection of the pulmonary trunk and its reconnection towards the left branch, effectively moving the pulmonary trunk away from the anomalous coronary artery [71]. This technique is nowadays only considered as an additional part of an unroofing procedure, and many objections have recently been advanced on the real effectiveness of this strategy in preventing compression phenomena.

2.4 Coronary Reimplantation

Coronary reimplantation can be performed by harvesting the aortic button of the anomalous coronary artery or by transecting it at the level of coronary takeoff. Necessary condition to perform translocation with aortic button is the absence of an intramural tract.

Bonilla-Ramirez et al. [72] recently reported their surgical experience with AAOCA repair in 61 patients comparing two groups of patients: unroofing repair in 74% and TAR repair (transection and reimplantation without aortic button) in 26%. The two groups of patients had similar intramural length of AAOCA (5 mm). At the last follow-up, 94% of patients who underwent TAR and 93% of patients who underwent unroofing were released to unrestricted exercise activities. The authors consider TAR a valuable alternative to unroofing when intramural segment lies below the commissure or when it is too short to adequately relocate the ostium into the appropriate sinus.

2.5 Anatomical Correction: The Ostioplasty Technique

In 2014, Vouhè et al. [73], from Necker Hospital, Paris, reported their first experience of "anatomical correction" for ALCA and ARCA by creating a neo-ostium at the level of the appropriate coronary sinus (the left sinus for the ALCA and the right sinus for the ARCA). The technique involves the creation of a neo-ostium using pericardial patch at the level of the aortic takeoff point of the anomalous coronary artery. The intramural segment and the slit-like ostium are left as they are, thus creating a double source of coronary flow: the native source and the neo-ostium. This technique, subsequently called "ostioplasty" by the same group, is the only one that allows to correct all the pathological characteristics (intramural and interarterial tract, the slit-like ostium, and the acute takeoff angle) of the ALCA and ARCA by virtue of the creation of a new ostium in the appropriate sinus.

Gaillard et al. (Necker Hospital, Paris) recently reported the medium-term outcome of 61 patients who underwent surgical repair of AAOCA [74]. Anatomical repair by ostioplasty [73] was used in 35 patients. Nineteen patients underwent coronary reimplantation without an aortic button (TAR) and 5 patients with intraseptal sub-pulmonic course underwent complete unroofing [68]. There was no early or late postoperative death. All patients with anatomical repair (ostioplasty) or septal release were free from ischemic symptoms at last follow-up. The authors pointed out the indications and contraindications for ostioplasty: The presence of a too short intramural segment, and therefore a juxta-commissural coronary takeoff, makes the creation of a neo-ostium in the appropriate sinus very difficult if not sometimes impossible. In these cases, and in particular for ARCA, the authors suggest the use of the traditional unroofing technique or a TAR technique, pointing out how the latter could be challenging and emphasizing the high risk of postoperative ischemic events it entails in small children.

Surgical repair of AAOCA is mandatory for particular anatomical subtypes and in the presence of specific symptoms and/or well-documented inducible ischemia. The superiority of one surgical technique over the other has not yet been demonstrated. However, surgical strategies avoiding commissural manipulation, as ostioplasty or reimplantation, may decrease the risk of developing postoperative complications like aortic insufficiency [75].

The optimal surgical strategy for AAOCA repair must therefore be selected on a case-by-case basis, according to the anatomical features of the coronary anomaly identified by advanced imaging study.

References

1. Cheezum MK, Liberthson RR, Shah NR, Villines TC, O'Gara PT, Landzberg MJ, Blankstein R. Anomalous aortic origin of a coronary artery from the inappropriate sinus of Valsalva. J Am Coll Cardiol. 2017;69(12):1592–608.
2. Maron BJ, Doerer JJ, Haas TS, Tierney DM, Mueller FO. Sudden deaths in young competitive athletes: analysis of 1866 deaths in the United States, 1980–2006. Circulation. 2009;119:1085–92.
3. Maron BJ. Sudden death in young athletes. N Engl J Med. 2003;349:1064–75.
4. Harmon KG, Drezner JA, Maleszewski JJ, et al. Pathogeneses of sudden cardiac death in national collegiate athletic association athletes. Circ Arrhythm Electrophysiol. 2014;7:198–204.
5. Angelini P, Cheong BY, Lenge De Rosen VV, Lopez A, Uribe C, Masso AH, Ali SW, Davis BR, Muthupillai R, Willerson JT. High-risk cardiovascular conditions in sports-related sudden death: prevalence in 5,169 schoolchildren screened via cardiac magnetic resonance. Tex Heart Inst J.
6. Davis JA, Cecchin F, Jones TK, Portman MA. Major coronary artery anomalies in a pediatric population: incidence and clinical importance. J Am Coll Cardiol. 2001;37:593–7.
7. Pelliccia A, Spataro A, Maron BJ. Prospective echocardiographic screening for coronary artery anomalies in 1,360 elite competitive athletes. Am J Cardiol. 1993;72:978–9.
8. Molossi S, Sachdeva S. Anomalous coronary arteries: what is known and what still remains to be learned? Curr Opin Cardiol. 2020;35:42–51.
9. Basso C, Maron BJ, Corrado D, Thiene G. Clinical profile of congenital coronary artery anomalies with origin from the wrong aortic sinus leading to sudden death in young competitive athletes. J Am Coll Cardiol. 2000;35:1493–501.
10. Eckart RE, Scoville SL, Campbell CL, et al. Sudden death in young adults: a 25-year review of autopsies in military recruits. Ann Intern Med. 2004;141:829–34.
11. Molossi S, Agrawal H, Mery CM, Krishnamurthy R, Masand P, Tejtel SKS, Noel CV, Qureshi AM, Jadhav SP, McKenzie ED, Fraser CD Jr. Outcomes in anomalous aortic origin of a coronary artery following a prospective standardized approach. Circ Cardiovasc Interv. 2020;eb;13(2):e008445.
12. Maron Barry J, Doerer Joseph J, Haas Tammy S, et al. Sudden deaths in young competitive athletes. Circulation. 2009;119:1085–92.
13. Angelini P. Coronary artery anomalies: an entity in search of an identity. Circulation. 2007;115:1296–305.

14. Molossi S, Martı'nez-Bravo LE, Mery CM. Anomalous aortic origin of a coronary artery. Methodist Debakey Cardiovasc J. 2019;15:111.
15. Johnson JN, Bonnichsen CR, Julsrud PR, Burkhart HM, Hagler DJ. Single coronary artery giving rise to an intraseptal left coronary artery in a patient presenting with neurocardiogenic syncope. Cardiol Young. 2011;21(5):572–6.
16. Mogensen UM, Grande P, Kober L, Kofoed KF. Anomalous origin of the left main coronary artery from the right sinus of Valsalva with a septal course: an explanation to disabling angina? Int J Cardiol. 2011;151:e74–6.
17. Glusko T, Seifert R, Brown F, Vigilance D, Irarte B, Teytelboym OM. Transeptal course of anomalous left main coronary artery originating from single right coronary orifice presenting as unstable angina. Radiol Case Rep. 2018;13:549–54.
18. Mainwaring RD, Hanley FL. Surgical treatment of anomalous left main coronary artery with an intraconal course. Congenit Heart Dis. 2019;00:1–7.
19. Basso C, Maron BJ, Corrado D, et al. Clinical profile of congenital coronary artery anomalies with origin from the wrong aortic sinus leading to sudden death in young competitive athletes. J Am Coll Cardiol. 2000;35:1493–501.
20. Gaudin R, Raisky O, Vouhé PR. Anomalous aortic origin of coronary arteries: 'anatomical' surgical repair. Multimed Man Cardiothorac Surg. 2014;
21. Escaned J, Cortés J, Flores A, et al. Importance of diastolic fractional flow reserve and dobutamine challenge in physiologic assessment of myocardial bridging. J Am Coll Cardiol. 2003;42:226–33.
22. Bourassa MG, Butnaru A, Lespérance J, Tardif J-C. Symptomatic myocardial bridges: overview of ischemic mechanisms and current diagnostic and treatment strategies. J Am Coll Cardiol. 2003;41:351–9.
23. Ishikawa Y, Akasaka Y, Akishima-Fukasawa Y, et al. Histopathologic profiles of coronary atherosclerosis by myocardial bridge underlying myocardial infarction. Atherosclerosis. 2013;226:118–23.
24. Frommelt PC, Berger S, Pelech AN, et al. Prospective identification of anomalous origin of left coronary artery from the right sinus of Valsalva using transthoracic echocardiography: importance of color doppler flow mapping. Pediatr Cardiol. 2001;22:327–32.
25. Lorber R, Srivastava S, Wilder TJ, et al. Anomalous aortic origin of coronary arteries in the young: echocardiographic evaluation with surgical correlation. JACC Cardiovasc Imaging. 2015;8:1239–49.
26. de Jonge GJ, van Ooijen PM, Piers LH, et al. Visualization of anomalous coronary arteries on dual-source computed tomography. Eur Radiol. 2008;18:2425–32.
27. Kacmaz F, Ozbulbul NI, Alyan O, et al. Imaging of coronary artery anomalies: the role of multidetector computed tomography. Coron Artery Dis. 2008;19:203–9.
28. Komatsu S, Sato Y, Ichikawa M, et al. Anomalous coronary arteries in adults detected by multislice computed tomography: presentation of cases from multicenter registry and review of the literature. Heart Vessel. 2008;23:26–34.
29. Lee S, Uppu SC, Lytrivi ID, et al. Utility of multimodality imaging in the morphologic characterization of anomalous aortic origin of a coronary artery. World J Pediatr Congenit Heart Surg. 2016;7:308–17.
30. Su JT, Chung T, Muthupillai R, et al. Usefulness of real-time navigator magnetic resonance imaging for evaluating coronary artery origins in pediatric patients. Am J Cardiol. 2005;95:679–82.
31. Aljaroudi WA, Flamm SD, Saliba W, et al. Role of CMR imaging in risk stratification for sudden cardiac death. JACC Cardiovasc Imaging. 2013;6:392–406.
32. Brothers JA, Whitehead KK, Keller MS, et al. Cardiac MRI and CT: differentiation of normal ostium and intraseptal course from slitlike ostium and interarterial course in anomalous left coronary artery in children. Am J Roentgenol. 2015;204:W104–9.

33. Brothers JA, McBride MG, Seliem MA, et al. Evaluation of myocardial ischemia after surgical repair of anomalous aortic origin of a coronary artery in a series of pediatric patients. J Am Coll Cardiol. 2007;50:2078–82.
34. Stout KK, Daniels CJ, Aboulhosn JA, Bozkurt B, Broberg CS, Colman JM, Crumb SR, Dearani JA, Fuller S, Gurvitz M, Khairy P, Landzberg MJ, Saidi A, Valente AM, Van Hare GF. 2018 AHA/ACC guidelines for the Management of Adults with Congenital Heart Disease. J Am Coll Cardiol. 2019;73(12):e81–e192.
35. Opolski MP, Pregowski J, Kruk M, Witkowski A, Kwiecinska S, Lubienska E, Demkow M, Hryniewiecki T, Michalek P, Ruzyllo W, Kepka C. Prevalence and characteristics of coronary anomalies originating from the opposite sinus of Valsalva in 8,522 patients referred for coronary computed tomography angiography. Am J Cardiol. 2013;111:1361_1367.
36. Mainwaring RD, Reddy VM, Reinhartz O, Petrossian E, MacDonald M, Nasirov T, Miyake CY, Hanley FL. Anomalous aortic origin of a coronary artery: medium-term results after surgical repair in 50 patients. Ann Thorac Surg. 2011;92:691_697.
37. Frommelt PC, Sheridan DC, Berger S, Frommelt MA, Tweddell JS. Ten-year experience with surgical unroofing of anomalous aortic origin of a coronary artery from the opposite sinus with an interarterial course. J Thorac Cardiovasc Surg. 2011;142:1046_1051.
38. Jegatheeswaran A, Devlin PJ, McCrindle BW, Williams WG, Jacobs ML, Blackstone EH, DeCampli WM, Caldarone CA, Gaynor JW, Kirklin JK, Lorber RO, Mery CM, St Louis JD, Molossi S, Brothers JA. Features associated with myocardial ischemia in anomalous aortic origin of a coronary artery: a congenital heart surgeons' society study. J Thorac Cardiovasc Surg. 2019;158:822_834 e823.
39. Angelini P. Novel imaging of coronary artery anomalies to assess their prevalence, the causes of clinical symptoms, and the risk of sudden cardiac death. Circ Cardiovasc Imaging. 2014;7:747–54.
40. Rajiah P, Setser RM, Desai MY, Flamm SD, Arruda JL. Utility of free-breathing, whole-heart, three-dimensional magnetic resonance imaging in the assessment of coronary anatomy for congenital heart disease. Pediatr Cardiol. 2011;32:418–25.
41. Angelini P. Is echocardiography adequate to identify the severity of anomalous coronary arteries? JACC Cardiovasc Imaging. 2016;9:898–9.
42. Angelini P, Flamm SD. Newer concepts for imaging anomalous aortic origin of the coronary arteries in adults. Catheter Cardiovasc Interv. 2007;69:942–54.
43. Angelini P. Sudden death and coronary anomalies: the importance of a detailed description. Tex Heart Inst J. 2011;38:544–6.
44. Angelini P, Uribe C, Monge J, Tobis JM, Elayda MA, Willerson JT. Origin of the right coronary artery from the opposite sinus of Valsalva in adults: characterization by intravascular ultrasonography at baseline and after stent angioplasty. Catheter Cardiovasc Interv. 2015;86:199–208.
45. Warnes CA, Williams RG, Bashore TM, Child JS, Connolly HM, Dearani JA, Del Nido P, Fasules JW, Graham Jr TP, Hijazi ZM, Hunt SA, King ME, Landzberg MJ, Miner PD, Radford MJ, Walsh EP, Webb GD. ACC/AHA 2008 guidelines for the Management of Adults with congenital heart disease: executive summary: a report of the American College of Cardiology/American Heart Association task force on practice guidelines (writing committee to develop guidelines for the management of adults with congenital heart disease). Circulation. 2008;118(23):2395–451.
46. Pflederer T, Marwan M, Ropers D, Daniel WG, Achenbach S. CT angiography unmasking catheter-induced spasm as a reason for left main coronary artery stenosis. J Cardiovasc Comput Tomogr. 2008;2:406–7.
47. Baumgartner H, De Backer J, Babu-Narayan SV, Budts W, Chessa M, Diller GP, Lung B, Kluin J, Lang IM, Meijboom F, Moons P, Mulder BJM, Oechslin E, Roos-Hesselink JW, Schwerzmann M, Sondergaard L, Zeppenfeld K, ESC Scientific Document Group. ESC guidelines for the management of adult congenital heart disease. Eur Heart J. 2021;42(6):563–645.

48. Cheezum MK, Ghoshhajra B, Bittencourt MS, et al. Anomalous origin of the coronary artery arising from the opposite sinus: prevalence and outcomes in patients undergoing coronary CTA. Eur Heart J Cardiovasc Imaging. 2017;18:224–35.
49. Brothers J, Carter C, McBride M, Spray T, Paridon S. Anomalous left coronary artery origin from the opposite sinus of Valsalva: evidence of intermittent ischemia. J Thorac Cardiovasc Surg. 2010;140:e27–9.
50. Uebleis C, Groebner M, von Ziegler F, Becker A, Rischpler C, Tegtmeyer R, Becker C, Lehner S, Haug AR, Cumming P, et al. Combined anatomical and functional imaging using coronary CT angiography and myocardial perfusion SPECT in symptomatic adults with abnormal origin of a coronary artery. Int J Cardiovasc Imaging. 2012;28:1763–74.
51. Said SM, Cetta F. Pulmonary root mobilization and modified Lecompte Maneuver for trans-septal course of the left Main coronary artery. World Journal for Pediatric and Congenital Heart Surgery. 2020;11(6):792–6.
52. Agrawal H, Mery C, Krishnamurthy R, et al. Stress myocardial perfusion imaging in anomalous aortic origin of a coronary artery: results following a standardized approach. J Am Coll Cardiol. 2017;69(11_S):1616.
53. Greenwood JP, Maredia N, Younger JF, et al. Cardiovascular magnetic resonance and single-photon emission computed tomography for diagnosis of coronary heart disease (CE-MARC): a prospective trial. Lancet. 2012;379:453–60.
54. Noel Cory V, Krishnamurthy R, Silvana M, et al. Cardiac MR stress perfusion with regadenoson or dobutamine in children single center experience in repaired & unrepaired congenital & acquired heart disease. Circulation. 2016;134(suppl_1):A19899–A119899.
55. Pflugi S, Roujol S, Akçakaya M, Kawaji K, Foppa M, Heydari B, Goddu B, Kissinger K, Berg S, Manning WJ, Kozerke S, Nezafat R. Accelerated cardiac MR stress perfusion with radial sampling after physical exercise with an MR-compatible supine bicycle ergometer. Magn Reson Med. 2015;74(2):384–95.
56. Agrawal H, Molossi S, Alam M, et al. Anomalous coronary arteries and myocardial bridges: risk stratification in children using novel cardiac catheterization techniques. Pediatr Cardiol. 2017;38:624–30.
57. Tonino PAL, De Bruyne B, Pijls NH, et al. Fractional flow reserve versus angiography for guiding percutaneous coronary intervention. N Engl J Med. 2009;360:213–24.
58. De Bruyne B, Bartunek J, Sys SU, et al. Simultaneous coronary pressure and flow velocity measurements in humans: feasibility, reproducibility, and hemodynamic dependence of coronary flow velocity reserve, hyperemic flow versus pressure slope.
59. Eckart RE, Shry EA, Burke AP, et al. Sudden death in young adults: an autopsy-based series of a population undergoing active surveillance. J Am Coll Cardiol. 2011;58:1254–61.
60. Krasuski RA, Magyar D, Hart S, et al. Long-term outcome and impact of surgery on adults with coronary arteries originating from the opposite coronary cusp. Circulation. 2011;123:154–62.
61. Frescura C, Basso C, Thiene G, et al. Anomalous origin of coronary arteries and risk of sudden death: a study based on an autopsy population of congenital heart disease. Hum Pathol. 1998;29:689–95.
62. Kaushal S, Backer CL, Popescu AR, et al. Intramural coronary length correlates with symptoms in patients with anomalous aortic origin of the coronary artery. Ann Thorac Surg. 2011;92:986–91.
63. Sharma V, Burkhart HM, Dearani JA, et al. Surgical unroofing of anomalous aortic origin of a coronary artery: a single-center experience. Ann Thorac Surg. 2014;98:941–5.
64. Molossi S, Mery CM, Krishnamurthy R, et al. Standardized approach to patients with anomalous aortic origin of a coronary artery: results from the coronary anomalies program a Texas Children's hospital. J Am Coll Cardiol. 2015;65(10_S):A501.

65. Sachdeva S, Frommelt MA, Mitchell ME, et al. Surgical unroofing of intramural anomalous aortic origin of a coronary artery in the pediatric patients: single-center perspective. J Thorac Cardiovasc Surg. 2018;155(4):1760–8.
66. Vinnakota A, Stewart RD, Najm H, et al. Anomalous aortic origin of the coronary arteries: a novel unroofing technique in an adult cohort. Ann Thorac Surg. 2019;107(3):823–8.
67. Mostefa Kara M, Fournier E, Cohen S, et al. Anomalous aortic origin of coronary arteries: is the unroofing procedure always appropriate? Eur J Cardiothorac Surg. 2021;59(3):705–10.
68. Agati S, Secinaro A, Caldaroni F, et al. Perfusion study helps in the management of the intraseptal course of an anomalous coronary artery. World J pediatr Congenit Heart Surg. 2019;10(3):360–3.
69. Najm KH, Ahmad M. Transconal unroofing of anomalous left main coronary artery from right sinus with trans-septal course. Ann Thorac Surg. 2019;108(6):e383–6.
70. Mainwaring RD, Hanley FL. Surgical treatment of anomalous left main coronary artery with an intraconal course. Congenit Heart Dis. 2019;14(4):504–10.
71. Rodefeld MD, Culbertson CB, Rosenfeld HM, et al. Pulmonary artery translocation: a surgical option for complex anomalous coronary artery anatomy. Ann Thorac Surg. 2001;72(6):2150–2.
72. Bonilla-ramirez C, Molossi S, Sachdeva S, et al. Outcomes in anomalous aortic origin of a coronary artery after surgical reimplantation. J Thorac Cardiovasc Surg. 2021:S0022-5223/20)33455-3. https://doi.org/10.1016/j.jtcvs.2020.12.100.
73. Gaudin R, Raisky O, Vouhè P. Anomalous aortic origin of coronary arteries: "anatomical" surgical repair. Multimed Man Cardiothorac Surg. 2014;2014:mmt022. https://doi.org/10.1093/mmcts/mmt022.
74. Gaillard M, Pontailler M, Danial P, et al. Anomalous aortic origin of coronary arteries: an alternative to the unroofing strategy. Eur J Cardiothorac Surg. 2020;58(5):975–82.
75. Jegatheeswaran A, Devlin PJ, Williams WG, et al. Outcomes after anomalous aortic origin of a coronary artery repair: a congenital heart Surgeon's society study. J Thorac Cardiovasc Surg. 2020;160(3):757–771.e5.

Surgical Myocardial Revascularization with Cardiopulmonary Bypass

Giovanni Concistrè and Marco Solinas

Abbreviations

CABG	Coronary artery bypass grafting
LAD	Left anterior descending
CAD	Coronary artery disease
LIMA	Left internal mammary artery
PCI	Percutaneous coronary intervention

1 Introduction

Surgery for revascularization of the myocardium continues to be an effective and lasting means of managing patients with multivessel coronary artery disease. However, the recent evolution of intracoronary stents has enabled interventional cardiologists to treat coronary stenoses percutaneously with early results approaching those of surgical bypass procedures. This has had an impact on the number and types of patients who are referred for coronary artery bypass surgery. Therefore, our surgical patients are now generally older and have more comorbid conditions and more severe left ventricular dysfunction, and many have had previous catheter-based interventions. These patients are at increased surgical risk and may have poor surgical targets. To handle this group of patients, surgeons need to incorporate newer procedures into their practice, including off-pump surgery and

G. Concistrè (✉) · M. Solinas
Adult Cardiac Surgery Unit, Ospedale del cuore "G. Pasquinucci", Fondazione Toscana G. Monasterio, Massa, Italy
e-mail: solinas@ftgm.it

G. Concistrè (ed.), *Ischemic Heart Disease*,
https://doi.org/10.1007/978-3-031-25879-4_22

transmyocardial laser revascularization, and pursue such strategies as angiogenic and cell-based technology.

Ultimately, the goal in the operating room is to provide patients with grafts that have the best long-term patency. The LIMA has proven to be the gold standard of conduits. Its patency is better than 90% at 15 years, and its use has been proven to prolong patient survival. The in situ LIMA is the graft of choice to the LAD coronary artery. The in situ right internal thoracic artery has slightly lower patency compared with the in situ LIMA. In younger patients, this is an excellent choice of graft to the ramus intermedius, proximal obtuse marginal coronary artery, or mid- to distal right coronary artery.

2 History

A variety of surgical procedures have been developed over the last 70 years to treat the symptoms of obstructive CAD [1]. Myocardial revascularization began in the early 1900s with extracardiac operations, such as sympathetic denervation and thyroid ablation. Initial attempts by Beck and others abraded the exposed pericardial surface to induce inflammatory adhesions and neovascularization between the epicardium and the parietal pericardium. More than 60 years ago, an operation was developed by Vineberg in which the transected internal mammary artery was implanted in the myocardium. In the late 1950s and early 1960s, a few attempts at direct coronary endarterectomy were made. The question of who performed the first CABG is a subject of great debate, with claims of the first such operations reported decades later. Goetz performed the first well-documented CABG operation utilizing the right mammary artery and the right coronary artery employing a metal tube to connect the two in 1960. CABG began in earnest, however, in the late 1960s, along two parallel paths that included bypassing coronary artery obstructions using either the mammary artery as the bypass conduit or the reversed saphenous vein grafts from the leg. Each approach had early proponents, but the use of saphenous vein grafts became the dominant approach by the majority of cardiac surgeons in the 1970s. This preference was based on the perceived ease of use with the larger and technically less demanding saphenous vein grafts. Saphenous veins could be used to graft any coronary artery site, including arteries on the lateral and inferior wall of the heart. Mammary artery graft, however, especially the pedicled graft, was limited to anterior and proximal coronary artery sites. Although many of the earliest CABG procedures were limited to one or two distal coronary artery targets, multi-artery grafting was performed increasingly frequently as the procedure grew in popularity and effectiveness. By the late 1970s, just 10 years after the initiation of direct CABG, most patients were receiving multiple bypass grafts with anastomoses to the distal right and circumflex systems in addition to the LAD and proximal right coronary arteries. Some early proponents of the mammary artery graft persisted in the use of this conduit as a pedicled graft to the LAD.

By the mid-1980s, with CABG being carried out increasingly throughout the world and with 10- to 15-year follow-up experience available from the early group of bypass recipients, two extremely important observations were made. Many of the earliest patients to receive bypass grafts were returning 5–10 years after their operation, with recurrent angina and symptoms similar or even worse than the original complaints that had led to their initial bypass operation. On repeat catheterizations, many were found to have marked progression of atherosclerosis in their native coronary arteries and, even more alarming, severe obstructive atherosclerosis in the vein grafts that were used in the original procedure. A second unexpected observation was that, in patients who had mammary artery bypass grafts performed previously, graft atherosclerosis and premature graft occlusion were rarely encountered. This observation was even true in patients whose accompanying saphenous vein grafts were severely diseased and/or obstructed. These findings led to changes in the approach that was taken to CABG in the mid- to late 1980s, which have resulted in the current standard approach to CAB surgery. The majority of patients who undergo CABG surgery today receive a pedicled mammary graft to the LAD. Other required bypasses are constructed using reversed saphenous vein grafts, with proximal aortic anastomoses. This combination of LIMA plus two or more saphenous vein grafts can be described as the traditional, and most common, configuration for patients who have multiple coronary bypass grafting still today. That paradigm, however, is slowly changing based upon favorable data with the use of total arterial revascularization. The use of bilateral internal mammary grafts, skeletonized mammary arteries, radial artery grafts, as well as techniques of sequential anastomoses allows for complete arterial revascularization. The use of bilateral mammary grafts, however, does increase the risk of sternal wound infection, especially in diabetic patients.

The technique of hybrid coronary revascularization involves the use of minimally invasive techniques for the LIMA graft to the LAD and then the use of angioplasty/stenting to lesions in the right and circumflex artery distributions. This can be done at the time of CABG in a hybrid suite or in a staged fashion. The role of hybrid revascularization is discussed in Chapter 27.

A key feature in the current therapeutic approach to patients who undergo coronary bypass is the initiation of specific medications postoperatively to reduce progression of native artery and especially vein graft atherosclerosis. This secondary preventive approach includes the use of aspirin and other antiplatelet agents, lipid-lowering medications, and a variety of other drugs that affect baseline coronary artery tone and degree of vasodilation, heart rate, blood pressure, and even endothelial inflammatory susceptibility. Other important components of secondary prevention for patients who have a coronary bypass grafting procedure are weight loss and stress reduction, dietary compliance, exercise programs, and smoking cessation, whenever applicable.

Indications for CABG are discussed further in Chapter 17.

3 Preoperative Evaluation

All patients who are referred to a surgeon for consideration of CABG will have had a coronary angiogram performed. Often, however, the patient who is referred for CABG will require one or more additional studies. Assessment of global left ventricular function with calculation of the ejection fraction as well as assessment of regional ventricular function, using a perfusion study or 2D echocardiogram, may be helpful. Regional wall motion assessment may be especially important in situations in which coronary arterial branches are completely occluded and not visualized on coronary angiography. The presence of retained regional contractile function, as well as other signs of viability, should prompt an attempt at coronary artery identification and grafting in these areas. The surgeon should assess these studies and discuss his or her plans for bypass grafting with the patient before the procedure. Requests by cardiologists for consideration of bypass grafting should be seen as actual consultations for assessment of suitability for surgery, not prescriptions to perform specific operations according to the judgments made exclusively by the cardiologists or other physicians.

Another important component of preoperative assessment that requires the input of the surgeon is the availability of suitable conduits. Few CABG candidates have such severe peripheral vascular disease that the mammary artery is not suitable for use as a bypass conduit. A complete occlusion of the proximal left subclavian artery, however, such that a subclavian "steal" might occur, can be determined by the absence or marked reduction of blood pressure in the left arm. The diagnostic cardiologist should be expected to visualize the LIMA during coronary artery studies in patients with severe brachiocephalic arterial obstructive disease. A more common problem that causes unsuitability of the LIMA for grafting is seen in patients who have had prior anterior thoracic irradiation, especially those who have been radiated for mediastinal lymphoma. A frequent problem that is overlooked when referring patients for multivessel coronary artery grafting, however, is the absence of saphenous veins in those who have had saphenous vein stripping because of severe varicosities. In addition, varicosed saphenous veins may pose problems. In either situation, physical examination and ultrasound venous mapping should be undertaken preoperatively. The expanded use of arterial conduits makes this less of a problem today than in years past. The presence of significant peripheral vascular disease can alter the approach to lower extremity vein harvesting. Leg testing with calculation of arterial brachial indices is indicated. Evaluation for concomitant carotid artery disease by ultrasound is indicated in those with physical exam findings of a carotid bruit or a history of transient ischemic attack or stroke. Significant chronic obstructive pulmonary disease should be evaluated with preoperative pulmonary function tests, and an attempt at smoking cessation and medical optimization is paramount. An Allen's test and/or ultrasound of the radial artery in the nondominant arm can be performed.

4 Surgical Intervention

4.1 Incision

The incision is made from the midpoint of the sternal notch and sternal angle down to the tip of the xyphoid. Retraction in the sternal notch allows careful division of the clavicular–clavicular ligament. Careful attention is paid to the position of the innominate artery, which is typically superior and deep to this. After division and retraction, the edges of the sternum are carefully cauterized for hemostasis. A minimal amount of bone wax is used to stop bleeding in the marrow. The thymic tissues, subcutaneous tissue, and any muscle are divided up to the inferior edge of the brachiocephalic vein.

The graft materials, harvesting methods, and treatment of grafts are discussed in Chapter 24.

4.2 Establishment of Cardiopulmonary Bypass

The pericardium is divided into a T-shape. The remnant of thymic tissue and pericardial fat is divided in the midline until the inferior aspect of the left innominate vein is identified. Placement of pericardial retraction sutures to create a pericardial cradle improves exposure. The distal ascending aorta is inspected and manually palpated for soft nonatherosclerotic areas suitable for cannulation and cross-clamping. Systemic anticoagulation is achieved prior to arterial cannulation with intravenous administration of heparin. Two partial-thickness concentric diamond-shaped purse-string sutures using 3-0 Tevdek or polypropylene suture are placed in the distal ascending aorta. The aortic cannula is inserted and properly positioned, and the purse strings are tightened. The rubber tourniquet is secured to the aortic cannula with a heavy silk tie, and then the cannula is secured to the skin. The aortic cannula is then de-aired and connected to the arterial end of the pump tubing. The purse-string suture is tightened, and the tourniquet is secured to the venous cannula with a heavy silk tie. The venous line is then connected to the pump tubing. After ensuring that the appropriate activated clotting time target has been reached, cardiopulmonary bypass is initiated. An aortic root cannula for administration of cardioplegia and venting is placed in the ascending aorta. Retrograde cardioplegia may be used, particularly if there is aortic regurgitation, left main disease, severe proximal multivessel disease, or poor left ventricular function. Patients with aortic insufficiency that is not to be surgically addressed may benefit from the placement of a left ventricular vent catheter via the right superior pulmonary vein to avoid left ventricular distention.

Target vessels may be easier to identify before cardioplegic arrest while they are fully distended in their native state. Target locations are usually confirmed by visual inspection and epicardial examination with the location of planned distal anastomoses. Systemic cooling to between 28 and 34 °C is preferred by many surgeons, although it is our practice to perfuse patients normothermically. Cardioplegia may be administered warm, tepid (25 °C), or cold via antegrade or retrograde routes. Some surgeons even administer cardioplegia simultaneously both antegrade and retrograde. A sub-study of the CABG Patch Trial investigated the effect of cardioplegia type, temperature, and delivery route in 885 CAD patients with low ejection fraction (EF) (36%). Patients receiving crystalloid cardioplegia versus those receiving blood cardioplegia were found to have significantly more operative deaths (2% versus 0.3%), postoperative myocardial infarction (10% versus 2%), shock (13% versus 7%), and postoperative conduction defects (21.6% versus 12.4%). Despite a higher operative morbidity, no significant difference was demonstrated in early or late mortality between crystalloid and blood cardioplegia. Furthermore, patients receiving normothermic blood cardioplegia had less postoperative right ventricular dysfunction (10%) than those receiving cold blood (25%), or cold blood with warm reperfusion (30%). There was also no significant difference in early or late mortality with regard to temperature of blood cardioplegia. Finally, combined antegrade and retrograde cardioplegia delivery was associated with significantly less inotrope use (71% versus 84%), right ventricular dysfunction (23% versus 41%), and postoperative balloon pump use (12% versus 19%) than antegrade cardioplegia delivery alone [2].

4.3 Distal Anastomoses

Exposure of the coronary arteries for the distal anastomosis of the saphenous vein to the coronary arteries can be accomplished by a number of techniques. In our experience, static exposure of the distal right coronary artery and its posterior descending branch can be obtained by placing one traction stitch on the acute margin of the heart and one traction stitch under the proximal right coronary artery. Exposure of the left coronary branches is accomplished by two tapes. One tape is drawn through the transverse sinus and the other tape through an opening below the right inferior pulmonary vein behind the inferior vena cava. The traction of these tapes allows exposure of left cardiac wall. The technique for anastomosis to all the coronary arteries is essentially the same. The arteriotomy is made at the selected site. It is enlarged to a length of 5–7 mm with Potts scissors. The distal end of the conduit must be tailored to have an oblique, hood-shaped lumen with a circumference at least 25% larger than that of the arteriotomy. The distal anastomosis is started with 7-0 or 8-0 Prolene sutures, double armed with tapered needles. Traditionally, the vein or the thoracic artery is held by the assistant surgeon with two atraumatic forceps.

4.4 Proximal Anastomosis

Once an appropriate site for aortotomy is identified, the fatty tissue overlying the aorta is removed. An arteriotomy is created, and a 4–5 mm punch is used to create a circular aortomy. The size of the punch will vary depending on the size of the conduit graft. The proximal aspect of the conduit is beveled and then notched at the heel. A running 6-0 polypropylene suture is used in our experience. The long axis of the graft is aligned at an appropriate angle to the ascending aorta. Symmetry in the spacing of sutures is paramount to obtain a hemostatic anastomosis.

5 Outcome

5.1 Evidence for Outcomes in CABG: Observational Studies

CABG is perhaps unique in medicine with the volume of short-term and long-term outcome data accumulated over the years. In 1988, the Society of Thoracic Surgeons database was started to assess short-term (30-day) mortality outcomes for CABG in response to non-risk-adjusted mortality being reported in local papers by Medicare. This database effort has become the flagship clinical database program in medicine; currently, >95% of all hospitals in which open-heart surgery is performed currently participate in this database. Over 150 observational analysis manuscripts have been published from this database program. At a national level, these studies have documented the remarkable decline in 30-day mortality and, to a lesser extent, morbidity in the face of a relentless increase in the preoperative risk status of the patients coming to CABG. These studies have also documented, through a series of quality improvement studies funded by the Agency for Healthcare Research and Quality, the importance of preoperative beta-blocker use and internal mammary artery use on acute mortality, as well as the opportunity and importance of secondary prevention medications following isolated CABG. Over the past several years, these national data have also documented that mortality for CABG has reached an asymptote of 1.8–2.0% nationally by the Society of Thoracic Surgeons National Database data. Not surprisingly, at this level of infrequency of outcomes, additional improvements will be more difficult to achieve, perhaps requiring developments that change CABG in a paradigm-shifting manner. Other critically important information has been generated from regional database activities, beginning with the Northern New England Cardiac Surgery studies, and including the New York State database analyses. Other studies from the Virginia Cardiac Surgery Quality Improvement project, the Michigan Society of Thoracic and Cardiovascular Surgery, and the Washington State COAP program have generated additional considerable observational evidence about the processes and outcomes of CABG. Importantly, these national/regional observational analyses were limited in that most did not capture long-term outcome data. The NY State databases for PCI and CABG allowed for long-term follow-up analysis of the comparison of these two procedures, which suggested a long-term survival benefit with CABG vs. PCI. Two reports from the Duke University Clinical Cardiology database over 25 years both suggested improved survival with CABG vs. PCI or medical therapy in patients with more severe anatomic disease [3].

5.2 Evidence for Outcomes in CABG: Randomized Trials

The limitations of observational dataset analyses are inherent site and selection confounding bias that cannot be addressed without the rigor of a randomized design. As PCI emerged as an alternative therapy to CABG for ischemic heart disease, a number of inferiority-design trials in low-risk surgical patients documented equivalent short-term outcomes. Several of these trials, such as the ARTS trial, had longer term outcomes reported as well [4]. Overall, however, these trials mostly excluded patients with more severe disease by anatomic classification, while including patients with lower predicted surgical risk. To address these trial design issues, the Synergy between Percutaneous Coronary Intervention with Taxus and Cardiac Surgery (SYNTAX) and Future Revascularization Evaluation in Patients with Diabetes (FREEDOM) trials were designed and executed over the past 5–7 years [5, 6]. In SYNTAX, the anatomic construct for revascularization reached its apogee with the development and use of the SYNTAX score to classify patient's SIHD based on anatomic severity. In FREEDOM, 83% of patients had at least moderately severe three-vessel disease in both arms of the trial. Both trials have recently reported 5-year results, with important and perhaps surprisingly consistent results regarding late outcomes from CABG vs. PCI in "real world" and diabetic patients. There was a demonstrated long-term survival benefit seen in both SYNTAX and FREEDOM, statistically favoring CABG. In SYNTAX, this freedom from mortality was seen in patients with more severe anatomic disease, as indicated in the intermediate and high SYNTAX tertiles. In FREEDOM, the mortality benefit was seen across all three SYNTAX tertiles, probably because of the underlying severity of anatomic disease present in these patients. In both SYNTAX and FREEDOM, at 5 years, there was a decreased incidence of myocardial infarction in the CABG arms, as well.

References

1. Mueller RL, Rosengart TK, Isom OW. The history of surgery for ischemic heart disease. Ann Thorac Surg. 1997;63(3):869–78.
2. Flack JE 3rd, Cook JR, May SJ, Lemeshow S, Engelman RM, Rousou JA, Deaton DW. Does cardioplegia type affect outcome and survival in patients with advanced left ventricular dysfunction? Results from the CABG Patch Trial. Circulation. 2000;102(19 Suppl 3):III84–9.
3. Edwards FH, Shahian DM, Grau-Sepulveda MV, Grover FL, Mayer JE, O'Brien SM, DeLong E, Peterson ED, McKay C, Shaw RE, Garratt KN, Dangas GD, Messenger J, Klein LW, Popma JJ, Weintraub WS. Composite outcomes in coronary bypass surgery versus percutaneous intervention. Ann Thorac Surg. 2014;97(6):1983–8. discussion 1988-90
4. Patrick W, Serruys L, Ong ATL, van Herwerden LA, Sousa JE, Jatene A, Bonnier JJRM, Schönberger JPMA, Buller N, Bonser R, Disco C, Backx B, Hugenholtz PG, Firth BG, Unger F. Five-year outcomes after coronary stenting versus bypass surgery for the treatment of multivessel disease: the final analysis of the Arterial Revascularization Therapies Study (ARTS) randomized trial. J Am Coll Cardiol. 2005;46(4):575–81.

5. Mohr FW, Morice MC, Kappetein AP, Feldman TE, Ståhle E, Colombo A, Mack MJ, Holmes DR Jr, Morel MA, Van Dyck N, Houle VM, Dawkins KD, Serruys PW. Coronary artery bypass graft surgery versus percutaneous coronary intervention in patients with three-vessel disease and left main coronary disease: 5-year follow-up of the randomised, clinical SYNTAX trial. Lancet. 2013;381(9867):629–38. https://doi.org/10.1016/S0140-6736(13)60141-5.
6. Aggarwal B, Goel SS, Sabik JF, Shishehbor MH. The FREEDOM trial: in appropriate patients with diabetes and multivessel coronary artery disease, CABG beats PCI. Cleve Clin J Med. 2013;80(8):515–23. https://doi.org/10.3949/ccjm.80a.13030.

Surgical Myocardial Revascularization Without Cardiopulmonary Bypass

Paul Sergeant

1 Patient Selection

Nearly all coronary revascularization patients are perfect candidates for this approach. They are not unconditional perfect candidates but demand a very strict anaesthesia as well as surgical pathway in combination with an appropriate conceptual, simulation, and organizational learning process. This selection is not conditional of extensive experience, but conditional of following a strict proven conceptual pathway. Any deviation from such a strict conceptual pathway will reduce this list considerably and maybe even exclude nearly all patients.

From a ventricular function perspective, there is no issue in low ejection fraction, hypertrophic left ventricle, aortic valve regurgitation, and mitral valve regurgitation. Only a functional mitral valve regurgitation, present only during active ischaemia, is very difficult to manage.

From an anatomical perspective, left main stenosis, an intramural LAD, a diffusely diseased LAD, or a calcified aorta create specific expertise and management but are no obstacles.

From an approach perspective, a normal repeat CABG procedure is possible in off-pump mode but to use a previously constructed arterial graft as inflow will create an additional ischaemic possibility. A history of deep wound infection will most certainly mandate the use of the extracorporeal circulation.

P. Sergeant (✉)
Gasthuisberg University Hospital, Leuven, Belgium
e-mail: paul.sergeant@uz.kuleuven.ac.be

G. Concistrè (ed.), *Ischemic Heart Disease*,
https://doi.org/10.1007/978-3-031-25879-4_23

From a haemodynamic perspective, same-day infarct patients with an index under 2l/M^2 can be operated in off-pump mode, maybe with the support of an IABP. But if the index is under 1l/M^2 or if there are signs of reduced saturation or runs of ventricular arrythmia, then the safety of the extracorporeal circulation is preferable.

2 Criteria for Optimal Exposure

The criteria are described in Table 1.

Table 1 The essential criteria for optimal exposure

Stress	No stress for patient, surgeon, or anaesthesiologist
Anatomy	All coronary vessels, including intramural and intra-septal pathways
Anastomosis	A perfect anastomosis by a resident trained in OSATS-based simulation
Heart rate	Physiological heart rates for patient and surgeon
Cardiac output	Physiological cardiac outputs for patient
Filling pressures	Physiological filling pressures in arterial and venous systems
Mitral incompetence	No new or increase of existing incompetence
Aortic incompetence	No new or increase of existing incompetence
Inotropic medication	Normal physiology without inotropic support
Conversion rates	4 and 5 sigma rates
Outcomes	Annihilation of early risk and no loss of late outcome benefit

3 Conditioning of the Patient Before Exposing the Different Sides of the Heart

These patient selection and optimal exposure criteria cannot be reached without conditions. So, the proposed methodologies in the next sections demand a very strict preparation of the patient, starting with a surgical team approach and a continued team interaction with an equal respect for nurse, anaesthesiologist, and surgeon. Although it seems possible to perform CABG with locoregional anaesthesia, we select general anaesthesia as the preferred method. The basic anaesthesia access is arterial and venous lines; the basic monitoring is pulmonary artery monitoring of pressures and curves, multi-lead ST monitoring, as well as visual observations of shape, colour, and contractile waves of the heart. Ischaemia prevention and monitoring are based on mandatory shunting, a strict understanding of the surgical phases with additional ischaemic risk, ST-segment monitoring, as well as PA pressure and curve shape monitoring. The body temperature remains within normothermic ranges, without drift below 36 °C. This is achieved through strict temperature management from the hospital bed, during anaesthesia, and until draping. All gasses and fluids are heated, and the mattress is heated. The operating-room temperature is secondary to the patient's temperature drift. Filling remains within a physiologic range; where needed, the legs only are elevated; and all displacements of the heart are very controlled. Trendelenburg position is considered outdated since it increases central venous pressures outside of a physiological range and decreases the venous cerebral return. Physiologic pressures are maintained without the use of inotropy; only selective vasoconstriction can compensate the vasodilatation observed in the very warm patient. Anticoagulation is complete with an ACT above 400 and mandatory check every 15 min. PVCs caused by manipulation are inacceptable; all PVCs are therefore considered early warning signals of possible ischaemia and treated as such. Potassium is maintained above 4 mmol/L, beta-blocking adjusts tachycardia, and pacing is installed when the patient has a documented LBBB/RBBB/LAHB/AFib.

4 The Exposure of the Anterolateral Wall

We normally perform a complete sternotomy. It is possible to reduce skin incision, certainly in the cranial part and with women. This does not considerably increase the difficulty. The sternal retractor is placed with the transverse bar at the top of the chest (Fig. 1), creating thereby an optimal retraction in the lower part of the mediastinum. This positioning will allow a very low positioning of the anastomotic stabilizer over the diaphragm (see later) and the stabilization of the hand of the surgeon during the anastomotic phase.

Our approach is driven by the use of both ITA arteries in nearly all procedures. We open both pleural cavities (only after harvesting both IMA) to allow maximum length and mobility of these grafts. The opening of the right chest is not used for enucleating the heart, since this will distort and strangulate the inflow of the two caval veins.

The pericardium is opened after the pre-elevation of both ITA arteries. Five different incision lines (Fig. 2) are performed. Line no. 1 is a midline incision. Line nos. 2 and 3 follow the diaphragm. Line nos. 4 and 5 are created at the level of the pulmonary valve and go down to the level of the phrenic nerves, where they follow a short horizontal track.

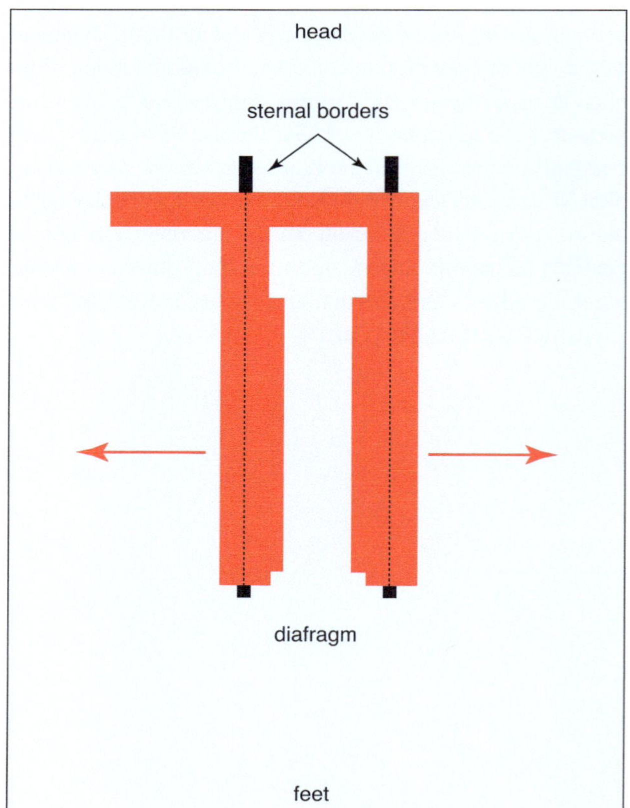

Fig. 1 The positioning of the sternal retractor

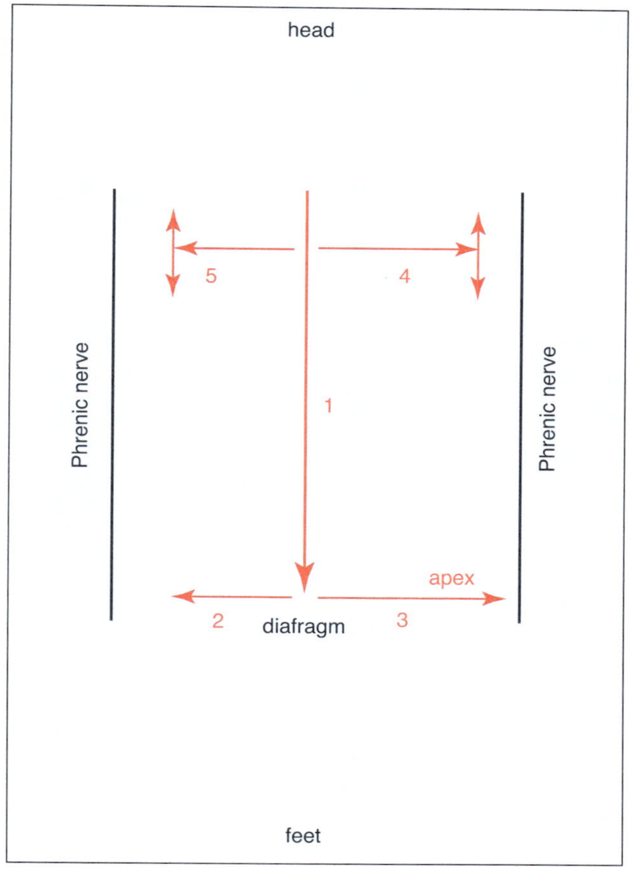

Fig. 2 The incision of the pericardium

The LAD, and its septal and diagonal tributaries, is the coronary system with the largest outflow area. Therefore, this area is always vascularized first and preferably with an in situ arterial graft. If diagonal anastomoses are needed, then they are performed in a sequential fashion on that same graft and before the LAD.

At this moment, we see mostly the right ventricle and some sections of the LAD.

To expose the left anterolateral wall, we start by suspending the left pericardium to the chest wall. If we plan to do the proximal right coronary, this will be released, and the right pericardium only will be suspended. So let us return to the left anterolateral wall. We will avoid touching the left ventricle with the hands or instruments, other than the stabilizer, to avoid even a single PVC. It is possible to stabilize the LAD now over a large portion, but we prefer to improve the visualization even more before attempting the anastomoses of the anterolateral wall. To do that, we place a series of silk stitches, parallel and above the phrenic nerve, from the top towards the diaphragm, to gradually lift the left ventricle and expose the LAD and its branches. The separate stitches are also fixed to the sternal wall.

Fig. 3 The stabilization of the anastomotic region: the anastomotic stabilizer

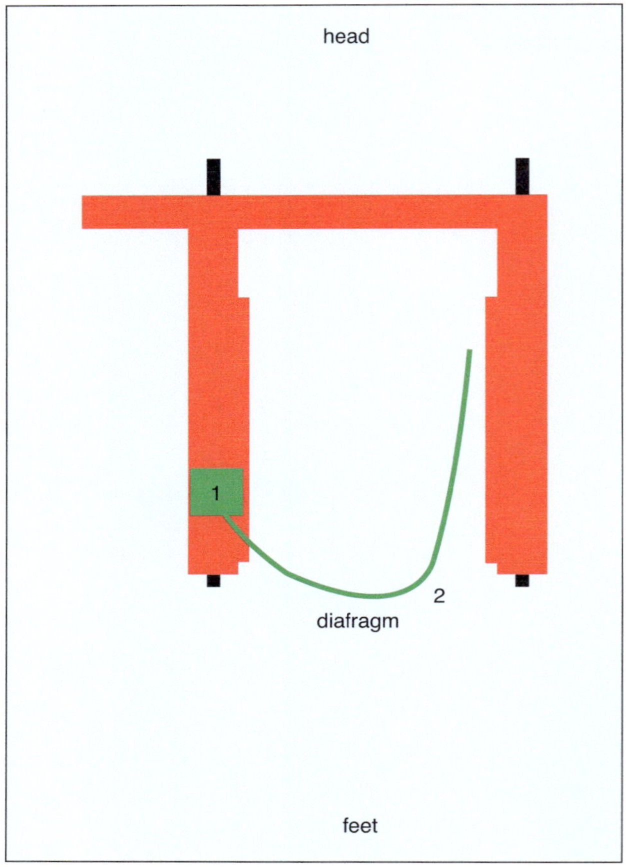

At this moment, we bring in the anastomotic stabilizer. It is fixed to the sternal retractor on the lower part of the right arm and makes a curve (Fig. 3), low above the diaphragm, and is then positioned in the anastomotic region. The stabilizer suctions the anterior wall and is then slightly lifted, so that absolutely no pressure is exercised on the anastomotic region of the ventricle. The hand of the surgeon, holding the needle holder, can rest on this arm.

Usually, there is still insufficient stabilization; therefore, a secondary stabilization is performed. This is obtained (Fig. 4) by placing everting retracting stitches with a 4-0

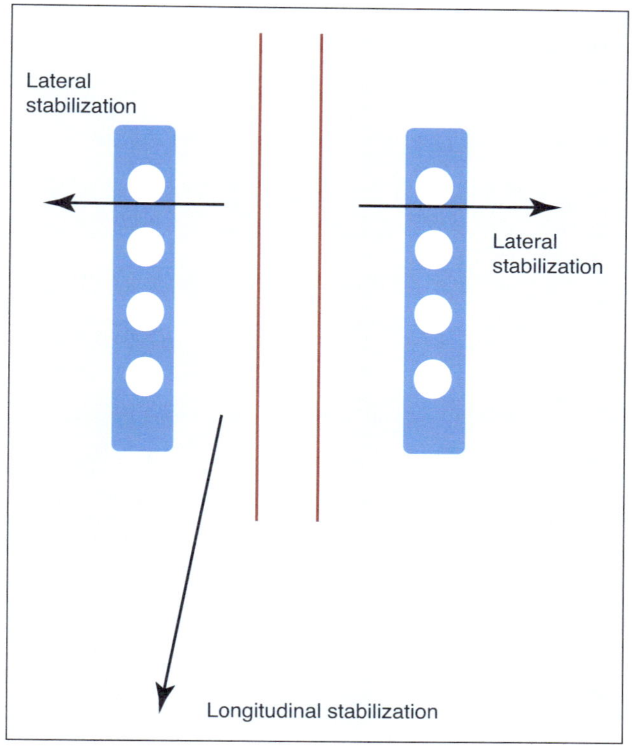

Fig. 4 The secondary stabilization

suture on both sides if the residual instability is laterolateral, and proximal or distal if the instability is longitudinal.

Now, optimal visualization and stabilization are obtained to place the shunt and perform the sequential or unique anastomosis. The appropriate shunting and anastomotic techniques are not part of this manuscript.

The anastomotic stabilizer should not be placed on top of a coronary vessel; even touching or bending a coronary artery can induce ischaemia. Where needed, one or both branches can be spread to adapt to the local situation. This will decrease the stabilization, but this can be recuperated by the secondary stabilization. In addition, some wax can occlude a suction hole, where it crosses an artery or a cavity (Fig. 5).

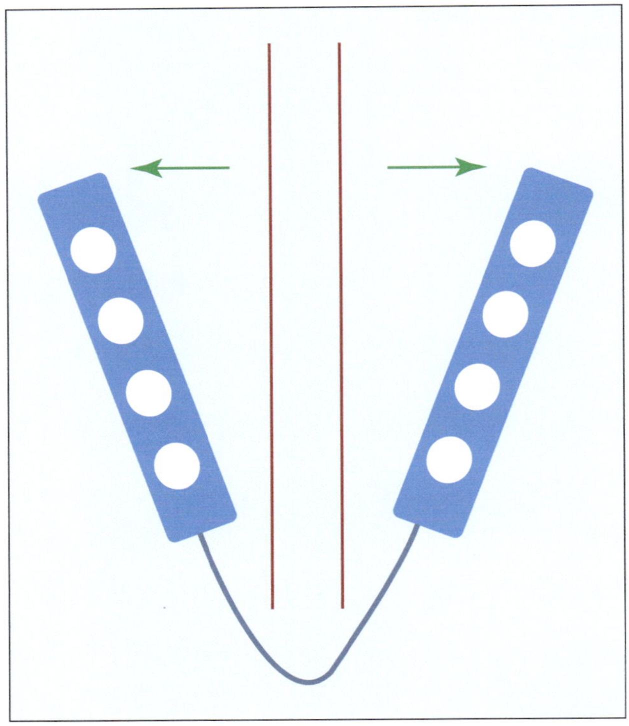

Fig. 5 Spreading one or both branches of the stabilizer

5 The Exposure of the Posterolateral Wall

Several methods (Table 2) have been proposed to enucleate the heart out of the pericardium; each of these methods delivers a leverage, induces hemodynamic consequences, and proposes a visibility on the posterolateral area of the heart. In this manuscript, we will not describe each method, but focus on the method with the best leverage, the least haemodynamic consequence, and the best visibility.

Table 2 Different enucleating methods (+++ very good, ++ good, + average, −−− totally inacceptable, −− inacceptable, − not good)

Method	Leverage	Haemodynamics	Visibility
Retrocardiac sponge/prosthesis	+	+	−
Cross-your-heart tapes	+++	−−−	++
Anastomotic stabilizer as enucleator	+	+	+
Apical positioner (suction cap)	++	+	++
Apical positioner (suction surface)	++	++	++
Deep stitch in lateral posterior pericardium	+	−−	+
Deep tape under the left atrium (ULA)	+++	+++	++
Deep tape ULA with apical positioner (surface)	+++ **Preferred**	+++ **Preferred**	+++ **Preferred**

Table 3 The components of Newton's second law

The centre of the mass to be elevated and rotated	G
The distance of the middle of the front wheel to the centre of the mass	b
The distance between the centre of the mass and the hands lifting the wheelbarrow	c

The exposure of the posterolateral wall demands two movements of the left ventricle, namely a rotational movement out of the cavity and an elevation movement. In fact, this is exactly what a wheelbarrow does with a load. Newton in his second law studies this effect (Table 3).

Newton describes that if the distance b is 0, there will be no lift, only rotation. The longer the distance b, the higher the lift. This has considerable consequences. So, the closer we will bring the anchoring stitch to the bottom of the heart on the left pericardium, the better the lift. But it is possible to move even further, namely under the left atrium closer to the right superior pulmonary vein. There are some issues in placement, but we will discuss this later. In addition, we have documented that nearly all anchor placements outside of the left atrial quadrangle induce mitral valve incompetence by breaking the atrioventricular axis. One needs to measure the pulmonary artery pressures to observe this.

To lift the heart, we can use three possible structures.

The first one is the posterior pericardial wall. This wall is fixed to the posterior side of the pericardium and will only lift minimally.

The second possibility is to use sutures and have the heart lay on the sutures. This will be much better, but a suture has only a small contact zone with the cardiac surface and is at risk of creating abrasion.

The third possibility and our preferred one is a wide, wet tape that is anchored under the left atrium. The larger and wet contact zone annihilates the risk of abrasion and spreads the leverage movement during rotation and lifting. Some units even use warm fluids to wet the tapes.

Step 1:

Interface with anaesthesia and request permission to start the process. The conditioning of the patient should be perfect, as the filling of the patient, no ischaemia, and physiological values for the ions. See the applications "CABG OPCAB training" and "MyCVsurgery" for videos and graphical depictions of every step involved.

Step 2:

Have a small sponge in the right hand. Place the left hand in the chest and take the ventricle out of its pocket, in a gentle move and without compressing the ventricle, so that it can continue to fill and empty. Pass the ventricle from the left hand to the right hand and keep the small sponge between the heart and the right hand. Scoop with the fingers of the left hand under the left atrium and between the two inferior pulmonary veins: with one finger if it is a small older lady, and with up to three fingers where possible. Lift the scooped left atrium upwards.

This movement separates the left atrial wall from the posterior mediastinum under that left atrium. That posterior mediastinal wall becomes visible. Make sure not to squeeze the heart under the left forearm. Indeed, if you do not allow the heart to fill, it will not eject. Practise this manoeuvre having the aorta cannulated.

Step 3:

Place a 1 Prolene 100 cm long polypropylene suture in the pulmonary quadrant, under the left atrium, as high up as possible and as close as possible to the right superior pulmonary vein. Beware of the route of oesophagus. Do not anchor into the pulmonary inflow veins; their structure is not solid enough.

Bring the needle out of the chest and return the heart gently to its physiologic position. These complete steps 2 and 3; together, it should only need 5–7 s. Allow the haemodynamic situation to return to normal. After some experience, this can be done without reduction of filling and ejection.

Step 4:

Place a long and stiff tourniquet around the previously inserted 1 Prolene suture, place a long and wet sponge through the open eye of the tourniquet, and divide it into two equal lengths of sponge, creating a two-pronged or two-armed structure.

Step 5:

Interface again with anaesthesia, and request permission for the second manoeuvre. Use the left hand to displace the left ventricle, and use a solid forceps in the right hand to push the sponge down in the open space, all the way down to the anchor point. The first assistant or scrub nurse follows downwards with the tourniquet and affixes it with a solid clamp.

Place one prong of the sponge more upwards and one more downwards, so that the mass of the ventricle is centred in the middle between both, as in a cradle. The surgeon returns the heart to its physiologic position. This manoeuvre should take less than 3–4 s. Allow the haemodynamic situation to return to normal.

Step 6:

Interface again for the third time with anaesthesia and agree on starting the actual enucleation process. The anaesthesiologist monitors the monitoring systems as well as the surgical field. The surgeon monitors only the surgical field. In the past, a Google Glass-type monitoring system was used by the surgeon. It was conceptually incorrect; each medical profession should monitor its own domain. The two prongs should be separated around 4 cm from one another and the mass of the left ventricle around halfway in between. If the distance between the two sponge prongs is too close, the ventricle will slide one way or the other; if it is too wide, the ventricle will not enucleate.

Step 7:

Very slowly elevate and pull the two prongs towards the left side of the chest, with the intention of giving as much space as possible to the left ventricle to enucleate. The heart is slowly elevated, and the prongs are repeatedly adjusted in function of the pathway followed by the left ventricle to maintain optimal control. Not a single premature ventricular contraction should be observed.

The anaesthesiologist is given time to respond to changes in filling, by elevating the legs. Trendelenburg is considered outdated to avoid cerebral venous congestion. If needed, additional volume or selective vasoconstrictors are given. The whole process should take a few minutes and should result in a full erectile left ventricle.

Step 8:

If the ventricular shape is rather oblong, it is possible to observe an axial instability of the erectile left ventricle. This creates PVCs and even minor haemodynamic consequences.

If the ventricular shape is round, the airspace between the left ventricular wall and the sternal retractor is minimal and sometimes even absent. Both issues are solved by placing a tri-appendage apical positioner.

In fact, we use an apical positioner in nearly all cases to facilitate the procedure for the surgeon with lesser experience. The negative suction, needed to control the movement of the heart, can be reduced from the proposed −400 mm Hg to −200 mmHg, because the ventricle is completely supported from the bottom-up. If too much elevation tension is applied, it is preferable for the positioner to disconnect from the ventricle.

The positioner is placed in the zone left lateral to the LAD with two appendages pointing towards and the third away from the LAD. The LAD is avoided as is the diaphragmatic surface of the right ventricle because the suction will disconnect at the first manipulation of the positioner.

The movement of the positioner will be longitudinal to optimize longitudinal axis. The exact reference is the diaphragmatic surface of the right ventricle. This surface must be physiologically flat. The rectilinear ventricular axis will be maintained, and all bending of the ventricular axis is avoided.

The movement of the positioner will be lateral to optimize the exposure of the different vessels, avoiding an unnecessary simultaneous exposure of all the lateral, posterior, and inferior vessels.

Step 9:

The position on the retractor depends on the anastomotic targets. For all targets from the intermediary (angularis) coronary vessel to the second lateral branch, the positioner is fixed at the most inferior part of the right arm of the retractor and the anastomotic stabilizer, just above. Make sure that the ventricular shape is not touching and is not deformed by the anastomotic stabilizer (Fig. 6).

For all targets beyond the second lateral up to the posterior descending coronary vessel, it is preferable to fix the positioner on the superior part of the right or left arm of the sternal retractor. Otherwise, the arm of the positioner comes in the airspace needed for visioning the anastomotic area.

The branches of the stabilizer will always point downwards towards the posterior mediastinum. Please observe that the curvatures of the heart are respected in all directions. This will preserve the haemodynamic stability.

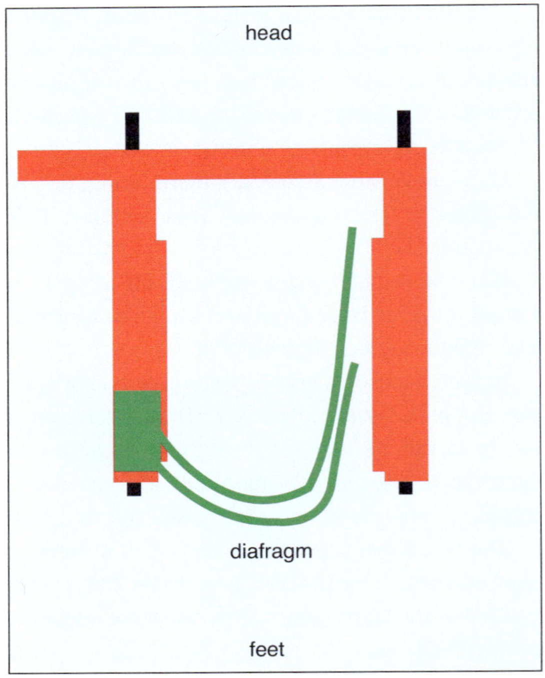

Fig. 6 The positioning of the apical positioner for all anastomoses to the deeper anterolateral vessels

Step 10:

In the presence of severe left ventricular hypertrophy, the airspace is often very reduced. It is possible to increase this airspace by transforming the two arms of the stabilizer into a spoon shape, creating a linear inwards curvature.

This 10-step enucleation method was developed in the research lab, studying the contractility and relaxation of a sheep heart during different alternatives.

6 The Exposure of the Proximal Right Coronary Artery

Moderate lesions of the proximal right have very good results after being treated by stenting, but severe stenosis or proximal occlusion mandates specific surgical steps. Indeed, the right proximal coronary is often a very diffusely disease vessel, with an internal diameter up to and sometimes larger than 3 mm. It also perfuses a large part of the right and sometimes left ventricular mass.

Temporary occlusion of the right coronary vessel can lead to total atrioventricular block. The conduction safety is improved by the mandatory placement, before the start of the anastomosis, of atrioventricular pacing wires and their testing. The ischaemic safety is improved by completing the RCA anastomosis at the end of the grafting sequence when all other grafts are opened. Shunting is mandatory, and the largest possible shunts need to be available in the operating theatre.

The left-sided pericardial suspension is brought down, and the right pericardial section is retracted. It might also be easier for the surgeon to perform the anastomosis from the left side of the table.

7 Conclusion

It is perfectly possible to visualize and stabilize all sections of the coronary system that are normally revascularized. It is essential to follow strict conditioning of the patient and to monitor every possible haemodynamic and ischaemic variation using real-time methods. Finally, the very reduced airspace, as observed in off-pump CABG, forces the surgeon to move from parachuted to non-parachuted anastomotic techniques. This is outside of the scope of this manuscript.

Graft Materials, Harvesting Methods, and Treatment of Grafts in Surgical Myocardial Revascularization

Rahk Margaryan

Abbreviations

CABG	Coronary artery bypass grafting
CAD	Coronary artery disease
ePTFE	Extended polytetrafluoroethylene
EVH	Endoscopic vein harvesting
EC	Endothelial cells
GVS	Great saphenous vein
OVH	Open vein harvesting
OM	Obtuse margin branch

Coronary artery bypass grafting (CABG) remains the "holy grail" of revascularization for stable multivessel coronary artery disease (CAD) [1, 2]. The most widely used conduits are autologous internal thoracic arteries, radial arteries, and saphenous veins, which provide excellent mechanical stability and natural antithrombogenicity [3]. Only simple search on PubMed Central gives us an idea on how many articles had been published on a single argument of this chapter since 60s of the last century (see Fig. 1).

In this chapter, we first describe the conduit, then harvesting techniques, conduit treatment after harvest, and best target for a given graft.

R. Margaryan (✉)
Ospedale del Cuore "G. Pasquinucci"; Fondazione Toscana G. Monasterio, Massa, Italy
e-mail: margaryan@ftgm.it

G. Concistrè (ed.), *Ischemic Heart Disease*,
https://doi.org/10.1007/978-3-031-25879-4_24

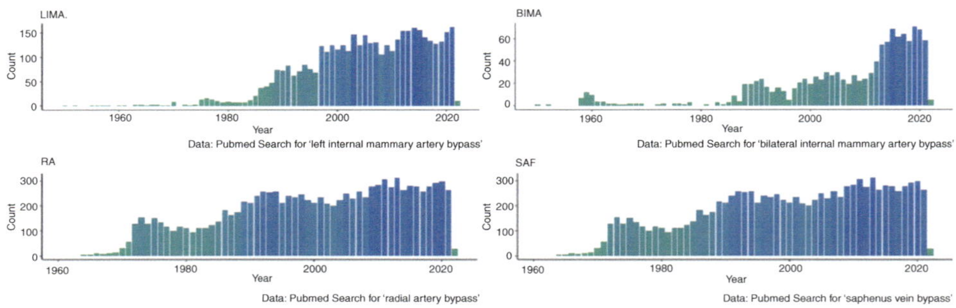

Fig. 1 PubMed search for all main conduit terms by year

1 Graft Materials

Graft material are classified into three main groups:

1.1 Arterial Grafts

- Left/right internal thoracic/mammary artery (LIMA/RIMA)
- Radial artery (RA)
- Right gastroepiploic artery (GAS)
- Inferior epigastric artery
- Other rare arterial grafts

1.2 Venous Grafts

- Greater saphenous vein (GVS)
- Short saphenous vein (SSV)
- Cephalic vein (CEV)

1.3 Alternative Conduits for CABG

- ePTFE
- Dacron
- Biological prosthesis
- Other types of materials

1.4 Left Internal Mammary Artery (LIMA)/Left Internal Thoracic Artery (LITA)

Vineberg et al. were the first to recognize the properties of internal mammary artery (IMA) and used it for myocardial revascularization in 1945 [4]. It was documented that it is usually spared from atherosclerosis and reasoned that its branches could form collaterals with myocardial arterioles. They injected contrast medium in postmortem specimens demonstrating connections between the implant and the coronary arteries. ITAs have unique molecular mechanisms to combat atherosclerosis formation, and that is why it is considered superior to other grafts for revascularization purposes [5]. LIMA originates from subclavian artery just above and behind the sternal end of the clavicle. The artery descends vertically 1 cm lateral to the sternal border, behind the first six costal cartilages. LIMA is widely used these days, especially for the anastomosis with LAD. After dividing the sternum, a retractor is placed to lift the left sternal edge. The operating table can be elevated and rotated to expose LIMA properly and harvest it. LIMA can be harvested as pedicle graft (along with internal thoracic veins, fat, muscles, and pleura) or skeletonized vessel. Skeletonized LIMA is supposed to preserve the venous drainage of the sternum, and it is often preferred when there is suspicion of sternal healing and wound infection. All small branches of LIMA are clipped. The proximal end of the LIMA is kept attached to the subclavian artery, and then after giving heparin, the distal end is ligated and divided. In the same way as LIMA is harvested, RIMA can also be harvested if it is needed for grafting. Harvesting of the internal mammary artery during CABG surgery using a skeletonized technique was associated with a higher rate of graft occlusion and worse clinical outcomes than the traditional pedicled technique [6]. While the long-term survival of patients was not different between groups, the rate of adverse cardiovascular events was consistently higher in the skeletonized group and the difference was associated with surgeon-related factors. Further evidence on the outcome of skeletonized ITA is needed [7]. After internal mammary takedown, it is usually treated with hot papaverine solution 50 mg in 100 ml physiological solution. The use of intraluminal papaverine entails a high frequency of vessel wall injury. Intraluminal papaverine solution administered once or twice in addition to external papaverine exposure is a predictor of high flow compared with only external papaverine exposure and provides a more effective distal dilation [8]. Lately, minimally invasive harvesting of LIMA/RIMA is becoming widespread [9]. Coronary surgeons can rapidly become proficient in robotic assisted endoscopic LIMA harvest, with significant improvement in operative times evident within the first 20 cases completed. These data may be useful in designing appropriate training programs for newer surgeons seeking to gain experience in robotic assisted coronary surgery [10]. Valdis et al. have demonstrated that a virtual robotic simulation curriculum can significantly improve the efficiency and quality of learning in robotic cardiac surgery. Further evaluation of this curriculum is required for its widespread implementation in surgical training [11].

1.5 Right Internal Mammary Artery

Right internal mammary artery (RIMA) inherits all the same abovementioned features and is usually considered as a second conduit. Some surgeons prefer RIMA on DA when LIMA is not available, or it is used for other important left-sided vessels. When bypassing with RIMA, preference should be given to grafting arteries with a high-grade stenosis or occlusion, to grafting left rather than right coronary arteries, and to using in situ rather than free ITA grafts [12]. Passing the RITA to the left, either anterior to the aorta or through the transverse sinus, does not influence the graft patency [13]. Its length can be predicted as shown in our latest research [14].

1.6 Bilateral Internal Mammary Artery

BIMA grafting is associated with enhanced overall long-term outcomes compared with LIMA grafting. While the BIMA patients demonstrate an increased incidence of DSWI (rather slight increase), the survival benefits and other morbidity advantages outweigh this short-term risk [15]. Target importance has a major role as defined by Bakaeen and colleges [16]. In BIMA grafting, bypassing multiple important targets (>75% of heart length) to maximize myocardium supplied by ITAs improved long-term survival. In patients with a nondominant LAD, selecting an important target for the second ITA lowered operative mortality [16]. Bilateral internal thoracic artery grafting produces improved survival compared with single internal thoracic artery grafting during the second postoperative decade, and the magnitude of that benefit increases through 20 postoperative years [17]. Both internal mammary arteries can be harvested in direct vision in sternotomy and thoracotomy, and endoscopic and robotic harvesting is becoming more popular due to increase of minimally invasive revascularization interventions [18]. Step-by-step harvesting techniques could be found in multimedial manual of cardiothoracic surgery by Mateo Marín-Cuartas et al.

2 Radial Artery

Second most commonly used artery is the radial artery (RA). It is usually harvested from nondominant hand. The RA arises from the bifurcation of the brachial artery in the cubital fossa and terminates by forming the deep palmar arch in the hand. The main concern using RA is blood supply to the wrist and hand. Before using the radial artery, we should assess the patency and collateral blood circulation from the ulnar artery. It can be assessed clinically by Allen's and modified Allen's tests. This can also be assessed by preoperative arterial ultrasound. The radial artery can be harvested by open conventional method or endoscopically. The radial artery should be flushed and kept in a solution prepared with Ringer's lactate (500 ml), sodium nitroprusside (50 mg), and heparinized blood (30 ml). Conventionally, radial artery is harvested openly, but in record years, more groups are adopting endoscopic harvesting [19] and reporting its noninferiority.

3 Right Gastroepiploic Artery

It is very rarely used as an arterial graft when other conduits are not available or intended complete arterial revascularization in the absence of other conduits. To harvest this artery, the midline incision over the sternum is extended to the upper abdomen, and the abdominal cavity is opened. There are two gastroepiploic arteries: left and right. Both arteries participate in the stomach vascularization and are collateral blood circulation with other blood vessels of the stomach. Harvesting right gastroepiploic artery as conduit does not compromise stomach blood supply. Branches of this artery to the stomach and omentum are ligated and divided. This artery is positioned either anteriorly or posteriorly to the duodenum and stomach, depending on the tension on graft. A circular opening is made in the diaphragm, medial to the inferior vena cava, and the gastroepiploic artery is passed through this opening to anastomose it with RCA or PDA coronary arteries.

4 Venous Grafts

4.1 Greater Saphenous Vein

The greater saphenous vein (GVS) is the most commonly used conduit for CABG. The greater saphenous vein of the lower extremity is the best choice of this type of graft based on the following:

- There are two independent types of low-extremity vein system, and removal of superficial one does not jeopardize the venous flow from the leg.
- Position, diameter, and length of the GSV are in constant pattern, which simplifies its harvest.

Usually, a single long segment is harvested. About 12–15 cm segment may be needed for diagonal branch, about 20–24 cm length for OM branches, and 18–22 cm length for RCA and PDA coronary arteries. Poor quality and veins with varicosities should be avoided.

GSV is harvested in two different ways:

- Directly by single full incision or through multiple incisions
- Endoscopic vein harvest

Conventional saphenous vein graft preparation with low-pressure distension and harvesting the vein with a surrounding pedicle yielded similar graft wall thickness after 12 months, but low pressure was associated with fewer adverse events [20]. This means that even after perfect harvesting, one needs to be careful not to damage the graft with extensive distension. No-touch SVG grafts have excellent patency similar to that of RA grafts after 8 years, over 80%. In addition, no-touch grafts can be used in situations that are not ideal for RA grafts due to the absence of reaction on competitive flow [21]. In the endoscopic vein harvest (EVH) patients, harvesting time increased, and incision closure time decreased in comparison with open vein harvesting (OVH). The hospital stay was declared as 5.5 ± 2.4 days in the EVH group versus 9.5 ± 2.7 days in the OVH group. Leg wound complications were significantly reduced in the EVH group in comparison with the OVH group [22]. Zenati et al. did not find a significant difference between open vein graft harvesting and endoscopic vein graft harvesting in the risk of major adverse cardiac events [23].

4.2 Short Saphenous Vein

In rare cases, when not enough conduits are available, some surgeons have to use short saphenous vein. It can be harvested by positioning the patient in prone or supine position.

4.3 Cephalic Vein

Even though we have not used the vein as an alternative graft, this can be used in case when other grafts need it. The cephalic vein can be harvested from the wrist up to the shoulder. The walls of the vein are thinner than the saphenous veins, and long-term patency is also lesser than saphenous veins [24].

5 Alternative Conduits for CABG

5.1 ePTFE

PTFE is an inert fluorocarbon polymer and subsequently made more microporous by extrusion and sintering to form expanded PTFE (ePTFE). This polymer is nonbiodegradable with an electronegative luminal surface that is antithrombotic and is now widely used for lower limb bypass grafts (7–9 mm) with excellent results. Cardiac surgeons have used ePTFE grafts, though reluctantly, in many centers. These grafts are rigid compared with the elastic host artery [25]. The poor mechanical characteristics (compliance) and the lack of endothelial cells (ECs) lining the lumen of such graft materials are the significant factors contributing to their poor patency [26].

5.2 Dacron

Dacron is a type of polyester in the form of multiple filaments either woven or knitted into vascular grafts [27]. Dacron has been used as an alternative to autologous grafts, but it has shown poor patency rates when used in small diameter sizes or in low-flow locations [28]. In 1976, Sauvage reported a successful adult case with a knitted Dacron vascular graft (4 cm long and 3.5 mm in diameter) between the aorta and right coronary artery [29]. The graft was angiographically patent up to 16 months after surgery. At that time, the literature showed only two other successful uses of aortocoronary Dacron prostheses, both of which were placed in children with coronary anomalies [30, 31]. These three successful prostheses were short and used as interposition grafts between the ascending aorta and the proximal end of the coronary artery with high flow.

5.3 Biologic Prosthesis

Some biologic vascular grafts have been applied in the coronary artery position; however, most of them have failed because of thrombogenicity and degenerative changes. Like some other artificial small-diameter vascular grafts showing excellent antithrombogenicity in in vitro studies, no long-term results or patencies have been reported so far for their use in CABG. A human umbilical vein (HUV) graft (Biograft, Meadox Medicals, Oakland, NJ, USA; 4 mm internal diameter) demonstrated angiographic graft patency rate of 46% (6/13) at 3–13 months [32]. In another report, treated bovine IMA graft (Biocor BIMA Biograft, Biocor laboratory, 4 and 5 mm of internal diameter) was implanted in the coronary artery position of 20 patients [33]. Graft patency was confirmed in only two patients at 6 months. However, no long-term results or other patient information has been reported so far. Perloff et al. implanted two glutaraldehyde-tanned polyester mesh-supported sheep connective tissue tubes (6 mm diameter) for left and right main coronary artery bypasses in one patient [34]. They confirmed patency angiographically at 19 months. Dialdehyde starch-treated bovine artery grafts (Bioflow, BioVascular Inc., St. Paul, MN, USA) were used over the past few years outside of the USA and Japan [35]. Only one long-term follow-up clinical report was available, and it revealed graft patency rates of 16% (3/19) at 3–23 months [36]. This is much lower than the reported patency rates for PTFE grafts. Furthermore, the graft has a tendency for dilatation due to degenerative changes, as has been reported in a coronary artery position in a canine study [37].

5.4 Harvesting Methods

5.4.1 Graft Management in Surgical Myocardial Revascularization (Table 1)

Table 1 Strategies to optimize utilization and outcomes of multiarterial revascularization

Patient selection	Patient age <70 years Life expectancy >10 years Hemodynamically stable
Conduit selection	Right internal thoracic artery • BMI <30 kg/m^2 • HbA1c <7% Radial artery • Intact palmar arch • No dissection/instrumentation
Target selection	Important vessel (>75% reach toward ventricular apex) >1.5 mm caliber >80% proximal stenosis
Surgeon selection	O:E operative mortality and complications <1.0 Prioritize complete revascularization Facile with right internal thoracic artery and radial harvest Expertise in composite and sequential grafts
Practice drivers	Implement effective surgical site infection bundle Establish multiarterial revascularization quality metric Target referral to committed surgeons Educate physicians and patients Upgrade guideline recommendations Increase the evidence base

BMI = body mass index; HbA1c = hemoglobin A1c; O:E = ratio of observed to expected [38]

Length and diameter of mostly used conduits are given in the study of Martinez-Gonzalez et al. [39]

References

1. Neumann F-J, Sousa-Uva M, Ahlsson A, Alfonso F, Banning AP, Benedetto U, et al. 2018 ESC/EACTS Guidelines on myocardial revascularization. European Heart Journal. Available from: https://academic.oup.com/eurheartj/advance-article/doi/10.1093/eurheartj/ehy394/5079120
2. 2021 ACC/AHA/SCAI guideline for coronary artery revascularization: A report of the American College of Cardiology/American Heart Association joint committee on clinical practice guidelines | journal of the American College of Cardiology. Available from: https://www.jacc.org/doi/10.1016/j.jacc.2021.09.006?_ga=2.113540548.255118602.1643044109-1910640928.1643044109
3. Angelini GD, Newby AC. The future of saphenous vein as a coronary artery bypass conduit. European Heart Journal. 1989;10(3):273–80. https://doi.org/10.1093/oxfordjournals.eurheartj.a059476.
4. Vineberg A, Miller G. Treatment of coronary insufficiency. Canadian Medical Association Journal. 1951;64(3):204–10. Available from: https://www.ncbi.nlm.nih.gov/pmc/articles/PMC1821866/

5. Otsuka F, Yahagi K, Sakakura K, Virmani R. Why is the mammary artery so special and what protects it from atherosclerosis? Annals of Cardiothoracic Surgery. 2013;2(4):519–26. https://doi.org/10.3978/j.issn.2225-319X.2013.07.06.
6. Lamy A, Browne A, Sheth T, Zheng Z, Dagenais F, Noiseux N, et al. Skeletonized vs Pedicled Internal Mammary Artery Graft Harvesting in Coronary Artery Bypass Surgery: A Post Hoc Analysis From the COMPASS Trial. JAMA cardiology. 2021; https://doi.org/10.1001/jamacardio.2021.1686.
7. Gaudino M, Audisio K, Rahouma M, Chadow D, Cancelli G, Soletti GJ, et al. Comparison of Long-term Clinical Outcomes of Skeletonized vs Pedicled Internal Thoracic Artery Harvesting Techniques in the Arterial Revascularization Trial. JAMA cardiology. 2021;6(12):1380–6. https://doi.org/10.1001/jamacardio.2021.3866.
8. Dregelid E, Heldal K, Resch F, Stangeland L, Breivik K, Svendsen E. Dilation of the internal mammary artery by external and intraluminal papaverine application. The Journal of Thoracic and Cardiovascular Surgery. 1995;110(3):697–703. Available from: https://www.sciencedirect.com/science/article/pii/S002252239570101X
9. Lysenko AV, Bedzhanyan AL, Lednev PV, Salagaev GI, Belov YV. Endoscopic harvesting of internal mammary artery for coronary artery bypass grafting. Khirurgiia. 2018;11:96–9. https://doi.org/10.17116/hirurgia201811196.
10. Hemli JM, Henn LW, Panetta CR, Suh JS, Shukri SR, Jennings JM, et al. Defining the learning curve for robotic-assisted endoscopic harvesting of the left internal mammary artery. Innovations (Philadelphia, PA). 2013 Oct;8(5):353–8. https://doi.org/10.1097/IMI.0000000000000017.
11. Valdis M, Chu MWA, Schlachta CM, Kiaii B. Validation of a Novel Virtual Reality Training Curriculum for Robotic Cardiac Surgery: A Randomized Trial. Innovations (Philadelphia, PA). 2015 Dec;10(6):383–8. https://doi.org/10.1097/IMI.0000000000000222.
12. Buxton BF, Ruengsakulrach P, Fuller J, Rosalion A, Reid CM, Tatoulis J. The right internal thoracic artery graft–benefits of grafting the left coronary system and native vessels with a high grade stenosis. European Journal of Cardio-Thoracic Surgery: Official Journal of the European Association for Cardio-Thoracic Surgery. 2000;18(3):255–61. https://doi.org/10.1016/s1010-7940(00)00527-3.
13. Brown JA, Sultan I. Just go with the Flow: Coronary Targets may Dictate Right Internal Mammary Artery Patency More than Inflow Configuration. The Annals of Thoracic Surgery. 2021; https://doi.org/10.1016/j.athoracsur.2021.09.076.
14. Margaryan R, Latta DD, Bianchi G, Martini N, Gori A, Solinas M. Double mammary in situ: Predicting feasibility of right mammary artery in situ for circumflex coronary artery system. medRxiv. 2021.; Available from: https://www.medrxiv.org/content/early/2021/09/04/2020.12.05.20243964
15. Lytle BW, Blackstone EH, Loop FD, Houghtaling PL, Arnold JH, Akhrass R, et al. Two internal thoracic artery grafts are better than one. The Journal of Thoracic and Cardiovascular Surgery. 1999;117(5):855–72. https://doi.org/10.1016/S0022-5223(99)70365-X.
16. Bakaeen FG, Ravichandren K, Blackstone EH, Houghtaling PL, Soltesz EG, Johnston DR, et al. Coronary Artery Target Selection and Survival After Bilateral Internal Thoracic Artery Grafting. Journal of the American College of Cardiology. 2020;75(3):258–68. https://doi.org/10.1016/j.jacc.2019.11.026.
17. Lytle BW, Blackstone EH, Sabik JF, Houghtaling P, Loop FD, Cosgrove DM. The effect of bilateral internal thoracic artery grafting on survival during 20 postoperative years. The Annals of Thoracic Surgery. 2004;78(6):1. https://doi.org/10.1016/j.athoracsur.2004.05.070.
18. Tarui T, Ishikawa N, Watanabe G. A Novel Robotic Bilateral Internal Mammary Artery Harvest Using Double Docking Technique for Coronary Artery Bypass Grafting. Innovations (Philadelphia, Pa). 2017;12(1):74–6. https://doi.org/10.1097/IMI.0000000000000331.

19. Van Linden A, Hecker F, Lehmann-Grube J, Arsalan M, Richter M, Matzke B, et al. Randomized Trial of 2 Endoscopic Radial Artery Harvesting Devices-Immunofluorescence Assessment. The Annals of Thoracic Surgery. 2020;110(3):897–902. https://doi.org/10.1016/j.athoracsur.2019.12.063.
20. Angelini GD, Johnson T, Culliford L, Murphy G, Ashton K, Harris T, et al. Comparison of alternate preparative techniques on wall thickness in coronary artery bypass grafts: The HArVeST randomized controlled trial. Journal of Cardiac Surgery. 2021;36(6):1985–95. https://doi.org/10.1111/jocs.15477.
21. Dreifaldt M, Mannion JD, Geijer H, Lidén M, Bodin L, Souza D. The no-touch saphenous vein is an excellent alternative conduit to the radial artery 8 years after coronary artery bypass grafting: A randomized trial. The Journal of Thoracic and Cardiovascular Surgery. 2021;161(2):624–30. https://doi.org/10.1016/j.jtcvs.2019.09.177.
22. Mubarak Y, Abdeljawad A. Leg Wound Complications: A Comparison Between Endoscopic and Open Saphenous Vein Harvesting Techniques. The Heart Surgery Forum. 2021;24(4):E604–10. https://doi.org/10.1532/hsf.3915.
23. Zenati MA, Bhatt DL, Bakaeen FG, Stock EM, Biswas K, Gaziano JM, et al. Randomized Trial of Endoscopic or Open Vein-Graft Harvesting for Coronary-Artery Bypass. The New England Journal of Medicine. 2019;380(2):132–41. https://doi.org/10.1056/NEJMoa1812390.
24. Wijnberg DS, Boeve WJ, Ebels T, van Gelder IC, van den Toren EW, Lie KI, et al. Patency of arm vein grafts used in aorto-coronary bypass surgery. European Journal of Cardio-Thoracic Surgery: Official Journal of the European Association for Cardio-Thoracic Surgery. 1990;4(9):510–3. https://doi.org/10.1016/1010-7940(90)90176-z.
25. Tai NR, Salacinski HJ, Edwards A, Hamilton G, Seifalian AM. Compliance properties of conduits used in vascular reconstruction. The British Journal of Surgery. 2000;87(11):1516–24. https://doi.org/10.1046/j.1365-2168.2000.01566.x.
26. Berger K, Sauvage LR, Rao AM, Wood SJ. Healing of arterial prostheses in man: its incompleteness. Annals of Surgery. 1972;175(1):118–27. https://doi.org/10.1097/00000658-197201000-00018.
27. Xue L, Greisler HP. Biomaterials in the development and future of vascular grafts. Journal of Vascular Surgery. 2003;37(2):472–80. https://doi.org/10.1067/mva.2003.88.
28. Soldani G, Losi P, Bernabei M, Burchielli S, Chiappino D, Kull S, et al. Long term performance of small-diameter vascular grafts made of a poly(ether)urethane-polydimethylsiloxane semi-interpenetrating polymeric network. Biomaterials. 2010;31(9):2592–605. https://doi.org/10.1016/j.biomaterials.2009.12.017.
29. Sauvage LR, Schloemer R, Wood SJ, Logan G. Successful interposition synthetic graft between aorta and right coronary artery. Angiographic follow-up to sixteen months. The Journal of Thoracic and Cardiovascular Surgery. 1976;72(3):418–21.
30. Hallman GL, Cooley DA, Mcnamara DG, Latson JR. Single Left Coronary Artery with Fistula to Right Ventricle: Reconstruction of Two-Coronary System with Dacron Graft. Circulation. 1965;32:293–7. https://doi.org/10.1161/01.cir.32.2.293.
31. Cooley DA, Hallman GL, Bloodwell RD. Definitive surgical treatment of anomalous origin of left coronary artery from pulmonary artery: indications and results. The Journal of Thoracic and Cardiovascular Surgery. 1966;52(6):798–808.
32. Silver GM, Katske GE, Stutzman FL, Wood NE. Umbilical vein for aortocoronary bypass. Angiology. 1982;33(7):450–3. https://doi.org/10.1177/000331978203300704.
33. Vrandecic MO. New graft for the surgical treatment of small vessel diseases. The Journal of Cardiovascular Surgery. 1987;28(6):711–4.
34. Perloff LJ, Christie BA, Ketharanathan V, Field PL, Milne PY, MacLeish DG, et al. A new replacement for small vessels. Surgery. 1981;89(1):31–41.

35. Suma H, Wanibuchi Y, Terada Y, Fukuda S, Saito T, Isshiki T, et al. Bovine internal thoracic artery graft. Successful use at urgent coronary bypass surgery. The Journal of Cardiovascular Surgery. 1991;32(2):268–70.
36. Mitchell IM, Essop AR, Scott PJ, Martin PG, Gupta NK, Saunders NR, et al. Bovine internal mammary artery as a conduit for coronary revascularization: long-term results. The Annals of Thoracic Surgery. 1993;55(1):120–2. https://doi.org/10.1016/0003-4975(93)90485-z.
37 Tomizawa Y, Moon MR, DeAnda A, Castro LJ, Kosek J, Miller DC. Coronary bypass grafting with biological grafts in a canine model. Circulation. 1994;90(5 Pt 2):II160–6.
38. Chikwe J, Adams DH. State-of-the-art revascularization. Journal of the American College of Cardiology. 2020;75(3):269–72. Available from: https://www.jacc.org/doi/10.1016/j.jacc.2019.12.005
39. Martínez-González B, Reyes-Hernández CG, Quiroga-Garza A, Rodríguez-Rodríguez VE, Esparza-Hernández CN, Elizondo-Omaña RE, et al. Conduits used in coronary artery bypass grafting: A review of morphological studies. Annals of Thoracic and Cardiovascular Surgery. 2017;23(2):55–65. Available from: https://www.ncbi.nlm.nih.gov/pmc/articles/PMC5422630/

Total Arterial Revascularization, Techniques, and Results

Massimo Lemma

1 Arteries vs. Veins

The long history of CABG started just over 100 years ago, since Alexis Carrel in 1910 first described the concept of operating on the coronary circulation [5]. With his pioneering work, CABG entered an evolutionary journey that led it to be the standard of care for treating stable patients with multivessel coronary artery disease.

After Carrel, many other visionary surgeons developed techniques aimed at myocardial revascularization. The first graft used in humans was the LITA, as early as 1945 by Arthur Vineberg, who implanted it directly in the left ventricular myocardium, a technique later called "Vineberg procedure" [3]. Also, the first successful suture technique, CABG operation, was performed with a LITA graft. In 1964, Kolesov, with specially designed magnifying glasses and scissors, grafted the LITA to the left circumflex artery in a patient who remained free of angina during 3 years of follow-up [6].

However, the era of CABG with the prevalent use of the SV was just round the corner. In 1967, while working at the Cleveland Clinic, Rene' Favaloro reported the use of SV graft in direct coronary surgery in 180 patients [7], establishing an important landmark that brought to the birth of modern surgical myocardial revascularization. Paradoxically, although at its origin coronary surgery began with arterial grafts, the SV with its technical ease of harvest, its robust handling characteristics, and its versatility as an aortocoronary graft simplified the conduct of the operation and allowed for widespread reproducibility, establishing the current primacy of mixed venous and arterial grafting achieved by blending the use of LITA for LAD coronary artery and the SV for the targets on the circumflex and right coronary artery.

M. Lemma (✉)
Jilin Heart Hospital, Changchun, China
e-mail: dr.lemma@jlheart.org

G. Concistrè (ed.), *Ischemic Heart Disease*,
https://doi.org/10.1007/978-3-031-25879-4_25

LITA started to be frequently used by surgeons as early as the 1970s, but it was not until the mid-1980s that its importance to favorably influence the clinical outcome was recognized. Loop and colleagues from the Cleveland Clinic [8] were the first to report better outcomes over 10 years with the use of the LITA when compared to SV grafting alone. Following the obvious benefits of single LITA grafting to LAD, many groups postulated that BITA harvesting would further improve outcomes. The use of BITA was first described by Suzuki in 1973 [9], and in 1999, Bruce Lytle from the Cleveland Clinic confirmed that it was associated with greater survival and reduced need for repeat revascularization when compared to SITA grafting [10]. In his historical paper, he stated that "it has been the position of some coronary artery surgeons that the consideration of multiple arterial grafting could be ignored because no clear evidence existed that outcomes were improved for any patient subsets. That position is no longer tenable." However, after more than 20 years, the proportion of BITA currently used in North America is less than 5% [4] with a trend constant over time, based on the assumption that:

1. BITA is not supported by a level of evidence A, namely data derived from multiple randomized clinical trials or meta-analyses, making its use not scientifically supported "sensu stricto."
2. BITA is more technically demanding and time consuming, requiring for an in situ RITA to cross the mediastinum midline to reach the LAD or circumflex systems.
3. BITA is associated with a greater incidence of sternal wound complications particularly in patients with severe airway disease, obesity, and diabetes [11].

To overcome the problems related to BITA but at the same time recognizing the superiority of arteries over the SV, other arterial grafts were subsequently proposed. In 1971, Alain Carpentier used first the RA for CABG, reporting early graft failure rates and significant intimal hyperplasia, evidences that led to its abandoning for many years to follow [12]. It was nearly 20 years later that Christophe Acar, from the same Carpentier's group, reported excellent RA patency results on early postoperative angiography, using a different harvesting technique (pedicled vs. skeletonized) and preventing treatment to address RA spasm (pharmacological vs. mechanical vasodilation). It is worth to note that the renewed interest in the RA by the Carpentier's group was a consequence of serendipity, the accidental angiographic finding of a patent RA graft carried out 15 years before and found occluded at postoperative control [13]. Further multiple reports of positive RA outcomes coupled with its several favorable anatomical features (length, size, wall quality, constant uniform caliper) and easiness of harvesting led to RA widespread adoption, putting it in competition with the RITA as the second arterial graft of choice [14].

Also, the RGEA, the inferior epigastric artery, and the ulnar artery have been tested as coronary grafts. Of these, only the RGEA still has a few enthusiast supporters, particularly in Japan, who advocate multiple arterial grafting with only in situ grafts [15]. The need to open the abdominal cavity for harvesting, the complexity linked to the transdiaphragmatic route, the additional procedural length, and its nearly exclusive use on the distal branches of the right coronary artery have limited its widespread adoption.

2 Should We Pursue TAR?

As previously mentioned, the majority of cardiac surgical procedures performed worldwide are isolated CABG. Data extrapolated from the STS Adult Cardiac Surgery Database, 2019, show that by adding the number of isolated CABG to combined CABG procedures (CABG plus mitral valve and aortic valve), CABG makes up 63% of all typologies recorded [16]. Regrettably, TAR accounts for approximately only 2% of all multivessel CABG [17], while the use of more than one arterial graft ranges, according to the main series of Europe and North America, between 3.9% and 34.2% [18]. All the remaining CABG are performed by much the same technique that was developed more than 30 years ago, namely bypass LITA-LAD plus SV grafts to all non-LAD targets.

After the Cleveland Clinic report on BITA in 1999, other papers suggested that a second arterial conduit is associated with improved survival, graft patency, freedom from reoperation, and less incidence of major adverse cardiovascular events [19, 20], but this favorable data have not been confirmed by randomized studies [21–23] and also the recent intention-to-treat analysis of the ART found no difference in survival between patients receiving SITA or BITA at 10-year follow-up [24]. The available data suggest an improvement in clinical outcome for the use of more than one arterial graft, but there is little evidence to support a further benefit for TAR, considering the favorable differences seen in observational series probably due to treatment allocation biases [25].

The lack of a strong scientific evidence supporting the compelling use of arterial grafts was cited by almost one-third of UK surgeons when asked what issues limited the use of BITA in clinical practice [26], while for those surgeons convinced by the available evidence base, the factor limiting the use of arterial grafts seems related to the increased complexity of the procedure and its potential complications. Regrettably, the quality metrics which both surgeons and hospitals are usually held accountable are based on 30-day outcomes, and the very good results achievable 1 month after surgery by the traditional LITA-LAD plus SV graft strategy distract attention from the benefits of the more technically challenging TAR procedure that will not become evident until much later follow-up. Under these circumstances, TAR is considered only in patients with reasonable life expectancy [27] and in patients with poor vein quality independently of age.

3 Which Strategy for TAR?

The aim of TAR is to bypass all patient's graftable coronary arteries with significant lumen stenosis using only arterial grafts. It is a complex surgical procedure, more demanding if compared to single LITA + SV CABG, whose correct execution is influenced by technical, patient, and logistic factors, all of which are decisive for obtaining good results. As a consequence, both a good clinical and surgical sense is of paramount importance to choose the strategy that allows to give patients the maximum of expected benefits while running the minimum of risks.

3.1 Surgeon's Technical Skill and Team Readiness for TAR

Knowing that the evidence supporting better clinical outcomes with TAR is slim and that TAR is more technically demanding if compared to standard CABG, surgeons should remember that only making a procedure more complex does not automatically make it better and that deciding to increase the surgical complexity in the name of possible future benefits, they will be directly accountable for the potential short-term side effects of this choice. It follows that surgeons must have a realistic idea of both their technical skills and the readiness of the entire team regarding TAR patients' management. An alive patient with ITA and SV is a very good result, but a catastrophe after a complex TAR is not and has no excuses when it is due to blatant lack of team experience and/or surgical bravado. In other words, both the surgeon and the team must be specifically trained before establishing a TAR program.

3.2 Patient's Clinical Presentation

Patients who are most likely to benefit from a TAR are relatively young, with little or no comorbidity, good left ventricular function, and clinical stability. Based on the experience of both the surgeon and the team, it is possible in specific cases to derogate from one or more of these indications but is seldom a good idea to perform TAR in emergency or highly unstable patients, when prognosis is mainly related to revascularization quickness than to its durability. The same is true also for patients with significantly reduced left ventricular systolic function who could need high doses of vasoactive drugs in the postoperative period, increasing the risk of potential generalized arterial graft vasospasm, a catastrophic complication that must be carefully prevented.

3.3 Coronary Artery Anatomy

Coronary artery anatomy seems to represent a key factor for proper patient selection, being generally accepted that the cutoff stenosis for arterial graft is higher than that for the SV. It has been reported that RGEA and RA are much less tolerant than ITA to the detrimental effect of chronic competitive coronary flow [28], and it is usually recommended to use the RA only if the native coronary artery stenosis is sub-occlusive (>70–90%) [29]. This postulation has been recently weakened by Royse et al. who reported angiographic results of 76 symptomatic patients (belonging to a larger group of 464 patients) who underwent TAR with composite LITA-RA-Y graft between 1996 and 1999, showing that grafting any coronary artery with a greater than 50% stenosis with LITA-RA-Y graft had acceptable rates of graft patency at a mean of 5.8 years postoperatively (LAD 94%, circumflex 90%, right coronary artery 74%) [30]. The same report gives also the opportunity to subject to revaluation of a second generally accepted assumption, namely that ITA grafts and LITA-Y grafts have higher vulnerability to competitive flow from native coronary arteries [31].

3.4 Second Arterial Graft Selection: RITA vs. RA

With LITA being the ideal graft for LAD, RITA has consequently been the second arterial graft of choice after LITA for many surgeons and for many years, even in the absence of robust data supporting its use. The only large RCT on the use of single ITA vs. bilateral ITA grafting is ART, which compared single and bilateral ITA grafting in 3102 patients. In ART, there was no statistically significant difference in survival (HR, 0.96 [95% CI, 0.82–1.12]) or event-free survival (HR, 0.90 [95% CI, 0.79–1.03]) at 10 years. However, BITA harvesting was linked to a significant higher rate of sternal wound complications, particularly in patients with morbid obesity, diabetes mellitus, and chronic obstructive pulmonary disease [24]. Several authors have reported a correlation between BITA harvesting and increased incidence of sternal wound complications, finding in the pedicled technique the main responsible for the greater sternal devascularization. Benedetto et al. have reported fewer sternal wound infections if ITA skeletonization is used [32], and other authors have reported reduced pain, dysesthesia, and improved sternal blood flow with the same technique [33].

The bad news is that ITA skeletonization seems to be associated with a greater risk of major adverse cardiac events and repeat revascularization compared with the pedicle technique after a mean follow-up of 2 years from surgery, as reported by Lamy et al. in a post hoc analysis of the Cardiovascular Outcomes for People Using Anticoagulation Strategies (COMPASS) clinical trial [34]. Similar results are found in the retrospective analysis of the ART trial at 10 years done by Gaudino, who reports a significant higher incidence of MACE in the skeletonized group compared with the pedicled group (HR, 1.25; 95% CI, 1.06–1.47; P = .01) and a numerically greater number of deaths in the skeletonized cohort [35]. The difference in outcomes could be explained with the diversity of surgical harvesting technique between pedicled ITA and skeletonized ITA, the latter requiring direct manipulation of the artery that results to be more traumatic for the vessel wall causing intramural hematoma, dissection, and early thrombosis.

RA as the second arterial graft could be the ideal solution to overcome the decision-making stall generated by BITA harvesting, namely to use pedicled ITA grafts with good patency but increased risk of sternal wound complications or skeletonize the ITAs with higher risk of late graft occlusion but lower risk of sternal wound complications.

Contemporary myocardial revascularization guidelines consider RITA as class II and RA as class I indication [36], with the latter having a higher level and amount of evidence supporting improved patency rate and clinical outcomes compared to SV. It is overall recognized that the RA may improve CABG outcomes. A recent systematic review and meta-analysis has compared the clinical outcomes of patients undergoing isolated CABG with RA versus SV at a median follow-up of 10 years finding that RA was associated with a statistically significant reduction of the incidence of a composite outcome of death, myocardial infarction, or repeat revascularization (220 vs. 237 total events; 41 vs. 47 events per 1000 patient-years; hazard ratio, 0.73 [95% CI, 0.61–0.88]; $P < .001$) [37]. A further network meta-analysis from the same author has then analyzed 149,902 patients comparing the clinical results of RA, RITA, and SV, finding that the use of SV was associated with higher long-term mortality compared with the RA (incidence rate ratio, 1.23; 95% CI, 1.12–1.34) and RITA (incidence rate ratio, 1.26; 95% CI, 1.17–1.35) while there were no differences for any outcome between RA and RITA [38]. Eventually, the RA has been compared with the free RITA in addition to LITA-LAD in the Radial Artery Patency and Clinical Outcomes (RAPCO) trial. A total of 394 patients <70 years of age were assigned to receiving a RA or free RITA to compare the long-term patency, finding that the 10-year patency rate of the RA was significantly higher than that of the free RITA (89% vs. 80%, HR 0.45 [95% CI, 0.23–0.88]) [39]. These data support the use of the RA as free conduit of choice to complement the LITA in CABG surgery.

From the technical point of view, the RA is more surgeon friendly compared to the RITA and it has been shown that surgeon's experience plays a key role for BITA but not for RA [4]. RA harvesting can be done simultaneously to LITA and has thicker wall and larger diameter than RITA, features that make it more accessible during the operation rendering coronary anastomosis easier and faster to perform, reducing operative time. Moreover, the average harvested length is longer for RA allowing anastomosis to any of the coronary arteries when used as composite graft on LITA [40].

3.5 Arterial Graft Optimization

Patients with three-vessel disease rarely receive TAR with only in situ grafts, namely harvesting BITA and right GEA. This strategy is generally 1) time consuming (three grafts' harvesting time); 2) technically demanding (need to cross the mediastinal midline with the RITA to reach LAD or the territory of distribution of the circumflex coronary artery and need to open the abdominal cavity for GEA harvesting and its routing through the diaphragm on the distal branches of the right coronary artery); and 3) at increased risk of complications (sternal dehiscence and/or infection after BITA harvesting or RITA or RGEA damage in case of sternum reopening or upper abdominal surgery in the follow-up period after CABG). Following all this, the exclusive use of in situ grafts has always had adoption by only a niche of enthusiast surgeons [41] and cannot be considered the approach of choice.

Alternative techniques to make TAR less time consuming, technically demanding, and prone to potential complications are needed, and the creation of composite Y/T graft between LITA and a second arterial graft, usually RITA or RA, represents the possible answer. Historically, the concept of anastomosing another bypass graft to in situ LITA was introduced by Mills to overcome the stroke risk in the presence of a severely atherosclerotic ascending aorta [42]. Later, this technique gained more popularity, and in 1994, Tector reported the first series of patients who received BITA using the T-graft technique [43]. A few years later, the RA was used with the left ITA as a composite Y-graft by Royse who has recently reported the 21-year survival comparison of LITA-RA Y-graft versus the more conventional LITA plus SV on ascending aorta finding that survival after LITA plus

SV was worse than LITA-RA Y-graft both for unmatched (Kaplan-Meier, $p < 0.001$) and propensity score-matched groups (Kaplan-Meier, $p = 0.043$; Cox hazard ratio: 1.3; 95% confidence interval: 1.0–1.6; $p = 0.038$) [44].

Many cardiac surgeons are skeptical about composite Y/T-grafts because of concerns on the adequacy of LITA as single inflow for all the left ventricular mass. It has however been shown that LITA is able to adapt its dimension to flow demand in the late postoperative period [45] with a vascular remodeling that increases the diameter on follow-up angiograms at 3–10 months postoperatively [46]. More recently, it has been shown that in composite Y/T-graft, the proximal LITA is able to actively adapt its dimension to the flow demand, probably through the release of endothelial vasoactive mediators such as nitric oxide (NO), in response to higher values of wall shear stress (WSS) [47]. This process of adaptation begins immediately after the Y/T connection for a passive increase of blood flow due to the lower vascular resistance in the Y/T-graft system, according to the Kirchhoff's second law $1/Rtot = 1/R1+1/R2$, where Rtot is the total system resistance and R1 and R2 are the resistances of each vessel. After a Y/T-graft connection, the LITA main stem passively provides more blood flow due to the lower vascular resistance of the two branches of the composite graft, causing an increase in WSS values. The resulting higher blood flow in turn stimulates the synthetic and secretory functions of endothelial cells, modulating the production of NO (vasodilator) and endothelin-1 (vasoconstrictor), two potent endothelium-derived vasoactive mediators, producing active LITA dilation and return of WSS numbers within the normal range. A significant increase in LITA diameter can be seen starting from 5 days after surgery and continuing up to 10–12 months postoperatively.

Practical advantages resulting from the use of LITA as a composite Y/T-graft are the increased efficiency of the second graft in terms of length and the reduced stroke risk incidence for less manipulation of the ascending aorta.

The increased efficiency of second graft length is intuitive, with the distance between the point of inflow (LITA) and the point of outflow (coronary artery) being shorter if compared to a standard graft bridging ascending aorta and coronary arteries. Composite grafts either in Y or T shape allow TAR in nearly all patients, with very few exceptions due to peculiar anatomical features like a combination of short chest and arms, multiple coronary targets with diffusely diseased coronary arteries, and left ventricular dilation. In this regard, it is useful to remember that RA is generally longer than RITA and that under these circumstances it should be considered the preferred graft [48].

The reduced incidence of operative cerebral stroke deriving from the reduced ascending aorta manipulation is particularly evident when Y/T-grafts are combined with off-pump CABG in the so-called anaortic CABG (no-touch ascending aorta CABG). A propensity-matched analysis reported a trend toward a significant reduction of in-hospital all-cause mortality associated with avoiding aortic clamping [49], and a network meta-analysis of 13 studies and 37,720 patients supports this result by showing significant reduction in mortality, stroke, and renal failure when the anaortic CABG is adopted [50].

3.6 Graft Spasm Prevention

Coronary artery, arterial, and venous grafts are all prone to spasm. Among grafts, arteries are considered more prone to spams than veins, and among arteries, RA more than ITA [51]. Many factors can trigger spasm during CABG like mechanical stimulation during graft harvesting, hypothermia, pharmacological stimulation (alpha-adrenoceptor agonists), and cardiopulmonary bypass use (increased endothelin concentration). Endothelial disfunction seems to play a decisive role in the onset of spasm, and patients who require coronary revascularization through CABG usually present multiple risk factors, which can interfere with normal endothelial function like obesity, hypertension, hypercholesterolemia, diabetes mellitus, and smoking [52]. The incidence of spasm after CABG is reported to be 0.43% of all operations, but due to the rapid hemodynamic compromise requiring immediate treatment, its angiographic evidence is considered to be largely underestimated [53]. Planning for TAR, prevention of graft spasm must be part of the routine management, like no-touch graft harvesting techniques (pedicle vs. skeletonization), protection and preservation of graft endothelium, and topical pharmacological treatment after graft harvesting for spasm prevention, to discard distal ITA bifurcation for coronary anastomosis and avoid the use of high-dose alpha-adrenoceptor agonists if not counterbalanced by adequate administration of systemic vasodilator agents [54].

4 Conclusion

The evolution of CABG surgery provides us with enough evidence as to why veins are less desirable than arteries as conduit, suggesting that TAR should be performed every day on patients who undergo CABG. This does not mean that SV has not a role anymore in CABG surgery but that many more patients who could benefit from TAR are currently inappropriately treated. At the same time, it warns us about the fact that when compared to a LITA + SV grafts, TAR is more time consuming and more technically demanding. It follows that the current low uptake of TAR is more related to a problem of surgical training than a lack of scientific evidence, and that it is mainly in this direction that the cardiac surgery community should work. The Randomized Comparison of the Clinical Outcome of Single vs. Multiple Arterial Grafts (ROMA) [55] trial is in progress and has gotten rid of the flaws of the ART trial. If this multicenter RCT will show better clinical outcomes with multiple arterial grafts, will the average cardiac surgeon be ready to embrace the change overnight?

References

1. Bachar BJ, Manna B. Coronary Artery Bypass Graft. In: StatPearls. StatPearls Publishing, Treasure Island (FL); 2020.
2. Marti MC, Bouchardy B, Cox JN. Aorto-coronary bypass with autogenous saphenous vein grafts: histopathological aspects. Virchows Arch A Pathol Pathol Anat. 1971;352:255–66.
3. Vineberg A, Munro DD, Cohen H, et al. Four years' clinical experience with internal mammary artery implantation in the treatment of human coronary artery insufficiency including additional experimental studies. J Thorac Surg. 1955;29:1–32. discussion 32-6
4. Schwann TA, Habib RH, Wallace A, et al. Operative Outcomes of Multiple-Arterial Versus Single-Arterial Coronary Bypass Grafting. Ann Thorac Surg. 2018;105:1109–20.
5. Carrel AVIII. On the Experimental Surgery of the Thoracic Aorta and Heart. Ann Surg. 1910;52:83–95.
6. Kolesov VI, Potashov LV. Surgery of coronary arteries [in Russian]. Eksp Khir Anesteziol. 1965;10(2):3–8.
7. Favaloro RG. Saphenous vein autograft replacement of severe segmental coronary artery occlusion: operative technique. Ann Thorac Surg. 1968;5:334–9.
8. Loop FD, Lytle BW, Cosgrove DM, et al. Influence of the internal-mammary-artery graft on 10-year survival and other cardiac events. New Engl J Med. 1986;314:1–6.
9. Suzuki A, Kay EB, Hardy JD. Direct anastomosis of the bilateral internal mammary artery to the distal coronary artery, without a magnifier, for severe diffuse coronary atherosclerosis. Circulation. 1973;48(1):III190–7.
10. Lytle BW, Blackstone EH, Loop FD, et al. Two internal thoracic artery grafts are better than one. J Thorac Cardiovasc Surg. 1999;117:855–72.
11. Kouchoukos NT, Wareing TH, Murphy SF, et al. Risks of bilateral internal mammary artery bypass grafting. Ann Thorac Surg. 1990;49:210–7.
12. Curtis JJ, Stoney WS, Alford WC Jr, et al. Intimal hyperplasia. A cause of radial artery aortocoronary bypass graft failure. Ann Thorac Surg. 1975;20:628–35.
13. Acar C, Jebara VA, Portoghese M, et al. Revival of the radial artery for coronary artery bypass grafting. Ann Thorac Surg. 1992;54:652–9.
14. Tranbaugh RF, Dimitrova KR, Lucido DJ, et al. The second best arterial graft: a propensity analysis of the radial artery versus the free right internal thoracic artery to bypass the circumflex coronary artery. J Thorac Cardiovasc Surg. 2014;147:133–42.
15. Suma H, Tanabe H, Takahashi A, Horii T, Isomura T, Hirose H, et al. Twenty years experience with the gastroepiploic artery graft for CABG. Circulation. 2007;116(11 Suppl):I188–91.
16. D'Agostino RS, et al. The society of thoracic surgeons adult cardiac surgery database: 2018 update on outcomes and quality. Ann Thorac Surg. 2018;105:1523.
17. Tatoulis J, Wynne R, Skillington PD, et al. Total arterial revascularization: achievable and prognostically effective—a multicenter analysis. Ann Thorac Surg. 2015;100:126875.
18. Gaudino M, Chikwe J, Falk V, Lawton JS, Puskas JD, Taggart DP. Transatlantic editorial: the use of multiple arterial grafts for coronary revascularization in Europe and North America. Eur J Cardiothorac Surg. 2020;57(6):10321037.

19. Lytle BW, Blackstone EH, Sabik JF, et al. The effect of bilateral internal thoracic artery grafting on survival during 20 postoperative years. Ann Thorac Surg. 2004;78:2005–12. discussion 2012-4
20. Takagi H, Goto SN, Watanabe T, et al. A meta-analysis of adjusted hazard ratios from 20 observational studies of bilateral versus single internal thoracic artery coronary artery bypass grafting. J Thorac Cardiovasc Surg. 2014;148:1282–90.
21. Goldstone AB, Chiu P, Baiocchi M, Wang H, Lingala B, Boyd JH, et al. Second arterial versus venous conduits for multivessel coronary artery bypass surgery in California. Circulation. 2018;137:1698–707.
22. Samadashvili Z, Sundt TM, Wechsler A, Chikwe J, Adams DH, Smith CR, et al. Multiple versus single arterial coronary bypass graft surgery for multivessel disease. J Am Coll Cardiol. 2019;74:1275–85.
23. Pu A, Ding L, Shin J, Price J, Skarsgard P, Wong DR, et al. Long-term outcomes of multiple arterial coronary artery bypass grafting: a population-based study of patients in British Columbia. JAMA Cardiol. 2017;2:1187–96.
24. Taggart DP, Benedetto U, Gerry S, et al. Bilateral versus single internal-thoracic-artery grafts at 10 years. N Engl J Med. 2019;380:437–46.
25. Gaudino M, Di Franco A, Rahouma M, et al. Unmeasured confounders in observational studies comparing bilateral versus single internal thoracic artery for coronary artery bypass grafting: a meta-analysis. J Am Heart Assoc. 2018;7(1):e008010.
26. Jayakumar S, Gasparini M, Treasure T, et al. Cardiothoracic Trainees Research Collaborative. How do surgeons decide? Conduit choice in coronary artery bypass graft surgery in the UK. Interact CardioVasc Thorac Surg. 2019;29:179–86.
27. ESC/EACTS Task Force on Myocardial Revascularization. Eur J Cardio-Thorac Surg 38, S1 (2010) S1 S52.
28. Spadaccio C, Glineur D, Barbato E, et al. Fractional flow reserve-based coronary artery bypass surgery: current evidence and future directions. JACC Cardiovasc Interv. 2020;13(9):1086–96.
29. Nakajima H, Kobayashi J, Toda K. A 10-year angiographic follow-up of competitive flow in sequential and composite arterial grafts. Eur J Cardiothorac Surg. 2011;40(2):399–404.
30. Royse AG, Brennan A, Pawns Z, et al. Patency when grafted to coronary stenosis more than 50% in LIMA-RA-Y grafts. Heart, Lung and Circulation. 2020;29(7):1101–7.
31. Gaudino M, Alessandrini F, Pragliola C, et al. Effect of target artery location and severity of stenosis on mid-term patency of aorta-anastomosed vs. internal thoracic artery-anastomosed radial artery grafts. Eur J Cardiothorac Surg. 2004;25(3):4248.
32. Benedetto U, Altman DG, Gerry S, et al. Arterial Revascularization Trial investigators. Pedicled and skeletonized single and bilateral internal thoracic artery grafts and the incidence of sternal wound complications: Insights from the Arterial Revascularization Trial. J Thorac Cardiovasc Surg. 2016;152(1):270–6.
33. Boodhwani M, Lam BK, Nathan HJ, et al. Skeletonized internal thoracic artery harvest reduces pain and dysesthesia and improves sternal perfusion after coronary artery bypass surgery: a randomized, double-blind, within-patient comparison. Circulation. 2006;114(8):766–73.
34. Lamy A, Browne A, Sheth T, et al. COMPASS Investigators. Skeletonized vs pedicled internal mammary artery graft harvesting in coronary artery bypass surgery: a post hoc analysis from the COMPASS Trial. JAMA Cardiol. 2021;6(9):1042–9.
35. Gaudino M, Audisio K, Rahouma M, et al; the ART Investigators. Comparison of long-term clinical outcomes of skeletonized vs pedicled internal thoracic artery harvesting techniques in the Arterial Revascularization Trial. JAMA Cardiol. Published online September 29, 2021.
36. Neumann F-J, Sousa-Uva M, Ahlsson A, et al. ESC/EACTS guidelines on myocardial revascularization. Eur Heart J. 2019;40(2):87165.

37. Gaudino M, Benedetto U, Fremes S, et al. Association of Radial Artery Graft vs Saphenous Vein Graft With Long-term Cardiovascular Outcomes Among Patients Undergoing Coronary Artery Bypass Grafting. A Systematic Review and Meta-analysis. JAMA. 2020;324(2):179–87.
38. Gaudino M, Lorusso R, Rahouma M, et al. Radial Artery Versus Right Internal Thoracic Artery Versus Saphenous Vein as the Second Conduit for Coronary Artery Bypass Surgery: A Network Meta-Analysis of Clinical Outcomes. J Am Heart Assoc. 2019;8:e010839.
39. Buxton BF, Hayward PA, Raman J, et al. Long-Term Results of the RAPCO Trials. Circulation. 2020;142:1330–8.
40. Lemma M, Gelpi G, Mangini A, et al. Myocardial Revascularization With Multiple Arterial Grafts: Comparison Between the Radial Artery and the Right Internal Thoracic Artery. Ann Thorac Surg. 2001;71:1969–73.
41. Tavilla G, Bruggemans EF, Putter H. Twenty-year outcomes of coronary artery bypass grafting utilizing 3 in situ arterial grafts. J Thorac Cardiovasc Surg. 2019;157(6):2228–36.
42. Mills NL. Physiologic and technical aspects of internal mammary artery coronary artery bypass grafts. Cardiothorac Surg. 1982;48:119.
43. Tector AJ, Amundsen S, Schmahl TM, Kress DC, Peter M. Total revascularization with T grafts. Ann Thorac Surg. 1994;57:339.
44. Royse AG, Brennan AP, Jared Ou-Young J, et al. 21-Year survival of left internal mammary artery radial arteryY graft. J Am Coll Cardiol. 2018;72:133240.
45. Walpoth BH, Schmid M, Schwab A, et al. Vascular adaptation of the internal thoracic artery graft early and late after bypass surgery. J Thorac Cardiovasc Surg. 2008;136:87683.
46. Gurne O, Chenu P, Polidori C, et al. Functional evaluation of internal Mammary artery bypass grafts in the early and late postoperative periods. J Am Coll Cardiol. 1995;25:11208.
47. Lemma M, Innorta A, Pettinari M, et al. Flow dynamics and wall shear stress in the left internal thoracic artery: composite arterial graft versus single graft. Eur J Cardiothorac Surg. 2006;29:4738.
48. Lemma M, Mangini A, Gelpi G, et al. Is it better to use the radial artery as a composite graft? Clinical and angiographic results of aorto-coronary versus Y-graft. Eur J Cardiothorac Surg. 2004;26:110–7.
49. Börgermann J, Hakim K, Renner A, et al. Clampless off-pump versus conventional coronary artery revascularization: a propensity score analysis of 788 patients. Circulation. 2012;126(suppl 1):S176–82.
50. Zhao DF, Edelman JJ, Seco M, et al. Coronary artery bypass grafting with and without manipulation of the ascending aorta: a network meta-analysis. J Am Coll Cardiol. 2017;69:924–36.
51. He GW, Yang CQ, Starr A. Overview of the nature of vasoconstriction in arterial grafts for coronary operations. Ann Thorac Surg. 1995;59:676–83.
52. Fonseca DA, Entunes PE, Cotrim MD. Endothelium-dependent vasoactivity of the human internal mammary artery. Coronary Artery Disease. 2014;25:266–74.
53. Lorusso R, Crudeli E, Lucà F, et al. Refractory spasm of coronary arteries and grafted conduits after isolated coronary artery bypass surgery. Ann Thorac Surg. 2012;93(2):545–51.
54. He GW, Taggart DP. Antispastic management in arterial grafts in coronary artery bypass grafting surgery. The Annals of thoracic surgery. 2016;102(2):659–68.
55. Gaudino M, Taggart D, Fremes S. The ROMA trial why it is needed. Curt Op Cardiol. 2018;33(6):622–6.

Management of Patients with Concomitant Coronary and Carotid Artery Disease

Giuseppe Santarpino, Dario Fina, Chiara Simeone, Anna Nicoletti, and Giuseppe Nasso

1 Introduction

1.1 Stroke Following Coronary Artery Bypass Grafting

In patients undergoing CABG, there are many factors that may account for the occurrence of an ischemic event [1]: (i) embolization caused by aortic manipulation (e.g., aortic atheroma); (ii) cannulation, decannulation, total/partial clamping, and construction of proximal anastomoses on the aorta; (iii) alterations in blood coagulation during extracorporeal circulation or pressure changes (too high or too low) during the perioperative phase; and (iv) perioperative rhythm abnormalities, in particular due to the onset of atrial fibrillation. Obviously, all these factors are even more critical in patients with characteristics that suggest a higher risk, such as advanced age or a history of previous stroke. In these circumstances, diagnostic techniques may be suggested that can help guide the surgical strategy (e.g., aortic no-touch technique, Y-grafts [2], computed tomography for imaging of the aorta, or direct ultrasound examination of the aorta during the intraoperative phase [3]).

G. Santarpino (✉) · D. Fina · C. Simeone · A. Nicoletti · G. Nasso
Città di Lecce Hospital, GVM Care & Research, Lecce, Italy

Department of Experimental and Clinical Medicine, Magna Graecia University, Catanzaro, Italy

Department of Cardiac Surgery, Paracelsus Medical University, Nuremberg, Germany

Anthea Hospital, GVM Care & Research, Bari, Italy
e-mail: santarpino@unicz.it; gnasso@gvmnet.it

G. Concistrè (ed.), *Ischemic Heart Disease*,
https://doi.org/10.1007/978-3-031-25879-4_26

1.2 Coronary Artery Disease and Carotid Artery Stenosis

Based on the aforementioned reasons, it is easy to understand how the presence of carotid artery stenosis is only one of the several factors that may play a role in the occurrence of stroke after coronary artery bypass surgery. Carotid artery stenosis is associated with an increased risk of stroke, which more often develops if bilateral carotid occlusion is present [4]. It is estimated that 14% of postoperative strokes are due to carotid artery stenosis, whereas nearly 90% are due to the other causes listed above.

Therefore, to date, no clear indications exist regarding carotid screening before coronary artery bypass surgery, perioperative treatment of carotid artery stenosis, and best treatment modality of carotid artery stenosis (carotid endarterectomy vs. stenting) [1].

Preoperative carotid screening can be useful for assessing the overall atherosclerotic burden, but in some conditions (young patients, single-vessel coronary artery disease, no neurological history, urgent indication for CABG), there is no need/indication for postponing cardiac surgery after a carotid Doppler examination is performed as carotid screening does not protect the patient from the risk of stroke more than not doing it [1].

Furthermore, in the event of a significant stenosis, there is ongoing debate on carotid artery revascularization, especially if performed for prophylactic purposes in an asymptomatic patient. It is not clear whether concurrent carotid endarterectomy and CABG can reduce the risk of stroke, unless the patient has severe bilateral injuries or a history of prior stroke or transient ischemic attack [5].

In the event of coexisting coronary artery disease and carotid stenosis, the guidelines recommend that every patient should undergo evaluation by a multidisciplinary team, always involving a neurologist, and treatment decisions should be made on an individual basis.

Given the high prevalence of the association between coronary and carotid artery disease, this issue becomes extremely relevant [6]. Data from epidemiological studies demonstrate that 5–9% of patients with coronary artery disease show significant associated carotid disease, and 39–61% of patients with significant carotid disease show ischemic heart disease [7].

1.3 Coronary Artery Bypass Grafting and Carotid Revascularization

When selecting the best treatment option for patients with both coronary and carotid artery disease and evaluating also advantages and disadvantages, the following two aspects should be considered: (i) timing (if treatment of carotid artery disease should be performed before, concomitantly, or after CABG) and (ii) revascularization technique (on-pump vs. off-pump CABG, and carotid endarterectomy vs. stenting).

A recent review of the literature compared either strategy, without demonstrating however a clear advantage of one technique over the others [8]. Notwithstanding this, several important data could be derived: (i) a history of previous stroke is the most significant risk factor for stroke after bypass surgery [4, 8–10]; (ii) there is no evidence supporting prophylactic carotid endarterectomy; therefore, this procedure should be restricted to patients with severe bilateral lesions or a history of previous stroke [8–11]; (iii) the treatment strategy (carotid endarterectomy vs. stenting) should be discussed with a multidisciplinary team; and (iv) considering the multiple factors that may contribute to the occurrence of stroke, off-pump CABG has been shown to reduce the risk of stroke in patients with coronary artery disease associated with severe carotid stenosis [12].

In summary, each treatment strategy has advantages and disadvantages:

(i) A staged approach with CABG followed by carotid revascularization results in a higher risk of stroke.
(ii) A staged approach with carotid revascularization followed by CABG results in a higher risk of myocardial infarction.
(iii) A staged approach with carotid artery stenting under dual-antiplatelet therapy followed by CABG after ≥1 month results in an even higher risk of myocardial infarction [13, 14].
(iv) Synchronous carotid endarterectomy and CABG are associated with a higher risk of cardiac and cerebrovascular events than synchronous carotid artery stenting and CABG [15]. However, it is also true that CABG performed after carotid artery stenting when the patient is on dual-antiplatelet therapy is associated with a higher risk of intraoperative bleeding [16, 17].
(v) A staged approach with carotid artery stenting followed by CABG on the same day seems to confer a low risk of stroke [18, 19].
(vi) In patients with asymptomatic carotid artery stenosis, a staged approach with CABG followed by carotid endarterectomy is the treatment strategy that is associated with the highest risk for stroke and death, with an eightfold higher risk than performing carotid endarterectomy before or concomitantly with CABG [20].

2 Summary of the Relevant Recommendations from the Vascular, Cardiologic, and Cardiac Surgery Guidelines

The reference guidelines in the setting of concomitant coronary and carotid artery disease are the following:

- 2017 ESC Guidelines on the diagnosis and treatment of peripheral arterial diseases, in collaboration with the European Society for Vascular Surgery (ESVS), with reference to the specific section on “Carotid artery disease in patients scheduled for CABG” [7]
- 2017 ESC Guidelines on the diagnosis and treatment of peripheral arterial diseases, in collaboration with the European Society for Vascular Surgery (ESVS)—Web Addenda [21]

– 2018 ESC/EACTS Guidelines on myocardial revascularization, with reference to the specific section on "Prevention of stroke associated with carotid artery disease and myocardial revascularization" [22]

Specifically, the points concerning our area of interest can be summarized as follows:

(1) The main recommendation that was given a Class I indication is the importance of an individualized approach after discussion with a multidisciplinary team, including a neurologist.
(2) In patients with symptomatic carotid artery disease, i.e., with recent (<6 months) history of transient ischemic attack/stroke after bypass surgery, carotid endarterectomy should be considered in the presence of a 50–99% carotid stenosis [23, 24], whereas carotid revascularization is not recommended in patients with carotid stenosis <50%, including those with a previous cerebral ischemic event.
(3) Patients with asymptomatic carotid artery disease should be evaluated in an even more "tailored" way:
    – Routine prophylactic carotid revascularization is not recommended in asymptomatic patients with a 70–99% carotid stenosis, and CABG should be performed with no other associated carotid procedures.
    – Carotid revascularization combined with CABG may be considered in asymptomatic patients with bilateral 70–99% carotid stenosis or 70–99% carotid stenosis and contralateral occlusion, in the presence of one or more characteristics of increased risk of stroke, i.e., intraplaque hemorrhage, large echolucent plaques on ultrasound imaging, spontaneous embolization on transcranial Doppler, internal hypoechoic areas, and stenosis progression (>20%). All these features may be an indication for carotid revascularization also in asymptomatic patients. Several clinical characteristics (contralateral stroke) or imaging findings (ipsilateral silent infarction, lipid-rich necrotic core on magnetic resonance angiography) are also included among those factors that increase the risk of stroke.
(4) Systematic screening for carotid stenosis in patients with coronary artery disease is not recommended. However, it is recommended in patients scheduled for CABG with a recent (<6 months) history of transient ischemic attack/stroke. Vice versa, screening for carotid artery stenosis is not indicated in patients requiring urgent CABG with no recent history of cerebral ischemia. In patients with no recent history of transient ischemic attack/stroke, an ultrasound scan of the carotid arteries may be considered in those aged ≥70 years or with multivessel coronary artery disease, peripheral vasculopathy, or carotid bruit on clinical auscultation.

3 What Is New?

In addition to the latest guidelines, a number of studies have provided useful information with potential behavioral changes in the care and periprocedural management of this patient population.

3.1 Tzoumas et al. Vascular 2020 [25]

Type of study. Meta-analysis.

Aim. To compare synchronous vs. staged carotid artery stenting and CABG.

Summary. The simultaneous approach was associated with an increased risk of 30-day stroke compared to the staged strategy. However, the other outcome measures (mortality, myocardial infarction, acute kidney injury, postoperative bleeding, and atrial fibrillation) did not differ between the two groups.

Take-home message. Only four studies fulfilled the predetermined eligibility criteria, the sample size was small, and the results were based mainly on data derived from one single study. Little information was provided on the off-pump approach for CABG and timing of the synchronous or staged procedure. In summary, staged carotid artery stenting followed by CABG does not seem to be associated with a higher risk of bleeding in patients on dual-antiplatelet therapy but should be evaluated on an individual basis (e.g., are coronary lesions such that the patient can wait? And for how long?).

3.2 Giannopoulos et al. Ann Vasc Surg 2020 [26]

Type of study. Meta-analysis.

Aim. To compare synchronous carotid endarterectomy and CABG versus staged carotid artery stenting and CABG.

Summary. There were no significant differences in the rates of perioperative transient ischemic attack/stroke and myocardial infarction between groups. However, the simultaneous procedure had a significantly higher risk of 30-day mortality.

Take-home message. On the basis of data derived from the aforementioned two meta-analyses, at present, coronary artery stenting followed by CABG seems to be the more safe strategy in terms of lower risk of stroke and death.

3.3 Santarpino et al. Eur J Vasc Endovasc Surg 2018 [27]

Type of study. Post hoc analysis of data from a prospective multicenter observational study on 2813 patients.

Aim. To evaluate the prognostic impact on untreated asymptomatic carotid artery stenosis in patients undergoing isolated CABG.

Summary. In untreated asymptomatic patients, only carotid artery stenoses ≥90% are an independent predictor of postoperative stroke but rates of stroke in these patient subsets are low (7.0%).

Take-home message. Asymptomatic severe carotid artery stenosis has a low prevalence and, if left untreated, is associated with a relatively low risk of stroke. Therefore, preoperative screening for asymptomatic carotid artery stenosis before CABG may not be justified. This is largely consistent with current guidelines, but there remain specific asymptomatic patient subsets for whom carotid screening is recommended (elderly patients, multivessel coronary artery disease, known peripheral vasculopathy).

3.4 Weimar et al. Stroke 2017 [28]

Type of study. Prospective randomized trial.

Aim. To compare the safety and efficacy of synchronous carotid endarterectomy and CABG vs. isolated CABG in patients with asymptomatic high-grade carotid artery stenosis.

Summary. The rate of any stroke or death in the intention-to-treat population was 12/65 (18.5%) in patients receiving synchronous carotid endarterectomy and CABG as compared with 6/62 (9.7%) in patients receiving isolated CABG.

Take-home message. Also, this study confirms the validity of current guidelines showing that in patients with unilateral asymptomatic high-grade carotid artery stenosis, the combined approach of carotid endarterectomy and CABG is not superior to isolated CABG.

3.5 Zhang et al. Thorac Cardiovasc Surg 2017 [29]

Type of study. Systematic review.

Aim. To compare synchronous vs. staged carotid artery stenting and CABG.

Summary. The observed overall death/stroke/myocardial infarction rate was 8.5% in the staged group and 4.8% in the synchronous group.

Take-home message. This study compared 3 years earlier the same treatment strategy as Tzoumas et al. [28], coming to exactly opposite results: in the present study, the synchronous approach was safer than the staged approach, whereas in the Tzoumas experience, the staged strategy performed better. Both studies, however, agree on the need for an individual patient evaluation and that further studies are warranted to define the best treatment for this patient population.

3.6 Yang et al. ANZ J Surg 2016 [30]

Type of study. Single-center prospective study.

Aim. To compare hybrid or staged revascularization by carotid artery stenting and off-pump CABG in patients with concomitant carotid and coronary artery disease.

Summary. The incidence of stroke, myocardial infarction, or death at 30 days was 10% in the hybrid group and 5.1% in the staged group, though without reaching statistical significance due to the small sample size. The effect of the off-pump technique was not apparent.

Take-home message. Although no significant differences were observed between groups, this study should be considered in favor of the staged approach as incidence rates were twice as high in the hybrid group compared to the staged group.

3.7 Shama et al. Ann Thorac Surg 2014 [31]

Type of study. Meta-analysis.

Aim. To compare synchronous vs. staged carotid endarterectomy and CABG.

Summary. This analysis recorded comparable outcomes with the combined and staged approach, suggesting that the two strategies can be used interchangeably in clinical practice, with each having specific applications according to specific clinical conditions.

Take-home message. In this meta-analysis, which is not mentioned in current guidelines, the authors leave the door open to both strategies emphasizing the need for a tailored approach to the patient, in line with the conclusions reached later by Zhang and Tzoumas who compared synchronous vs. staged carotid artery stenting and CABG.

3.8 Oakes and Eichenbaum. Anesthesiol Clin 2014 [32]

Type of study. Review.

Aim. To provide an overview on the surgical approaches for carotid and coronary revascularization.

Summary. The authors underlined how the adoption of "protective" techniques (e.g., better diagnostic stratification for atheromatous disease, off-pump surgery) has contributed to the reduction in overall rates of perioperative stroke over time. They also reported that a significant proportion of perioperative strokes after CABG is multifactorial in origin (e.g., due to embolic phenomena, hypoperfusion, intracardiac thrombi, hemorrhage, or often "unclassified").

Take-home message. As the general population ages, the prevalence of severe carotid atherosclerotic disease is increasing in the patient population scheduled for CABG. Estimates suggest that significant carotid stenosis (>70%) is now present in approximately 10% of the CABG population. As a result, the need to manage patients with significant concurrent carotid and coronary artery stenosis is likely to become more common in the future. Although many questions still remain about the optimal surgical approach to this high-risk patient population, it is clear that these patients, when they do present in the surgical room, pose important clinical anesthetic challenges.

3.9 Gopaldas et al. Ann Thorac Surg 2011 [33]

Type of study. Analysis of data from the U.S. Nationwide Inpatient Sample database.

Aim. To compare staged vs. synchronous carotid endarterectomy and CABG.

Summary. Among 6153 patients who underwent carotid endarterectomy before or after CABG and 16,639 patients who underwent both procedures on the same day, no significant differences in mortality or neurologic complications were recorded. Staged procedures were associated with an increased risk of overall complications and higher hospital charges than synchronous procedures. On-pump CABG was associated with higher stroke rates in the synchronous group.

Take-home message. In this study, off-pump CABG was associated with a reduced risk stroke, which could be even better with the aortic "no-touch" technique, though no studies have been conducted in combination with carotid endarterectomy. The staged procedure was found to be associated with an increased risk of complications. However, since 2011, the date of publication of this study, much has changed in antiplatelet/pharmacological and anesthetic protocols, so that the potential complications in the interval between the two procedures can be significantly reduced, such as also the risk of bleeding during antiplatelet therapy.

4 Future Perspectives and Conclusions

On the basis of the available evidence, there is no univocal consensus on the strategy to be adopted in patients with concomitant coronary and carotid artery disease. Most of the studies in this setting are small case series and, except for some more larger registry studies, most often data are derived from reviews and meta-analyses. Despite the high prevalence of stroke in this patient population, it seems that there is no interest in conducting a randomized controlled trial dedicated to evaluating the best treatment for these patients, likely because of the lack of attention on this matter by the manufacturers of carotid stents and vascular prostheses.

In conclusion, the following suggestions and checkpoints are provided:

- Nowadays, the typical patient scheduled to undergo CABG most often presents with polyvascular disease and/or diabetes, or extracoronary vasculopathy. Therefore, carotid screening is mandatory except for emergency conditions or in patients with no history of previous stroke.

- Both in symptomatic and asymptomatic patients, also with unilateral carotid stenosis >50%, the indication for carotid revascularization should always be individualized after discussion within a multidisciplinary team, including a neurologist.
- Carotid artery stenting before CABG, even if performed on the same day, seems to be the best approach that is associated with a favorable risk/benefit ratio, but the decision of the most appropriate treatment option should be made based on the individual patient and available resources and skills.
- Presence of a hybrid room for the combined procedure?
- Specific expertise in carotid artery surgery? Use of vascular shunts? Procedure performed under locoregional anesthesia?
- Use of protective systems during carotid artery stenting?
- CABG performed on-pump or off-pump? Aortic no-touch technique? Preoperative screening for aortic plaques?
- Willingness to change procedural standards (e.g., simultaneous transcarotid artery revascularization with flow reversal) [34]?

Several issues remain to be addressed regarding indications, optimal timing, and technical considerations in patients with combined coronary and carotid artery disease. However, no definite answer on the best (and above all safer) treatment approach to be adopted in this patient population will be available until a randomized controlled trial comparing the different strategies is conducted and all the characteristics of the study patients are well described.

References

1. Masabni K, Raza S, Blackstone EH, Gornik HL, Sabik JF 3rd. Does preoperative carotid stenosis screening reduce perioperative stroke in patients undergoing coronary artery bypass grafting? J Thorac Cardiovasc Surg. 2015;149:1253–60.
2. Lee R, Matsutani N, Polimenakos AC, Levers LC, Lee M, Johnson RG. Preoperative noncontrast chest computed tomography identifies potential aortic emboli. Ann Thorac Surg. 2007;84:38–41.
3. Biancari F, Santini F, Tauriainen T, Bancone C, Ruggieri VG, Perrotti A, Gherli R, Demal T, Dalén M, Santarpino G, Rubino AS, Nardella S, Nicolini F, Zanobini M, De Feo M, Onorati F, Mariscalco G, Gatti G. Epiaortic ultrasound to prevent stroke in coronary artery bypass grafting. Ann Thorac Surg. 2020;109:294–301.
4. Naylor AR, Bown MJ. Stroke after cardiac surgery and its association with asymptomatic carotid disease: An updated systematic review and meta-analysis. Eur J Vasc Endovasc Surg. 2011;41:607–24.
5. Naylor AR. Does the risk of post-CABG stroke merit staged or synchronous reconstruction in patients with symptomatic or asymptomatic carotid disease? J Cardiovasc Surg. 2009;50:71–81.
6. Lin JC, Kabbani LS, Peterson EL, Masabni K, Morgan JA, Brooks S, Wertella KP, Paone G. Clinical utility of carotid duplex ultrasound prior to cardiac surgery. J Vasc Surg. 2016;63:710–4.
7. Aboyans V, Ricco JB, Bartelink MEL, Bjorck M, Brodmann M, Cohnert T, Collet JP, Czerny M, De Carlo M, Debus S, Espinola-Klein C, Kahan T, Kownator S, Mazzolai L, Naylor AR, Roffi M, Rother J, Sprynger M, Tendera M, Tepe G, Venermo M, Vlachopoulos C, Desormais I, ESC

Scientific Document Group. 2017 ESC Guidelines on the Diagnosis and Treatment of Peripheral Arterial Diseases, in collaboration with the European Society for Vascular Surgery (ESVS): Document covering atherosclerotic disease of extracranial carotid and vertebral, mesenteric, renal, upper and lower extremity arteries. Endorsed by: The European Stroke Organization (ESO). The Task Force for the Diagnosis and Treatment of Peripheral Arterial Diseases of the European Society of ESC/EACTS Cardiology (ESC) and of the European Society for Vascular Surgery (ESVS). Eur Heart J. 2018;39:763–816.

8. Naylor AR, Mehta Z, Rothwell PM, Bell PR. Carotid artery disease and stroke during coronary artery bypass: a critical review of the literature. Eur J Vasc Endovasc Surg. 2002;23:283–94.
9. Schoof J, Lubahn W, Baeumer M, Kross R, Wallesch CW, Kozian A, Huth C, Goertler M. Impaired cerebral autoregulation distal to carotid stenosis/occlusion is associated with increased risk of stroke at cardiac surgery with cardiopulmonary bypass. J Thorac Cardiovasc Surg. 2007;134:690–6.
10. Stamou SC, Hill PC, Dangas G, Pfister AJ, Boyce SW, Dullum MK, Bafi AS, Corso PJ. Stroke after coronary artery bypass: incidence, predictors, and clinical outcome. Stroke. 2001;32:1508–13.
11. Naylor AR. Delay may reduce procedural risk, but at what price to the patient? Eur J Vasc Endovasc Surg. 2008;35:383–91.
12. Lamy A, Devereaux PJ, Prabhakaran D, Taggart DP, Hu S, Paolasso E, Straka Z, Piegas LS, Akar AR, Jain AR, Noiseux N, Padmanabhan C, Bahamondes JC, Novick RJ, Vaijyanath P, Reddy S, Tao L, Olavegogeascoechea PA, Airan B, Sulling TA, Whitlock RP, Ou Y, Ng J, Chrolavicius S, Yusuf S, Investigators CORONARY. Off-pump or on-pump coronary-artery bypass grafting at 30 days. N Engl J Med. 2012;366:1489–97.
13. Randall MS, McKevitt F, Cleveland TJ, Gaines PA, Venables GS. Is there any benefit from staged carotid and coronary revascularization using carotid stents? A single-center experience highlights the need for a randomized controlled trial. Stroke. 2006;37:435–9.
14. Van der Heyden JSM, Bal ET, Ernst JM, Ackerstaff RG, Schaap J, Kelder JC, Schepens M, Plokker HW. Staged carotid angioplasty and stenting followed by cardiac surgery in patients with severe asymptomatic carotid artery stenosis: early and long-term results. Circulation. 2007;116:2036–342.
15. Shishehbor MH, Venkatachalam S, Sun Z, Rajeswaran J, Kapadia SR, Bajzer C, Gornik HL, Gray BH, Bartholomew JR, Clair DG, Sabik JF 3rd, Blackstone EH. A direct comparison of early and late outcomes with three approaches to carotid revascularization and open heart surgery. J Am Coll Cardiol. 2013;62:1948–56.
16. Durand DJ, Perler BA, Roseborough GS, Grega MA, Borowicz LM Jr, Baumgartner WA, Yuh DD. Mandatory versus selective preoperative carotid screening: a retrospective analysis. Ann Thorac Surg. 2004;78:159–66.
17. Aboyans V, Lacroix P. Indications for carotid screening in patients with coronary artery disease. Presse Med. 2009;38:977–86.
18. Versaci F, Del Giudice C, Scafuri A, Zeitani J, Gandini R, Nardi P, Salvati A, Pampana E, Sebastiano F, Romagnoli A, Simonetti G, Chiariello L. Sequential hybrid carotid and coronary artery revascularization: immediate and mid-term results. Ann Thorac Surg. 2007;84:1508–13.
19. Chiariello LNP, Pellegrino A, Saitto G, Chiariello GA, Russo M, Zeitani J, Versaci F. Simultaneous carotid artery stenting and heart surgery: expanded experience of hybrid surgical procedures. Ann Thorac Surg. 2015;99:1291–7.
20. Illuminati G, Ricco JB, Calio F, Pacile MA, Miraldi F, Frati G, Macrina F, Toscano M. Short-term results of a randomized trial examining timing of carotid endarterectomy in patients with severe asymptomatic unilateral carotid stenosis undergoing coronary artery bypass grafting. J Vasc Surg. 2011;54:993–9.
21. Halliday A, Bax JJ. 2017 ESC Guidelines on the diagnosis and treatment of peripheral arterial diseases, in collaboration with the European Society for Vascular Surgery (ESVS)-Web Addenda. Eur J Vasc Endovasc Surg. 2018;55:1–22.

22. Neumann FJ, Sousa-Uva M, Ahlsson A, Alfonso BAP, Benedetto U, Byrne RA, Collet JP, Falk V, Head SJ, Juni P, Kastrati A, Koller A, Kristensen SD, Richter DJ, Seferovic PM, Sibbing D, Stefanini GG, Windecker S, Yadav R, Zembala MO. ESC/EACTS Guidelines on myocardial revascularization. Eur Heart J. 2018;2019(40):87–165.
23. Naylor AR, Cuffe RL, Rothwell PM, Bell PR. A systematic review of outcomes following staged and synchronous carotid endarterectomy and coronary artery bypass. Eur J Vasc Endovasc Surg. 2003;25:380–9.
24. Paraskevas KI, Nduwayo S, Saratzis AN, Naylor AR. Carotid stenting prior to coronary bypass surgery: an updated systematic review and meta-analysis. Eur J Vasc Endovasc Surg. 2017;53:309–19.
25. Tzoumas A, Giannopoulos S, Charisis N, Texakalidis P, Kokkinidis DG, Zisis SN, Machinis T, Koullias GJ. Synchronous versus staged carotid artery stenting and coronary artery bypass graft for patients with concomitant severe coronary and carotid artery stenosis: a systematic review and meta-analysis. Vascular. 2020;28:808–15.
26. Giannopoulos S, Texakalidis P, Charisis N, Jonnalagadda AK, Chaitidis N, Giannopoulos S, Kaskoutis C, Machinis T, Koullias GJ. Synchronous carotid endarterectomy and coronary artery bypass graft versus staged carotid artery stenting and coronary artery bypass graft for patients with concomitant severe coronary and carotid stenosis: a systematic review and meta-analysis. Ann Vasc Surg. 2020;62:463–473.e4.
27. Santarpino G, Nicolini F, De Feo M, Dalén M, Fischlein T, Perrotti A, Reichart D, Gatti G, Onorati F, Franzese I, Faggian G, Bancone C, Chocron S, Khodabandeh S, Rubino AS, Maselli D, Nardella S, Gherli R, Salsano A, Zanobini M, Saccocci M, Bounader K, Rosato S, Tauriainen T, Mariscalco G, Airaksinen J, Ruggieri VG, Biancari F. Prognostic impact of asymptomatic carotid artery stenosis in patients undergoing coronary artery bypass grafting. Eur J Vasc Endovasc Surg. 2018;56:741–8.
28. Weimar C, Bilbilis K, Rekowski J, Holst T, Beyersdorf F, Breuer M, Dahm M, Diegeler A, Kowalski A, Martens S, Mohr FW, Ondrášek J, Reiter B, Roth P, Seipelt R, Siggelkow M, Steinhoff G, Moritz A, Wilhelmi M, Wimmer-Greinecker G, Diener HC, Jakob H, Ose C, Scherag A, Knipp SC. CABACS Trial Investigators. Safety of simultaneous coronary artery bypass grafting and carotid endarterectomy versus isolated coronary artery bypass grafting: a randomized clinical trial. Stroke. 2017;48:2769–75.
29. Zhang J, Xu RW, Fan X, Ye Z, Liu P. A systematic review of early results following synchronous or staged carotid artery stenting and coronary artery bypass grafting. Thorac Cardiovasc Surg. 2017;65:302–10.
30. Yang T, Zhang L, Wang X, Dong H, Jiang X, Sun H. Revascularization by carotid artery stenting and off-pump coronary artery bypass. ANZ J Surg. 2016;86:602–7.
31. Sharma V, Deo SV, Park SJ, Joyce LD. Meta-analysis of staged versus combined carotid endarterectomy and coronary artery bypass grafting. Ann Thorac Surg. 2014;97:102–9.
32. Oakes DA, Eichenbaum KD. Perioperative management of combined carotid and coronary artery bypass grafting procedures. Anesthesiol Clin. 2014;32:699–721.
33. Gopaldas RR, Chu D, Dao TK, Huh J, LeMaire SA, Lin P, Coselli JS, Bakaeen FG. Staged versus synchronous carotid endarterectomy and coronary artery bypass grafting: analysis of 10-year nationwide outcomes. Ann Thorac Surg. 2011;91:1323–9.
34. Williams Z, Olivere LA, Gilmore B, Weissler H, Cox MW, Long C, Shortell CK, Schroder J, Southerland KW. Safety and feasibility of simultaneous transcarotid revascularization with flow reversal and coronary artery bypass grafting for concomitant carotid artery stenosis and coronary artery disease. Vasc Endovasc Surg. 2020;54:395–9.

Minimally Invasive Myocardial Revascularization

Giovanni Concistrè and Marco Solinas

Abbreviations

CABG	Coronary artery bypass grafting
LAD	Left anterior descending coronary artery
MIDCAB	Minimally invasive direct coronary artery bypass
OPCABG	Off-pump coronary artery bypass grafting
PCI	Percutaneous coronary intervention

1 Introduction

After the first description of a beating-heart anastomosis between the mammary artery and a coronary artery by Kolesov [1], this concept was not established in clinical reality for decades. Since the reintroduction of MIDCAB into the spectrum of surgical revascularization in the 1990s by Calafiore [2] and Subramanian [3], this technique has been further developed. Today, it is a representative part of the cardiac surgical program in some institutions. MIDCAB has been mainly used in patients with proximal stenosis of LAD. In these patients, often interventional treatment with PCI appears risky or impossible due to complex lesions, close relationship to the main stem or other coronary arteries, or total occlusion of the target vessel. In other patients, repeated interventions at the LAD remained without long-standing success.

G. Concistrè (✉) · M. Solinas
Adult Cardiac Surgery Unit, Ospedale del cuore "G. Pasquinucci",
Fondazione Toscana G. Monasterio CNR—Regione Toscana, Massa, Italy
e-mail: solinas@ftgm.it

G. Concistrè (ed.), *Ischemic Heart Disease*,
https://doi.org/10.1007/978-3-031-25879-4_27

Besides its original intention for revascularization of the LAD, MIDCAB can be a useful part of hybrid procedures in patients with multivessel disease where a major coronary surgery procedure would not be well tolerated. Although multivessel disease is a predictor of elevated mortality after CABG, the MIDCAB procedure can be performed as a standalone procedure with acceptable results in midterm morbidity and mortality, even though formally incomplete revascularization may remain [4]. Several studies and our own experience proved that in selected patients with main stem stenosis or multivessel disease, MIDCAB can be safely performed [5]. Complete revascularization can be achieved by a hybrid approach with accompanying PCI [5, 6].

2 Patient Selection

Patients for the MIDCAB approach should be selected carefully. The ideal candidate would have severe stenosis or complete occlusion of the proximal LAD. It is important that the distal LAD is visualized either by collateral filling or by computed tomographic angiography in cases in which the patient has complete occlusion. Obesity is a relative contraindication. Although the LIMA takedown is technically possible in obese patients, the pressure placed on the wound edges by the retractor can lead to tissue necrosis and wound infections. Similarly, female patients with large breasts are at increased risk of wound necrosis. All contraindications are summarized in Table 1.

Table 1 Absolute and relative contraindications to MIDCAB

Absolute contraindications	Relative contraindications
Hemodynamic instability	Obesity
Emergency cases	Significant left ventricular dysfunction
Cardiogenic shock	Significant left ventricular dilatation
Ischemic arrythmias	Previous sternotomy
Acute myocardial infarction	Previous left-chest surgery
	Chest wall deformities
	Previous left-chest irradiation
	Pulmonary hypertension
	Intramyocardial coronary artery
	Heavily calcified vessel
	Small target vessel
	Occluded coronaries without good filling via collaterals

3 Surgical Technique

Standard monitoring is applied, and temperature management as for OPCABG is applied. Since single-lung ventilation is used, a double-lumen tube or bronchus blocker is applied to provide selective right-lung ventilation. Two defibrillator pads are accurately placed across the chest wall to guarantee effective electric conduction. The patient is placed in a supine position with an air sac under the left scapula, elevating the left chest slightly in order to achieve optimal exposure of the working field. Prior to the incision, main landmarks (sternum and intercostal spaces) have to be identified, which can be difficult, especially in obese patients.

An oblique 5–7 cm long skin incision is made 2 cm laterally from the left sternal border to the inferior margin of the left nipple (Fig. 1).

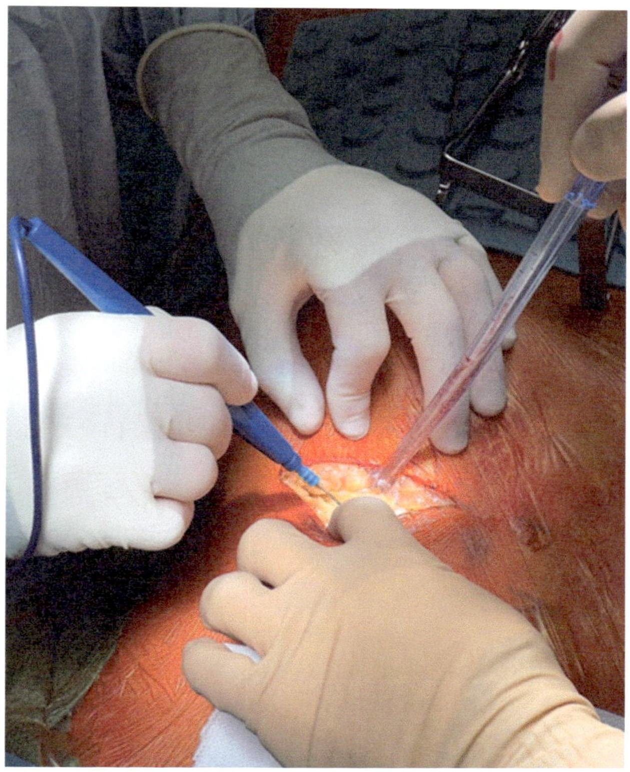

Fig. 1 Incision at left fourth intercostal space

After subcutaneous tissue division, the upper edge of the fifth rib is prepared, dividing the intercostal muscles over a length larger than the incision itself, which decreases tension and rib fracture risk. Preparation of the lower edge of the fourth rib has to be avoided because of the underlying intercostal pedicle. The fourth intercostal space is identified and opened. A small rib retractor is inserted through the thoracotomy, avoiding wide opening to prevent excessive stretching and damaging of the LIMA. A tissue pad is positioned into the pleural space to retract the lung. The left internal mammary lateral vein and artery are identified in the fatty tissue adjacent to the wall pleura; the vein is interrupted between clips and the artery is progressively harvested, under the vein itself, in a skeletonized fashion with hemoclips. The retractor is progressively opened wide enough to allow 4–5 cm of LIMA harvesting proximally and distally. The ribs must be retracted progressively to avoid fractures that would result in excessive postoperative pain and bleeding. We usually proceed to LAD search and analysis prior to complete LIMA harvesting in order to avoid a useless procedure in the case of an intramural or extremely calcified LAD, which would necessitate a conversion to sternotomy. Before pericardium opening, a flap of mediastinal fatty tissue is prepared to cover and protect the anastomotic site at the end of the operation, as described further on. The pericardium is then opened in a T- or cross-shape fashion. Usually, the LAD is immediately visible and, in cases of calcifications, digital palpation helps to localize the anastomosis site. Sometimes, the LAD course is very medial and close to the sternum or, when the heart is dilated or hypertrophic, the LAD may be located more laterally. In all cases, properly placed pericardial stay sutures will help to expose the anastomotic site. Be aware that in cases of a very lateral LAD, an extra length of LIMA is required, as described further on.

Whenever LAD identification is difficult or uncertain, we suggest checking its correct position by lifting the ventricular apex and following the LAD course. The LAD follows the interventricular septum, which is easily localized with digital palpation at the edge of the right ventricle. After LAD identification, LIMA harvesting is then completed. The LIMA is harvested under direct vision with the aid of special retractors. The mammary retractor is inserted in the thoracotomy, replacing the rib retractor. The ribs have to be retracted progressively to avoid fractures. If the exposure is poor, the incision can be slightly lengthened.

Usually, the LIMA is harvested under good vision, from distal to proximal, close to the subclavian vein, with the skeletonized technique. We use a long cautery blade, a long or endoscopic clip applier, and long fine or endoscopic forceps (20 cm shaft). This is the key point of the whole operation, and particular attention is necessary to avoid artery injuries, hematomas, or bleeding in the proximal part, which are all difficult to control. The LIMA must be harvested as proximal as possible, ideally close to the subclavian vein, but in any case, the LIMA should lean without tension on the medial mediastinum (Fig. 2).

Serious complications of too short harvesting can be mammary angulation, kinking, or even avulsion, and it can result in fatal outcomes. Sometimes, especially in cases of a lateral LAD or distal anastomotic target, evaluating the proper LIMA length can be difficult. We suggest a simple trick: before the LIMA distal cut, try to pull the artery gently

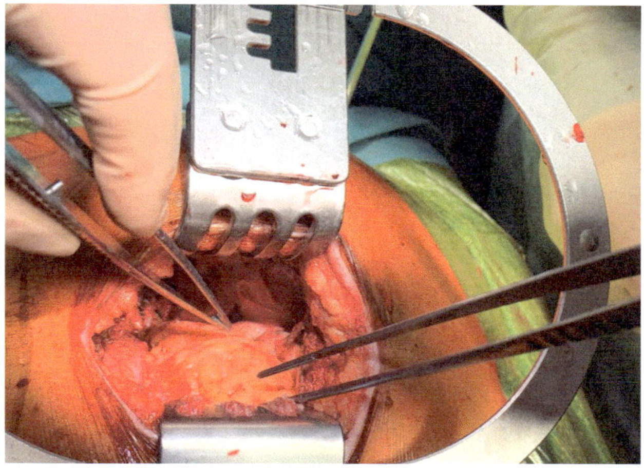

Fig. 2 Left internal mammary artery harvesting

toward the LAD. If you are able to reach the LAD, the LIMA is long enough; if the LAD is still more lateral, you will probably need more LIMA length. When the LIMA is too short, we generally harvest a more distal segment in the fifth intercostal space, through the same skin incision, for 3–4 additional centimeters, before making the distal cut. After harvesting the LIMA, a small retractor is inserted through the thoracotomy. The internal mammary artery is clipped, cut distally, checked for adequate flow, and clipped distally to check the adequate length. Then the distal end is secured with a holding stitch and prepared for anastomosis. The LIMA-LAD end-side anastomosis is performed on a beating heart using suction or a pressure stabilizer and a CO_2 blower. An Octopus Nuvo Suction Stabilizer (Medtronic, Minneapolis, MN, USA), inserted in the sixth intercostal space at the hemi-clavicular line, has been used. The anastomosis is then performed after proximal coronary rubber snaring or intracoronary shunt, familiar from off-pump surgery (parachute technique, an 8-0 polypropylene suture) (Fig. 3).

In cases of a large diagonal branch to be grafted, the anastomosis can be done either sequentially with the left mammary or with a Y-graft (vein/radial) originating from it. In the sequential setting, the diagonal is anastomosed first followed by the LAD. In the Y-graft setting, the Y-anastomosis is performed first, then the LAD, and the diagonal at the end. The anastomosis is checked for residual bleeding.

At the end of the procedure, protamine is given. The pericardium is closed with single sutures attaching the fatty pad margin to the medial portion of the pericardium to protect the anastomosis site from lung rubbing, which can cause malpositioning and/or clip avulsion. A chest tube is inserted with care on the upper edge of the sixth or seventh rib to avoid injury of the intercostal pedicle. No tube is inserted into the pericardium. The tissue pad is removed from the chest, and the anesthesiologist is asked to inflate the left lung. The lung inflation must be carefully monitored to avoid any accidental LIMA stretching in this phase. Note that the LIMA should be positioned medially, leaning without tension on the medial mediastinum, and allowing the lung to inflate above it, without any interference.

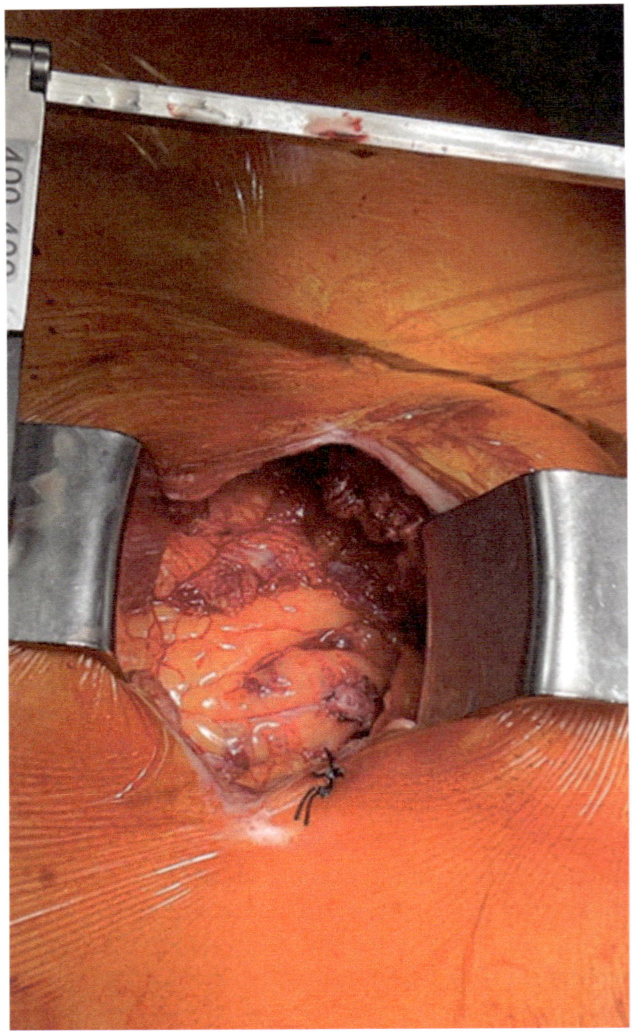

Fig. 3 LIMA-LAD anastomosis

The intercostal space is closed with one or two braided suture single stitches through the ribs (not around them) to avoid injuring the intercostal pedicle. Any rib fractures should be consolidated with more stitches. It is important to re-approximate the intercostal space properly to avoid subsequent lung herniation that would lead to a thoracoplasty.

A long-acting anesthetic agent is used for local infiltration of the intercostal space to minimize postoperative pain. We leave a towel in the thorax for bleeding control until it is closed. The incision is checked for bleeding from the ribs, muscles, and subcutaneous tissue. The pectoral muscle is then closed with one line of running suture followed by a second and third line for the subcutaneous tissue. The skin is closed with an absorbable running suture [7].

4 Outcomes

The keys to management of these patients are analgesia and early mobilization. Many patients are extubated on the table, but if a period of postoperative ventilator support is required, the endotracheal tube is changed to a single-lumen tube. Bronchoscopy before extubation is not mandated but has become part of our routine to clear secretions from the bronchial tree. Nonsteroidal anti-inflammatory medications are used in addition to narcotics. Intravenous fluids are restricted, and patients are usually allowed to get out of bed on the same evening. Monitoring lines and chest tubes are removed on the second postoperative day, and patients ambulate aggressively. Once pain is well controlled with oral medications, patients are discharged home usually on the fourth or fifth postoperative day.

The overall reported results of MIDCAB have been excellent [8–16]. Procedural success is high (98%). Operative mortality is 1% in most series. Reoperation rates for bleeding vary from 1 to 3%. Chest wound complications occur in 2–3%, and pulmonary complications are seen in 1–3% of patients. Angiographic patency in the early postoperative period and at 6 months has been excellent, and reintervention for ischemic events has been unusual [17].

MIDCAB is an attractive option for patients who would like to avoid a sternotomy. It is experiencing resurgence with the growth of hybrid revascularization. With careful planning and teamwork in the operating room, it can be accomplished safely and with excellent patency rates.

References

1. Kolessov VI. Mammary artery-coronary artery anastomosis as method of treatment for angina pectoris. J Thorac Cardiovasc Sug. 1967;54:535–44.
2. Calafiore AM, Di Giammarco G, Teodori G, et al. Left anterior descending coronary artery grafting via left anterior small thoracotomy without cardiopulmonary bypass. Ann Thorac Surg. 1996;61:1658–65.
3. Subramanian VA, Sani G, Benetti FJ, et al. Minimally invasive coronary artery bypass surgery: a multi-center report of preliminary clinical experience. Circulation. 1995;92:1645.
4. Lichtenberg A, Klima U, Paeschke H. Impact of multivessel coronary artery disease on outcome after isolated minimally invasive bypass grafting of the left anterior descending artery. Ann Thorac Surg. 2004;78:487–91.
5. Holzhey DM, Jacobs S, Mochalski M, et al. Minimally invasive hybrid coronary artery revascularization. Ann Thorac Surg. 2008;86:1856–60.
6. Wittwer T, Cremer J, Boonstra P, et al. Myocardial hybrid revascularization with minimally invasive direct coronary artery bypass grafting combined with coronary angioplasty: preliminary results of a multicenter study. Heart. 2000;83:58–63.
7. Repossini A, Baudo M, D'Alonzo M, Petruccelli R, Rosati F. MIDCAB Tips and tricks for a successful procedure. Multimed Man Cardiothorac Surg. 2020 May;22:2020.
8. Mack MJ, Magovern JA, Acuff TA, et al. Results of graft patency by immediate angiography in minimally invasive coronary artery surgery. Ann Thorac Surg. 1999;68:383–90.

9. Calafiore AM, Vitolla G, Mazzei V, et al. The LAST operation: Techniques and results before and after the stabilization era. Ann Thorac Surg. 1998;66:998–1001.
10. Doty JR, Fonger JD, Salazar JD, et al. Early experience with minimally invasive direct coronary artery bypass grafting with the internal thoracic artery. J Thorac Cardiovasc Surg. 1999;117:873–80.
11. Diegeler A, Matin M, Falk V, et al. Quality assessment in minimally invasive coronary artery bypass grafting. Eur J Cardiothorac Surg. 1999;16(suppl 2):S67–72.
12. Repossini A, Moriggia S, Cianci V, et al. The LAST operation is safe and effective: MIDCABG clinical and angiographic evaluation. Ann Thorac Surg. 2000;70:74–8.
13. Cremer JT, Wittwer T, Boening A, et al. Minimally invasive coronary artery revascularization on the beating heart. Ann Thorac Surg. 2000;69:1787–91.
14. Moussa I, Oetgen M, Subramanian V, et al. Frequency of early occlusion and stenosis in bypass grafts after minimally invasive direct coronary arterial bypass surgery. Am J Cardiol. 2001;88:311–3.
15. Holzhey DM, Jacobs S, Mochalski M, et al. Seven year follow-up after minimally invasive direct coronary artery bypass: Experience with more than 1300 patients. Ann Thorac Surg. 2007;83:108–14.
16. Mehran R, Subramanian V, Mack M, et al. Angiographic patency of LIMA-LAD anastomosis after MIDCAB compared to conventional CABG: Results from the POEM trial. J Am Coll Cardiol. 2001;37(suppl A):12a.
17. Ramachandra CR. Minimally invasive direct coronary artery bypass: technical considerations. Semin Thoracic Surg. 23:216–9.

Redo CABG: History, Epidemiology, Surgical Treatment, and Outcomes

Armin Darius Peivandi, Andreas Rukosujew, and Angelo Maria Dell'Aquila

1 Background, History, and Epidemiology

Since René Favaloro and colleagues first performed CABG, the treatment of coronary artery disease has undergone ongoing changes including new revascularization techniques and indications [1]. A consequence of this development was the performance of repeated revascularization in patients who had previously undergone CABG surgery. After redo CABG operations peaked in the early 1990s, their number has more than halved since then [2, 3]. While this development is in accordance with an overall decrease in CABG operations [4], three specific reasons have been identified to contribute to this trend [5]. First, medical therapy of coronary artery disease has significantly improved. This includes most prominently the introduction of the statin therapy [6, 7] in conjunction with antiplatelet regimen [8]. Second, the use of the LITA as a bypass graft for the LAD and a trend towards TAR techniques have enhanced long-term outcomes of CABG, making the need for revascularization less common. [9]. Third, an increasing number of PCI as another revascularization technique after previous CABG has become more common [5].

An analysis of the data from the Society of Thoracic Surgeons Adult Cardiac Surgery Database showed a decrease of the percentage of redo CABG from 6% in 2000 to 3.4% in 2009 [10]. This investigation also revealed that patients undergoing redo surgery of the coronary arteries were older and sicker than patients undergoing first-time CABG. Advanced age, male sex, diabetes, hypercholesterolemia, chronic obstructive pulmonary disease, hypertension, peripheral vascular disease, and preoperative arrythmias were found to be more common in this group [10].

A. D. Peivandi · A. Rukosujew · A. M. Dell'Aquila (✉)
Department of Cardiothoracic Surgery, University Hospital Muenster, Muenster, Germany
e-mail: armindarius.peivandi@ukmuenster.de; andreas.rukosujew@ukmuenster.de; angelo.dellAquila@ukmuenster.de

G. Concistrè (ed.), *Ischemic Heart Disease*,
https://doi.org/10.1007/978-3-031-25879-4_28

Another study, analyzing data from the National Inpatient Sample database, found a total decrease in redo CABG with no changes on the proportion of reoperations from 2002 to 2016. According to this study, recently published in the Journal of the American Heart Association, the current rate of redo CABG lays at around 2.2% (2016) [11]. In Europe, however, redo rates have been reported even lower as per a recent publication on trends of CABG in the UK states. In this study, redo CABG accounted for 0.2% of CABG operations from 2015 to 2016 [12]. This high variation in the rate of redo CABG reflects the high variation in referral to CABG surgery already observed in past guidelines on revascularization [13]. Regarding the risk factors for redo CABG, one retrospective study identified the following predictors: prior PCI, dyslipidemia, diabetes, and hypertension [3]. However, due to this high variation in the indication to redo CABG and scarce literature on this specific topic, caution must be advised when interpreting those results.

2 Indications for Redo CABG

While repeated revascularization is less commonly needed after primary CABG in comparison to primary PCI (13.7% vs. 25.9% at 5 years) [14], three main indications may require repeated revascularization after previous CABG surgery: early graft failure, late graft failure, and disease progression. Specific recommendations for choice of treatment are given in the current consensus guidelines of the European Society of Cardiology (ESC) and the European Association of Cardio-Thoracic Surgery (EACTS) on coronary revascularization [15]: When early graft failure is detected in post-CABG coronary angiography, the guideline recommends the choice between emergency reoperation and PCI to be made in the heart team (Class I, Level C). According to the guideline, an unsuitable anatomy for PCI, multiple graft occlusions, and clear errors at the anastomosis rather require redo CABG. Other factors that should be taken into account include area at risk, clinical status, and feasibility of revascularization [15]. Only few studies have compared treatment strategies after perioperative myocardial infarction until now. These studies did not show significant differences when comparing treatment modalities [16–18]. A comparison of treatment strategies is however difficult and associated with confounders, as each treatment modality has its specific indications.

Regarding late graft failure, the guideline states that revascularization in disease progression and late graft failure should take place when severe symptoms are present despite medical therapy and when there is a large area of ischemia (Class I, Level B) [15]. In the AWESOME trial [19, 20], a total of 454 patients with medically refractory myocardial ischemia and risk factors for adverse outcomes with bypass were randomized to PCI (222) or CABG (232) group. Within these groups, only around 30% of patients (32% in CABG group, 30% in PCI group) had previously undergone CABG surgery. It was shown that survival rates in redo CABG vs. PCI at 3 years were similar (CABG: 73%; PCI: 76%). Hence, the guideline recommends PCI as the first choice over CABG if safe and anatomically feasible (Class IIa, Level C) [15]. However, in the abovementioned AWESOME trial,

PCI after initial CABG was associated with significantly more repeated revascularizations (survival free of repeated revascularizations: PCI 50%, CABG 60%) and significantly more unstable angina pectoris (survival free of unstable angina: PCI 43%, CABG 61%) [19, 20].

Therefore, one should consider CABG over PCI in patients with recurrent in-stent restenosis (Class IIa, Level C) [15].

In summary, conditions in favor of redo CABG are depicted in the following cases (adapted from the 2018 guidelines):

- Multiple graft occlusions
- Extensively diseased or occluded grafts
- Absence of patent arterial grafts
- Anatomy unsuitable for PCI
- Anastomosis error
- Recurrent in-stent stenosis

3 Operative Techniques

The operative technique of redo CABG is largely comparable to primary CABG although more challenging due to some technical aspects mainly related to the sternal reentry, graft selection, and availability.

According to the current guidelines, the internal thoracic artery remains the first choice for redo CABG if not used during primary operation (Class I, Level B) [15]. This recommendation is largely based on a study conducted by Sabik III et al. published in the Journal of the American College of Cardiology. This group was able to clearly show benefits of LITA grafting compared to saphenous vein grafting in redo CABG when used for LAD revascularization. Including a cohort of 3473 patients, they showed that hospital mortality was significantly lower, and early and late survival was higher in the LITA group. The group detected an absolute mortality risk reduction in the LITA group with a number needed to treat (NNT) of 16 [21].

Considering the advantages of arterial grafts, numerous techniques have been developed in order to "recycle" arterial grafts [22, 23]. In particular, a Y anastomosis can be performed on patent internal mammary; if stenosis of distal anastomosis occurs, arterial grafts can be re-anastomosed [22, 23]. Finally, arterial grafts can be distally removed and used for the revascularization of other vessels. All those techniques, however, must undergo a pre- and intraoperative critical evaluation in relation to the feasibility, the time required for performing this, and the patients' comorbidities. In fact, a careful surgical planning and enhanced expertise are of utmost importance for successful revascularization.

An additional tool for preoperative planning is offered by the use of multidetector computed tomographic angiography CT imaging [24]. To this regard, a study by Kamdar et al.

assessed the use of this diagnostic tool in reoperative planning. The study included a total of 167 patients. All of them had a history of previous CABG and were scheduled for redo CABG. In their study, significant correlation between high-risk findings detected through a multidetector computed tomographic angiography and preventive surgical strategies was found. High-risk findings included right ventricle/aorta to chest wall or CABG crossing midline in close proximity. As a consequence of those findings, change of operative strategy was adopted including non-midline approach, cardiopulmonary bypass initiation before incision, peripheral arterial and venous cannulation before sternotomy, deep hypothermic circulatory arrest, or a combination of all those preventive strategies [25]. Frequency of severe bleeding, graft injuries, and 1-month mortality as reported by the authors lay by 4.4%, 5%, and 2.5%, respectively [25].

As part of a careful surgical approach, a patent LIMA has to be preserved during redo CABG. According to a study conducted by Smith et al., a clamping of a patent LIMA graft during redo surgery is not associated with a survival benefit but rather with an increased risk of LIMA injury (7.9%). In their retrospective analysis, the group investigated 206 patients with patent LIMA-LAD grafts and found no significant difference in survival rates when comparing the clamping vs. the non-clamping group. Noteworthy in the non-clamping group, cardioplegia was given in shorter time intervals and the patients were cooled down to 28–32 °C [26].

4 Off-Pump vs. On-Pump Redo CABG

Recently, scientific focus has been lying on the question of on-pump vs. off-pump redo CABG. Many studies have suggested a benefit of redo off-pump surgery [27–29]. Bruno et al. conducted a propensity score-matched analysis in which they compared 10-year survival rates in patients operated on- and off-pump. In their retrospective study, 84 matched redo CABG patients were included in each group. There was no significant difference in 10-year survival between on-pump and off-pump CABG in their analysis. OPCAB, however, resulted in better outcomes in terms of in-hospital mortality and IABP implantation rates and showed a reduction in the composite outcome of their study (consisting of acute kidney injury, stroke, in-hospital mortality, and severe low cardiac output in need of IABP) [27]. In line with those results, another study analyzing data from the Japan Cardiovascular Surgery Database came to the same result of Bruno et al. In this study, 200 OPCAB patients were compared to 200 on-pump using a propensity matching to overcome biases deriving from the non-randomization. In addition to that, they were able to show a lower 30-day mortality in the OPCAB group. Moreover, composite mortality or major morbidities, prolonged ventilation, ICU stay, and blood transfusion rates were significantly lower in the off-pump group [29]. A recently published meta-analysis by Zhang et al. found the off-pump technique to be associated with a significantly reduced 30-day mortality. In their analysis, 21 redo CABG studies were included. In particular, all of them were observational studies, and of them 19 were retrospective and 2 prospective.

In this meta-analysis, moreover, they also identified other advantages of off-pump in comparison with conventional on-pump redo: postoperative new-onset atrial fibrillation, myocardial infarction, acute kidney injury, low cardiac output, blood transfusion, duration of mechanical ventilation, and ICU and hospital stay were significantly lower if redo was conducted off-pump. Although completeness of revascularization was not significantly different in both groups, there was a clear trend towards a more complete revascularization in on-pump patients (83% on-pump vs. 66.18% off-pump) [30]. In this setting, large prospective randomized controlled studies on this topic are needed in order to tease out the real benefit of off-pump surgery over the on-pump. Moreover, issues such as the benefit of completeness in revascularization over a more parsimonious approach are to be addressed through randomization. In this setting, other factors that in the observational studies are not accounted for relate to the individual surgical expertise and to the choice of procedure that can once more hardly depend on the technical feasibility and the status of native vessels.

5 Risk Factors and Outcomes

As already mentioned in the first paragraph, patients undergoing redo CABG operations are generally sicker when baseline characteristics are compared to patients referred to first-time CABG [31, 32]. In this setting, identification of risk factors for mortality after redo CABG is a crucial step for patient selection and planning of appropriate strategy.

In this regard, Elbadawi et al. found three main predictors of mortality among redo CABG: history of heart failure, chronic kidney disease, and electrolyte/fluid imbalances. In this analysis, a total of 46,820 redo CABG patients were compared with patients receiving primary CABG (n = 3,165,948). Data were retrieved from the National Inpatient Sample database in the United States. Redo CABG patients showed an increased in-hospital mortality (3.2% versus 1.9%). Additionally, they found that the adverse events of cardiac arrest, cardiogenic shock, and vascular and respiratory complications were higher in the redo group [11].

In another study, Gallo et al. analyzing the outcome of 126 redo CABG showed that redo CABG needed significantly more blood products during surgery. After propensity matching, redo CABG did not result in a significantly higher mortality when compared with first-time CABG (3.1% vs. 2.1%). Interestingly, most redo CABGs were performed in a period of 10 years or more after primary CABG [3].

In another report of the Japanese Association of Thoracic Surgery (JATS), operative mortality of redo CABG was more than three times higher than that of primary CABG (4.7% vs. 1.3% in 2010). Additionally, emergency redo was associated with increased 30-day mortality in comparison with elective redo (9.7% vs. 3.3%) [5]. Interestingly, data were reported as crude rates without performing adjustment.

In this setting, Bianco et al. did not report any significant difference in terms of 30-day or 1-year operative mortality between CABG and redo CABG (5.3% vs. 7.5% and 12.1%

vs. 14.8%, respectively) [33] after propensity score matching. However, blood product transfusion and delayed sternal closure were significantly higher for reoperative CABG group. In his study, 7265 of these patients with first-time CABG and 350 patients with reoperative CABG were included. The higher mortality rate of first-time CABG is due to the selection of patients with high-risk profile for matching with redo CABG that are more likely to have more comorbidities. On the other hand, results of redo surgery have substantially improved and the redo condition must not be seen as risk factors per se [32].

In summary, although challenging, redo CABG can be conducted safely with advanced operative techniques and a decreasing rate of adverse events and mortality [2, 3]. Nonetheless, numbers of redo CABG have decreased over time due to an improved medical therapy, arterial grafting in primary CABG, and an increase in PCI [5]. While current guidelines rather recommend PCI as the first choice after primary CABG [15], decision upon indication should be made in the heart team upon careful consideration of all factors. Large prospective RCTs on long-term results after redo CABG vs. PCI after primary CABG are still missing and desirable aims for the future. While studies indicate a benefit of the OPCAB technique in redo, patient safety should not be compromised and choice of method should be based on surgical experience. Finally, the use of multidetector computed tomographic angiography CT imaging is an important tool for accurate planning of surgical strategy and therefore its use is advisable.

References

1. Favaloro RG. Critical analysis of coronary artery bypass graft surgery: a 30-year journey. J Am Coll Cardiol. 1998;31(4 Suppl B):1B–63B. https://doi.org/10.1016/s0735-1097(97)00559-7.
2. Spiliotopoulos K, Maganti M, Brister S, Rao V. Changing pattern of reoperative coronary artery bypass grafting: a 20-year study. Ann Thorac Surg. 2011;92(1):40–6. https://doi.org/10.1016/j.athoracsur.2011.03.104.
3. Gallo M, Trivedi JR, Monreal G, Ganzel BL, Slaughter MS. Risk Factors and Outcomes in Redo Coronary Artery Bypass Grafting. Heart Lung Circ. 2020;29(3):384–9. https://doi.org/10.1016/j.hlc.2019.02.008. Epub 2019 Mar 4
4. Bowdish ME, D'Agostino RS, Thourani VH, Desai N, Shahian DM, Fernandez FG, Badhwar V. The Society of Thoracic Surgeons Adult Cardiac Surgery Database: 2020 Update on Outcomes and Research. Ann Thorac Surg. 2020;109(6):1646–55. https://doi.org/10.1016/j.athoracsur.2020.03.003. Epub 2020 Apr 2
5. Yaku H, Doi K. Redo coronary artery bypass grafting. Gen Thorac Cardiovasc Surg. 2014;62(8):453–60. https://doi.org/10.1007/s11748-014-0426-6. Epub 2014 Jun 7. PMID: 24906816
6. Doenst T, Bargenda S, Kirov H, Moschovas A, Tkebuchava S, Safarov R, Velichkov I, Diab M. Cardiac Surgery 2019 Reviewed. Thorac Cardiovasc Surg. 2020;68(5):363–76. https://doi.org/10.1055/s-0040-1713648. Epub 2020 Jun 27
7. Nissen SE, Tuzcu EM, Schoenhagen P, Crowe T, Sasiela WJ, Tsai J, Orazem J, Magorien RD, O'Shaughnessy C, Ganz P. Reversal of Atherosclerosis with Aggressive Lipid Lowering (REVERSAL) Investigators. Statin therapy, LDL cholesterol, C-reactive protein, and coronary artery disease. N Engl J Med. 2005;352(1):29–38. https://doi.org/10.1056/NEJMoa042000.

8. Sousa-Uva M, Head SJ, Milojevic M, Collet JP, Landoni G, Castella M, Dunning J, Gudbjartsson T, Linker NJ, Sandoval E, Thielmann M, Jeppsson A, Landmesser U. 2017 EACTS Guidelines on perioperative medication in adult cardiac surgery. Eur J Cardiothorac Surg. 2018;53(1):5–33. https://doi.org/10.1093/ejcts/ezx314.
9. Diegeler A, Thiele H, Falk V, Hambrecht R, Spyrantis N, Sick P, Diederich KW, Mohr FW, Schuler G. Comparison of stenting with minimally invasive bypass surgery for stenosis of the left anterior descending coronary artery. N Engl J Med. 2002;347(8):561–6. https://doi.org/10.1056/NEJMoa013563.
10. Ghanta RK, Kaneko T, Gammie JS, Sheng S, Aranki SF. Evolving trends of reoperative coronary artery bypass grafting: an analysis of the Society of Thoracic Surgeons Adult Cardiac Surgery Database. J Thorac Cardiovasc Surg. 2013;145(2):364–72. https://doi.org/10.1016/j.jtcvs.2012.10.051.
11. Elbadawi A, Hamed M, Elgendy IY, Omer MA, Ogunbayo GO, Megaly M, Denktas A, Ghanta R, Jimenez E, Brilakis E, Jneid H. Outcomes of Reoperative Coronary Artery Bypass Graft Surgery in the United States. J Am Heart Assoc. 2020;9(15):e016282. https://doi.org/10.1161/JAHA.120.016282. Epub 2020 Jul 21. PMID: 32691683; PMCID: PMC7792259
12. Ohri SK, Benedetto U, Luthra S, Grant SW, Goodwin AT, Trivedi U, Kendall S, Jenkins DP. Coronary artery bypass surgery in the UK, trends in activity and outcomes from a 15-year complete national series. Eur J Cardiothorac Surg. 2021;1:ezab391. https://doi.org/10.1093/ejcts/ezab391. Epub ahead of print
13. Authors/Task Force members, Windecker S, Kolh P, Alfonso F, Collet JP, Cremer J, Falk V, Filippatos G, Hamm C, Head SJ, Jüni P, Kappetein AP, Kastrati A, Knuuti J, Landmesser U, Laufer G, Neumann FJ, Richter DJ, Schauerte P, Sousa Uva M, Stefanini GG, Taggart DP, Torracca L, Valgimigli M, Wijns W, Witkowski A. 2014 ESC/EACTS Guidelines on myocardial revascularization: The Task Force on Myocardial Revascularization of the European Society of Cardiology (ESC) and the European Association for Cardio-Thoracic Surgery (EACTS)Developed with the special contribution of the European Association of Percutaneous Cardiovascular Interventions (EAPCI). Eur Heart J. 2014;35(37):2541–619. https://doi.org/10.1093/eurheartj/ehu278. Epub 2014 Aug 29
14. Parasca CA, Head SJ, Milojevic M, Mack MJ, Serruys PW, Morice MC, Mohr FW, Feldman TE, Colombo A, Dawkins KD, Holmes DR Jr, Kappetein PA, SYNTAX Investigators. Incidence, Characteristics, Predictors, and Outcomes of Repeat Revascularization After Percutaneous Coronary Intervention and Coronary Artery Bypass Grafting: The SYNTAX Trial at 5 Years. JACC Cardiovasc Interv. 2016;9(24):2493–507. https://doi.org/10.1016/j.jcin.2016.09.044.
15. Neumann FJ, Sousa-Uva M, Ahlsson A, Alfonso F, Banning AP, Benedetto U, Byrne RA, Collet JP, Falk V, Head SJ, Jüni P, Kastrati A, Koller A, Kristensen SD, Niebauer J, Richter DJ, Seferovic PM, Sibbing D, Stefanini GG, Windecker S, Yadav R, Zembala MO, ESC Scientific Document Group. 2018 ESC/EACTS Guidelines on myocardial revascularization. Eur Heart J. 2019;40(2):87–165. https://doi.org/10.1093/eurheartj/ehy394. Erratum in: Eur Heart J. 2019 Oct 1;40(37):3096
16. Thielmann M, Massoudy P, Jaeger BR, Neuhäuser M, Marggraf G, Sack S, Erbel R, Jakob H. Emergency re-revascularization with percutaneous coronary intervention, reoperation, or conservative treatment in patients with acute perioperative graft failure following coronary artery bypass surgery. Eur J Cardiothorac Surg. 2006;30(1):117–25. https://doi.org/10.1016/j.ejcts.2006.03.062. Epub 2006 May 24
17. Davierwala PM, Verevkin A, Leontyev S, Misfeld M, Borger MA, Mohr FW. Impact of expeditious management of perioperative myocardial ischemia in patients undergoing isolated coronary artery bypass surgery. Circulation. 2013;128(11 Suppl 1):S226–34. https://doi.org/10.1161/CIRCULATIONAHA.112.000347.

18. Preußer MJ, Landwehrt J, Mastrobuoni S, Biancari F, Dakkak AR, Alshakaki M, Martens S, Dell'Aquila AM. Survival results of postoperative coronary angiogram for treatment of perioperative myocardial ischaemia following coronary artery bypass grafting: a single-centre experience. Interact Cardiovasc Thorac Surg. 2018;26(2):237–42. https://doi.org/10.1093/icvts/ivx317.
19. Sedlis SP, Ramanathan KB, Morrison DA, Sethi G, Sacks J, Henderson W. Department of Veterans Affairs Cooperative Study #385, Angina With Extremely Serious Operative Mortality Evaluation (AWESOME) Investigators. Outcome of percutaneous coronary intervention versus coronary bypass grafting for patients with low left ventricular ejection fractions, unstable angina pectoris, and risk factors for adverse outcomes with bypass (the AWESOME Randomized Trial and Registry). Am J Cardiol. 2004;94(1):118–20. https://doi.org/10.1016/j.amjcard.2004.03.041.
20. Morrison DA, Sethi G, Sacks J, Henderson WG, Grover F, Sedlis S, Esposito R. Investigators of the Department of Veterans Affairs Cooperative Study #385, Angina With Extremely Serious Operative Mortality Evaluation. Percutaneous coronary intervention versus repeat bypass surgery for patients with medically refractory myocardial ischemia: AWESOME randomized trial and registry experience with post-CABG patients. J Am Coll Cardiol. 2002;40(11):1951–4. https://doi.org/10.1016/s0735-1097(02)02560-3.
21. Sabik JF 3rd, Raza S, Blackstone EH, Houghtaling PL, Lytle BW. Value of internal thoracic artery grafting to the left anterior descending coronary artery at coronary reoperation. J Am Coll Cardiol. 2013;61(3):302–10. https://doi.org/10.1016/j.jacc.2012.09.045.
22. Dohi M, Doi K, Okawa K, Yaku H. Upgrading redo coronary artery bypass graft by recycling in situ arterial graft. Ann Thorac Surg. 2014;98(1):311–4. https://doi.org/10.1016/j.athoracsur.2013.09.066.
23. Nwaejike N, Tennyson C, Mosca R, Venkateswaran R. Reusing the patent internal mammary artery as a conduit in redo coronary artery bypass surgery. Interact Cardiovasc Thorac Surg. 2016;22(3):346–50. https://doi.org/10.1093/icvts/ivv338. Epub 2015 Dec 15. PMID: 26669852; PMCID: PMC4986558
24. Imran Hamid U, Digney R, Soo L, Leung S, Graham AN. Incidence and outcome of re-entry injury in redo cardiac surgery: benefits of preoperative planning. Eur J Cardiothorac Surg. 2015;47(5):819–23. https://doi.org/10.1093/ejcts/ezu261. Epub 2014 Jul 9
25. Kamdar AR, Meadows TA, Roselli EE, Gorodeski EZ, Curtin RJ, Sabik JF, Schoenhagen P, White RD, Lytle BW, Flamm SD, Desai MY. Multidetector computed tomographic angiography in planning of reoperative cardiothoracic surgery. Ann Thorac Surg. 2008;85(4):1239–45. https://doi.org/10.1016/j.athoracsur.2007.11.075.
26. Smith RL, Ellman PI, Thompson PW, Girotti ME, Mettler BA, Ailawadi G, Peeler BB, Kern JA, Kron IL. Do you need to clamp a patent left internal thoracic artery-left anterior descending graft in reoperative cardiac surgery? Ann Thorac Surg. 2009;87(3):742–7. https://doi.org/10.1016/j.athoracsur.2008.12.050.
27. Bruno VD, Zakkar M, Rapetto F, Rathore A, Marsico R, Chivasso P, Ascione R. Early health outcome and 10-year survival in patients undergoing redo coronary surgery with or without cardiopulmonary bypass: a propensity score-matched analysis. Eur J Cardiothorac Surg. 2017;52(5):945–51. https://doi.org/10.1093/ejcts/ezx137. PMID: 28505298; PMCID: PMC5848803
28. Usta E, Elkrinawi R, Ursulescu A, Nagib R, Mädge M, Salehi-Gilani S, Franke UF. Clinical outcome and quality of life after reoperative CABG: off-pump versus on-pump - observational pilot study. J Cardiothorac Surg. 2013;5(8):66. https://doi.org/10.1186/1749-8090-8-66. PMID: 23561396; PMCID: PMC3622626
29. Dohi M, Miyata H, Doi K, Okawa K, Motomura N, Takamoto S, Yaku H, Japan Cardiovascular Surgery Database. The off-pump technique in redo coronary artery bypass grafting reduces mortality and major morbidities: propensity score analysis of data from the Japan Cardiovascular

Surgery Database†. Eur J Cardiothorac Surg. 2015;47(2):299–307. https://doi.org/10.1093/ejcts/ezu081. Epub 2014 Mar 12

30. Zhang P, Wang L, Zhai K, Huang J, Wang W, Ma Q, Liu D, Gao B, Li Y. Off-pump versus on-pump redo coronary artery bypass grafting: a systematic review and meta-analysis. Perfusion. 2021;36(7):724–36. https://doi.org/10.1177/0267659120960310. Epub 2020 Oct 4
31. Mohamed MO, Shoaib A, Gogas B, Patel T, Alraies MC, Velagapudi P, Chugh S, Sharma K, Mohamed W, Murphy GJ, Kwok CS, Rashid M, Bagur R, Mamas MA. Trends of repeat revascularization choice in patients with prior coronary artery bypass surgery. Catheter Cardiovasc Interv. 2021;98(3):470–80. https://doi.org/10.1002/ccd.29234. Epub 2020 Sep 5
32. Sabik JF 3rd, Blackstone EH, Houghtaling PL, Walts PA, Lytle BW. Is reoperation still a risk factor in coronary artery bypass surgery? Ann Thorac Surg. 2005;80(5):1719–27. https://doi.org/10.1016/j.athoracsur.2005.04.033.
33. Bianco V, Kilic A, Gleason TG, Aranda-Michel E, Habertheuer A, Humar R, Wang Y, Navid F, Sultan I. Long-term Outcomes After Reoperative Coronary Artery Bypass Grafting. Ann Thorac Surg. 2021;111(1):150–8. https://doi.org/10.1016/j.athoracsur.2020.04.092. Epub 2020 Jun 6

Surgical Complications After Acute Myocardial Infarction: Ventricular Septal Defect and Free Wall Rupture

Alina Gallo and Silvia Solari

Abbreviations

AMI	Acute myocardial infarction
CABG	Coronary artery bypass grafting
CPB	Cardiopulmonary bypass
ECMO	Extracorporeal membrane oxygenation
FWR	Free wall rupture
IABP	Intra-aortic balloon pump
LAD	Left anterior descending coronary artery
LV	Left ventricle
LVEF	Left ventricular ejection fraction
LVFWR	Left ventricular free wall rupture
MCS	Mechanical circulatory support
MI	Myocardial Infarction
PCI	Percutaneous coronary intervention
PTFE	Polytetrafluoroethylene
PET	Polyethylene terephthalate
RCA	Right coronary artery
RV	Right ventricle

A. Gallo (✉)
Department of Cardiac Surgery, Azienda Ospedaliera SS. Antonio e Biagio e Cesare Arrigo, Alessandria, Italy
e-mail: alina.gallo@ospedale.al.it

S. Solari
Department of Cardio-Thoracic Surgery, Cliniques de L'Europe, Bruxelles, Belgium
e-mail: s.solari@europehospitals.be

G. Concistrè (ed.), *Ischemic Heart Disease*,
https://doi.org/10.1007/978-3-031-25879-4_29

STEMI	ST-elevation myocardial infarction
ST	Sutured repair
SLT	Sutureless repair
VA-ECMO	Veno-arterial extracorporeal membrane oxygenation
VSD	Ventricular septal defect

1 Postischemic Ventricular Septal Defect

1.1 Historical Note

Postischemic ventricular septal defect (VSD) refers to a rupture of the interventricular wall that occurs secondary to a transmural myocardial infarction (MI) after complete occlusion of a coronary artery.

This concept of interventricular septal rupture was first introduced in 1847 by Latham [1] after postmortem examination and upon antemortem evaluation by Brumm in 1923 [2]; however, the first procedure to repair postischemic VSD was published more than a century later by Cooely and Colleagues, in 1957 [3]. Thence, it was quickly realized that surgical treatment, despite very high mortality, provided greater probability of survival and that it should be offered to as many patients as possible rather than only to those who survived the first weeks after a myocardial infarction. Modern concepts in VSD surgery were quickly introduced, and many surgical approaches were proposed, including the left transventricular (Kay and Dubost, 1969 [4, 5] and Kitamura in 1970 [6]) or the right transatrial (Filgueir and colleagues, 1986 [7]). Further, David and colleagues [8] added the concept of excluding the infarcted zone during septal repair and, in 1987, described the use of three oval patches in the autologous pericardium: the first to close the VSD and the free wall infarcted area, the second to close the VSD from the right, and the third to cover the epicardial surface of the VS.

1.2 Natural History

A recent report from the JAMA (2020) once again confirmed cardiac diseases to be the foremost cause of death in the United States, with a worrying increase by 4.8%. This is the largest increase from 2012 [9] and could be associated, to some extent, with the COVID-19 pandemic, which was the third leading cause of death in 2020. The COVID-19 pandemic greatly disrupted health systems and increased fear among patients requiring health care. The incidence of VSD, which is a mechanical complication of MI, had reduced from 1–2% to 0.2% [10] due to the advent of early myocardial reperfusion strategies; however, the COVID-19 pandemic has led to its recrudescence because of delayed access to tertiary care among patients experiencing angina.

1.3 Morphology of VSD

VDS typically occurs as a consequence of a transmural acute myocardial infarction (AMI) that is limited to a segment of the interventricular septum, secondary to complete occlusion of a coronary artery. Depending on the extent of the MI, VSD can occur between a few hours and the first 2 weeks after the MI.

The left anterior descending coronary artery (LAD) and the right coronary artery (RCA) are the most common arteries involved; they lead to 42% and 46%, respectively, of all postinfarction VSD [11]. Concomitant lesions in collateral circulation are also commonly observed. Occlusion of the LAD results in an apical septal defect because it supplies the anterior portion of septum; similarly, the dominant RCA supplies most of the inferior portion of the septum; hence, its occlusion leads to an infero-basal VSD.

The morphology of an anterior VSD is significantly different from that of a posterior VSD, and this is crucial for determining the setup of the cardiac team for evaluating treatment timing and management. Notably, these differences are well described by the radiological and cardiology group of the Bristol Royal Infirmary [12]. The morphology of both anterior and posterior VSDs has been investigated by echocardiography, magnetic resonance [MRI], and electrocardiographically gated computed tomography [CT] imaging to identify anatomic features most suitable for percutaneous closure, and the results show (i) that VSDs due to occlusion of the LAD (LAD-VSD) are smaller than those due to RCA obstruction, (ii) that they are wider in the left side of the septum, and (iii) that they undergo a smaller size change between systolic and diastolic phases. Further, the distance from the defect to the myocardium, which is 5 mm thick and pragmatically provides an adequate seal against percutaneous occlusion, is greater in anterior and apical VDS than in posterior ones.

LAD-VSDs are significantly more likely to be simple or entirely intraseptal; in contrast, RCA-VSDs are generally complex with the septum torn from the free wall of the heart or associated with an intramyocardial dissection that can progress to free wall rupture. Thus, this chapter deviates from the current consensus in which VSDs are classified as simple when there is a direct connection between the two ventricles and complex when they have a serpiginous course [13].

1.4 Pathophysiology, Clinical Features, and Diagnosis

Disruption of the ventricular septum results in a left-to-right shunt and a sudden decrease in forward left ventricular (LV) stroke volume, apart from right ventricle (RV) volume and pressure overload and secondary left-side overload due to greater venous pulmonary return. Pulmonary and systemic vascular resistance affects shunt fraction, and the pulmonary-to-systemic blood flow ratio (Qp/Qs) is usually ≥ 2.0.

RV dysfunction greatly impacts prognosis, and it occurs when the inferior RV basal wall is involved due to an inferior infarct or severe ischemia, along with a sudden increase in pulmonary blood flow from the left-to-right shunt [14]. The size of the defect and biventricular function affect the degree of the left-to-right shunt, hemodynamic changes, clinical presentation, and prognosis of the patient.

A harsh pansystolic murmur at the lower left sternal border, a thrill (in 50% of the cases), and a clinical history of transmural AMI should lead to a suspicion of a post-infarct VSD as concomitant secondary mitral regurgitation could worsen clinical presentation. Patients with VSD may be relatively hemodynamically stable or present with various degrees of hemodynamic instability, including cardiogenic shock that requires mechanical ventilation, intra-aortic balloon counterpulsation (IABP), inotropes, diuretics, and nitrates. In relatively stable patients, it is very important to detect any early signs of hemodynamic deterioration and act before multi-organ failure develops. Once an electrocardiogram (ECG) has established a diagnosis of STEMI, two-dimensional echocardiography, either transthoracic or transesophageal, is highly sensitive and specific for differentiating between VSD and mitral papillary muscle rupture, calculating VSD size, quantifying left-to-right shunt, analyzing RV and LV function, and evaluating wall motion abnormalities and mitral and tricuspid valves.

A Swan-Ganz catheter, coronary angiogram, and ventriculography are invasive studies, and the cardiac team should decide whether the patient can tolerate these tests or if only a coronary angiogram with minimal contrast injection should be acquired. Complete coronary revascularization during surgery for postinfarction VSD might improve long-term outcomes among patients, but it does not affect early outcomes and, therefore, should not be a priority in patients in cardiogenic shock [15]. Cardiac MRI and CT scan can play a substantial role in planning interventional percutaneous closure in hemodynamically stable patients.

1.5 Indications and Timing of Surgery

Postinfarction VSD has a broad range of clinical presentations that can help the cardiac team in recommending the best time for surgery. In the early phase after MI (72 h), the infarcted myocardium is fragile and the infarcted zone shows inward migration of macrophages, monocytes, and neutrophils, metalloproteinase activity, tissue breakdown, and an inflammatory response that leads to the expansion of infarcted areas. Notably, proliferation of connective tissue begins only about three weeks after the infarction [16]. Thus, while the best time to operate would be after the necrotic muscle has healed, rapid onset of clinical deterioration with acute heart failure or cardiogenic shock in most cases precludes any delay in surgery.

The European Society of Cardiology recommends early surgery in patients who are nonresponsive to aggressive heart failure treatments because of a high mortality rate (20–40%) and greater risk of recurrent ventricular rupture; thus, delayed elective surgery should only be considered in very stable patients, with or without pharmacologic help, IABP, or mechanical support [17]. In contrast, the 2013 American Heart Association guidelines recommend emergency surgery even in stable patients because of the excessive risk of hemodynamic collapse in case of VSD enlargement, which has a mortality rate of 20–87% [18].

Results from several publications indicate that time elapsed between VSD occurrence and surgery is a factor that directly affects survival. For example, Arnaoutakis et al. report a mortality rate of 54% when surgery was performed within seven days from VSD detection, while it reduced to 18% if surgery was postponed to after the first week [19]. Similarly, Malhotra et al. show that delaying surgery by as little as 3 days can help reduce mortality from 76% to 18%. A retrospective study of data from the Japanese National Database also confirmed a more favorable outcome if surgery was delayed; specifically, mortality rate was 13.2% among patients undergoing elective surgery while it was 56.0% among patients requiring emergency surgery and 80.5% in salvage patients [19]. Such a high mortality in the cluster of patients undergoing emergency surgery is understandable not only because of the technical difficulties in grafting a patch on to an infarcted, friable, and weak area, but also due to hemodynamic compromise, cardiogenic shock, and multiple-organ failure that necessitated the decision for surgery.

The time interval between VSD and surgical repair is also a good indicator of the severity of the cardiac damage as a short duration is indicative of severe ischemia, poor coronary collateral circulation, and difficulty of the heart and its adaptive systems to cope with hemodynamic changes [20]. In this scenario, the importance of the heart team, composed of a cardiac surgeon, cardiac intensivist, cardiologist, and hemodynamist, is strongly emphasized, and they, together, must analyze the patient's history, clinical presentation, risk factors, comorbidities, hemodynamic situation, echocardiogram, and hemodynamic calculations to recommend an individualized optimal treatment strategy for each patient. Patient age and comorbidities can greatly influence the therapeutic approach used and timing of surgery; however, in the presence of severe cardiogenic shock with rapid deterioration of the patient, surgical repair remains the only effective treatment. Risk factors associated with lower survival are older age, obesity, female gender, no-smoking history, no prior angina or MI, COPD, renal failure, FE <30%, preoperative shock, three-vessel disease, longer CPB and cross-clamping time, and inferior-basal defects. Emergency/salvage status is a strong risk factor for intra- and perioperative death [21].

1.6 Surgical Techniques

The main treatment goals in a patient with VSD are to reduce the left-to-right shunt by limiting afterload, improve coronary perfusion with IABP and nitroglycerin (where possible), maintain organ perfusion (MAP and SVR), and use opioids to limit stress and sympathetic stimulation triggered by pain or invasive procedures.

Surgery is performed to close the communication between the left and right ventricles.

Concomitant myocardial revascularization should be considered if multiple coronary vessel disease is simultaneously present, which is seen in more than 50% of the patients with post-MI VSD. The advantage of this strategy lies in bringing oxygenated blood from the areas surrounding the transmural infarction to affected areas of the myocardium for potential recovery and ensuing reduction in the infarcted area. However, revascularization of the occluded coronary artery responsible for the VSD is not useful because the affected myocardium is no longer viable and because the vessel often remains trapped in the suture line of the ventriculotomy. Further, performing coronary artery bypass graft (CABG) surgery during post-MI VSD repair does not significantly increase short- and long-term survival, and the risks associated with prolonged cardiopulmonary bypass time must be weighed.

The principles of VSD repair surgery are as follows: incise the ventricle in the infarcted area, use one or more patches (in polyester or pericardium) to cover the defect, close the septal communication by passing the stitches on the septum and away from the infarcted friable area, use interrupted sutures with pledgets and/or continuous sutures to reduce tension on the patch, exclude the infarcted area in the free wall, and ensure minimal tissue debridement. Almost all patients who require surgery also have IABP support. Hence, cardiopulmonary bypass is established with bicaval cannulation, but some hospitals—once mitral valve surgery has been ruled out—directly cannulate the right atrium. Once extracorporeal circulation is initiated, the patient is subjected to moderate hypothermia (28°C) and cardioplegia is administered, initially warm, anterograde, and into the aortic root, and then retrograde and into the coronary venous sinus.

Predominantly used techniques in anterior VSD repair are amputation of the apex, infarctectomy and closure (Daggett's technique), modified Daggett's technique, David infarct exclusion technique and its modifications (single or double patch), and sandwich technique.

If the VSD is due to a distal occlusion of the anterior descending coronary artery, only the apical septum may be affected, and in this case, a simple amputation of the ventricular apex can be performed, including the involved portion of the septum and the apical portion of the RV. The apex is then reconstructed using two PTFE felt strips on either side of the septum and two more strips adjacent to the left and right apical endocardium. Heavy mattress sutures are applied through these four felt layers to approximate the left and right apical endocardium and to close the breaches.

The Daggett's technique of infarctectomy and closure involves a two-patch repair and has been applied and modified over time to reduce patch tension and VSD recurrence. Anterior exposure is through the infarcted myocardium. Interrupted pledgeted sutures are first placed at the base of the septum through the healthy tissue and subsequently through the "first" patch, which is cut to length to complete the VSD repair. Depending on the quality of the superior septal tissue, sutures are passed on the left or the right ventricular free wall, adjacent to the septum. Two patches are used to reconstruct the septum, the anterior wall may be separated or connected, and the septum patch can also be brought out of the anterior ventriculotomy and later anchored to the sutures placed to secure the second patch; the latter is used to close the anterior infarcted free wall of the VS (patch-to-patch junction of the septum and the anterior wall) [22, 23].

The modified Daggett's technique involves three patches instead of two: specifically, one to close the VDS and a double internal and external composite patch to close the left ventriculotomy. Fibrin glue is used to seal the two patches and reduce the risk of bleeding [24].

In the infarct-excluding, single-patch David technique, the infarcted septum is exposed through an anterior ventriculotomy that runs parallel to the LAD vessel. The infarcted septum and myocardium free wall are excluded using a large patch of bovine pericardium or a collagen- or gelatin-impregnated polyester patch and deep bites are taken through healthy tissue. Both interrupted pledgeted sutures and continuous suture may be used to reduce tension on the patch. The ventriculotomy is closed without an infarctectomy, using two strips of PTFE felt or buttressed sutures in the pericardium [25, 26]. This technique can also be applied to posterior defects, but here, the heart is lifted, and the incision is made parallel to the posterior descending coronary artery. Next, a triangle-shaped patch is placed such that one vertex is anchored to the fibrous annulus of the mitral valve, its medial margin attached to the non-infarcted septum adjacent to the defect, and its lateral margin fixed to the free wall of the LV adjacent to the posterior papillary muscle. The ventriculotomy is then closed with a double strip of Teflon.

The double patch or "sandwich technique" is another well-described VSD repair procedure where the defect is corrected using a double patch on both the left and right sides of the septum. The ventricle can be approached from either the left or the right side. Separate stitches are passed into the first patch, then through the healthy septum around the defect, and subsequently into the second patch. Some authors prefer autologous pericardium stabilized in 0.6% glutaraldehyde, while others have used bovine pericardium or a composite of Dacron or Teflon patches covered with autologous or heterologous pericardium for the surface in contact with blood. The use of glue, such as gelatin-resorcin-formalin (GRF) glue (Cardial, Technopole, Saint-Étienne, France) or BioGlue (CryoLife Inc., Kennesaw, Georgia, USA), injected into the space between the two patches, has also been described and may help prevent a residual left-to-right shunt.

A modification of this technique involves combining the double patch with the exclusion of the infarcted area of the left ventricular free wall. Here, the second patch is shaped such that some tissue is available to both close the left-side defect and exclude the infarcted area, according to David's technique. The LV incision line is double-suture closed using the felt sandwich method and 3-0 polypropylene sutures [27–29].

1.7 Percutaneous Closure

In the era of interventional cardiology, any possibility to nonsurgically close a postischemic VSD represents an attractive alternative, especially in those patients who are poor candidates for surgery. However, compared to those treated with open surgery, outcomes are not significantly different among these patients because 30-day or in-hospital mortality after percutaneous closure is around 32%, despite a procedural success rate of approximately 89%. Moreover, mortality after percutaneous closure is strictly correlated with preoperative status—in-hospital or 30-day mortality is 88% in patients in cardiogenic shock compared to 38% in more stable patients. Importantly, these rates reflect surgical mortality of a procedure performed in the first 14 days after MI [30, 31]. Thus, the cardiac team has a decisive role in selecting the most appropriate treatment strategy for the patient, and the percutaneous transcatheter option can be considered as (i) an alternative to surgery, (ii) to close a residual postsurgical defect or (iii) as a bridge-to-surgery for reducing the shunt and enabling hemodynamic stabilization, and exclusively in centers where appropriate expertise exists.

A widely used specific device is the Amplatzer P.I. Muscular VSD Occluder (St. Jude Medical, St. Paul, MN, USA), which consists of two discs of nitinol wire that are deployed on the sides of the septum and are connected by a 10 mm stem (waist). The length of the stem ranges between 18 and 24 mm and provides nominal size to the device. Ideally, the discs should match the 5 mm septal thickness to provide adequate seal and the defect size should be <25 mm on both sides of the septum (optimally <15 mm). Further, the device should be oversized when possible (even up to 150%), there should be adequate septal "rim," and it should not hinder the tricuspid subvalvular apparatus. Unfortunately, these optimal features are found in less than one-half of all cases, i.e., the defects are often wider and asymmetric, and the septum is too thin to ensure adequate sealing [12]. Additionally, VSD Occluder device use requires double-antiplatelet therapy for 6 months, followed by only aspirin.

Technically, the procedure uses femoral arterial access to insert a soft wire that is passed through the VSD and captured in the pulmonary artery, which is then externalized by a snare advanced from the femoral or jugular vein. Through this arteriovenous rail, the device delivery sheath is advanced through the defect from the venous side and then released at the defect site under transesophageal echocardiographic guidance. Procedural complications that predominantly affect survival are arrhythmias (third-degree atrioventricular block, ventricular fibrillation/tachycardia, bradycardia, atrial fibrillation), device embolization, ventricular rupture, device-related hemolysis, recurrence of septal defect due to ongoing necrosis and tissue instability in early closure, and vascular access-related complications. Other methods include percutaneous/surgical hybrid closure via thoracotomy, which affords greater direct visualization of the defect and simpler crossing, or direct deployment of the device during open surgery [32].

1.8 Role of Mechanical Circulatory Support

The deployment of short-term mechanical circulatory support (MCS) devices is gaining ground in the management of postischemic VSD as it allows modification of two of the most determining factors of mortality, viz., pre-procedural time and cardiogenic shock.

Current European guidelines do not recommend the systematic use of IABP in cardiogenic shock (class III, level of evidence B), but its use should be considered in hemodynamically unstable patients and in cardiogenic shock related to postinfarction mechanical complications (class IIa, level of evidence C) [33, 34].

The use of IABP in postischemic VSD is well established and is indicated for stabilization of the VSD patient as it can not only reduce afterload and left-to-right shunt but also enable diastolic augmentation and improve coronary perfusion. However, its effects on cardiac output are modest and may not be sufficient to ensure good peripheral perfusion in the presence of severe left-right or biventricular dysfunction due to the infarction or if a large left-right interventricular shunt already exists (Fig. 1a).

Technological progress has delivered advanced MCS devices capable of providing hemodynamic support to critically ill patients with postischemic VSD, and these include the veno-arterial (VA) extracorporeal membrane oxygenation (ECMO), the Impella (Abiomed, Danvers, Massachusetts), the TandemHeart (LivaNova, London, UK), and other ventricular assist devices (VADs), including the total artificial heart (TAH). Combined with minimally invasive implantation using the percutaneous technique, such technological progress allows the potential use of these devices as a bridge-to-surgery or bridge-to-decision strategy in patients with advanced hemodynamic instability or even in more stable patients who must undergo high-risk procedures like percutaneous closure of the VSD. In the first group of patients, the heart team has to identify the pathophysiology underlying cardiogenic shock, i.e., whether it is related to extensive myocardial infarction, the presence of a large VSD with a severe left-to-right shunt, or a combination of the two. In such situations, treatment choices depend on whether it is more appropriate to initiate MCS to gain time as a bridge-to-surgery/decision, which allows time for the infarcted tissue to stabilize and the organs to recover, or to perform early surgery and use intraoperative MCS as a bridge for postoperative recovery (days to weeks) that can then not only reduce tension from sutures and the patch but also thereby lower the risk of VSD recurrence. Another aspect to consider when choosing the MCS device is the type of ventricular dysfunction, i.e., whether left (Impella CP, TandemHeart), right (Impella RP, right configuration TandemHeart, and Protek Duo), or biventricular (VA-ECMO, Bipella). In unrepairable VSD or VSD due to end-stage organ failure, TAH or HeartMate6 (two HeartMate3 as BiVAD) may be employed as a bridge-to-transplantation or -destination option.

Choice of an MCS device must consider device-related hemodynamic effects on the VSD and possible complications due to their interaction. Even though using two different devices can solve some problems, the complexity of subsequent patient management and accessibility to resources can become limitations (Fig. 1f,g,h). The VA ECMO certainly ensures good perfusion and oxygenation of organs and reduces pulmonary congestion due to pulmonary overflow; however, greater afterload and presence of a natural venting port, such as the VSD, reduce aortic valve opening and increase thrombotic risk of the coronary arteries and at the aortic root, apart from worsening the left-to-right shunt (Fig. 1b, e).

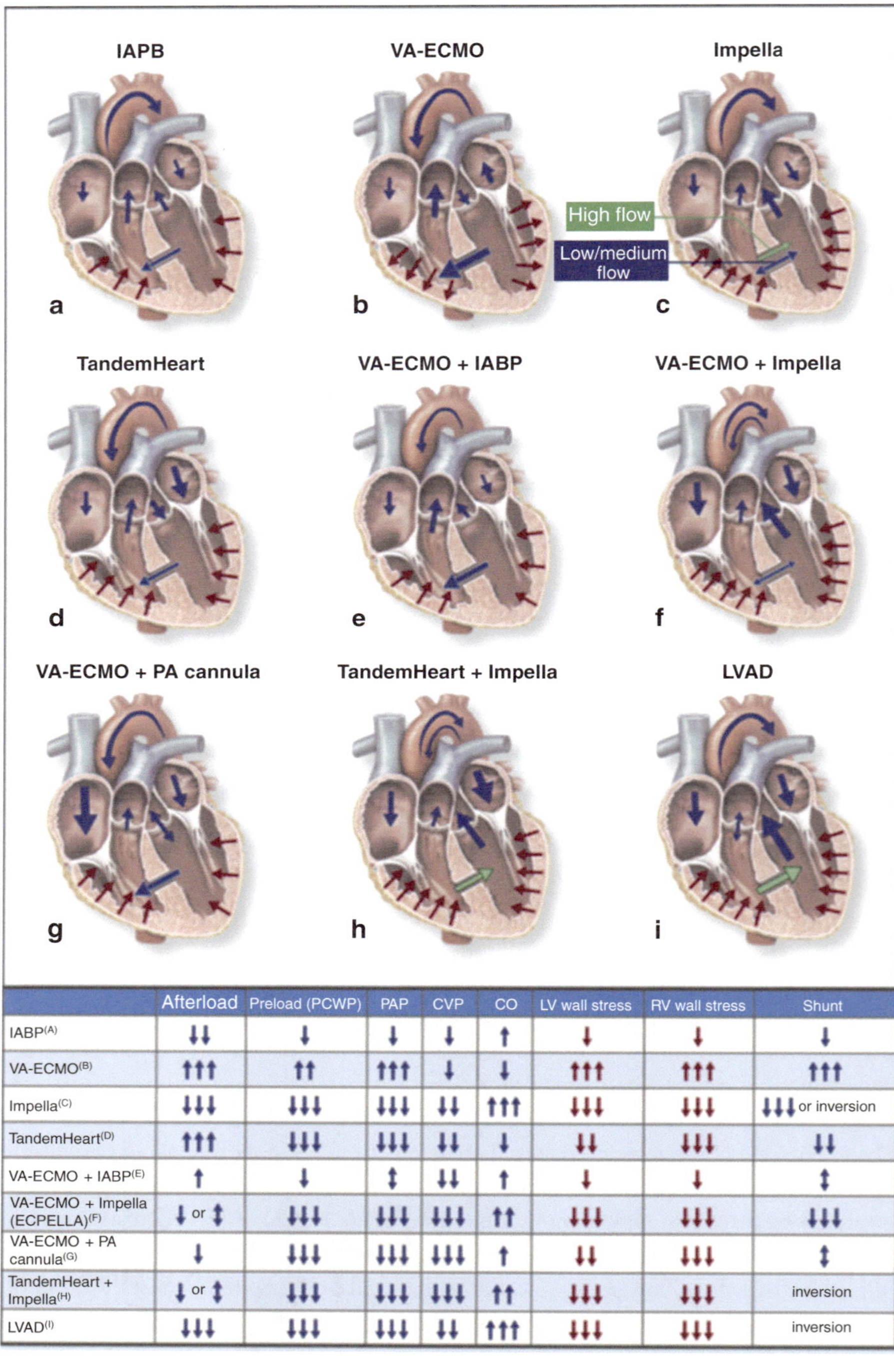

	Afterload	Preload (PCWP)	PAP	CVP	CO	LV wall stress	RV wall stress	Shunt
IABP(A)	↓↓	↓	↓	↓	↑	↓	↓	↓
VA-ECMO(B)	↑↑↑	↑↑	↑↑↑	↓	↓	↑↑↑	↑↑↑	↑↑↑
Impella(C)	↓↓↓	↓↓↓	↓↓↓	↓↓	↑↑↑	↓↓↓	↓↓↓	↓↓↓ or inversion
TandemHeart(D)	↑↑↑	↓↓↓	↓↓↓	↓↓	↓	↓↓	↓↓↓	↓↓
VA-ECMO + IABP(E)	↑	↓	↕	↓↓	↑	↓	↓	↕
VA-ECMO + Impella (ECPELLA)(F)	↓ or ↕	↓↓↓	↓↓↓	↓↓↓	↑↑	↓↓↓	↓↓↓	↓↓↓
VA-ECMO + PA cannula(G)	↓	↓↓↓	↓↓↓	↓↓↓	↑	↓↓	↓↓↓	↕
TandemHeart + Impella(H)	↓ or ↕	↓↓↓	↓↓↓	↓↓↓	↑↑	↓↓↓	↓↓↓	inversion
LVAD(I)	↓↓↓	↓↓↓	↓↓↓	↓↓	↑↑↑	↓↓↓	↓↓↓	inversion

Fig. 1 Hemodynamic effects of MCSs on postinfarction VSD pathophysiology (Ronco D et al. J Am Coll Cardiol Intv. 2021;14(10):1053–66)

The Impella, if properly installed with a moderate flow that does not invert the shunt through the VSD, guarantees good unloading of the LV and, consequently, of the RV. Its isolated use is optimal in the presence of good RV function and if the VSD is posterior because it facilitates the transcatheter procedure and leads to less manipulation of the infarcted area by the pigtail catheter (Fig. 1c).

In large anterior VSDs, the tandem heart may be suitable, again in conjunction with IABP, for promoting aortic valve opening [35] (Fig 1d). When defining a patient's tailored treatment strategy, it is important to consider MCS-related complications, including hemolysis, major bleeding, thromboembolic events, and ischemic stroke; of these, bleeding is the complication that predominantly affects in-hospital mortality.

In summary, postischemic VSD is a very serious complication that needs immediate intervention by highly experienced professionals. Multidisciplinary clinical evaluation of the patient by cardiac surgeon, cardiologist, intensive care anesthesiologist, hemodynamist, and radiologist permits the development of an optimal treatment strategy tailored for that patient, while also taking into account the skills and expertise of each specialist and available resources. The mortality rate of this condition can be modified in the future only by an interplay of surgical correction, percutaneous transcatheter closure, and hemodynamic stabilization using MCS, along with IABP support and optimal medical therapy. Thus, it is mandatory that these patients are referred to tertiary hub centers where they have a better chance of survival.

2 Free Wall Rupture

2.1 Introduction

Another life-threatening mechanical complication of acute myocardial infarction (AMI) is free wall rupture (FWR), and available literature indicates that it is the most common cause of death after acute infarction, just behind acute cardiac failure, and that it accounts for up to 20% of all early deaths [36]. However, its incidence has decreased over the years, probably due to increased availability of emergency revascularization treatments such as percutaneous coronary intervention (PCI). Multiple reports show no significant difference in outcomes among the various revascularization techniques used [37, 38]. Data from contemporary registries shows that FWR incidence stands at around 0.01–0.5% [39, 40], but despite its rarity, this complication portends an ominous prognosis as it is associated with an extremely high mortality rate (39-92%) [41–43]. Recognized risk factors include first transmural AMI in elderly patients, arterial hypertension, long episode of angina with delayed hospital assistance, and persistent ST-segment elevation [44].

2.2 Clinical Presentation

FWR usually occurs in the first 48 hours after the onset of AMI symptoms [45], but late rupture can occur up to 7 days later in 30% of the patients [46]. FWR is more often a gradual process that begins as small areas of necrosis or an incomplete rupture characterized by epicardial extravasation or slow bleeding that may be temporarily sealed by a clot or pericardial adhesion. These areas lead to hematomas that gradually dissect the necrotic myocardium into the pericardium, which results in tamponade and cardiogenic shock. This phenomenon is the so-called *oozing presentation* [47]. Less frequently, an abrupted rupture, characterized by active bleeding and a macroscopic tear in the infarcted area, may quickly result in sudden death from exsanguination [48] or tamponade—this is the so-called *blowout phenomenon* [49]. Clinical variables that appear to be highly significantly, but not specifically, associated with FWR include hypotension, recurrent or persistent chest pain, and syncope. Further, although transient electromechanical dissociation is very specific, it is not sensitive [50].

Two-dimensional (2-D) cardiac ultrasonography is clearly the most sensitive (>90%) and expeditious modality for diagnosing FWR [43, 46, 51–53], and typical ultrasonographic findings indicative of rupture are pericardial effusion and echogenic pericardial thrombus. A case series described by Lopez-Sendon [50] reported that a pericardial effusion of >5 mm was 100% sensitive for a diagnosis of subacute ventricular wall rupture; in contrast, according to the SHOCK Trail Registry, an effusion on echocardiography was seen in only 75% of our patients with rupture or tamponade. Further, as invasive tests such as ventriculography are very insensitive, they are, therefore, not recommended.

2.3 Preoperative Time and Surgical Techniques

Rupture occurs most commonly on the lateral or the antero-apical wall of the LV and in the middle of the ventricle, along the longitudinal axis from the base to the apex [52]. In SHOCK Trial Registry, the right coronary artery was less frequently the culprit in patients with rupture or tamponade, which more often led to a rupture of the lower ventricular septum [54, 55]. Early treatment, beginning with the recognition of signs and symptoms, is key to positive outcome. In the series reported by Nappi and colleagues, emergency surgery was performed with a time interval of 20 minutes to 3 hours between LV-FWR and skin incision (mean, 101.4 min; SD = 61 min) [56]; in contrast, in the cohort described by Matteucci et al., this interval was 4.7 ± 6 hours [38]. As some patients may be in cardiogenic shock at the time of surgery or suffer cardiac arrest at presentation, preoperative support with intra-aortic balloon pump (IABP) or extracorporeal membrane oxygenation (ECMO) may be needed [38, 39, 44, 57]. As IABP can improve coronary blood flow and decrease intracavity pressure in the left ventricle, it can either inhibit infarct extension or reduce the incidence of transition from oozing to blowout rupture [58]. Moreover, according to Lemura et al., IABP also appears to prevent re-rupture following surgery [59].

In contrast, the implantation of a veno-arterial (VA) ECMO is still controversial due to a lack of large datasets and poor/discouraging results published to date. An interesting meta-analysis published by Matteucci and colleagues failed to identify any specific indications for the use of VA-ECMO in the postoperative period because, first, few patients were provided postoperative VA-ECMO support and it was not possible to accurately identify factors that determine the need for mechanical support, besides CPB weaning failure, in these few patients. Second, none of the studies have focused on indications and management strategies such as weaning due to myocardial recovery or bridge-to-heart transplant or -long-term left ventricular assist device [60].

Several surgical techniques have been proposed over time, and these can be easily classified as suture techniques (ST) and suture-less techniques (SLT). One of the first techniques adopted was probably the most intuitive, and its purpose was to close the tear using two horizontal mattress sutures bolstered by PTFE felt strips. This approach, known as *direct closure or linear closure*, was first described by Montegut in 1972 [61]. An over-and-over suture can be added to approximate the edges of the PTFE felts to achieve satisfactory hemostasis [54]. However, better results have been reported after covering the ventricular tear and surrounding infarct area with a patch secured to the cardiac surface with stitches, sutures, or surgical glue [62]. Further, whenever a large necrotic area is encountered, a more complex *resection and patching technique* should be preferred to avoid the risk of distortion and alteration of organ anatomy. This is a somewhat less "popular" technique, probably because of its complexity; yet it remains the procedure of choice in cases of acute massive ruptures (blowout type) or if a concomitant interventricular defect is present. Procedurally, the first step is to excise the necrotic tissue and particular attention should be paid to preserving as much myocardial tissue as possible. Nonetheless, the entire infarcted area should be removed because it is highly fragile; this also allows adequate anchoring of the sutures. Subsequently, myocardial tissue is replaced by a prosthetic patch, tailored to recreate the geometry of the left ventricle, and sutured with pledgeted interrupted sutures. A continuous polypropylene running suture may be added to achieve hemostasis [53].

More recently, the availability of tissue adhesives and surgical glues has allowed wide use of SLT, namely the *patch covering techniques,* whose major advantage lies in avoiding transmural stiches. Here, a prosthetic patch (autologous or heterologous pericardium, PTFE, or PET) is applied above the ventricular wall to cover the area of hematoma and muscle necrosis, and it is crucial that the patch overlaps onto the healthy myocardium. A good amount of surgical glue is injected between the ventricular wall and the patch, and a slight compression is applied to evenly distribute the glue and promote adequate patch adherence until it becomes firmly attached and hemostatic. As stated above, a wide range of synthetic and biological glues can be used for this purpose, and this technique should be preferably used if the tear is sealed or the lesion is of the oozing type. If a small tear or limited bleeding occurs, a polypropylene single suture could be added to graft the patch to the epicardium before injecting the glue and special caution should be paid to avoid coronary involvement. Some authors also describe the use of SLT for actively bleeding lesions, provided that patients are on CPB with total decompression of the heart [63, 64]. Notwithstanding these advantages, the risk of rupture recurrence and pseudoaneurysm formation remains, which, in our opinion, is a real concern. Recent reports describe a trend to shift toward the use of patches coated with human fibrinogen and human thrombin such as TachoComb® or TachoSil®. Similar to the initial ST patches, an overlap onto surrounding healthy myocardium that is not involved in the necrotic process is needed to allow better anchoring and to avoid re-rupture [62]. This surgical approach, particularly when reserved for patients with the oozing-type rupture, has shown satisfactory clinical results [65, 66]. Thus, SLT is simple and fast and can be accomplished without CPB. Advantageously, the avoidance of CPB implies a significant reduction in the potential for postoperative bleeding.

2.4 Results

As mentioned above, early mortality due to FWR ranges between 39 and 92% and it includes every patient who died as a consequence of FWR, independent of whether medical or surgical treatment was provided. Despite meagre literature, medical management appears futile as it results in a mortality of up to 90% [67], but is nonetheless limited to a few patients [68]. According to a majority of investigators, surgical repair is considered the treatment of choice as it has a survival rate of 17–36% [38, 60, 69]. Extremely critical preoperative status is the main factor responsible for such a high mortality rate, given that Matteucci and colleagues reported preoperative LVEF, cardiac arrest, and ECMO support to be independent predictors of early mortality [38]. A higher operative mortality rate is related to blowout-type rupture, rather than the oozing type, because the former has a severe and acute course [60] that demands superior surgical techniques for a positive outcome. In fact, a trend toward a higher operative mortality and postoperative bleeding has been reported in patients undergoing ST surgery, but no significant differences in surgical outcomes have been shown between ST and SLT in literature.

Concomitant surgical revascularization remains debated, and according to available reports, simultaneous CABG could reduce the risk of operative mortality, albeit not significantly [70]. Currently, data from a modest number of patients who have undergone concomitant CABG is available for statistical analysis because they were stable enough to tolerate coronary angiography. However, it is still not clear if reduced mortality risk is a consequence of an unavoidable selection bias or if concomitant revascularization is a real protective factor. Further analysis is needed.

A topic worthy of further discussion is the use of MCS such as IABP and ECMO. While extensively employed in the perioperative period, insertion of IABP failed to demonstrate any protective effect in terms of operative mortality [60]. Next, even though ECMO was identified as an independent predictor of early mortality, probably due to the extremely severe hemodynamic status of the patients receiving ECMO support [38], the "2017 ESC Guidelines for the management of acute myocardial infarction in patients presenting with

ST-segment elevation" support the use of ECMO only in cases of hemodynamic deterioration due to mechanical complications post-AMI [71].

In summary, FWR is a rare but life-threatening event that can complicate acute AMI. Prompt diagnosis is the key, and surgical management is the gold standard of treatment. Preoperative clinical conditions and type of presentation (blowout vs. oozing) directly affect postoperative outcome.

References

1. Latham PM. Lectures on subjects connected with clinical medicine comparing diseases of the heart, vol. 2. London: Longmans, Brown, Green and Longmans; 1845. p. 168.
2. Brunn F. Zur Diagnostic der envorbenen Ruptur der Kammerscheidewand des Herzens. Wien Arch Finn. Med. 1923;6:533.
3. Cooley DA, Belmonte BA, Zeis LB, Schnur S. Surgical repair of ruptured interventricular septum following acute myocardial infarction. Surgery. 1957;41(6):930–7.
4. Kay JH. Discussion of paper by Iben et al. Ann Thorac Surg. 1969;8:252–62.
5. Dubost C. Discussion of paper by Iben AB et al. Ann Thorac Surg. 1969;8:252–62.
6. Kitamura S, Mendez A, Harold Kay JH. Ventricular septal defect following myocardial infarction. J Thorac Cardiovasc Surg. 1971;61(2):186–99. https://doi.org/10.1016/S0022-5223(19)42246-0.
7. Filgueira JL, Battistessa SA, Estable H, Lorenzo A, Cassinelli M, Scola R. Delayed repair of an acquired posterior septal defect through a right atrial approach. Ann Thorac Surg. 1986;42(2):208–9. https://doi.org/10.1016/s0003-4975(10)60521-8.
8. David TE, Feindel CM, Ropchan GV. Reconstruction of the left ventricle with autologous pericardium. J Thorac Cardiovasc Surg. 1987;94(5):710–4. https://doi.org/10.1016/S0022-5223(19)36184-7.
9. Ahmad FB, Anderson RN. The leading causes of death in the US for 2020. JAMA. 2021;325(18):1829–30. https://doi.org/10.1001/jama.2021.5469.
10. GUSTO investigators. An international randomized trial comparing four thrombolytic strategies for acute myocardial infarction. N Engl J Med. 1993;329(10):673–82. https://doi.org/10.1056/NEJM199309023291001.
11. Menon V, Webb JG, Hillis LD, Sleeper LA, Abboud R, Dzavik V, Slater JN, Forman R, Monrad ES, Talley JD, Hochman JS. Outcome and profile of ventricular septal rupture with cardiogenic shock after myocardial infarction: a report from the SHOCK Trial Registry. Should we emergently revascularize Occluded Coronaries in cardiogenic shocK? J Am Coll Cardiol. 2000;36(3):1110–6. https://doi.org/10.1016/s0735-1097(00)00878-0.
12. Hamilton MCK, Rodrigues JCL, Martin RP, Manghat NE, Turner MS. The in vivo morphology of post-infarct ventricular septal defect and the implications for closure. JACC Cardiovasc Intv. 2017;10(12):1233–43. https://doi.org/10.1016/j.jcin.2017.03.042.
13. Lewis AJ, Burchell HB, Titus JL. Clinical and pathologic features of postinfarction cardiac rupture. Am J Cardiol. 1969;23(1):43–53. https://doi.org/10.1016/0002-9149(69)90240-9.
14. Kouchoukos NT, Blackstone EH, Hanley FL, Kirklin JK. Postinfarction ventricular septal defect. Kirklin/Barrat-Boyes cardiac surgery, vol. I. 3rd ed. Churchill Livingstone; 2003. p. 456.
15. Cox FF, Plokker HW, Morshuis WJ, Kelder JC, Vermeulen FE. Importance of coronary revascularization for late survival after postinfarction ventricular septal rupture. A reason to perform coronary angiography prior to surgery. Eur Heart J. 1996;17(12):1841–5. https://doi.org/10.1093/oxfordjournals.eurheartj.a014801.

16. Sutton MG, Sharpe N. Left ventricular remodeling after myocardial infarction: pathophysiology and therapy. Circulation. 2000;101(25):2981–8. https://doi.org/10.1161/01.cir.101.25.2981.
17. Task Force on the management of ST-segment elevation acute myocardial infarction of the European Society of Cardiology (ESC), Steg PG, James SK, Atar D, Badano LP, Blömstrom-Lundqvist C, Borger MA, Di Mario C, Dickstein K, Ducrocq G, Fernandez-Aviles F, Gershlick AH, Giannuzzi P, Halvorsen S, Huber K, Juni P, Kastrati A, Knuuti J, Lenzen MJ, Mahaffey KW, Valgimigli M, Van't Hof A, Widimsky P, Zahger D. ESC Guidelines for the management of acute myocardial infarction in patients presenting with ST-segment elevation Task Force on the management of ST-segment elevation acute myocardial infarction of the European Society of Cardiology (ESC). Eur Heart J. 2012;33(20):2569–619. https://doi.org/10.1093/eurheartj/ehs215.
18. O'Gara PT, Kushner FG, Ascheim DD, Casey DE Jr, Chung MK, de Lemos JA, Ettinger SM, Fang JC, Fesmire FM, Franklin BA, Granger CB, Krumholz HM, Linderbaum JA, Morrow DA, Newby LK, Ornato JP, Ou N, Radford MJ, Tamis-Holland JE, Tommaso CL, Tracy CM, Woo YJ, Zhao DX. 2013 ACCF/AHA guideline for the management of ST-elevation myocardial infarction: executive summary: a report of the American College of Cardiology Foundation/American Heart Association Task Force on Practice Guidelines. J Am Coll Cardiol. 2013;61(4):485–510. https://doi.org/10.1016/j.jacc.2012.11.018.
19. Arnaoutakis GJ, Zhao Y, George TJ, Sciortino CM, McCarthy PM, Conte JV. Surgical repair of ventricular septal defect after myocardial infarction: outcomes from the Society of Thoracic Surgeons National Database. Ann Thorac Surg. 2012;94(2):436–43. https://doi.org/10.1016/j.athoracsur.2012.04.020.
20. Malhotra A, Patel K, Sharma P, Wadhawa V, Madan T, Khandeparkar J, Shah K, Patel S. Techniques, timing & prognosis of post infarct ventricular septal repair: a Re-look at old dogmas. Braz J Cardiovasc Surg. 2017;32(3):147–55. https://doi.org/10.21470/1678-9741-2016-0032.
21. Crenshaw BS, Granger CB, Birnbaum Y, Pieper KS, Morris DC, Kleiman NS, Vahanian A, Califf RM, Topol EJ. Risk factors, angiographic patterns, and outcomes in patients with ventricular septal defect complicating acute myocardial infarction. GUSTO-I (global utilization of streptokinase and TPA for occluded coronary arteries) Trial Investigators. Circulation. 2000;101(1):27–32. https://doi.org/10.1161/01.cir.101.1.27.
22. Arnaoutakis GJ, Conte JV. Repair of postinfarct ventricular septal defect: anterior apical ventricular septal defect. Oper Tech Thorac Cardiovasc Surg. 2014;19(1):96–114. https://doi.org/10.1053/j.optechstcvs.2014.03.002.
23. Daggett WM, Guyton RA, Mundth ED, Buckley MJ, McEnany MT, Gold HK, Leinbach RC, Austen WG. Surgery for post-myocardial infarct ventricular septal defect. Ann Surg. 1977;186(3):260–71. https://doi.org/10.1097/00000658-197709000-00004.
24. Nakajima M, Tsuchiya K, Inoue H, Naito Y, Mizutani E. Ann Thorac Surg. 2003;75(1):301–2. https://doi.org/10.1016/s0003-4975(02)03929-2.
25. David TE, Armstrong S. Surgical repair of postinfarction ventricular septal defect by infarct exclusion. Semin Thorac Cardiovasc Surg. 1998;10(2):105–10. https://doi.org/10.1016/s1043-0679(98)70003-6.
26. David TE, Dale L, Sun Z. Postinfarction ventricular septal rupture: repair by endocardial patch with infarct exclusion. J Thorac Cardiovasc Surg. 1995;110(5):1315–22. https://doi.org/10.1016/S0022-5223(95)70054-4.
27. Yamasaki T, Fujita S, Kaku Y, Katagiri J, Hiramatsu T. Modified double patch repair with infarct exclusion technique for ventricular septal perforation: a case study. J Cardiothorac Surg. 2018;13(1):17. https://doi.org/10.1186/s13019-018-0708-7.

28. Isoda S, Imoto K, Uchida K, Nishimura K, Karube N, Suzuki S, Masuda M. 'Sandwich Technique' via a right ventricle incision to repair postinfarction ventricular septal defects. J Card Surg. 2015;30(6):488–93. https://doi.org/10.1111/jocs.12546.
29. Salehi-Ardebili S, Mehdizade H, Askari B. Report of five cases: sandwich repair for post infarction ventricular septal rupture with right ventricular approach. Egypt Heart J. 2020;16:11. https://doi.org/10.1186/s43044-020-00048-2.
30. Schlotter F, de Waha S, Eitel I, Desch S, Fuernau G, Thiele H. Interventional post-myocardial infarction ventricular septal defect closure: a systematic review of current evidence. EuroIntervention. 2016;12(1):94–102. https://doi.org/10.4244/EIJV12I1A17.
31. Thiele H, Kaulfersch C, Daehnert I, Schoenauer M, Eitel I, Borger M, Schuler G. Immediate primary transcatheter closure of postinfarction ventricular septal defects. Eur Heart J. 2009;30(1):81–8. https://doi.org/10.1093/eurheartj/ehn524.
32. Jones BM, Kapadia SR, Smedira NG, Robich M, Tuzcu EM, Menon V, Krishnaswamy A. Ventricular septal rupture complicating acute myocardial infarction: a contemporary review. Eur Heart J. 2014;35(31):2060–8. https://doi.org/10.1093/eurheartj/ehu248.
33. Ponikowski P, Voors AA, Anker SD, Bueno H, Cleland JG, Coats AJ, Falk V, González-Juanatey JR, Harjola VP, Jankowska EA, Jessup M, Linde C, Nihoyannopoulos P, Parissis JT, Pieske B, Riley JP, Rosano GM, Ruilope LM, Ruschitzka F, Rutten FH, van der Meer P, Authors/Task Force Members, Document Reviewers. ESC Guidelines for the diagnosis and treatment of acute and chronic heart failure: the Task Force for the diagnosis and treatment of acute and chronic heart failure of the European Society of Cardiology (ESC). Developed with the special contribution of the Heart Failure Association (HFA) of the ESC. Eur J Heart Fail. 2016;18(8):891–975. https://doi.org/10.1002/ejhf.592.
34. Ibanez B, James S, Agewall S, Antunes MJ, Bucciarelli-Ducci C, Bueno H, Caforio ALP, Crea F, Goudevenos JA, Halvorsen S, Hindricks G, Kastrati A, Lenzen MJ, Prescott E, Roffi M, Valgimigli M, Varenhorst C, Vranckx P, Widimský P, ESC Scientific Document Group. 2017 ESC Guidelines for the management of acute myocardial infarction in patients presenting with ST-segment elevation: the Task Force for the management of acute myocardial infarction in patients presenting with ST-segment elevation of the European Society of Cardiology (ESC). Eur Heart J. 2018;39(2):119–77. https://doi.org/10.1093/eurheartj/ehx393.
35. Ronco D, Matteucci M, Ravaux JM, Marra S, Torchio F, Corazzari C, Massimi G, Beghi C, Maessen J, Lorusso R. Mechanical circulatory support as a bridge to definitive treatment in post-infarction ventricular septal rupture. JACC Cardiovasc Intv. 2021;14(10):1053–66. https://doi.org/10.1016/j.jcin.2021.02.046.
36. Slater J, Brown RJ, Antonelli TA, et al. Cardiogenic shock due to cardiac free-wall rupture or tamponade after acute myocardial infarction: A report from the SHOCK trial registry. J Am Coll Cardiol. 2000;36(Suppl A):1104–9. https://doi.org/10.1016/S0735-1097(00)00846-9.
37. Tripathi B, Aggarwal V, Abbott JD, Kumbhani DJ, Giri J, Kalra A, Sardar P, Chatterjee S. Mechanical complications in ST-elevation myocardial infarction (STEMI) based on different reperfusion strategies. Am J Cardiol. 2021;156:79–84. https://doi.org/10.1016/j.amjcard.2021.06.012.
38. Matteucci M, Kowalewski M, De Bonis M, Formica F, Jiritano F, Fina D, Meani P, Folliguet T, Bonaros N, Sponga S, Suwalski P, De Martino A, Fischlein T, Troise G, Dato GA, Serraino GF, Shah SH, Scrofani R, Antona C, Fiore A, Kalisnik JM, D'Alessandro S, Villa E, Lodo V, Colli A, Aldobayyan I, Massimi G, Trumello C, Beghi C, Lorusso R. Surgical treatment of post-infarction left ventricular free-wall rupture: A multicenter study. Ann Thorac Surg. 2021;112(4):1186–92. https://doi.org/10.1016/j.athoracsur.2020.11.019.
39. Elbadawi A, Elgendy IY, Mahmoud K, Barakat AF, Mentias A, Mohamed AH, Ogunbayo GO, Megaly M, Saad M, Omer MA, Paniagua D, Abbott JD, Jneid H. Temporal trends and outcomes

of mechanical complications in patients with acute myocardial infarction. JACC Cardiovasc Intv. 2019;12(18):1825–36. https://doi.org/10.1016/J.JCIN.2019.04.039.
40. French JK, Hellkamp AS, Armstrong PW, Cohen E, Kleiman NS, O'Connor CM, Holmes DR, Hochman JS, Granger CB, Mahaffey KW. Mechanical Complications After Percutaneous Coronary Intervention in ST-Elevation myocardial infarction (from APEX-AMI). Am J Cardiol. 2010;105(1):59–63. https://doi.org/10.1016/J.AMJCARD.2009.08.653.
41. Figueras J, Alcalde O, Barrabés JA, Serra V, Alguersuari J, Cortadellas J. Lidón RMChanges in hospital mortality rates in 425 patients with acute ST-elevation myocardial infarction and cardiac rupture over a 30-year period. Circulation. 2008;118(25):2783–9. https://doi.org/10.1161/CIRCULATIONAHA.108.776690.
42. López-Sendón J, Gurfinkel EP, Lopez de Sa E, Agnelli G, Gore JM, Steg PG, Eagle KA, Cantador JR, Fitzgerald G, Granger CB, Global Registry of Acute Coronary Events (GRACE) Investigators, E L de S, et al. Factors related to heart rupture in acute coronary syndromes in the Global Registry of Acute Coronary Events. Eur Heart J. 2010;31(12):1449–56. https://doi.org/10.1093/EURHEARTJ/EHQ061.
43. Slater J, Brown RJ, Antonelli TA, Menon V, Boland J, Col J, Dzavik V, Greenberg M, Menegus M, Connery C, Hochman JS. Cardiogenic shock due to cardiac free-wall rupture or tamponade after acute myocardial infarction: a report from the SHOCK Trial Registry. J Am Coll Cardiol. 2000;36:1. https://doi.org/10.1016/S0735-1097(00)00845-7.
44. Antunes MJ. Left ventricular free wall rupture: A real nightmare. J Card Surg. 2021;36(9):3334–6. https://doi.org/10.1111/jocs.15697.
45. Figueras J, Cortadellas J, Soler-Soler J. Left ventricular free wall rupture: clinical presentation and management. Heart. 2000;83(5):499–504. https://doi.org/10.1136/heart.83.5.499.
46. Raitt MH, Kraft CD, Gardner CJ, Pearlman AS, Otto CM. Subacute ventricular free wall rupture complicating myocardial infarction. Am Heart J. 1993;126(4):946–55. https://doi.org/10.1016/0002-8703(93)90711-H.
47. Daikoku S, Haze K, Ogawa H, Kawaguchi M, Nonogi H, Fukami K, Sumiyoshi T, Hiramori K. Clinical and anatomical features of acute myocardial infarction associated with double rupture of the interventricular septum and ventricular free wall. J Cardiol. 1991;21(2):229–36.
48. Balakumaran K, Verbaan CJ, Essed CE, Nauta J, Bos E, Haalebos MM, Penn O, Simoons ML, Hugenholtz PG. Ventricular free wall rupture: sudden, subacute, slow, sealed and stabilized varieties. Eur Heart J. 1984;5(4):282–8. https://doi.org/10.1093/OXFORDJOURNALS.EURHEARTJ.A061653.
49. Shozawa T, Masuda H, Sageshima M, Kawamura K, Okada E, Saito N. Classification of cardiac rupture complicated in myocardial infarction. Pathological study of 32 cases. Acta Pathol Jpn. 1987;37(6):871–86. https://doi.org/10.1111/J.1440-1827.1987.TB00438.X.
50. López-Sendón J, González A, López de Sá EL, Coma-Canella I, Roldán I, Domínguez F, Maqueda I, Martín JL. Diagnosis of subacute ventricular wall rupture after acute myocardial infarction: sensitivity and specificity of clinical, hemodynamic and echocardiographic criteria. J Am Coll Cardiol. 1992;19(6):1145–53. https://doi.org/10.1016/0735-1097(92)90315-E.
51. Pollak H, Diez W, Spiel R, Enenkel W, Mlczoch J. Early diagnosis of subacute free wall rupture complicating acute myocardial infarction. Eur Heart J. 1993;14(5):640–8. https://doi.org/10.1093/eurheartj/14.5.640.
52. Sutherland FWH, Guell FJ, Pathi VL, Naik SK. Postinfarction ventricular free wall rupture: strategies for diagnosis and treatment. Ann Thorac Surg. 1996;61(4):1281–5. https://doi.org/10.1016/0003-4975(95)01160-9.
53. Reardon MJ, Carr CL, Diamond A, Letsou GV, Safi HJ, Espada R, Baldwin JC. Ischemic left ventricular free wall rupture: prediction, diagnosis, and treatment. Ann Thorac Surg. 1997;64(5):1509–13. https://doi.org/10.1016/S0003-4975(97)00776-5.

54. Cobbs BW, Hatcher CR, Robinson PH. Cardiac rupture: three operations with two long-term survivals. JAMA. 1973;223(5):532–5. https://doi.org/10.1001/jama.223.5.532.
55. Núñez L, de la Llana R, López Sendón J, Coma I, Gil Aguado MG, Larrea JL. Diagnosis and treatment of subacute free wall ventricular rupture after infarction. Ann Thorac Surg. 1983;35(5):525–9. https://doi.org/10.1016/S0003-4975(10)60426-2.
56. Nappi G, De Santo LS, Torella M, Della Corte A, Maresca L, Romano G, Cotrufo M. Treatment strategies for postinfarction left ventricular free wall rupture: stabilization with peri-operative IABP and off-pump repair. Int J Artif Organs. 2003;26(4):346–50. https://doi.org/10.1177/039139880302600410.
57. Formica F, Mariani S, Singh G, D'Alessandro S, Messina LA, Jones N, Bamodu OA, Sangalli F, Paolini G. Postinfarction left ventricular free wall rupture: A 17-year single-centre experience. Eur J Cardiothorac Surg. 2018;53(1):150–6. https://doi.org/10.1093/ejcts/ezx271.
58. Kamohara K, Minato N, Ikeda K, Rikitake K, Takarabe K. Life-saving strategy for left ventricular free wall rupture after acute myocardial infarction. Infarction-covering repair on the ruptured site under the beating heart. Jpn J Thorac Cardiovasc Surg. 2000;48(5):291–4. https://doi.org/10.1007/BF03218141.
59. Iemura J, Oku H, Otaki M, Kitayama H, Inoue T, Kaneda T. Surgical strategy for left ventricular free wall rupture after acute myocardial infarction. Ann Thorac Surg. 2001;71(1):201–4. https://doi.org/10.1016/S0003-4975(00)02211-6.
60. Matteucci M, Formica F, Kowalewski M, Massimi G, Ronco D, Beghi C, Lorusso R. Meta-analysis of surgical treatment for postinfarction left ventricular free-wall rupture. J Card Surg. 2021;36(9):3326–33. https://doi.org/10.1111/jocs.15701.
61. Montegut FJ. Left ventricular rupture secondary to myocardial infarction: report of survival with surgical repair. Ann Thorac Surg. 1972;14(1):75–8. https://doi.org/10.1016/S0003-4975(10)65202-2.
62. Matteucci M, Fina D, Jiritano F, Meani P, Blankesteijn WM, Raffa GM, Kowaleski M, Heuts S, Beghi C, Maessen J, Lorusso R. Treatment strategies for post-infarction left ventricular free-wall rupture. Eur Heart J Acute Cardiovasc Care. 2019;8(4):379–87. https://doi.org/10.1177/2048872619840876.
63. Lachapelle K, DeVarennes B, Ergina PL, Cecere R. Sutureless patch technique for postinfarction left ventricular rupture. Ann Thorac Surg. 2002;74(1):96–101. https://doi.org/10.1016/S0003-4975(02)03581-6.
64. Kagaya S, Aida H, Chida Y. Successful repair of a blow-out type left ventricular free wall rupture after acute myocardial infarction using a viscous diisocyanate Prepolymer. Kyobu Geka. 2019;72(13):1061–5.
65. Raffa GM, Tarelli G, Patrini D, Settepani F. Sutureless repair for postinfarction cardiac rupture: a simple approach with a tissue-adhering patch. J Thorac Cardiovasc Surg. 2013;145(2):598–9. https://doi.org/10.1016/J.JTCVS.2012.08.049.
66. Bergman R, Jainandunsing JS, Woltersom BD, den Hamer IJ, Natour E. Sutureless management of left ventricle wall rupture; a series of three cases. J Cardiothorac Surg. 2014;9(1):136. https://doi.org/10.1186/S13019-014-0136-2.
67. Blinc A, Noč M, Pohar B, Černič N, Horvat M. Subacute rupture of the left ventricular free wall after acute myocardial infarction. Three cases of long-term survival without emergency surgical repair. Chest. 1996;109(2):565–7. https://doi.org/10.1378/CHEST.109.2.565.
68. Vo AT, Nguyen TT, Tran TT, Nguyen DH. Conservative treatment of postinfarction left ventricular free wall rupture. Case Rep Cardiol. 2020;2020:8832578. https://doi.org/10.1155/2020/8832578.
69. Okamura H, Kimura N, Mieno M, Matsumoto H, Yuri K, Yamaguchi A. Sutureless repair for postinfarction left ventricular free wall rupture. J Thorac Cardiovasc Surg. 2019;158(3):771–7. https://doi.org/10.1016/J.JTCVS.2019.01.124.

70. Mantovani V, Vanoli D, Chelazzi P, Lepore V, Ferrarese S, Sala A. Post-infarction cardiac rupture: surgical treatment. Eur J Cardiothorac Surg. 2002;22(5):777–80. https://doi.org/10.1016/S1010-7940(02)00485-2.
71. Ibanez B, James S, Agewall S, et al. ESC Guidelines for the management of acute myocardial infarction in patients presenting with ST-segment elevation: the Task Force for the management of acute myocardial infarction in patients presenting with ST-segment elevation of the European Society of Cardiology (ESC). Eur Heart J. 2017;119-177:1. https://doi.org/10.1093/EURHEARTJ/EHX393.

Surgical Ventricular Remodeling in Ischemic Cardiomyopathy

Serenella Castelvecchio, Laura Perfetti, Lucia Ramputi, and Lorenzo Menicanti

Abbreviations

HF	Heart failure
LV	Left ventricular
SVR	Surgical ventricular reconstruction
EF	Ejection fraction
CMR	Cardiac magnetic resonance
RFP	Restrictive filling pattern

1 Introduction

Estimates suggest that about 23 million people are affected by HF. Approximately 50% of these cases are heart failure with LV dysfunction and reduced ejection fraction, which remains a substantial cause of mortality and morbidity [1, 2]. Coronary heart disease plays a pivotal role in the development of LV dysfunction [3, 4]. The improved survival post-myocardial infarction is counterbalanced by an increase in the percentage of people at risk of developing HF, with greater involvement of women than men: 46% women versus 22% men, respectively, develop HF within 6 years of acute MI and for these people the prognosis is poor. HF, in turn, is related to adverse LV remodeling, defined as an increase in LV volume and a deterioration of LV geometry and function, standing therefore as the main target of therapeutic interventions beyond optimal medical therapy [5, 6]. Surgical

S. Castelvecchio · L. Perfetti · L. Ramputi · L. Menicanti (✉)
Department Cardiac Surgery, I.R.C.C.S. Policlinico San Donato, Milan, Italy
e-mail: Serenella.Castelvecchio@grupposandonato.it; laura.perfetti@grupposandonato.it; Lucia.Ramputi@grupposandonato.it; Lorenzo.Menicanti@grupposandonato.it

G. Concistrè (ed.), *Ischemic Heart Disease*,
https://doi.org/10.1007/978-3-031-25879-4_30

treatments include myocardial revascularization, mitral valve repair or replacement, and SVR otherwise combined according to specific conditions.

SVR is aimed to reduce the left ventricle through the resection of the scar tissue in selected patients predominantly symptomatic for HF, and it must be conducted in centers with high level of expertise. This review will outline the rationale to reconstruct the left ventricle, the technique, the indications, and the main results to the best of our knowledge acquired in more than 20 years of surgical experience and dedicated research.

2 Left Ventricular Remodeling

A change in the ventricular architecture as a result of a myocardial injury is referred to as LV adverse remodeling, and it is linked with increased mass and volume as well as changed geometry, which in turn affects cardiac function (Fig. 1) [7, 8]. Because of increased wall stress, both the infarcted and non-infarcted myocardium are involved [9]. On a histological level, the increased mass is due to a combination of myocyte hypertrophy and apoptosis and replacement fibrosis. After the myocardial insult, LV dilatation serves as a compensatory mechanism in an attempt to preserve stroke volumes while the EF decreases after loss of contractile tissue [9]. Yet, more often, the remodeling process affects the remote, non-infarcted regions, primarily guided by eccentric hypertrophy, which is liable for increased mass, further chamber enlargement, and geometric distortion. Geometric changes cause structural abnormalities of the myocytes and of the myocardium, which aggravate cardiac

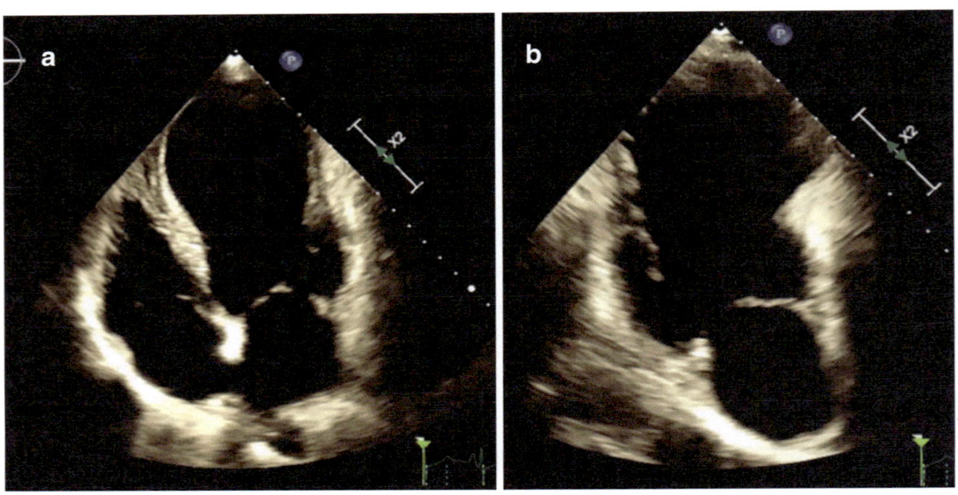

Fig. 1 Anterior LV remodeling after a previous anterior MI in apical four-chamber view (**a**) and two-chamber view (**b**) showing an extensive involvement of the anterior and posterior septum and of the apex

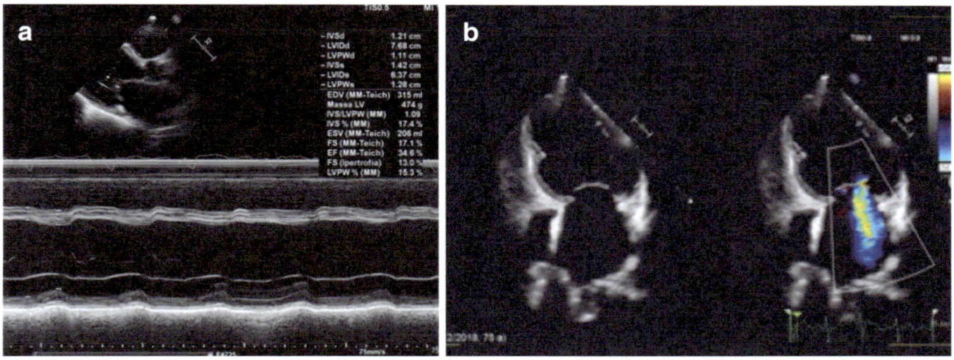

Fig. 2 Ischemic mitral regurgitation. (**a**) PLAX view: LV internal diameter is increased; (**b**) apical four-chamber view: the shape of the ventricle is spherical due to the presence of MR

function and increase neurohormonal activation. In turn, this may make the cardiovascular system less receptive to normal homeostatic control mechanism [7–9].

In ischemic cardiomyopathy, a series of structural changes are put in action to compensate for the increased load from the akinetic or dyskinetic regions. Anterior myocardial infarction mainly involves the LV apex, determining changes at the anterior, inferoseptal, and septal components [10]. In order to maintain a stable ratio (i.e., a stable sphericity index, or short ration to long axis), the elongation and widening of the ventricle develop harmoniously. Yet, when developing secondary mitral regurgitation, as a result of chamber dilatation and distortion leading to displacement of the papillary muscles, leaflet tethering, and annular dilatation, the sphericity index is anomalous and the ventricle is more spherical [10]. Therefore, the conicity index is more used to estimate the apex's conical shape and its modification after MI [10].

LV remodeling after an inferior MI, on the other hand, is quite different. The broadening of the short axis rather than the long one leads to an increase in the sphericity index and accounts for the more frequent occurrence and the more severe degree of MR (Fig. 2) (50–60% vs. 20–25% of patients with anterior MI). For these patients with MR and ischemic HF, the life expectancy is significantly reduced [11, 12].

3 Rationale for Surgical Reshaping of Failing Ventricles

As known, myocardial fibers are arranged in a spiral manner. Fiber orientation is an objective of transmural location, with fiber being placed mostly longitudinally in the endocardial region, circumferentially in the midwall, and again longitudinally over the epicardial surface. This double-layered alignment builds a dual helix [13, 14]. The myofiber sheets do not run parallel to one another in the LV wall, but instead diverge, causing angulations relative to the plane of the epicardial surface. This angulation helps to preserve geometry and maintain tension's distribution respectively at a longitudinal, radial, and circumferential level. Because there is such a strong link between form and function, any change in angulation induced by fiber disruption, fibrosis, or scarring will have an impact on the ventricle's features and functionality. Indeed, for a given fiber contractile status, the ejection fraction changes according to the shape of the ventricle, being low in a spherical ventricle and high in an elliptical shape [15].

The aim of SVR is to exclude the scar tissue from left ventricle and to reduce ventricle's volume to a physiological one and to an elliptical shape. In accordance with Laplace's law, the reduction in chamber radius lowers myocardial systolic and diastolic wall stresses and has the prospect to conduce to reverse remodeling, which in turn enhances cardiac function [16]. Moreover, since the regions far from the scar tissue—abovementioned remote regions—may be ischemic but viable, according to the extension of coronary artery disease, myocardial revascularization combined with SVR as complete as possible has the potential to promote functional recovering.

Lastly, in the presence of secondary MR, SVR per se has the potential of improving valve competence by reducing LV volumes and papillary muscle distance or decreasing internal diameters (especially in case of posterior remodeling). Alternatively, SVR allows the surgeon to repair the mitral valve at the time of the LV opening [17].

4 "One Solution Does Not Fit All!": How to Select the Right Patient

The diagnostic workup aimed to establish if a patient is eligible for SVR has profoundly changed over the past 10 years because of the widespread new imaging techniques and laboratory test in the daily clinical practice. Furthermore, the center's experience has allowed to optimize the patient selection integrating clinical parameters, imaging, and laboratory tests obtained before surgery and at predefined follow-up time points.

The roadmap includes the following:

- **Clinical evaluation**: history of previous MI; predominant symptoms of HF and/or presence of ventricular arrythmias and/or angina needing surgical revascularization if the previous conditions are present [18].
- **Multimodality imaging evaluation**: a complete ***transthoracic 2D echocardiogram*** with color Doppler is the first imaging step, providing accurate information of wall thickness, LV geometry, systolic and diastolic chamber dimensions and volumes, global cardiac function, and a complete evaluation of mitral valve apparatus [18, 19]. Appropriate candidates should have a dilated left ventricle (left ventricular end-systolic volume index—LVESVI—greater than 60 ml/m^2): small ventricles have a higher likelihood for diastolic function worsening [20]. Regional LV asynergy, either dyskinetic or akinetic, should be detectable; when LV asynergy is severe and diffuse, SVR should be performed only if regions remote from the scar show detectable contraction. To this aim, CMR represents nowadays the gold standard imaging technique for planning the

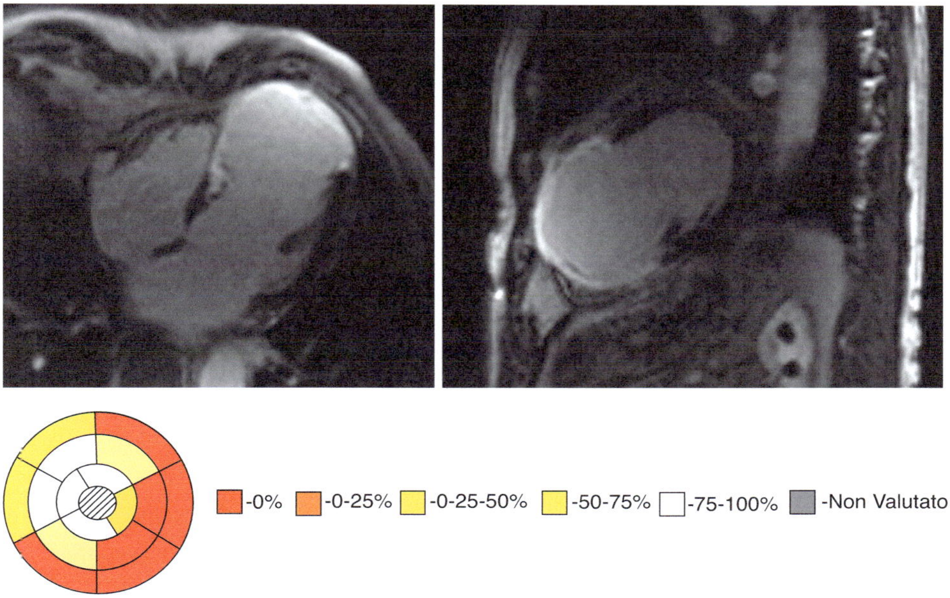

Fig. 3 Contrast-enhanced cardiac magnetic resonance. Late gadolinium enhancement (LGE) images show extensive antero-apical ventricular remodeling in four- and two-chamber view surrounded by transmural fibrosis with different degrees of transmurality (%)

surgical procedure when not contraindicated [21]. CMR allows to evaluate the structure and function of right and left ventricle of any shape and size and has the ability to forecast the prognosis of LV functional recovery when myocardial fibrosis is found also in the remote regions [22]. The greatest advantage of CMR is the recognition through LGE of the myocardial scar in terms of location, extension, and percentage of transmurality (Fig. 3). Our group have found that the presence of LGE in the proximal anterior LV segments is linked to a negative response to SVR in terms of reverse remodeling, which in turn has a negative impact on the survival, while LGE extension appears to be unrelated to the outcome [22].

- **Laboratory test**: Baseline measurements of N-terminal pro-B-type natriuretic peptide (NT-proBNP) have been included in the preliminary evaluation for prognostication. We have recently reported that the combination of high levels of NT-proBNP and RFP—in the meaning of severe diastolic dysfunction—allows a better prognostic stratification of this population, being associated with the highest risk of all-cause death or HF hospitalizations within 36-month follow-up after SVR [23].

According to our experience, suggested contraindications to the SVR should include right ventricular dilatation and dysfunction; a severe diastolic impairment, defined as an E/A ratio >2, likely associated with high NYHA class and mitral insufficiency [18]; and a baseline geometric pattern of LV remodeling, indicated by very low relative wall thickness (RWT <0.25), which has been resulted to be significantly associated with persistent restrictive diastolic pattern after the operation [24].

5 The SVR Technique

Dor and colleagues first described the procedure in 1984 [25]. Over the following years, the surgical technique for the reconstruction of the LV ventricle has been refined, but essentially there are four variations of the procedure:

- Linear closure by Jatene [26]
- Modified linear closure by Mickleborough [27]
- Circular closure with a patch by Dor and Menicanti [28]
- Double-cerclage closure without a patch by McCarthy [29]

In the recent years, due to an extensive use of percutaneous coronary interventions, and improved medical treatment, the phenotype of the LV dyskinetic aneurysm has disappeared in favor of a global LV dilatation without a neck and a well-defined transitional zone. This, in turn, has led to a change in the above techniques to suit the new anatomy.

Since 2001 in our center, SVR has been performed under total cardiac arrest with antegrade crystalloid or cold-blood cardioplegia [18]. First CABG is accomplished, when necessary, to ensure a complete myocardial revascularization. After that, the surgical techniques differ according to the site of the previous MI and LV remodeling and presence of MR [18].

6 Details of the Technique for Anterior Remodeling

The ventricle is opened incising parallel to the left anterior descending artery, starting from the middle of the ventricle proceeding toward the apex. The cavity is examined, and thrombi are excised if present. In case of MR, the valve is repaired through the opening with a double-armed stich at the posterior annulus, from trigone to trigone, and the mitral orifice is undersized with a 26 mm valve sizer [30]. From 2001 to standardize the procedure, we introduced the use of a mannequin (Chase Medical, Richardson, TX, USA). The device has different sizes, and the correct one is chosen according to the body surface area of the patient. The mannequin has a conical shape and, once inserted in the cavity, is inflated with saline; the base is positioned below the mitral annulus and the apex, toward the portion of the cavity that should be excluded indicating where the new apex will be placed. The device is useful as both a shaper to remodel the apex and as a sizer to ensure an elliptical shape. If the scarred tissue involves also the inferior wall, a suture plicating the inferior dilatation is conducted from the base of the papillary muscles and works its way up to the point indicated by the sizer's apex. The ventricle is remodeled using the mannequin as a scaffold. A second suture begins proximally, where the dilatation occurs. This point can be located rather high up, just a few millimeters from the aortic valve. The suture connects the two rims of scar responsible for the dilatation, bringing the lateral wall to the septum. In this way, going deep into the septum at the transitional border, a complete exclusion of scarred tissue is obtained. When the suture reaches the new apex, the mannequin is deflated and removed before closing the cavity. The remaining tissue is closed over to ensure hemostasis. As above described, we previously performed SVR with the aid of a patch to close the LV cavity; the patch is now being discontinued because it can cause an abnormal shortening of the longitudinal diameter, promoting in turn the sphericalization of the ventricle.

7 Details of the Technique for Posterior Remodeling

There is a scarcity of data on surgical correction for LV dilatation caused by inferior MI [31]. Posterior remodeling can develop as a result of either the classic posterior aneurysm, which causes a bulging of the inferior wall, or a more widespread LV dilatation. Usually, the surgical treatment for posterior aneurysm involves the use of a patch to close the neck of dilatation. We abandoned the use of the patch because while using the mannequin as a scaffold, it was evident that there is not a deficiency of tissue and the dilatation is mainly determined by an increase of length and extension of the scar; therefore, the use of patch is not indicated and it is possible to exclude the diseased tissue connecting directly the two rims of scarred tissue. In case of a broader posterior remodeling, the surgical treatment is more complex because of the relationship between the scar and the dilatation. We use two different techniques to treat such kind of dilatation [18]:

- If the dilatation is in between the papillary muscles, the wall is opened at the scar level, parallel to the posterior descending artery. The two papillary muscles are drawn near by a 2-0 Prolene suture excluding the enlarged zone.
- If the dilatation is in between the papillary muscles and the septum, the wall is opened and then the suture is brought past the posteromedial papillary muscles, bringing the posterior wall against the septum.

8 Outcomes

The results of SVR have been reported reasonably good and consistent by several groups, generally in agreement that SVR improves LV systolic function, NYHA functional class, and 5-year survival by a reduction in ventricular volumes and an increase in EF not only in patients with classic dyskinetic aneurysm but also in dilated ischemic cardiomyopathy and severe LV dysfunction (Fig. 4) [32–36]. Also, the levels of natriuretic peptides signifi-

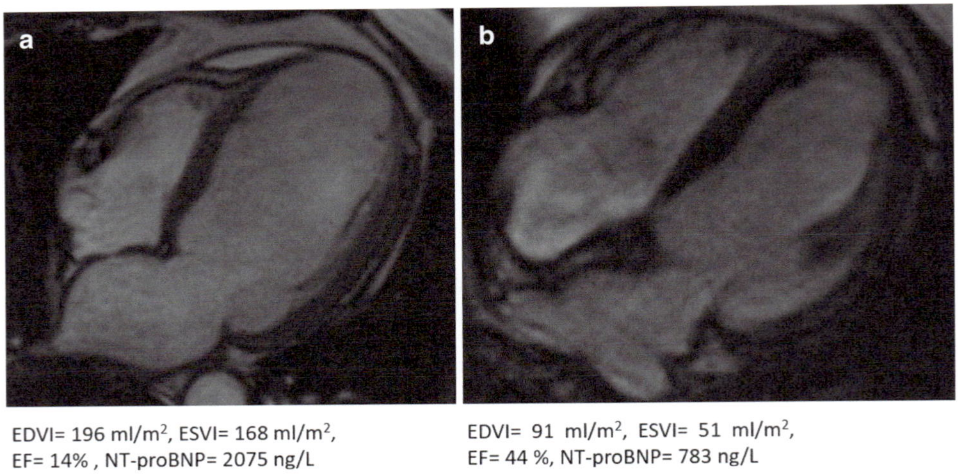

Fig. 4 CMR images from a patient with extensive LV remodeling before (**a**) and after SVR (**b**) showing significant LV volume reduction, improved EF, and an important decrease in circulating levels of NT-proBNP

cantly decrease after the operation, likely reflecting the volume reduction and associated improving in myocardial wall stress [37]. The most common risk factors for mortality across studies include advanced age (>75 years), high NYHA functional class, preoperative high LVESVI, low EF, severity of MR, and restrictive filling pattern [33, 38, 39]. The rate of rehospitalization after SVR has also been reported as low among different series, although results must be interpreted with caution because of different definition or statistical methods of analysis (all-causes versus cardiac causes, different length of follow-up, first rehospitalization versus total numbers, considering mortality or first hospitalization as competing events). Overall, the rate of hospital readmission varies from 15% over just 1 year [39–41] to 22% after 5 years [33].

Our group recently investigated the correlation between sex and surgical outcomes in ischemic HF patients undergoing SVR [42]. We included in the analysis all our 648 patients, of whom 17% were women and 83% men. All patients underwent SVR, and 90% of them received also CABG. Although women were older and more symptomatic and with a higher mortality risk, in the long term, the outcomes were equivalent in both sexes. The estimated mortality was 19.1% in women and 12.2% in men at 2 years, 23.4% in women and 18.8% in men at 4 years, and 41.8% in women and 36.2% in men at 8 years. Within 8 years after surgery, the crude cumulative incidence of all-cause hospitalization as the first event was 37.8% in women and 35.8% in men. The probability of all-cause and hospitalizations was not statistically different between sexes. The large number of female patients involved in this study and the long-term follow-up make this analysis one of the most representative in the field.

8.1 CABG Alone Versus CABG Plus SVR

The role of CABG combined or not with SVR in HF patients with LV systolic dysfunction has been investigated in the STICH trial [43]. The trial failed to show an additional survival benefit of the SVR over isolated CABG, although the combined procedure resulted in a significant greater reduction in LVESVI, reflecting a more extensive reverse remodeling. The relatively small percentage in LVESVI reduction observed in the combined group raised concerns on the extent of the SVR procedure that was applied in this trial, in the meaning of selection criteria. Our group hypothesized that the lack of benefit in terms of survival in the SVR group observed in the STICH trial might be a result of the inadequate volume reduction, which left the patients in the two arms at identical risk [44]. Indeed, a further post hoc analysis from the STICH trial showed that a postoperative LVESVI of 70 ml/m^2 or lower resulted in improved survival compared with CABG alone [45]. In agreement with these results, the latest ESC/EACTS guidelines on myocardial revascularization recommend SVR at the time of CABG in selected patients operated in centers with a high level of surgical expertise (class of recommendation IIb; level of evidence B) [11]. The major limitations of the STICH trial have been discussed in previous reports [18, 46]. We believe that the main limitation of this trial relates to the heterogeneous population of patients enrolled with moderate symptoms of either angina or HF, small volumes, and lack of clear evidence of scar tissue (cardiac MRI was not mandatory), along with poor standardization of the surgical procedure across more than 120 centers all over the world, with different degrees of surgical skills.

An ongoing analysis aimed to compare the outcomes of patients with postinfarction LV dysfunction and HF treated by SVR in one of the centers with the largest worldwide experience with the outcomes of patients enrolled in the STICH trial hopefully will do more clarity [47].

9 Future Directions

9.1 Biomechanical Insights

Assessment of strain—a measurement of myocardial deformation for quantification of regional and global LV function—reflects myocardial systolic function more directly than conventional echocardiographic parameters, firstly the EF, and allows to measure mechanical dispersion as a parameter of homogeneous LV contraction. Our group has recently investigated the role of real-time 3D transthoracic echocardiography (RT3DTTE) to better understand the mechanisms of LV functional recovery after SVR [48]. Applying this advanced tool, we showed that LV longitudinal strain improves after SVR mostly in the basal region, outlining the likely role of the remote myocardium in enhancing LV function volume reduction. Furthermore, mechanical dispersion improvement after LV surgery indicates a more homogeneous myocardial contraction. Of note, both isolated SVR and SVR combined with CABG improved LV strain, pointing out the additional advantage of extensive surgical reverse remodeling in improving LV performance. Further investigations, along with multidisciplinary approach and specialized training, are needed to ensure that this approach can be effective in monitoring global and local changes in LV function in patients undergoing surgery.

10 Conclusions

Beyond criticisms, surgical ventricular reconstruction still represents an important advancement in the surgical management of patients suffering from ischemic HF. Although many surgeons are reluctant toward the procedure which has been substantially abandoned, a renewed interest in this procedure has emerged from recent editorials and reviews. Action by the surgical community is needed to standardize the surgical procedure and design future studies that will enroll appropriately selected patients in a multidisciplinary approach shared with cardiologists, imaging experts, and researchers.

References

1. Yancy CW, Jessup M, Bozkurt B, Butler J, Casey DE Jr, Colvin MM, et al. 2017 ACC/AHA/HFSA focused update of the 2013 ACCF/AHA guideline for the Management of Heart Failure: a report of the American College of Cardiology/American Heart Association task force on clinical practice guidelines and the Heart Failure Society of America. Circulation. 2017;136:e137–61.
2. Van der Bijl P, Abou R, Goedemans L, Gersh BJ, Holmes DR Jr, Ajmone Marsan N, et al. Left ventricular post-infarct Remodeling: implications for systolic function improvement and outcomes in the modern era. JACC Heart Fail. 2020;8:131–40.
3. Heidenreich PA, Albert NM, Allen LA, Bluemke DA, Butler J, Fonarow GC, et al. Forecasting the impact of heart failure in the United States: a policy statement from the American Heart Association. Circ Heart Fail. 2013;6:606–19.
4. Engelfriet PM, Hoogenveen RT, Boshuizen HC, Van Baal PH. To die with or from heart failure: a difference that counts: is heart failure underrepresented in national mortality statistics? Eur J Heart Fail. 2011;13:377–83.
5. Felker GM, Shaw LK, O'Connor CM. A standardized definition of ischemic cardiomyopathy for use in clinical research. J Am Coll Cardiol. 2002;39:210–8.
6. Zannad F, Agrinier N, Alla F. Heart failure burden and therapy. Europace. 2009;11(Suppl 5):v1–9.
7. Konstam MA, Kramer DG, Patel AR, Maron MS, Udelson JE. Left ventricular remodeling in heart failure: current concepts in clinical significance and assessment. J Am Coll Cardiol Img. 2011;4:98–108.
8. Cohn JN, Ferrari R, Sharpe N. Cardiac remodeling-concepts and clinical implications: a consensus paper from an international forum on cardiac remodeling. J Am Coll Cardiol. 2000;35:569–82.
9. Pfeffer MA, Braunwald E. Ventricular remodeling after myocardial infarction. Experimental observations and clinical implications. Circulation. 1990;81:1161–72.

10. Di Donato M, Dabic P, Castelvecchio S, RESTORE Group, et al. Left ventricular geometry in normal and post-anterior myocardial infarction patients: sphericity index and "new" conicity index comparisons. Eur J Cardiothorac Surg. 2006;29(Suppl 1):S225–30.
11. Neumann FJ, Sousa-Uva M, Ahlsson A, Alfonso F, Banning AP, Benedetto U, et al. 2018 ESC/EACTS guidelines on myocardial revascularization: the task force on myocardial revascularization of the European Society of Cardiology (ESC) and the European Association for Cardio-Thoracic Surgery (EACTS) developed with the special contribution of the European Association of Percutaneous Cardiovascular Interventions (EAPCI). Eur Heart J. 2018;00:1–96.
12. Kumanohoso T, Otsuji Y, Yoshifuku S, Matsukida K, Koriyama C, Kisanuki A, et al. Mechanism of higher incidence of ischemic mitral regurgitation in patients with inferior myocardial infarction: quantitative analysis of left ventricular and mitral valve geometry in 103 patients with prior myocardial infarction. J Thorac Cardiovasc Surg. 2003;125:135–43.
13. Streeter DD Jr, Spotnitz HM, Patel DP, Ross J Jr, Sonnenblick EH. Fiber orientation in the canine left ventricle during diastole and systole. Circ Res. 1969;24:339–47.
14. Greenbaum RA, Ho SY, Gibson DG, Becker AE, Anderson RH. Left ventricular fibre architecture in man. Br Heart J. 1981;45:248–63.
15. Delepine S, Furber AP, Beygui F, Prunier F, Balzer P, Le Jeune JJ, et al. 3-D MRI assessment of regional left ventricular systolic wall stress in patients with reperfused MI. Am J Physiol Heart Circ Physiol. 2003;284:H1190–7.
16. Di Donato M, Sabatier M, Toso A, Barletta G, Baroni M, Dor V, et al. Regional myocardial performance of non-ischemic zones remote from anterior wall left ventricular aneurysm. Effects of aneurysmectomy. Eur Heart J. 1995;16:1285–92.
17. Menicanti L, Di Donato M, Frigiola A, Buckberg G, Santambrogio C, Ranucci M, et al. RESTORE group. Ischemic mitral regurgitation: intraventricular papillary muscle imbrication without mitral ring during left ventricular restoration. J Thorac Cardiovasc Surg. 2002;123:1041–50.
18. Castelvecchio S, Pappalardo OA, Menicanti L. Myocardial reconstruction in ischaemic cardiomyopathy. Eur J Cardiothorac Surg. 2019;55(Suppl 1):i49–56.
19. Menicanti L, Castelvecchio S. Left ventricular reconstruction. In: Chan LR, Kron IL, Spray TL, editors. Mastery of cardiothoracic surgery. 3rd ed. Philadelphia: Wolters Kluwer Health; 2014. p. 519–31.
20. Castelvecchio S, Menicanti L, Ranucci M, Di Donato M. Impact of surgical ventricular restoration on diastolic function: implications of shape and residual ventricular size. Ann Thorac Surg. 2008;86:1849–54.
21. Karamitsos TD, Francis JM, Myerson S, Selvanayagam JB, Neubauer S. The role of cardiovascular magnetic resonance imaging in heart failure. J Am Coll Cardiol. 2009;54:1407–24.
22. Castelvecchio S, Careri G, Ambrogi F, Camporeale A, Menicanti L, Secchi F, et al. Myocardial scar location as detected by cardiac magnetic resonance is associated with the outcome in heart failure patients undergoing surgical ventricular reconstruction. Eur J Cardiothorac Surg. 2018;53:143–9.
23. Toso A, Castelvecchio S, Menicanti L, Volpe M, Fantini F. Prognostic value of natriuretic peptides and restrictive filling pattern before surgical ventricular restoration. J Thorac Cardiovasc Surg. 2020;15:S0022–5223(20)32827.
24. Fantini F, Toso A, Menicanti L, Moroni F, Castelvecchio S. Restrictive filling pattern in ischemic cardiomyopathy: insights after surgical ventricular restoration. J Thorac Cardiovasc Surg. 2021;161:651–60.
25. Dor V, Kreitmann P, Jourdan J, et al. Interest of physiological closure (circumferential plasty on contractile areas) of left ventricle after resection and endocardiectomy for aneurysm or akinetic zone. Comparison with classical technique about a series of 209 left ventricular resections. J Cardiovasc Surg. 1985;26:73.
26. Jatene AD. Left ventricular aneurysmectomy. J Thorac Cardiovasc Surg. 1985;89:321.

27. Mickleborough LL, Carson S, Ivanov J. Repair of dyskinetic or akinetic left ventricular aneurysm: results obtained with a modified linear closure. J Thorac Cardiovasc Surg. 2001;121:675.
28. Menicanti L, Di Donato M. The Dor procedure: what has changed after fifteen years of clinical practice? J Thorac Cardiovasc Surg. 2002;124(5):886–90.
29. O'Neill JO, Starling RC, McCarthy PM, Albert NM, Lytle BW, Navia J, et al. The impact of left ventricular reconstruction on survival in patients with ischemic cardiomyopathy. Eur J Cardiothorac Surg. 2006;30(5):753–9.
30. Menicanti L, Di Donato M, Frigiola A, Buckberg G, Santambrogio C, Ranucci M, the RESTORE Group, et al. Ischemic mitral regurgitation: intraventricular papillary muscle imbrication without mitral ring during left ventricular restoration. J Thorac Cardiovasc Surg. 2002;123:1041–50.
31. Menicanti L, Dor V, Buckberg GD, Athanasuleas CL, Di Donato M, the RESTORE Group. Inferior wall restoration: anatomic and surgical considerations. Semin Thorac Cardiovasc Surg. 2001;13:504–13.
32. Dor V, Sabatier M, Di Donato M, Maioli M, Toso A, Montiglio F. Late hemodynamic results after left ventricular patch repair associated with coronary grafting in patients with postinfarction akinetic or dyskinetic aneurysm of the left ventricle. J Thorac Cardiovasc Surg. 1995;110:1291–301.
33. Athanasuleas CL, Buckberg GD, Stanley AW, Siler W, Dor V, Di Donato M, et al. RESTORE group. Surgical ventricular restoration in the treatment of congestive heart failure due to post-infarction ventricular dilation. J Am Coll Cardiol. 2004;44:1439–45.
34. Menicanti L, Castelvecchio S. Left ventricular reconstruction concomitant to coronary artery bypass grafting: when and how? Curr Opin Cardiol. 2011;26:523–7.
35. Di Donato M, Toso A, Dor V, Sabatttier M, Barletta G, Menicanti L, et al. RESTORE group. Surgical ventricular restoration improves mechanical intraventricular dyssynchrony in ischemic cardiomyopathy. Circulation. 2004;109:2536–43.
36. Ribeiro GA, da Costa CE, Lopes MM, Albuquerque AN, Antoniali F, Reinert GA, et al. Left ventricular reconstruction benefits patients with ischemic cardiomyopathy and non-viable myocardium. Eur J Cardiothorac Surg. 2006;29:196–201.
37. Castelvecchio S, Baryshnikova E, Pina IL, Ambrogi F, Milani V, Tramarin R, et al. Longitudinal profile of NT-proBNP levels in ischemic heart failure patients undergoing surgical ventricular reconstruction: the biomarker plus study. Int J Cardiol. 2018;260:24–30.
38. Witkowski TG, ten Brinke EA, Delgado V, Ng AC, Bertini M, Marsan NA, et al. Surgical ventricular restoration for patients with ischemic heart failure: determinants of two-year survival. Ann Thorac Surg. 2011;91:491–8.
39. Di Donato M, Castelvecchio S, Kukulski T, Bussadori C, Giacomazzi F, Frigiola A, et al. Surgical ventricular restoration: left ventricular shape influence on cardiac function, clinical status, and survival. Ann Thorac Surg. 2009;87:455–61.
40. Hobbs RD, Assi A, Bolling SF, Patel HJ, Deeb GM, Romano MA, et al. Long-term survival and echocardiographic findings after surgical ventricular restoration. Ann Thorac Surg. 2019;107:1754–60.
41. Athanasuleas CL, Stanley AW Jr, Buckberg GD, Dor V, DiDonato M, Blackstone EH. Surgical anterior ventricular endocardial restoration (SAVER) in the dilated remodeled ventricle after anterior myocardial infarction. RESTORE group. Reconstructive Endoventricular surgery, returning torsion original radius elliptical shape to the LV. J Am Coll Cardiol. 2001;37:1199–209.
42. Castelvecchio S, Milani V, Volpe M, Citarella M, Ambrogi F, Boveri S, et al. Comparable outcomes between genders in patients undergoing surgical ventricular reconstruction for ischaemic heart failure. ESC Heart Fail. 2021;8:291–9.
43. Jones RH, Velazquez EJ, Michler RE, Sopko G, Oh JK, O'Connor CM, et al. STICH hypothesis 2 investigators. Coronary bypass surgery with or without surgical ventricular reconstruction. N Engl J Med. 2009;360:1705–17.

44. Di Donato M, Castelvecchio S, Menicanti L. End-systolic volume following surgical ventricular reconstruction impacts survival in patients with ischemic dilated cardiomyopathy. Eur J Heart Fail. 2010;12:375–81.
45. Michler RE, Rouleau JL, Al-Khalidi HR, Bonow RO, Pellikka PA, Pohost GM, el. STICH trial investigators. Insights from the STICH trial: change in left ventricular size after coronary artery bypass grafting with and without surgical ventricular reconstruction. J Thorac Cardiovasc Surg. 2013;146:1139–45.
46. Buckberg GD, Athanasuleas CL, Wechsler AS, Beyersdorf F, Conte JV, Strobeck JE. The STICH trial unravelled. Eur J Heart Fail. 2010;12(10):1024–7.
47. Gaudino M, Castelvecchio S, Rahouma M, Robinson NB, Audisio K, Soletti GJ, et al. Results of surgical ventricular reconstruction in a specialized center and in comparison to the STICH trial: rationale and study protocol for a patient-level pooled analysis. J Card Surg. 2021;36(2):689–92.
48. Castelvecchio S, Frigelli M, Sturla F, Milani V, Pappalardo OA, Citarella M, et al. Elucidating the mechanisms underlying left ventricular function recovery in patients with ischemic heart failure undergoing surgical remodeling: a 3-dimensional ultrasound analysis. J Thorac Cardiovasc Surg. 2021;S0022–5223(21):00381–0.

Mitral Regurgitation from Ischemic Heart Disease

Giacomo Bianchi

1 Mitral Valve Functional Anatomy

Mitral valve is a complex structure that separates the left ventricle from the left atrium. It is composed (Fig. 1) by two leaflets, the anterior and posterior, which are attached at their hinge ends to the mitral annulus, and at their free edge to chordae tendineae which in turn attach to papillary muscles. Three orders of chordae tendineae are detectable: the chordae tendineae at the free edge and body of the valve leaflets (*first order*) prevent excessive movement of the valve leaflets into the left atrium during left ventricular systole and are therefore essential for valve competency; the *secondary order* chordae attach to the body of the valve leaflets from papillary muscles; the *tertiary order* chordae attach to the body of the valve leaflets directly from the mitral annulus and the left ventricle.

The papillary muscles are usually organized into two groups, the posteromedial and anterolateral papillary muscles, and are attached to the left ventricle wall approximately one-third distance from the apex and two-thirds from the annulus. The anterolateral papillary muscle usually attaches to the left ventricle at the junction between the septum and the posterior wall while the posteromedial papillary muscle usually attaches on the lateral wall of the left ventricle. The anterior and posterior leaflets approximate and overlap each other at their free edges and commissures, forming a surface of coaptation of about 7–9 mm. This surface of coaptation between the free edges of the two leaflets is essential for valve competency. The normal coaptation line lies parallel to the posterior annulus [1].

An anatomic alteration of one of these elements and which is accompanied by mitral insufficiency is termed *primary mitral insufficiency*. When mitral insufficiency is an

G. Bianchi (✉)
Ospedale del Cuore, Fondazione Toscana "G. Monasterio", Massa, Italy
e-mail: gbianchi@ftgm.it

G. Concistrè (ed.), *Ischemic Heart Disease*,
https://doi.org/10.1007/978-3-031-25879-4_31

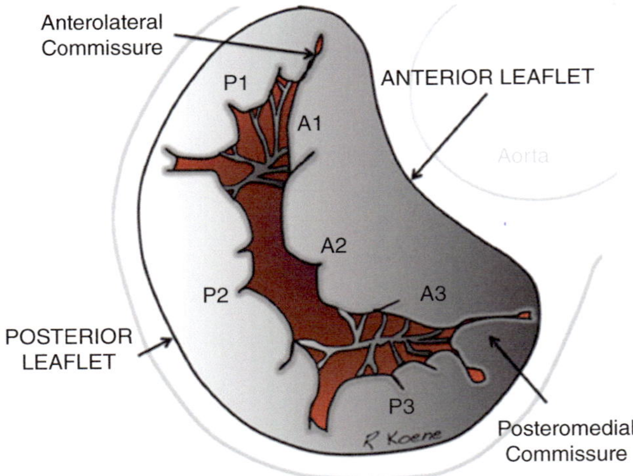

Fig. 1 Mitral valve anatomy

epiphenomenon of heart muscle disease, regardless the etiology, it is called *secondary* or *functional mitral insufficiency* (FMR).

FMR is the result of incomplete mitral leaflet coaptation in the setting of LV systolic dysfunction and dilatation with or without annular dilatation (e.g., dilated cardiomyopathy or ischemic cardiomyopathy) [2–4]. Left ventricular systolic dysfunction and dilatation also may be associated with longstanding mitral regurgitation caused by severe chronic LV volume overload. Most commonly, the etiology of nonischemic cardiomyopathy is unknown or idiopathic; the second most common cause is advanced valvular disease. FMR occurs in 40% of patients with heart failure caused by dilated cardiomyopathy [5].

Functional Ischemic mitral regurgitation (fIMR), a subset of FMR, is becoming widely appreciated as the population ages, and more patients survive acute myocardial infarction. In those with acute infarction, IMR occurs in approximately 15% of patients with anterior wall involvement and up to 40% of patients with an inferior infarct [6]. Generally, the severity of mitral regurgitation is related to the size of the area of LV akinesia or dyskinesia. The pathophysiology of IMR can be attributed to changes in global and regional LV function or geometry, alterations in mitral annular geometry, abnormal leaflet motion and malcoaptation, increased interpapillary distance, and papillary muscle malalignment leading to apical tethering of the leaflets with restricted systolic leaflet motion (type IIIb) [6–8]. Because of the interdependence of the elements constituting the valvular-ventricular complex in IMR, perturbation of any component, such as LV systolic function and geometry, annular geometry, leaflet motion and morphology, and papillary and chordal relationship, may result in mitral regurgitation.

2 Pathophysiology of Functional Ischemic Mitral Regurgitation

It is the result of complex ventricular and annular geometric adaptation, due to the close relationships between the ventricular myocardium, papillary muscles, and chordae tendineae, which is consequently reflected in the movement and morphology of the mitral leaflets.

Functional ischemic mitral regurgitation has been reported in a variable proportion of patients after acute myocardial infarction (AM), depending on the infarct area. The incidence of acute IMR varies according to the culprit lesion; this is due to the location of the papillary muscles and their supply by the coronary arteries and their specific branches.

It complicates approximately 15% of anterior infarcts but can reach 40% in inferior infarcts. The anteropapillary muscle because the anterolateral papillary muscle often has double irrigation (left anterior descending artery, LAD; and branches of circumflex artery, Cx), while the posteromedial papillary muscle only from the posterior descending artery (PD).

An elegant experimental study illustrated that mitral area does not change in case of acute LAD occlusion and varies little in case of distal branch occlusion of Cx, whereas it is significantly increased in case of Cx occlusion proximal to the second obtuse marginal [7].

During acute ischemia, the papillary-annular distances change, which reflects repositioning or dislocation of the papillary muscle tips with respect to the mitral annulus. This process can also contribute to apical tenting of the leaflets during systole [9]. With proximal circumflex artery occlusion and resulting fIMR in an ovine model, the interpapillary distance and LV end-diastolic volume both increase. There is also increased mitral annular area and displacement of both (but predominantly the posteromedial) papillary muscle tips away from the septal annulus throughout ejection and at end-systole [10]. Posteromedial papillary muscle tip displacement probably results from failure of the ischemic papillary muscle to shorten during systole, lengthening of the ischemic papillary muscle over time, and dyskinesia of the ischemic LV wall subtending the papillary muscle. Since posterior papillary muscle displacement in the apical and posterior directions also occurs in sheep that did not develop substantial degrees of fIMR, the additional posteromedial papillary muscle displacement in the lateral direction is a dominant factor in the development of fIMR.

Acute fIMR from proximal left circumflex artery occlusion experimentally results in delayed valve closure in early systole (termed *leaflet loitering*) and increased leaflet edge separation throughout ejection in three leaflet coaptation sites across the valve, specifically near the anterior commissure, the valve center, and near the posterior commissure [11]. In addition, there is lateral displacement of the central scallop of the posterior leaflet, suggesting that inter-scallop malcoaptation and septal-lateral annular dilatation, can contribute to fIMR in certain circumstances.

Chronic fIMR is also associated with posterior leaflet displacement in the posterior direction and lateral displacement of both leaflets. When the position of each leaflet edge is assessed independently, the anterior leaflet is not displaced apically after inferior infarction, although with more time and further remodeling, apical restriction of this leaflet may occur [10]. A strong echocardiographic determinant of leaflet tenting height is the distance from the tips of the papillary muscles to the saddle horn of the anterior annulus; LV end-diastolic volume is only weakly correlated with tenting height [12]. Recent human observations have revealed that in some patients with fIMR, there is growth or elongation of the leaflets associated with leaflet thickening that compensates for the larger orifice area and minimizes the amount of mitral regurgitation. In others, however, the leaflets do not become larger and cannot coapt normally across the large orifice, which causes more leaks [13].

In the past, the leaflet morphology in patients with fIMR was considered normal, but further analyses have shown the leaflets to be biochemically different, with extracellular matrix changes associated with altered cardiac dimensions. Mitral leaflets in heart failure have altered intrinsic structural properties suggesting that the permanently distended and fibrotic tissue is unable to stretch sufficiently to cover the valve orifice and that mitral regurgitation in these patients is not purely functional [14, 15].

Although left ventricular dilation and dysfunction are less pronounced in the inferior infarct than in the anterior infarct, the incidence and severity of mitral insufficiency are greater in inferior infarcts.

Over time, as the left ventricle dilates and changes shape after the ischemic event (postinfarction remodeling), the degree of fIMR progresses [16, 17]. Geometric changes associated with ventricular remodeling, such as posteromedial papillary muscle dislocation in the lateral axis, may lead to leaflet tenting, as reflected by a larger distance from the middle of the anterior annulus (saddle horn on echocardiography) to the posteromedial papillary muscle tip, and increased annular diameter [8, 17]. At the ventricular level, myocardial infarction associated with chronic fIMR is associated with greater adverse perturbations in LV systolic torsion and diastolic recoil than myocardial infarction without chronic fIMR [10]. These abnormalities may be linked to more LV dilatation, which possibly reduces the effectiveness of fiber shortening on torsion generation. Altered LV torsion and recoil may contribute to the "ventricular disease" component of chronic fIMR, with increased gradients of myocardial oxygen consumption adversely affecting cardiac efficiency and impaired early diastolic filling [10]. Additionally, in a subacute model of fIMR (less than 7 weeks), there is an equivalent increase in LV end-diastolic volume in those with mild mitral regurgitation compared to those with more severe mitral regurgitation, coupled with unchanged end-diastolic and end-systolic remodeling strains, including systolic circumferential, longitudinal, and radial strains; these findings in aggregate argue against an intracellular (cardiomyocyte) mechanism for the LV dysfunction [18]. Instead, differences in subepicardial shear strains suggest a causal role of altered interfiber interactions, and the mechanical impairment may be in extracellular matrix between the fibers and the microtubules in the cytoskeleton that couple cardiomyocyte shortening to LV wall thickening.

3 Imaging of Ischemic Functional Mitral Regurgitation

3.1 Echocardiography

Echocardiography is the most important noninvasive imaging technique for evaluating the presence and severity of functional ischemic mitral regurgitation. Its spatial resolution is sufficient to yield the necessary anatomical and morphological detail and hence accurately assess the mechanism of MR, and the temporal resolution combined with various Doppler techniques allows for in-depth physiological evaluation and ascertainment of the hemodynamic significance of the lesion. In the setting of fIMR, the echocardiography is key both in the early phase postinfarction and also in chronic ischemic mitral valve assessment (Fig. 2). In the early post AMI, fIMR can be silent is highly prognostically significant. One study used color Doppler echocardiography to show mild MR in 29% and moderate-severe MR in 6% of patients within 48 h of admission with AMI. Any degree of MR was associated with increased 1 year mortality [19]. In another study of 300 consecutive patients after non-ST elevation MI showed that MR was present in 42% within the first week. Again, MR was a predictor of outcome over 14 months' follow-up [20]. The echocardiogram has three main focuses: (1) confirm the diagnosis; (2) evaluate the severity of MR by qualitative and quantitative methods; and (3) identification of prognostic features.

The approach, due to the complex and dynamic nature of mitral valve, should include the 2D evaluation along with 3D imaging and speckle-tracking technique, to provide an in-depth morphological assessment of valve anatomy and ventricular geometry, focusing on the effects of ischemic remodeling. Table 1 reported the criteria to define severe functional IMR.

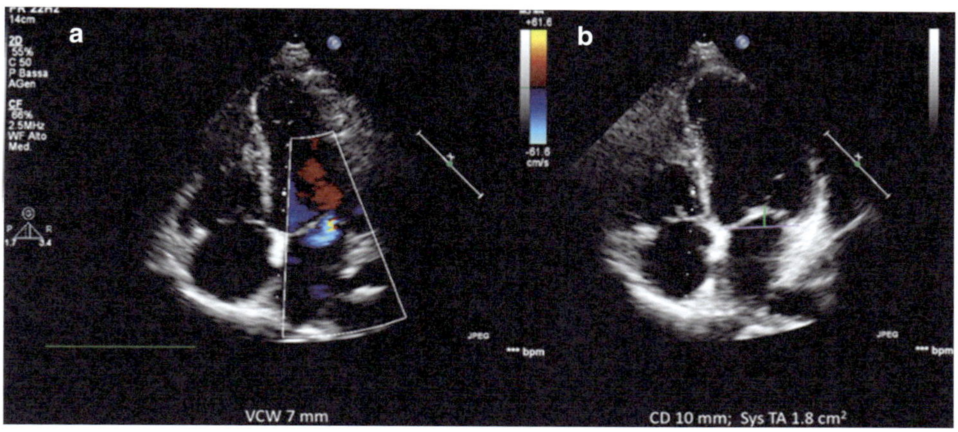

Fig. 2 Transthoracic Echocardiogram (TTE). (**a**) color doppler analysis; (**b**) measures to predict reparability. *VCW* vena contracts width, *CD* coaptation depth, *Sys TA* systolic tenting area

Table 1 Echo criteria for severe fIMR

Qualitative	
Mitral valve morphology	Flail leaflet/ruptured papillary muscle
Color flow regurgitant jet	Very large central or eccentric jet adhering, swirling and reaching the posterior wall of the left atrium
Continuous wave signal of regurgitant jet	Dense/triangular
Flow convergence zone	Large
Semi-quantitative	
Vena contracta width (mm)	>7 (>8 for biplane)
Pulmonary vein flow	Systolic flow reversal
Inflow	E-wave dominant >1.5 m/s
TVI mitral/TVI aortic	>1.4
Quantitative	
EROA (mm^2)	>20
Regurgitant volume (mL/beat)	>30
Cardiac chamber enlargement	Left ventricle, left atrium

Table 2 Echo predictors of surgical annuloplasty failure

Echo predictors of failure after undersizing annuloplasty for severe IMR
Coaptation depth >1 cm
Systolic tenting area >2.5 cm^2
Posterior mitral leaflet angle >45°
Distal anterior mitral leaflet angle >25°
LV end-diastolic diameter >65 mm

Echocardiography is also useful in providing prognostic parameters after surgical correction, in particular predictors of failure, as shown in Table 2.

A particular type of echocardiography, stress echocardiography, is useful in unmasking underlying ischemic disease and therefore is related to increased mitral regurgitation from baseline. Physical exercise mimics the situations patients find themselves in when they experience symptoms and induces ischemia that may exacerbate leaflet tethering by causing increased LV dilatation or inducing a segmental wall motion abnormality, increasing the MR; finally, there is the opportunity to document exercise-induced pulmonary hypertension which has prognostic importance and may influence the timing of intervention [21]. Furthermore, demonstration of contractile reserve by exercise stress testing can identify those more likely to have improved survival and functional capacity after mitral repair in patients with asymptomatic severe MR [22].

3.2 Magnetic Resonance Imaging

Magnetic resonance (CMR) is a complementary tool of multiple use in the setting of fIMR. While echocardiography is considered the gold standard for the diagnosis and quantification of MR, the CMR provides insights into the left ventricular size and function. The mitral valve structure can be assessed in 2-chamber, 3-chamber, and 4-chamber view; mitral valve stack images are used to localize the pathology to mitral leaflets scallops. In the LVOT view (3-chambers), useful parameters can be acquired: length of anterior and posterior leaflets; septal thickness; C-sept distance for LVOT obstruction and SAM risk after mitral valve repair; and aorto-mitral angle. In the 4-chamber view, the tenting area can be calculated as well as the coaptation distance and the posterior leaflet angle. As shown, these parameters have quite good overlap with echo-derived measures. As been said before, ventricular assessment is one of the strength points of CMR: in inferolateral MI, the infero-posterolateral left ventricular wall and the posteromedial papillary muscle (Carpentier type IIIb) are affected. In these patients, the posterior leaflet appears tethered to the infarcted wall, and the tenting pattern is asymmetrical. The MR jet is eccentric and posteriorly directed; in multivessel disease, the LV remodeling is more pronounced and the papillary muscle is displaced and dysfunctional; moreover, a fibrotic elongation of an infarcted papillary muscle will lead to prolapse of the corresponding segment of the mitral leaflet, resulting in various degree of MR at rest that eventually worsen during effort.

Furthermore, the CMR can calculate the MR volume subtracting the aortic forward stroke volume (AoSV) from LV stroke volume (LVSV); in turn the regurgitant fraction can also be calculated as the ratio between the mitral regurgitant volume and the LVSV (Fig. 3).

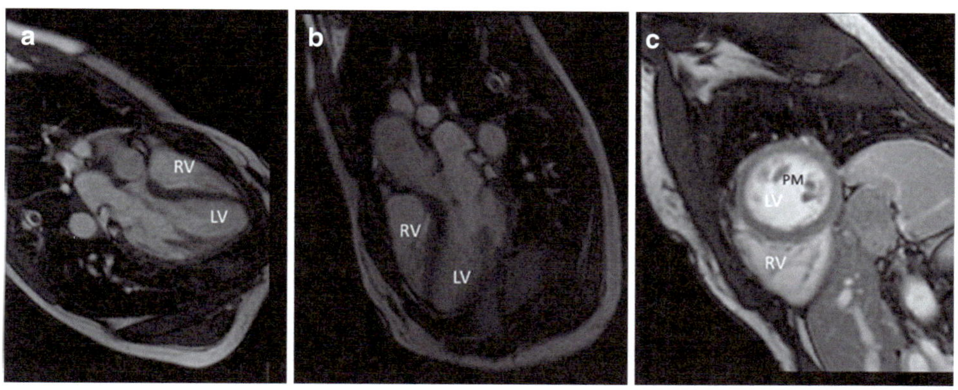

Fig. 3 MRI imaging of the heart. (**a** and **b**) Anatomical and functional assessment of the mitral valve. (**c**) RV and LV short axis for wall motion assessment, papillary muscle location, sphericity index. *RV* right ventricle, *LV* left ventricle

4 Treatment of Functional Ischemic Mitral Regurgitation

4.1 Resynchronization Therapy

Pathogenesis of functional mitral regurgitation (MR) involves multiple factors, including increased mitral leaflet tethering due to the outward displacement of the papillary muscles caused by global and regional left ventricular (LV) remodeling, decreased LV closing forces, and deformation of the whole mitral apparatus including the annulus [3].

The presence of global LV dyssynchrony may decrease the efficiency of LV contraction and, thus, decrease the LV closing force acting on the mitral leaflets; furthermore, dyssynchronous contraction of the papillary muscle insertion sites at the LV free wall may induce geometric distortion of the mitral valve apparatus.

Cardiac Resynchronization Therapy (CRT) can reduce the papillary muscle dyssynchrony and increase the rate of LV pressure, leading to an immediate decrease of fIMR after initiation of pacing. The effect is pacing-dependent, and recurrence of fIMR occurs when the CRT is stopped. Some degree of reverse LV remodeling has been described in the mid-long run [23]. The remodeling also correlates to the presence of viable myocardium, since large scar tissue and severe MR at baseline have been associated with lesser or no clinical response to CRT [24].

The CRT is indicated in symptomatic HF patients in functional class II–IV despite receiving optimal medical treatment, severe left ventricle systolic dysfunction with a left ventricular ejection fraction (LVEF) $\leq 35\%$ and presenting with a wide QRS on the ECG (QRS width ≥ 120 ms) preferably with a LBBB pattern. Patients with a baseline tenting area of $>3.8\ cm^2$ would benefit less from CRT since it is marker of an advance LV remodeling.

In responder patients, the reduction in MR severity with CRT typically occurs within the first days after starting CRT and can be expected even until the first 3-months follow-up. It is very unlikely to happen after that period. The use of CRT not only stratify responders, but also identify candidates for surgery after 3 months from device implantation when severe mitral regurgitation persists.

4.2 Bypass Grafting with or Without Mitral Valve Surgery

Reported hospital mortality in patients with IMR undergoing coronary artery bypass grafting (CABG) varies widely from 1.0% to 12.5%, due to differences in LV size and function [25, 26]. While percutaneous coronary intervention (PCI) continues to be offered to some patients at high risk for conventional open CABG, this modality often fails to address the persistently occluded coronary arteries common in IMR patients; a 28% rate of complete revascularization with PCI in this population has been reported, while complete revascularization by CABG offers better outcome [27]. LV contractile reserve may also play a role, in that successful CABG will restore viable LV segments in the region of papillary muscle attachment that may relieve tethering of the mitral valve. Recent work examining cardiac remodeling has revealed no change in MR grade among patients without improvement in LV function or LV size following isolated CABG for IMR, supporting the thesis that maximal restoration of perfusion to viable myocardium is prerequisite for successful remodeling [26].

Coronary revascularization alone in the setting of even moderate IMR leaves many patients with substantial residual mitral regurgitation and heart failure symptoms [28–30]. Immediately post-op, IMR is absent or mild in 73% and severe in 6%; on the other hand, by 6 weeks, only 40% of patients have absent or mild mitral regurgitation, and 22% have severe mitral regurgitation. Since CABG alone does not universally resolve IMR, valve repair has been proposed in these patients because it potentially can reduce cardiac morbidity and may improve long-term survival. In some studies, the combination of CABG and mitral valve repair does not emerge as a predictor of long-term survival. In CSTN study that compared CABG alone and CABG + mitral valve repair, although the death rate was lower in the second group (7.3% vs. 6.7% at 1 year) and also the rate of moderate or severe MR (31% vs. 11%), the addition of mitral valve surgery does not translate into a greater degree of LV reverse remodeling. In another study, the investigator identified the presence of viable myocardium and absence of LV dyssynchrony as factors for reliable improvement of moderate IMR [31].

In terms of best type of surgery, the LV status is the most important determinant of outcome, whether one undergoes repair or replacement. In the Cleveland Clinic experience, in the lower risk quintile, the valve repair conferred a survival advantage over replacement (58% at 5 years); in the higher risk quintile, the patients had similar poor prognosis with replacement actually conferred a small survival advantage [32]. In the Italian Study on the Treatment of Ischemic Mitral Regurgitation Trial using propensity score matching analysis to evaluate surgical outcomes of patients with chronic IMR and LV dysfunction (ejection fraction less than 40%), those who underwent mitral valve repair had an 8-year survival rate of 82% compared to 80% for those undergoing mitral valve replacement [33]. Further, LV function did not improve in group postoperatively, and mitral valve repair was a strong predictor of valve-related reoperation. The recent Cardiothoracic Surgical Trials Network multi-institutional randomized trial of 251 patients with severe IMR comparing complete rigid or semirigid ring annuloplasty with mitral valve replacement demonstrated no difference in LV reverse remodeling or survival at 12 months. The rate of recurrent or residual moderate or severe IMR 6 months postoperatively was 32.6% in the annuloplasty group versus 2.3% in the MVR group. Replacement provided a more durable correction of mitral regurgitation with no difference in clinical outcomes at this early follow-up period [34]. No significant between-group difference in left ventricular reverse remodeling or survival was found at 2 years follow-up; moreover, mitral regurgitation recurred more frequently in the repair group, resulting in more heart failure-related adverse events and cardiovascular admissions [35].

A compelling explanation for the generally poor long-term outcome of patients who undergo mitral valve repair for IMR is the presence of residual and/or recurrent mitral regurgitation postoperatively [36, 37]. Persistence of mitral regurgitation after annuloplasty is due predominantly to augmented posterior leaflet apical tethering with no improvement in anterior leaflet tethering and no increase in coaptation length; and higher preoperative LVED index may also predict recurrent mitral regurgitation [38, 39]. Data from the Cardiothoracic Surgical Trials Network severe IMR trial demonstrated a rate of recurrence of moderate regurgitation of 26% and of severe regurgitation of 4% at 6 months after mitral valve repair [39]. The presence of inferior basal aneurysm/dyskinesis was strongly associated with recurrent regurgitation and was a better predictor of recurrence than individual measures of leaflet tethering or LV remodeling, since it integrates both leaflet tethering and LV remodeling measure. In the Leiden experience with restrictive annuloplasty, distal anterior leaflet tethering and posterior leaflet tethering were independent predictors of recurrent mitral regurgitation [40].

4.3 Percutaneous Options for fIMR

Percutaneous mitral therapy could theoretically offer improved safety as compared to surgical MV surgery and may be suited for the treatment of higher risk FMR patients. In non-randomized trials, MitraClip showed good results with favorable 30-days and 6-months survival [41–43].

Although the COAPT randomized trial and MITRA-FR generated much expectation regarding transcatheter treatment of mitral pathology, these studies led to diametrically opposed results. The reason is the different types of patients enrolled, even if candidates for the same transcatheter or medical treatment. In MITRA-FR, the underlying cardiomyopathy (myocardial or LV disease) was likely the predominant cause of the heart failure and thus the main determinant of the poor clinical outcome. And in this context, the MR was probably more a bystander than an actor of the heart failure. On the other hand, in COAPT, heart failure was, in large part, related to the valvular disease (the MR was more severe), while LV disease (smaller size and higher LVEF) was less advanced. Hence in COAPT, MR was an important contributor to the heart failure and the clinical outcomes, whereas in MITRA-FR, the LV disease (dysfunction) was the main determinant of clinical outcomes. It has been proposed that MitraClip should be indicated in patients with at least moderate-to-severe (3+) secondary MR defined as EROA $\geq$30 mm^2 and/or regurgitant volume >45 mL, having an LVEF between 20% and 50% and LV end-systolic diameter <70 mm; furthermore they have to exhibit persistent heart failure symptoms (NYHA $\geq$ II) despite optimal (maximally tolerated) GDMT with cardiac resynchronization and coronary revascularization if appropriate. In these settings of "disproportionate" mitral regurgitation, as proposed by Grayburn et al., the transcatheter therapy is mostly effective [44].

References

1. Carpentier A, Adams D, Filsoufi F. Carpentier's reconstructive valve surgery. From valve analysis to valve reconstruction. Saunders Elsevier; 2010.
2. Nishimura RA, Otto CM, Bonow RO, et al. 2017 AHA/ACC focused update of the 2014 AHA/ACC guideline for the management of patients with valvular heart disease: a report of the American College of Cardiology/American Heart Association Task Force on Clinical Practice Guidelines. J Am Coll Cardiol. 2017;70:252–89.
3. Otsuji Y, Handschumacher MD, Liel-Cohen N, Tanabe H, Jiang L, Schwammenthal E, Guerrero JL, Nicholls LA, Vlahakes GJ, Levine RA. Mechanism of ischemic mitral regurgitation with segmental left ventricular dysfunction: three-dimensional echocardiographic studies in models of acute and chronic progressive regurgitation. J Am Coll Cardiol. 2001;37:641–8.
4. Grayburn PA, Carabello B, Hung J, Gillam LD, Liang D, Mack MJ, McCarthy PM, Miller DC, Trento A, Siegel RJ. Defining "severe" secondary mitral regurgitation: emphasizing an integrated approach. J Am Coll Cardiol. 2014;64:2792–801.
5. Ngaage DL, Schaff HV. Mitral valve surgery in non-ischemic cardiomyopathy. J Cardiovasc Surg. 2004;45:477–86.
6. Kumanohoso T, Otsuji Y, Yoshifuku S, Matsukida K, Koriyama C, Kisanuki A, Minagoe S, Levine RA, Tei C. Mechanism of higher incidence of ischemic mitral regurgitation in patients with inferior myocardial infarction: quantitative analysis of left ventricular and mitral valve geometry in 103 patients with prior myocardial infarction. J Thorac Cardiovasc Surg. 2003;125:135–43.
7. Timek TA, Lai DT, Tibayan F, et al. Ischemia in three left ventricular regions: insights into the pathogenesis of acute ischemic mitral regurgitation. J Thorac Cardiovasc Surg. 2003;125:559–69.
8. Ahmad RM, Gillinov AM, McCarthy PM, Blackstone EH, Apperson-Hansen C, Qin JX, Agler D, Shiota T, Cosgrove DM. Annular geometry and motion in human ischemic mitral regurgitation: novel assessment with three-dimensional echocardiography and computer reconstruction. Ann Thorac Surg. 2004;78:2063–2068; discussion 2068.
9. Kalra K, Wang Q, McIver BV, Shi W, Guyton RA, Sun W, Sarin EL, Thourani VH, Padala M. Temporal changes in interpapillary muscle dynamics as an active indicator of mitral valve and left ventricular interaction in ischemic mitral regurgitation. J Am Coll Cardiol. 2014;64:1867–79.
10. Tibayan FA, Rodriguez F, Zasio MK, Bailey L, Liang D, Daughters GT, Langer F, Ingels NB, Miller DC. Geometric distortions of the mitral valvular-ventricular complex in chronic ischemic mitral regurgitation. Circulation. 2003;108 Suppl 1:II116–21.
11. Glasson JR, Komeda M, Daughters GT, Bolger AF, Karlsson MO, Foppiano LE, Hayase M, Oesterle SN, Ingels NB, Miller DC. Early systolic mitral leaflet "loitering" during acute ischemic mitral regurgitation. J Thorac Cardiovasc Surg. 1998;116:193–205.
12. Yiu SF, Enriquez-Sarano M, Tribouilloy C, Seward JB, Tajik AJ. Determinants of the degree of functional mitral regurgitation in patients with systolic left ventricular dysfunction: a quantitative clinical study. Circulation. 2000;102:1400–6.
13. Chaput M, Handschumacher MD, Guerrero JL, Holmvang G, Dal-Bianco JP, Sullivan S, Vlahakes GJ, Hung J, Levine RA, Leducq Foundation MITRAL Transatlantic Network. Mitral leaflet adaptation to ventricular remodeling: prospective changes in a model of ischemic mitral regurgitation. Circulation. 2009;120:S99–103.
14. Grande-Allen KJ, Barber JE, Klatka KM, Houghtaling PL, Vesely I, Moravec CS, McCarthy PM. Mitral valve stiffening in end-stage heart failure: evidence of an organic contribution to functional mitral regurgitation. J Thorac Cardiovasc Surg. 2005;130:783–90.
15. Grande-Allen KJ, Borowski AG, Troughton RW, Houghtaling PL, Dipaola NR, Moravec CS, Vesely I, Griffin BP. Apparently normal mitral valves in patients with heart failure demonstrate

biochemical and structural derangements: an extracellular matrix and echocardiographic study. J Am Coll Cardiol. 2005;45:54–61.
16. Enomoto Y, Gorman JH, Moainie SL, Guy TS, Jackson BM, Parish LM, Plappert T, Zeeshan A, St John-Sutton MG, Gorman RC. Surgical treatment of ischemic mitral regurgitation might not influence ventricular remodeling. J Thorac Cardiovasc Surg. 2005;129:504–11.
17. Liel-Cohen N, Guerrero JL, Otsuji Y, Handschumacher MD, Rudski LG, Hunziker PR, Tanabe H, Scherrer-Crosbie M, Sullivan S, Levine RA. Design of a new surgical approach for ventricular remodeling to relieve ischemic mitral regurgitation: insights from 3-dimensional echocardiography. Circulation. 2000;101:2756–63.
18. Nguyen TC, Cheng A, Langer F, et al. Altered myocardial shear strains are associated with chronic ischemic mitral regurgitation. Ann Thorac Surg. 2007;83:47–54.
19. Feinberg MS, Schwammenthal E, Shlizerman L, et al. Prognostic significance of mild mitral regurgitation by color Doppler echocardiography in acute myocardial infarction. Am J Cardiol. 2000;86:903–7.
20. Perez de Isla L, Zamorano J, Quezada M, Almería C, Rodrigo JL, Serra V, García Rubira JC, Ortiz AF, Macaya C. Prognostic significance of functional mitral regurgitation after a first non-ST-segment elevation acute coronary syndrome. Eur Heart J. 2006;27:2655–60.
21. Lancellotti P, Magne J, Dulgheru R, Ancion A, Martinez C, Piérard LA. Clinical significance of exercise pulmonary hypertension in secondary mitral regurgitation. Am J Cardiol. 2015;115:1454–61.
22. le Polain de Waroux J-B, Pouleur A-C, Vancraeynest D, Pasquet A, Gerber BL, El Khoury G, Noirhomme P, Robert A, Vanoverschelde J-LJ. Early hazards of mitral ring annuloplasty in patients with moderate to severe ischemic mitral regurgitation undergoing coronary revascularization: the importance of preoperative myocardial viability. J Heart Valve Dis. 2009;18:35–43.
23. Sitges M, Vidal B, Delgado V, et al. Long-term effect of cardiac resynchronization therapy on functional mitral valve regurgitation. Am J Cardiol. 2009;104:383–8.
24. Sutton MGSJ, Plappert T, Hilpisch KE, Abraham WT, Hayes DL, Chinchoy E. Sustained reverse left ventricular structural remodeling with cardiac resynchronization at one year is a function of etiology: quantitative Doppler echocardiographic evidence from the Multicenter InSync Randomized Clinical Evaluation (MIRACLE). Circulation. 2006;113:266–72.
25. Tolis GA, Korkolis DP, Kopf GS, Elefteriades JA. Revascularization alone (without mitral valve repair) suffices in patients with advanced ischemic cardiomyopathy and mild-to-moderate mitral regurgitation. Ann Thorac Surg. 2002;74:1476–80; discussion 1480–1.
26. Kang D-H, Kim M-J, Kang S-J, Song J-M, Song H, Hong M-K, Choi K-J, Song J-K, Lee J-W. Mitral valve repair versus revascularization alone in the treatment of ischemic mitral regurgitation. Circulation. 2006;114:I499–503.
27. Ellis SG, Whitlow PL, Raymond RE, Schneider JP. Impact of mitral regurgitation on long-term survival after percutaneous coronary intervention. Am J Cardiol. 2002;89:315–8.
28. Aklog L, Filsoufi F, Flores KQ, Chen RH, Cohn LH, Nathan NS, Byrne JG, Adams DH. Does coronary artery bypass grafting alone correct moderate ischemic mitral regurgitation? Circulation. 2001;104:I68–75.
29. Lam B-K, Gillinov AM, Blackstone EH, Rajeswaran J, Yuh B, Bhudia SK, McCarthy PM, Cosgrove DM. Importance of moderate ischemic mitral regurgitation. Ann Thorac Surg. 2005;79:462–70; discussion 462–70.
30. Grossi EA, Crooke GA, DiGiorgi PL, Schwartz CF, Jorde U, Applebaum RM, Ribakove GH, Galloway AC, Grau JB, Colvin SB. Impact of moderate functional mitral insufficiency in patients undergoing surgical revascularization. Circulation. 2006;114:I573–6.

31. Penicka M, Linkova H, Lang O, Fojt R, Kocka V, Vanderheyden M, Bartunek J. Predictors of improvement of unrepaired moderate ischemic mitral regurgitation in patients undergoing elective isolated coronary artery bypass graft surgery. Circulation. 2009;120:1474–81.
32. Gillinov AM, Wierup PN, Blackstone EH, Bishay ES, Cosgrove DM, White J, Lytle BW, McCarthy PM. Is repair preferable to replacement for ischemic mitral regurgitation? J Thorac Cardiovasc Surg. 2001;122:1125–41.
33. Lorusso R, Gelsomino S, Vizzardi E, et al. Mitral valve repair or replacement for ischemic mitral regurgitation? The Italian Study on the Treatment of Ischemic Mitral Regurgitation (ISTIMIR). J Thorac Cardiovasc Surg. 2013;145:128–39; discussion 137–8.
34. Acker MA, Parides MK, Perrault LP, et al. Mitral-valve repair versus replacement for severe ischemic mitral regurgitation. N Engl J Med. 2014;370:23–32.
35. Goldstein D, Moskowitz AJ, Gelijns AC, et al. Two-year outcomes of surgical treatment of severe ischemic mitral regurgitation. N Engl J Med. 2016;374:344–53.
36. McGee EC, Gillinov AM, Blackstone EH, et al. Recurrent mitral regurgitation after annuloplasty for functional ischemic mitral regurgitation. J Thorac Cardiovasc Surg. 2004;128:916–24.
37. Zhu F, Otsuji Y, Yotsumoto G, et al. Mechanism of persistent ischemic mitral regurgitation after annuloplasty: importance of augmented posterior mitral leaflet tethering. Circulation. 2005;112:I396–401.
38. Lee LS, Kwon MH, Cevasco M, Schmitto JD, Mokashi SA, McGurk S, Cohn LH, Bolman RM, Chen FY. Postoperative recurrence of mitral regurgitation after annuloplasty for functional mitral regurgitation. Ann Thorac Surg. 2012;94:1211–6; discussion 1216–7.
39. Kron IL, Hung J, Overbey JR, et al. Predicting recurrent mitral regurgitation after mitral valve repair for severe ischemic mitral regurgitation. J Thorac Cardiovasc Surg. 2015;149:752–761.e1.
40. Ciarka A, Braun J, Delgado V, Versteegh M, Boersma E, Klautz R, Dion R, Bax JJ, Van de Veire N. Predictors of mitral regurgitation recurrence in patients with heart failure undergoing mitral valve annuloplasty. Am J Cardiol. 2010;106:395–401.
41. Auricchio A, Schillinger W, Meyer S, et al. Correction of mitral regurgitation in nonresponders to cardiac resynchronization therapy by MitraClip improves symptoms and promotes reverse remodeling. J Am Coll Cardiol. 2011;58:2183–9.
42. Franzen O, van der Heyden J, Baldus S, et al. MitraClip® therapy in patients with end-stage systolic heart failure. Eur J Heart Fail. 2011;13:569–76.
43. Taramasso M, Maisano F, Latib A, Denti P, Buzzatti N, Cioni M, La Canna G, Colombo A, Alfieri O. Clinical outcomes of MitraClip for the treatment of functional mitral regurgitation. EuroIntervention. 2014;10:746–52.
44. Grayburn PA, Sannino A, Packer M. Proportionate and disproportionate functional mitral regurgitation: a new conceptual framework that reconciles the results of the MITRA-FR and COAPT Trials. JACC Cardiovasc Imaging. 2019;12:353–62.

Cardiac Transplantation and Assist Devices for Ischemic Heart Disease

Andrea Montalto, Agostino La Marca, and Giuseppe Falivene

Abbreviations

ECMO	Extracorporeal membrane oxygenator
IABP	Intra-aortic balloon pump
p-LVAD	Percutaneous left ventricular assist devices
ST-MCS	Short-term mechanical circulation support

1 Introduction

The main determinant of favorable outcome in the patient suffering from ACS-STEMI complicated by cardiogenic shock is the promptness of treatment.

A recent meta-analysis of 12,675 STEMI patients in the context of the FITT-STEMI study emphasizes the strong negative impact of time delays on early mortality and short-term morbidity, especially in the context of STEMI with shock. In fact, in the ongoing shock, every 10 min of delay in treatment between 60 and 180 min from the first medical contact leads to an increase of 3.3 additional deaths per 100 patients treated.

Therefore, patients with STEMI complicated by cardiogenic shock constitute a selected group that derives the greatest benefits from the acceleration of all phases of the therapeutic process and from an early support and treatment.

A. Montalto · A. La Marca (✉)
Division of Cardiac Surgery, Ospedale S. Anna e S. Sebastiano, Caserta, Italy
e-mail: andrea.montalto@aorncaserta.it; agostino.lamarca@aorncaserta.it

G. Falivene
Division of Cardiac Surgery, Ospedale Monaldi, Naples, Italy

G. Concistrè (ed.), *Ischemic Heart Disease*,
https://doi.org/10.1007/978-3-031-25879-4_32

Emergency coronary angiography is indicated in all patients with acute heart failure or cardiogenic shock that complicates acute coronary syndrome.

Emergency percutaneous treatment of the culprit lesion has absolute and mandatory indication for patients with cardiogenic shock secondary to STEMI, regardless of the timing of the onset of symptoms. The infarct-related artery should be treated systematically during the initial procedure. Patients with extensive CAD involving territories far from the IRA have a worse prognosis after primary PCI; therefore, unfavorable determinants on the composite outcome (MACE) are persistent ischemia after PCI of the IRA and the incompleteness of revascularization with a multi-stage approach during hospitalization.

Emergency surgical revascularization (emergency-CABG) is recommended in the course of cardiogenic shock if the coronary anatomy is not amenable to percutaneous treatment. Residual myocardial ischemia in the context of AMI is the prerequisite for cardiogenic shock in patients with STEMI already treated with PCI. The further causes which provoke hemodynamic instability are mechanical complications: (1) acute mitral insufficiency due to papillary rupture; (2) post-infarct ISD; and (3) rupture of the free wall of the left ventricle. The SHOCK study demonstrated that in patients with AMI complicated by cardiogenic shock, the emergency revascularization with PCI or CABG improved long-term survival compared to medical therapy alone. A subanalysis of the same study shows overlapping survival rates in the two subgroups CABG vs. PCI. In the group of patients treated with CABG, however, multivessel involvement and the incidence of diabetes are higher. Therefore, the results from this non-randomized comparison suggest that CABG should be exclusively reserved for a selected subgroup of patients with cardiogenic shock secondary to AMI who have coronary anatomy unfavorable for PCI.

The routine use of the intra-aortic balloon pump in the context of cardiogenic shock secondary to ACS is not recommended. This patient population in relation to age, comorbidities, neurological status, life expectancy, and predictability of quality of life can be assisted with short-term mechanical circulatory support.

2 Purpose and Strategy

In the course of cardiogenic shock secondary to AMI, the priority is to promptly establish a circulation support that maintains cardiac output such as to allow optimal perfusion of the brain and peripheral organs. The optimization and stabilization of the hemodynamic pattern are necessary conditions to start making the next decision.

The patient suffering from cardiogenic shock, in the first instance, must be treated with inotropic support and ventilatory assistance; then he/she must be subjected to reperfusion/revascularization in the shortest possible time and finally it must be corrected any possible mechanical complications of AMI. The second decision level is determined by hemodynamic stability/instability. If conditions of hemodynamic stability exist, a weaning program is started, if vice versa there is hemodynamically instability it goes toward a short-term MCS program (mechanical assistance for the short-term circulation). The outcomes of the mechanical circulatory support can be twofold: (1) recovery of cardiac function and (2) no-recovery of cardiac function. In this second case, if there is a favorable neurological state and a preserved multi-organ function, it can be chosen between a destination therapy or a bridge to transplantation. If, on the other hand, an irreversible neurological deficit has already been established, the most appropriate program is a compassionate weaning.

3 Types of Support

ST-MCS can be considered in post-AMI refractory cardiogenic shock depending on the patient's age, neurological function, comorbidities, long-term expectation, and quality of life.

ST-MCS devices are as follows:

1. Intra-aortic balloon pump
2. Percutaneous left ventricular assist devices
3. Extracorporeal membrane oxygenator

1. IABP is an inexpensive device, easily implanted and equally safe in removal. Its hemodynamic benefit consists, firstly, in improving coronary diastolic perfusion cooling down the left ventricular workload by reducing the after load, and secondarily by increasing cardiac output moderately. The IABP-SHOCK II study (recruiting 600 patients) showed that the use of IABP did not reduce mortality at 30 days. Other recent reviews of studies have confirmed that the use of intra-aortic balloon pump, in spite of a modest immediate benefit on some hemodynamic parameters, does not present an improvement in survival. Therefore, the routine use of IABP in patients with AMI complicated by cardiogenic shock is not recommended.
2. p-LVAD with greater clinical experience at the moment are two devices: IMPELLA and TANDEM HEART. Impella is a transaortic microaxial pump that discharges the left ventricle directly providing a blood flow between 2.5 and 5.0 L/min. Tandem heart is a centrifugal assistance that discharges the left ventricle through a cannula introduced into the left atrium for transseptal puncture. These percutaneous devices have immediate hemodynamic benefits in terms of increased blood pressure, peripheral perfusion, and lactacidemia, at the expense of a modest increase in bleeding from the access site and an increased incidence of limb ischemia. However, extensive studies do not show a 30-day incidence of major adverse events in patients treated with p-LVAD compared to those treated with IABP.
3. ECMO is part of the ECLS procedures and in its configuration VA-ECMO is simply a reworked form of cardio-pulmonary bypass. The rationale for percutaneous VA-ECMO support is to drain the venous system through a major percutaneous access (femoral vein, jugular vein), and to re-introduce oxygenated and pressurized blood through

another percutaneous arterial access (femoral artery). The hemodynamic benefit of this circulatory support consists in decompressing the venous circulation; increasing coronary, cerebral, and peripheral perfusion; and finally optimizing oxygen delivery with additional blood oxygenation. As part of the percutaneous approach, the pathophysiological disadvantage consists in the impossibility of the left ventricular unloading in conjunction with an increase in the afterload. It is a relevant problem in the psychopathology of left ventricular refreshment that requires some resolution strategies. In patients in cardiac arrest secondary to AMI, observational studies indicate a better survival in patients treated with VA-ECMO than in those treated without it. Extensive meta-analysis of observational studies showed that in patients with post-AMI cardiogenic shock, the percutaneous VA-ECMO implant allows a 30-day survival, which is 33% higher than in patients treated with IABP. However, the scarceness of the patients treated does not allow definitive results.

4 Planning and Configuration

The use of ECLS during post-AMI cardiogenic shock can constitute a temporary cardiorespiratory support to compensate for mono-bi-ventricular dysfunction and obtain the inversion of the oxygen debt with optimization of organ perfusion and gas exchange while waiting for the evolution of cardiac injury.

An ECLS support in its most basic form consists of a centrifugal pump that extracts the blood from the patient's venous compartment, pushes it through a gas exchange device (oxygenator with hollow polymethylpentene fibers), and returns under pressure the oxygenated blood to the arterial tree of the patient. Centrifugal pumps are capable of developing flow rates up to 9 L/min and have a reduced traumatic impact on the corpuscular elements of the blood.

Conventional VA-ECMO requires the cannulation of a vein to drain the venous blood from the patient and of an artery to re-infuse oxygenated and pressurized blood into the patient. This starting structure can change because the drainage and reinfusion sites can and must vary according to the evolution of the patient's metabolic and hemodynamic parameters during ECLS. Therefore, there is not a standard and rigid configuration, but rather tailored and dynamic. This concept understood as hybrid ECLS presupposes a fluctuation in the cannulation strategy and in the configuration of the flows during the circulatory support. Hypoxemia, an inadequate flow rate, pulmonary stasis, left ventricular distention, peripheral ischemia are all unforeseeable occurrences at the start of assistance, but which must be diagnosed and corrected promptly. The need to switch to a different ECLS mode is not an error in the initial planning, but a necessity with respect to the dynamism of the patient's condition and the assistance performance.

In its basic configuration, an ECLS assistance consists of a venous drainage and an arterial reinfusion represented, respectively, by the vein and the femoral artery cannulated percutaneously. This VA-ECMO configuration may be inadequate for hemodynamic or metabolic reasons so requiring the transition to advanced configurations after implanting additional cannulas. ELSO reports document that hybrid-ECLS represents more than 2% of all ECLS run. The most frequent causes of an ECMO up grading are: (1) insufficient drainage; (2) pulmonary stasis; (3) left ventricular distention; (4) inadequate oxygenation.

The addition of a second drainage cannula through the right jugular vein in the right atrium can optimize venous return and decongest the right sections optimally. Through the same way, the cannula can selectively be inserted in the pulmonary artery and act as a vent through the pulmonary circulation to empty the left ventricle and prevent its distension. The same cannula, by reversing the flow and transforming it into arterial out-flow, can eject oxygenated blood through the pulmonary circulation and correcting differential aortic hypoxemia by supplying oxygenated blood to the coronary arteries and to the epiaortic vessels. Obviously an advanced configuration of the ECLS carries an increased risk of bleeding, infections, and thrombosis.

Therefore, a standard configuration during an ECLS does not exist, the drainage needs, the reinfusion capacity, the hemodynamic and metabolic state presuppose a dynamism in the cannulation sites and in the management of flows.

Different hemodynamic and structural scenarios may require a combination of devices. The most frequent combinations found in the clinical practice, although the small number of cases, are:

1. VA-ECMO + IABP
2. VA-ECMO + IMPELLA = ECMELLA

The contextual use of IABP and VA-ECLS stems from a practical criterion since IABP is the fastest and most widespread ST-MCS system, but also from a pathophysiological criterion since counter-pulsation makes the flow pulsatile and therefore: (1) reduces left ventricular postload, (2) reduces ventricular wall tension, (3) facilitates ventricular ejection, and (4) ultimately promotes ventricular unloading. The neutral results of the IABP-SHOCK II study have downgraded the routine use of the IABP alone in the course of shock to a III B recommendation class, therefore it is reasonable to think of the IABP implantation only as an initial prodrome for combined support.

The Impella is a catheter-based flow pump that percutaneously implanted allows uni-ventricular support while maintaining an intrinsic flow rate. The conjunction of Impella with ECMO offers the following advantages: rapid improvement of the hemodynamic and metabolic pattern that constitutes a weaning platform from ECLS and above all it allows the discharge of the left ventricle. Left ventricular distension occurs in at least 5% of ECLS and it is a negative prognostic factor on ventricular recovery. A VA-ECLS typically allows for effective drainage of the right side, but it may be ineffective in decompressing the left sections. A dysfunctional left ventricle, in the face of an increase in afterload, does not empty and there will be consequently blood stasis, thrombus formation, increased wall tension, sub-endocardial ischemia, and pulmonary congestion. Therefore, the left ventricular venting is decisive in the patient's prognosis during ECLS. The loss of flow pulsatility and the fixity in closure of the aortic valve are the two predictors of ventricular distention. Although there are less invasive measures to facilitate the left drainage of the heart, Impella in situ avoids this fatal pathophysiological mechanism in the bud.

When ECLS support is initiated in the course of post-AMI cardiogenic shock, the rationale is to ensure a compensatory extracorporeal flow to the native cardiac output such as to allow an optimal perfusion to fully support peripheral metabolic needs. The initial VA-ECLS flow can, at the beginning, be set at 4.5-5.0 L/min. or more on the basis of the metabolic and hemodynamic status of the patient, later it is progressively reduced since peripheral perfusion is supported by the native cardiac output due to the progressive recovery of the myocardium. The adequacy of the mechanical support to the circulation must be monitored by following the evolution of the hemodynamic and metabolic indices. In order to stabilize the hemodynamic and metabolic situation, concomitant with a recovery of cardiac function, a progressive weaning from the support with a gradual reduction of the flows is started. In fact, the persistence of high flows has deleterious effects both by causing hemolysis and thrombocytopenia, and by affecting an unfavorable increase in afterload. Therefore, the best relationship between the lowest flow and maximum perfusion in the necessary time for the myocardial recovery or the establishment of advanced therapeutic programs should always be sought.

Bibliography

1. Thiele H, Zeymer U, Neumann FJ, Ferenc M, Olbrich HG, Hausleiter J, de Waha A, Richardt G, Hennersdorf M, Empen K, Fuernau G, Desch S, Eitel I, Hambrecht R, Lauer B, Bohm M, Ebelt H, Schneider S, Werdan K, Schuler G, Intraaortic Balloon Pump in cardiogenic shock II (IABP-SHOCK II) Trial Investigators. Intra-aortic balloon counterpulsation in acute myocardial infarction complicated by cardiogenic shock (IABP-SHOCK II): final 12 month results of a randomised, open-label trial. Lancet. 2013;382:1638–45.
2. Thiele H, Zeymer U, Neumann FJ, Ferenc M, Olbrich HG, Hausleiter J, Richardt G, Hennersdorf M, Empen K, Fuernau G, Desch S, Eitel I, Hambrecht R, Fuhrmann J, Bohm M, Ebelt H, Schneider S, Schuler G, Werdan K, IABPSHOCK II Trial Investigators I-SIT. Intraaortic balloon support for myocardial infarction with cardiogenic shock. N Engl J Med. 2012;367:1287–96.
3. Unverzagt S, Buerke M, de Waha A, Haerting J, Pietzner D, Seyfarth M, Thiele H, Werdan K, Zeymer U, Prondzinsky R. Intra-aortic balloon pump counterpulsation (IABP) for myocardial infarction complicated by cardiogenic shock. Cochrane Database Syst Rev. 2015;3:CD007398.
4. Ouweneel DM, Schotborgh JV, Limpens J, Sjauw KD, Engstrom AE, Lagrand WK, Cherpanath TGV, Driessen AHG, de Mol B, Henriques JPS. Extracorporeal life support during cardiac arrest and cardiogenic shock: a systematic review and meta-analysis. Intensive Care Med. 2016;42:1922–34.
5. Burkhoff D, Cohen H, Brunckhorst C, O'Neill WW, TandemHeart Investigators Group. A randomized multicenter clinical study to evaluate the safety and efficacy of the TandemHeart percutaneous ventricular assist device versus conventional therapy with intraaortic balloon pumping for treatment of cardiogenic shock. Am Heart J. 2006;152:469.e1–8.

6. Seyfarth M, Sibbing D, Bauer I, Frohlich G, Bott-Flugel L, Byrne R, Dirschinger J, Kastrati A, Schomig A. A randomized clinical trial to evaluate the safety and efficacy of a percutaneous left ventricular assist device versus intra-aortic balloon pumping for treatment of cardiogenic shock caused by myocardial infarction. J Am Coll Cardiol. 2008;52:1584–8.
7. Thiele H, Jobs A, Ouweneel DM, Henriques JPS, Seyfarth M, Desch S, Eitel I, Poss J, Fuernau G, de Waha S. Percutaneous short-term active mechanical support devices in cardiogenic shock: a systematic review and collaborative metaanalysis of randomized trials. Eur Heart J. 2017;38:3523–31.
8. Acharya D, Loyaga-Rendon RY, Pamboukian SV, Tallaj JA, Holman WL, Cantor RS, Naftel DC, Kirklin JK. Ventricular assist device in acute myocardial infarction. J Am Coll Cardiol. 2016;67:1871–80.
9. Hochman JS, Sleeper LA, Webb JG, Dzavik V, Buller CE, Aylward P, Col J, White HD, SHOCK Investigators. Early revascularization and long-term survival in cardiogenic shock complicating acute myocardial infarction. JAMA. 2006;295(21):2511–5.
10. Abrams D, Garan AR, Abdelbary A, Bacchetta M, Bartlett RH, Beck J et al.; for The International ECMO Network (ECMONet) and The Extracorporeal Life Support Organization (ELSO). Position paper for the organization of ECMO program in adults patients. Intensive Care Med. 2018;44:717–29.
11. Brasseur A, Scolletta S, Lorusso R, Taccone FS. Hybrid extracorporeal membrane oxygenation. J Thorac Dis. 2018;10:S707–15.

Transmyocardial Laser Revascularization

Edoardo Zancanaro

Abbreviations

BMLR	Bone marrow laser revascularization
CABG	Coronary artery bypass grafting
CAD	Coronary artery disease
LIMA	Left internal mammary artery
PCI	Percutaneous coronary intervention
TEE	Transesophageal echocardiography
TMR	Transmyocardial laser revascularization
VEGF	Vascular endothelial growth factor

1 Introduction

CAD is a manifestation of atherosclerosis, which often leads to angina, myocardial infarction, congestive heart failure, and ultimately death. Currently, available options for treating CAD include lifestyle changes in conjunction with drug therapy (medical management), percutaneous coronary intervention (PCI), and CABG. Unfortunately, despite optimal therapy, there is a proportion of patients who have medically refractory angina who are not eligible for conventional revascularization or who has been underwent incompletely revascularized by CABG alone [1, 2]. The hallmark of this difficult patient population is the presence of diffuse CAD. It is estimated that 3% of patients presenting with CAD are not

E. Zancanaro (✉)
Adult Cardiac Surgery Unit, Ospedale del Cuore "G. Pasquinucci", Fondazione Toscana G. Monasterio CNR—Regione Toscana, Massa, Italy

G. Concistrè (ed.), *Ischemic Heart Disease*,
https://doi.org/10.1007/978-3-031-25879-4_33

candidates for conventional revascularization and that 15–25% of patients undergoing CABG will have one or more major target areas incompletely revascularized due to diffuse CAD [1]. Incomplete revascularization due to diffuse CAD is recognized as an independent predictor of operative mortality [3, 4] and is associated with decreased long-term freedom from cardiac death, acute myocardial infarction, and cardiac events. Diffuse CAD, when quantified, is a strong independent predictor of operative mortality, and the quality of distal target during CABG has been identified as a strong predictor of vein graft failure [5]. Transmyocardial laser revascularization (TMR) has yielded positive clinical results in these difficult subsets of patients.

2 History

In 1941, Schlesinger et al. observed that intramyocardial arterioles were not prone to arteriosclerosis. This prompted Vineberg to implant the left internal mammary artery (LIMA) directly onto the myocardium with the purpose of developing collaterals between the LIMA and the intramyocardial arterioles. Although the first patient to undergo the Vineberg procedure died 2 days later, the LIMA was found to be widely patent at autopsy. Vineberg later created an intramyocardial tunnel prior to LIMA implantation, and patency of these grafts was documented two decades later.

In 1965, Sen et al. studied the benefits of transmyocardial channels produced with needle punctures. Using a canine model, they placed numerous needle punctures in an ischemic area subtended by an occluded left anterior descending artery. They showed that the acupuncture-created channels resulted in decreased mortality, increased long-term survival, and decreased infarct size. Although patent channels were identified at 8 weeks, no evidence suggested that the channels had developed an endothelial cell lining, thus confirming successful re-arterialization.

In 1968, Sen et al. described marked improvements in patients with chronic angina following transmyocardial revascularization. These initial data supported attempts to improve myocardial perfusion by creating mechanisms for a direct flow of blood from the ventricular cavity to the myocardium, thus mimicking the anatomy of the reptilian heart, in which much of the myocardium is perfused with blood directly from the ventricular cavity.

During the next two decades, numerous studies were undertaken to evaluate the effects of needle-created transmyocardial channels in revascularizing ischemic myocardium. However, much of this research received little attention because it was not considered nearly as promising as the emerging techniques involving direct myocardial revascularization, such as CABG and angioplasty.

The development of laser energy sources in the 1980s stimulated investigators to restudy myocardial acupuncture. In 1981, Mirhoseini et al. demonstrated that the carbon dioxide laser could generate small transmyocardial channels in the ischemic myocardium of a dog. In 1983, Mirhoseini et al. used TMR on a patient with CAD, employing a carbon dioxide laser in conjunction with CABG to treat a hypokinetic area of the left ventricle. The patient did well with normal ventricular function demonstrated during a postoperative nuclear scan.

These initial clinical studies provided further impetus for the use of TMR. Since the early 1990s, carbon dioxide laser systems have been used to perform TMR in humans, with excellent results. Holmium:YAG TMR has also been approved by the FDA [6].

To date, more than 50,000 TMR procedures have been done worldwide, nearly one-third of them done in the USA alone. Over the past two decades, multiple studies have reported good-to-moderate outcomes.

3 Indication

Although no absolute indications have been described for the application of TMR, several studies have provided some necessary guidelines.

The initial non-randomized trials demonstrated that sole therapy TMR could be performed safely on patients with severe coronary artery disease who previously had no other options. The significant angina relief achieved in these patients led to prospective randomized controlled studies to further demonstrate the efficacy of TMR. In these pivotal trials, over 1000 patients were enrolled and randomized to receiving either TMR or medical management as treatment for their severe angina [6, 7].

The enrollment criteria for these sole therapy trials were as follows: patients had refractory angina that was not amenable to standard methods of revascularization. They had evidence of reversible ischemia based on myocardial perfusion scanning, and their left ventricular ejection fractions were greater than 25%.

Because the patients were equally randomized to the medical management group, there were no significant demographic differences between the TMR and the control groups for any of these trials. Three studies [6] employed a Holmium:yttrium-aluminum-garnet (Ho:YAG) laser and three others used a carbon dioxide (CO_2) laser. The average patient age was 62 years, and the majority were male (86%). While there were significant differences in the baseline distribution of patients according to Canadian Cardiovascular Society (CCS) Angina Class, the majority of the patients were in angina Class IV (61%) [8]. The ejection fractions for all of the patients were mildly diminished at 48 ± 10%. Many of the patients had suffered at least one previous myocardial infarction, and most had some prior revascularization, CABG and/or PCI. Two of the trials permitted a crossover from the medical management group to laser treatment for the presence of unstable angina that necessitated intravenous anti-anginal therapy for which they were unweanable over a period of at least 48 h [6, 8]. By definition, these crossover patients were less stable and significantly different than those who had been initially randomized to TMR or medical management alone.

A brief summary of all the indications published by the STS, ISMICS, and ACC/AHA is summarized in Table 1.

Table 1 Practice guidelines for patients undergoing sole therapy TMR and TMR + CABG

Society	Sole therapy TMR	TMR + CABG
ACC/AHA[a]	Class IIa, level of evidence: A	Class IIa, level of evidence: A
ISMICS[b]	Class I, level B evidence	Class IIa, level of evidence: B
ACCF/AHA[c]	n/a	Class IIb, level of evidence: B
STS[d]	Class I, level of evidence: A	Class IIA, level of evidence B
ACCF/AHA/ACP/AATS/PCNA/SCAI/STS[e]	Class IIb, level of evidence: B	Class IIb, level of evidence: B

[a]American College of Cardiology/American Heart Association
[b]International Society of Minimally Invasive Cardiothoracic Surgery (ISMICS)
[c]American College of Cardiology Foundation/American Heart Association
[d]The Society of Thoracic Surgeons
[e]American College of Cardiology Foundation/American Heart Association task force on practice guidelines, and the American College of Physicians, American Association for Thoracic Surgery, Preventive Cardiovascular Nurses Association, Society for Cardiovascular Angiography and Interventions, and Society of Thoracic Surgeons

4 Procedural Concepts

4.1 Procedural Technique

For sole therapy TMR, the patient is placed in a supine position with their left side slightly elevated. General anesthesia may be established using a double-lumen endotracheal tube or a bronchial blocker to help isolate the left lung. This facilitates the operation, particularly as most of the patients have pleural and mediastinal adhesions from previous bypass surgery. Additionally, a thoracic epidural catheter can be employed to provide postoperative pain control.

A left anterior thoracotomy in the fifth intercostal space is the usual incision site. Once the ribs are spread by a retractor, the pericardium is opened to expose the epicardial surface of the heart. Care must be taken to avoid previous bypass grafts. The left anterior descending artery is identified and used as a landmark for the location of the septum. The inferior and posterior lateral portions of the heart can be reached through this incision with a combination of manual traction, placement of packing behind the heart and with the use of a right-angled laser handpiece. Channels are created starting near the base of the heart and then serially in a line approximately 1 cm apart toward the apex, starting inferiorly and working superiorly to the anterior surface of the heart. As there is some bleeding from the channels, commencement of the TMR inferiorly keeps the anterior area clear and expedites the procedure. The number of channels created depends on the size of the heart and on the size of the ischemic area. Myocardium that is thinned by scar, particularly when the scar is transmural, should be avoided as TMR will be of no benefit to these regions and bleeding from channels in these areas may be problematic. The thoracotomy is then closed after the placement of a chest tube and in the majority of the cases, the patient is extubated in the operating room.

The CO_2 laser energy is delivered via hollow tubes and is reflected by mirrors to reach the epicardial surface, and 1-mm channels are made with a 15–20 J pulse. The firing of the laser is synchronized to occur on the r wave of the EKG to avoid arrhythmias. The transmural channel is created by a signal pulse in 40 ms and can be confirmed by transesophageal echocardiography (TEE). The vaporization of blood by the laser energy as the laser beam enters the ventricle creates an obvious and characteristic acoustic effect as noted on TEE.

The Ho:YAG laser achieves a 1-mm channel by manually advancing a fiber bundle through the myocardium while the laser fires. Typical pulse energies are 2 Js for this laser and at a rate of 5 pulses per second, 10–20 pulses are required to traverse the myocardium. Detection of transmural penetration is primarily by tactile sensation and then by auditory feedback.

4.2 Technical Instruments

While numerous devices, including ultrasound, cryoablation, radio frequency, heated needles, as well as hollow and solid needles have been used; none has engendered the same response that is seen with a laser. Additionally, numerous wavelengths of laser light have also been employed. These include xenon-chloride (XeCl), neodymium:YAG (ND:YAG), erbium:YAG (Er:YAG), and thulium-holmium-chromium:YAG lasers (THC:YAG). All of these devices have been explored experimentally but have not been pursued on a significant scale clinically.

Two laser-based systems have been approved by the FDA to deliver laser therapy to targeted areas of the left ventricle that cannot be revascularized using conventional methods: the holmium:yttrium-aluminum-garnet (Ho:YAG) laser system (CryoLife, Inc., Kennesaw, GA) and the carbon dioxide (CO_2) laser system (PLC Medical Systems, Franklin, MA), although the CO_2 laser has been discontinued [9]. The Ho:YAG system uses a 20-W-pulsed laser to deliver 7 W per laser pulse at a rate of 5 pulses per second through a 1-mm flexible fiber optic bundle. The hand piece allows the surgeon to position and stabilize the embedded fiber optic bundle against the epicardial surface.

4.3 Mechanism of Action

The mechanism of action should be explained throughout different points: the interaction between the laser and the tissue, the channel creation, the nervous system denervation, and the angiogenesis stimulation.

Concerning **laser–tissue interaction**: The result of any laser–tissue interaction is dependent on both laser and tissue variables. CO_2 has a wavelength of 10,600-nm, whereas Ho:YAG has a wavelength of 2120 nm. These infrared wavelengths are primarily absorbed in water and therefore rely on thermal energy to ablate tissue. One significant difference however is that the Ho:YAG laser is pulsed and the arrival of two successive pulses must be separated by time to allow for thermal dissipation, otherwise the accumulated heat will cause the tissue to explode under pressure. Such explosions create acoustic waves, which travel along the planes of lower resistance between muscle fibers and cause structural trauma as well as thermocoagulation. The standard operating parameters for the Ho:YAG laser are pulse energies of 1–2 Js and 6–8 W/pulse. The energy is delivered at a rate of 5 pulses/second through a flexible 1-mm optical fiber bundle. Despite the low energy level and short pulse duration, there are very high levels of peak power delivered to the tissue so that with each pulse there is an explosion. Additionally, the fiber is advanced manually through the myocardium and it is therefore impossible to know whether the channel is being created by the kinetic energy delivered via the mechanical effects of the fiber and whether there has been enough time for thermal dissipation prior to the next pulse.

In contrast, the CO_2 was used at an energy level of 15–20 Js/pulse with a pulse duration of 25–40 ms. At this level, the laser photons do not cause explosive ablation and the extent of structural damage is limited. Additionally, a transmural channel can be created with a single pulse. Confirmation of this transmurality is obtained by observing the vaporization of blood within the ventricle using TEE.

Finally, the CO_2 laser is synchronized to fire on the r wave and with its short pulse duration arrhythmic complications are minimized. The Ho:YAG device is unsynchronized and due to the motion of the fiber through the myocardium over several cardiac cycles, is more prone to ventricular arrhythmias.

Regarding **denervation**: The nervous system of the heart can function independent of inputs from extracardiac neurons to regulate regional cardiac function by reflex action. This intrinsic system contains afferent neurons, sympathetic efferent, postganglionic neurons, and parasympathetic efferent postganglionic neurons. Because of this complex system, it is difficult to demonstrate true denervation. However, several experimental studies have demonstrated that denervation may indeed play a role in Ho:YAG TMR [10].

Finally, **angiogenesis**: this mechanism fits the clinical picture of significant improvement in symptoms over time as well as a concomitant improvement in perfusion, as seen with the CO_2 laser. Numerous reports have demonstrated a histologic increase in neovascularization as a result of TMR channels. More molecular evidence of this angiogenic phenomenon was derived from work that demonstrated an upregulation of vascular endothelial growth factor (VEGF) messenger RNA, expression of FGF2, as well as matrix metalloproteinases following TMR [11].

5 Outcomes and Trials

In order to make a clear overview of different TMR outcomes, it has been proposed to divide the results into two categories: (1) TMR as a sole therapy and (2) TMR combined with CABG.

5.1 TMR as a Sole Therapy

The safety and effectiveness of TMR as sole therapy have been evaluated in five prospective, randomized trials [7]. Experimental designs and patient selection criteria were similar across the five trials. Study endpoints included operative (in-hospital/30 days) mortality and 1-year survival, improvement in angina class, myocardial perfusion, exercise tolerance, quality of life, cardiac-related hospitalization, and major adverse events. Aside from a variation in the number of patients enrolled, certain features made some trials unique. Whereas Allen et al. [6] only randomized patients with medically refractory CCS Class IV angina, Schofield and associates enrolled patients with primarily CCS Class III angina, which may have influenced results [12].

5.1.1 Operative Mortality

Operative mortality (in-hospital/30-day) for sole therapy TMR patients ranged from 1% to 5%. The lowest rate (1%) which was reported by Burkhoff et al. [13] was attributed to strict study enrollment criteria that excluded patients without at least one region of protected myocardium, left main stenosis >50%, or a change in angina symptoms or medication usage in the preceding 21 days prior to enrollment. Allen et al. [6] reported a reduced operative mortality rate from 5% overall to 2% in the last 100 consecutively randomized patients, attributable to refinement of surgical technique and improved patient selection.

A more recent, multicenter, nonrandomized post-approval study (PAS) showed that a total of 358 patients with stable CCS Class IV angina and preoperative ejection fraction of ≥25% underwent sole therapy TMR with the Ho:YAG laser system from 18 US centers. The primary endpoint, 30-day all-cause mortality, was significantly lower than the pre-market approval (PMA) study (2.2% vs. 5.3%; $p = 0.0033$). Univariate analyses identified only number of TMR channels (≥40 vs. 40 channels), to be a significant independent predictor of 30-day MACE (18.67% vs. 6.96%, $p = 0.0095$). Preoperative ejection fraction of ≤30% vs. >30% was the only significant predictor of operative mortality (11.1% vs. 1.5%; $p = 0.0167$).

5.1.2 Long-Term Survival

In a meta-analysis of randomized TMR trials conducted by the International Society of Minimally Invasive Cardiothoracic Surgery (ISMICS), Kaplan-Meier 1-year survival was similar between patients randomized to medical therapy versus TMR [14]. The effect on long-term survival is a key component in establishing the risk/benefit profile of any treatment. In a 5-year follow-up of randomized patients all with class IV angina, Allen [15] reported increased Kaplan-Meier survival in patients randomized to TMR versus maximal medical management (MM) (65% vs. 52%, $p = 0.05$). The annualized mortality rate after 1 year was 13% per year for medically managed patients compared to 8% per year for patients randomized to TMR ($p = 0.03$).

5.1.3 Angina Management

Important insight should be posed to angina improvement since TMR's primary indication is primarily the angina relief. Angina has been defined as decrease of two or more grade from the baseline.

Randomized trials have consistently demonstrated significant angina improvement following TMR when compared to continued medical management. In a meta-analysis of randomized controlled TMR trials conducted by ISMICS, forest plots of two class angina improvement depict the superiority of TMR versus maximal medical management at 1, 3, and 5-year follow-up [14]. Variations between trials with regard to angina relief efficacy may be attributable to patient's angina class at the time of enrollment. Schofield et al. [12] reported only a 25% 2-class angina improvement at 1-year compared to a 76% 2-class improvement reported by Allen et al. [6].

5.2 TMR Combined with CABG

One of the largest difficulties was analyzing the "TMR + CABG" cohort was for sure the bypasses conduit presence since they can create a more challenging anatomy to pursue the laser treatment.

Allen et al. [16] randomized 263 patients who had one or more ischemic areas not amenable to bypass grafting and who would be incompletely revascularized by CABG alone to either CABG + TMR ($N = 132$) or CABG alone ($N = 131$). Operative characteristics were similar between groups and patients were blinded as to whether they received TMR through 1 year. Significantly reduced operative mortality was observed following CABG + TMR compared to CABG alone (1.5% vs. 7.6%, $p = 0.02$) even though preoperative STS predicted mortality risk was comparable (6.3%, CABG/TMR vs. 6.6%, CABG alone, $p = 0.80$). Patients undergoing CABG/TMR required less postoperative inotropic support (30% vs. 55%, $p = 0.0001$) and had a greater 30-day freedom from major adverse cardiac events (97% vs. 91%, $p = 0.04$). Compared to CABG alone patients, CABG/TMR patients had a significantly better 1-year survival (95% vs. 89%, $p = 0.05$) and freedom from major adverse cardiac events, prospectively defined as death or myocardial infarction (92% vs. 86%, $p < 0.05$). The only multivariable predictor of the composite endpoint of death, MI, or recurrent class III/IV angina at 12 months, was being randomized to CABG alone (odds ratio 2.9; CI 1.4–6.2: $p = 0.04$).

Concerning angina relief, it was similar between CABG/TMR and CABG alone patients at 1-year with a trend toward better angina relief with CABG/TMR ($p = 0.2$). At

5-year follow-up, however, CABG/TMR patients had significantly lower mean angina scores compared to CABG alone patients (0.4 ± 0.7 vs. 0.7 ± 1.1, $p = 0.05$).

In a smaller prospective, randomized trial conducted at five U.S. Centers, Frazier et al. [17] randomized 49 patients who would be incompletely revascularized by CABG alone due to diffuse CAD to either CABG/TMR ($N = 22$) or CABG alone ($N = 27$). Patients were at high operative risk due to depressed ejection fraction (<0.35 [19%]), unstable angina (16%), preoperative intra-aortic balloon pump (18%), and prior CABG surgery (68%). A strong trend in reduced operative mortality was observed in the adjunctive TMR group compared to the CABG alone group (9% vs. 33%, $p = 0.09$). At 1 year, the rate of treatment failure (defined as death, repeat revascularization, or failure to improve by two or more angina classes) was non-significantly reduced in adjunctive TMR versus CABG alone patients (37% vs. 66%, $p = 0.3$). A 4-year follow-up of these randomized patients demonstrated a significant reduction in recurrent angina requiring percutaneous or repeat surgical revascularization in CABG/TMR versus CABG alone patients (0% vs. 24%, $p < 0.05$), even though the number of bypass grafts placed at the time of enrollment (3.1 ± 0.7 vs. 3.1 ± 0.8, $p = 0.85$) were similar between groups. The long-term freedom from treatment failure showed a strong trend favoring CABG/TMR patients at a mean of 4-year follow-up (39% vs. 14%, $p = 0.06$).

6 Future Perspectives

Although TMR's superiority over medical therapy has been demonstrated in randomized trials, its effectiveness is not 100%. In up to 25% of patients treated with sole therapy TMR, angina relief is not significantly improved at 1 year. To increase the angiogenic response and the associated clinical efficacy of TMR in treating ischemic heart disease, the potential synergy of combining TMR with a cell-based therapy has been evaluated (stem cell strategy will be described in the following chapter). Bone marrow laser revascularization (BMLR) describes the delivery of autologous bone marrow concentrate in conjunction with TMR channels into targeted ischemic tissue. It is hypothesized that the delivery of bone marrow derived stem cells to the laser-stimulated border zone surrounding the channels will significantly enhance the angiogenic response compared with TMR alone. Larger clinical trials will be required to validate the clinical benefit of combining TMR with cell therapy.

References

1. Muhkerjee D, Bhatt DL, Roe MT, Patel V, Ellis SG. Direct myocardial revascularization and angiogenesis – how many patients might be eligible? Am J Cardiol. 1999;84:598–600.
2. Weintraub WS, Jones EL, Craver JM, Guyton RA. Frequency of repeat coronary bypass or coronary angioplasty after coronary artery bypass surgery using saphenous venous grafts. Am J Cardiol. 1994;73:103–12.

3. Osswald BR, Blackstone EH, Tochtermann U, et al. Does the completeness of revascularization affect early survival after coronary artery bypass grafting in elderly patients? Eur J Cardiothorac Surg. 2001;20:120–6.
4. Allen KB. Holmium:YAG laser system for transmyocardial revascularization. Expert Rev Med Devices. 2006;3:137–46.
5. Lopes RD, Hafley GE, Allen KB, et al. Endoscopic versus open vein-graft harvesting in coronary-artery bypass surgery. N Engl J Med. 2009;361:235–44.
6. Allen KB, Dowling RD, Fudge TL, et al. Comparison of transmyocardial revascularization with medical therapy in patients with refractory angina. N Engl J Med. 1999;341:1029–36. [PubMed: 10502592]
7. Aaberge L, Nordstrand K, Dragsund M, et al. Transmyocardial revascularization with CO_2 laser in patients with refractory angina pectoris. Clinical results from the Norwegian randomized trial. J Am Coll Cardiol. 2000;35(5):1170–7. [PubMed: 10758957]
8. Frazier OH, March RJ, Horvath KA. Transmyocardial revascularization with a carbon dioxide laser in patients with end-stage coronary artery disease. N Engl J Med. 1999;341:1021–8. [PubMed: 10502591]
9. Jeevanandam V, Auteri JS, Oz MC, et al. Myocardial revascularization by laser-induced channels. Surg Forum. 1990;41:225–7.
10. Kwong KF, Kanellopoulos GK, Nikols JC, et al. Transmyocardial laser treatment denervates canine myocardium. J Thorac Cardiovasc Surg. 1997;114:883–90. [PubMed: 9434682]
11. Horvath KA, Chiu E, Maun DC, et al. Up-regulation of VEGF mRNA and angiogenesis after transmyocardial laser revascularization. Ann Thorac Surg. 1999;68:825–9.
12. Schofield PM, Sharples LD, Caine N, et al. Transmyocardial laser revascularization in patients with refractory angina: a randomised controlled trial. Lancet. 1999;353:519–24.
13. Burkhoff D, Schmidt S, Schulman SP, et al. Transmyocardial laser revascularisation compared with continued medical therapy for treatment of refractory angina pectoris: a prospective randomized trial. Lancet. 1999;354:885–90.
14. Cheng D, Diegeler A, Allen K, et al. Transmyocardial laser revascularization: a meta-analysis and systematic review of controlled trials. Innovations. 2006;1:295–313.
15. Allen KB, Dowling RD, Angell WW, et al. Transmyocardial revascularization: five-year follow-up of a prospective, randomized, multicenter trial. Ann Thorac Surg. 2004;77:1228–34.
16. Allen KB, Dowling RD, DelRossi AJ, et al. Transmyocardial laser revascularization combined with coronary artery bypass grafting: a multicenter, blinded, prospective, randomized, controlled trial. J Thorac Cardiovasc Surg. 2000;119:540–9.
17. Frazier OH, Boyce SW, Griffith BP, et al. Transmyocardial revascularization using a synchronized CO_2 laser as adjunct to coronary artery bypass grafting: results of a prospective, randomized multi-center trial with 12 month follow-up. Circulation. 1999;100:I248.

Stem Cells Therapy for Ischemic Heart Disease

Nicola Pradegan and Gino Gerosa

1 Introduction

With more than 17 million deaths worldwide each year, IHD caused by coronary artery disease is the most common cause of death and a major cause of hospital admission in developed countries. In Europe, IHD is the main cause of death among women >50 years of age and men [1, 2].

Conventional therapies have significantly reduced mortality of acute IHD, leaving an increasing number of patients with chronic IHD and/or HF without further treatment options. An increasing morbidity rate of this nature in an aging population is a huge burden for current society. HF is an expensive disease, both in terms of financial burden ($30 billion/year in medical expenditures in the US) and reduced quality of life and workdays lost [3]. Although HF survival has improved since 1979, the death rate remains very high, with more people dying of cardiac disease than cancer and chronic lower respiratory disease combined. Therapies aimed at restoring the billions of cardiomyocytes lost during myocardial infarction or damaged by nonischemic cardiomyopathies are sorely needed.

Among different medical strategies developed in the last decades to relieve symptoms, prevent disease progression, and improve survival and quality of life, stem cells therapy has emerged as a promising therapeutic approach to promote myocardial repair and regeneration. Cardiovascular disease is perhaps the field with the most clinical research on cell-based therapeutics, with over 200 clinical trials since 2001 examining multiple stem cell products for a diverse array of cardiac syndromes. Despite this extensive body of

N. Pradegan · G. Gerosa (✉)
Cardiac Surgery Unit, Cardiac-Thoracic-Vascular Sciences and Public Health Department, Padova University Hospital, Padova, Italy
e-mail: gino.gerosa@unipd.it

G. Concistrè (ed.), *Ischemic Heart Disease*,
https://doi.org/10.1007/978-3-031-25879-4_34

research, stem cell therapy has yet to transition from research to practice, as there is no definitive evidence of an efficacious cell product.

With this chapter, we aim to overview the biology of stem cell types used in cardiovascular research, and current preclinical and clinical applications regarding stem cells use in acute and chronic IHD.

2 Stem Cells Source

Stem cells are undifferentiated cells defined by their capacity for both self-renewal and ability to differentiate into other mature cell types. While embryonic stem cells are the prototypical pluripotent stem cells, capable of becoming any other cell type in an embryo, there are numerous stem cells populations found in adult tissues. These adult stem cells have a more limited differentiation potential and generally exist to maintain tissue homeostasis and replenish lost cells from that particular tissue. Some of these adult stem cells can naturally (albeit rarely) transdifferentiate to form cells outside of their original tissue of origin.

Several studies have shown that various cell types exerted beneficial effects on cardiac repair. Overall stem cells effect is summarized in Fig. 1.

- **Skeletal myoblast** was the first cell type to be clinically tested, but the efficacy was unsatisfactory mainly due to the high incidence of arrhythmias [4].
- **Bone marrow-derived mononuclear cell** contains the undifferentiated HSC and MSC as well as other committed cells in various stages of maturation. Its abundance and easy

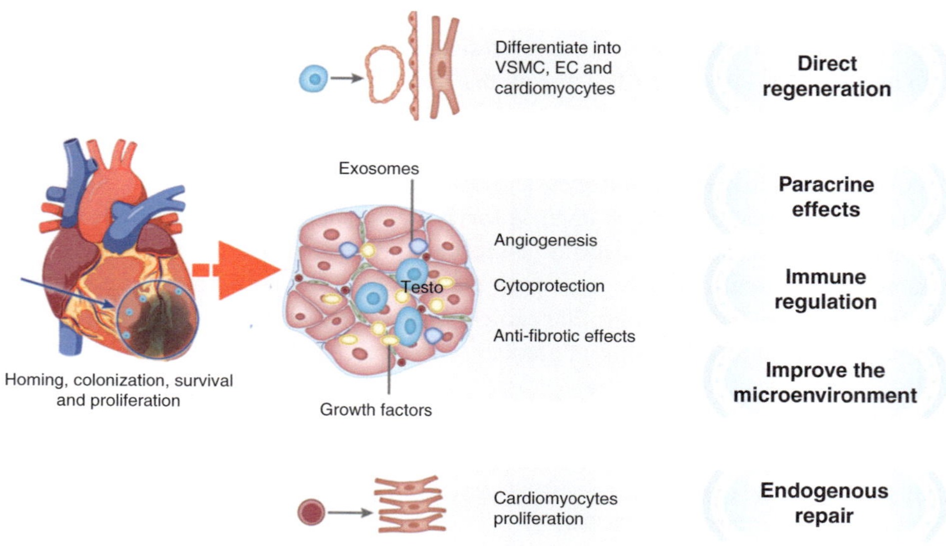

Fig. 1 Stem cells effect on cardiac remodeling and function

accessibility allow for autologous implantation without expansion in tissue culture, which avoids the decline of stem cell differentiation and migration ability, and reduces the incidence of immune rejection. Preclinical studies show discordant results in terms of angiogenesis and left ventricle function among different animal models [5–10]. Clinically, BMMNCs have been evaluated both for AMI and ischemic heart failure. In AMI, intracoronary delivery of autologous BMMNCs were evaluated in the REPAIR-AMI clinical trial: this was a large, phase III, double-blinded, placebo-controlled study designed to determine the therapeutic efficacy of BMMNCs. There were 204 patients randomized to receive either cells or placebo 3–7 days following AMI. Initial results at 4-months were encouraging, with LVEF significantly improved in the BMMNC-treated group by 5.5% on average, whereas the placebo-treated group exhibited a 3.0% in increase in LVEF. At 1-year, there were some encouraging signs. There were fewer myocardial infarctions, less need for repeat revascularization and fewer incidences of death in the BMMNC compared to the placebo group [11]. However, a longer follow-up analysis (5-year follow-up) found out that, despite a preserved benefit on mortality, improvement in LVEF was not maintained [12]. These mid-term results were also highlighted by other clinical experiences which did not find any significant improvement of myocardial function after BMMNCs administration in AMI (e.g., TIME trial [13], LateTIME trial [14], SWISS AMI trial [15], BOOST-2 trial [16], MiHeart/AMI trial [17]). In patients with post-ischemic HF, results have been more promising: in fact, a recent meta-analysis reports a mean improvement of 4.33% in LVEF as well as reductions in left ventricle volumes after MBBNCs injection in patients with post-ischemic HF [18]. This analysis suggested that overall BMMNCs for post-ischemic cardiomyopathy appear to produce positive effects on cardiac function and remodeling.

- **Hematopoietic stem cell** has multiple differentiation potentials and can be autologously transplanted, but they are limited in abundance, which leads to poor efficacy [19].
- **Endothelial progenitor cells** are isolated from peripheral blood and bone marrow and can give rise to vascular cells. Clinical application of EPC transplantation is expected to increase the capillary density and subsequently improve the microcirculation around the transplanted sites in infarcted heart. Studies have showed that EPC transplantation can also improve heart function, but its effect is restricted, which may result from its weak differentiation ability [20].
- **Embryonic stem cells** have strong proliferation and differentiation capabilities, but it has ethical controversies and high risks of teratoma formation, which create hurdles to its clinical translation [21].
- **Induced pluripotent stem cells** can differentiate into multiple cell types, are anti-inflammatory, and have therapeutic potential to repair tissues following ischemic disease. They have great proliferative capacity and might have the potential to be a major source for cardiac repair, but preclinical studies are needed to assess potential tumor formation and other safety issues [22, 23].

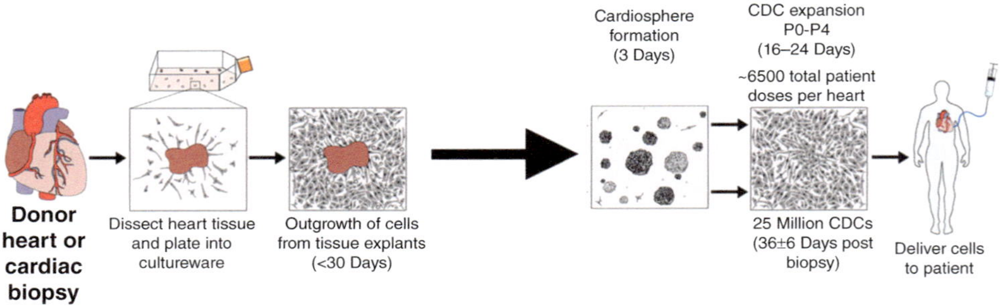

Fig. 2 Laboratory pathway to obtain cardiosphere-derived cells

- **Cardiosphere-derived cells**: The discovery of small clusters of heart cells expressing stem cell antigens (originally called "side population"—SP) capable of symmetric (self to identical self) or asymmetric (self to differentiated daughter progeny) division prompted the enthusiastic declaration that in situ, adult stem cells exist and such cells might have therapeutic potential. These in situ stem cells have been obtained by cardiac biopsies and then expanded in particular cultures to generate the CDCs (Fig. 2), which have clonogenic potential and express markers indicative of progenitor/stem cell identity [24]. To date, several trials have already tested this new population of cells. The CADUCEUS trial was the first to determine if intracoronary injection of autologous CDCs to patients soon after myocardial infarction was safe [25]. At 1 year of follow-up, CDC-treated patients had smaller scar sizes, increased viable myocardium, and improved regional function compared to control patients. A subsequent study using allogenic CDCs also confirmed the positive outcomes in terms of ventricular function improvement (even if no difference was found in terms of scar size) [26]. These results are hypothesized to be caused by the paracrine anti-inflammatory, immunomodulatory, and anti-fibrotic effect of these cells on the injured area rather than a CDC differentiation into local new myocardial cells [27].
- **Mesenchymal stem cells** are isolates by multiple tissues (e.g., bone marrow, adipose tissue, dental pulp, umbilical cord) and can be expanded in vitro. Among the different cells studied for these purposes, MSCs are the most widely studied because of their abundancy, their easy retrieval and their immune exemption [28]. This type of cell is known since early 70s, and it has been called with different names (osteogenic stromal cell, stromal stem cell, mesenchymal stem cell, mesenchymal progenitor/precursor cell, multipotent mesenchymal stromal cell). It is now called MSC because of the hypothesis that postnatal MSC might generate all mesoderm-derived tissues (including myocardium). However, the formation of similar differentiated similar cells is still a point of controversy. The main and most studied source of MSCs for cardiac regeneration is bone marrow (Fig. 3 summarizes the process to obtain bone marrow MSCs); however, further studies have demonstrated favorable results in terms of LVEF improve-

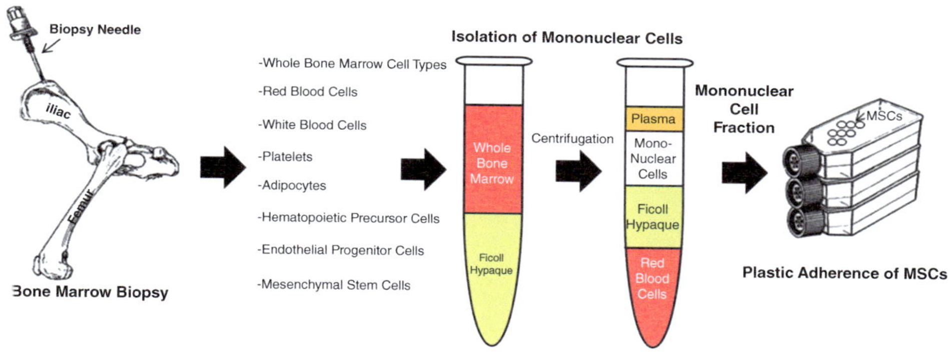

Fig. 3 Isolation of bone marrow mesenchymal stem cells

ment, perfusion, and remodeling for MSCs isolated from adipose tissue and umbilical cord in large-animal models [29, 30]. Particularly, adipose-derived MSCs can differentiate into cardiomyocytes, endothelial cells, and vascular smooth muscle cells and exhibit immunomodulatory properties that can protect other cell types (e.g., endothelial progenitor cells) from rejection.

3 MSCs Mechanisms of Action

MSCs favor cardiac repair by means of fibrosis reduction (Fig. 4), angiogenesis stimulation, and ventricular function improvement. The mechanism of action is heterogeneous and includes engraftment and heterocellular coupling (stem and somatic cell intercommunication) [31] and paracrine mediated signaling [32]. Figure 5 summarizes all the mechanisms of action. The initial idea that MSCs differentiate and directly remuscularize a scarred myocardial area has been disconfirmed since multiple studies have shown that cardiomyocyte replacement by MSCs is low and does not represent a therapeutically meaningful mechanism of MSC action [33, 34]. Regarding paracrine signaling, MSCs release a variety of growth factors, with variability according to MSC tissue source. Besides, MSC secretion also includes exosomes and extracellular vesicles containing mRNA, miRNA and non-protein encoding RNA, peptides, and other bioactive compounds, which produce a wide variety of effects on target tissues (e.g., angiogenesis, reduction of infarct size, cardiac function preservation, and anti-arrhythmic effect) [35]. Further studies are required to determine the extent and duration of these effects. Heterocellular coupling through gap junctions allows for the transfer of small molecules and plays a role in coordinating activities between neighboring cells during tissue function. Mitochondrial transfer is also allowed through these gap junctions, and it is involved in rescuing damaged cells, reducing the ischemia-reperfusion injury [36].

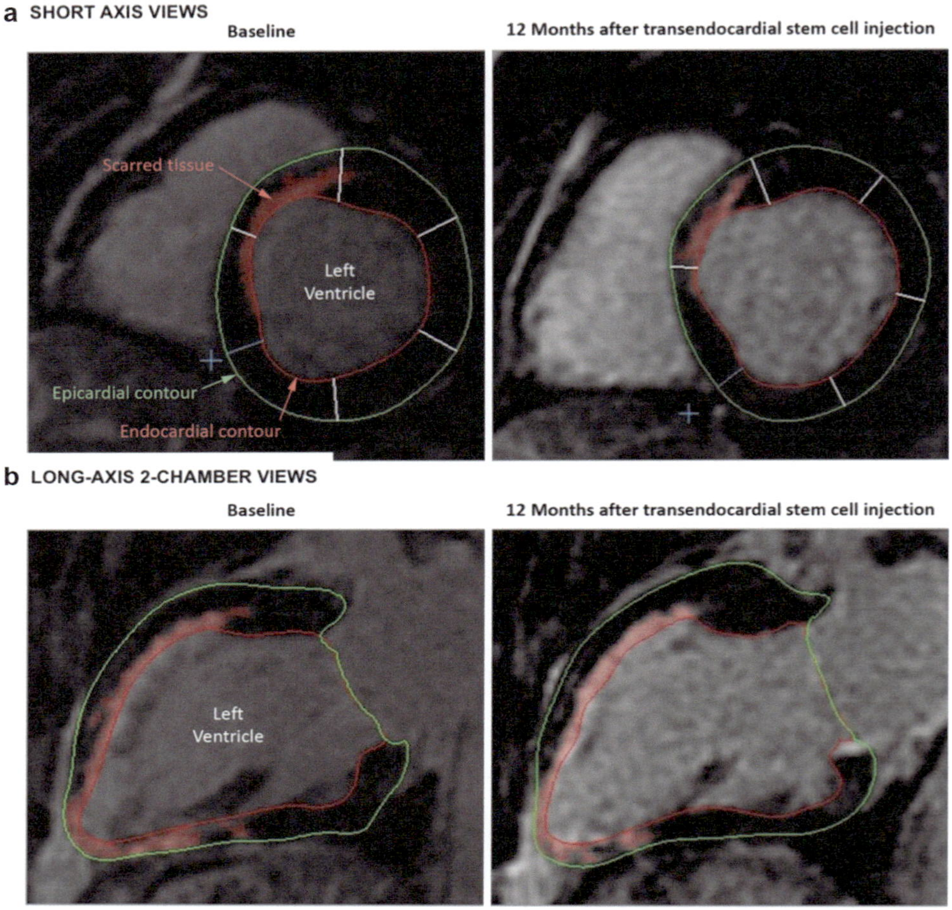

Fig. 4 Cardiac magnetic resonance showing mesenchymal stem cells effect on myocardial fibrosis on short-axis view (**a**) and long-axis 2-chamber view (**b**)

Regarding the immunomodulatory action, MSCs lack surface molecules which can activate the immune system. Furthermore, they reduce the expression of proinflammatory cytokines and lymphocytes proliferation.

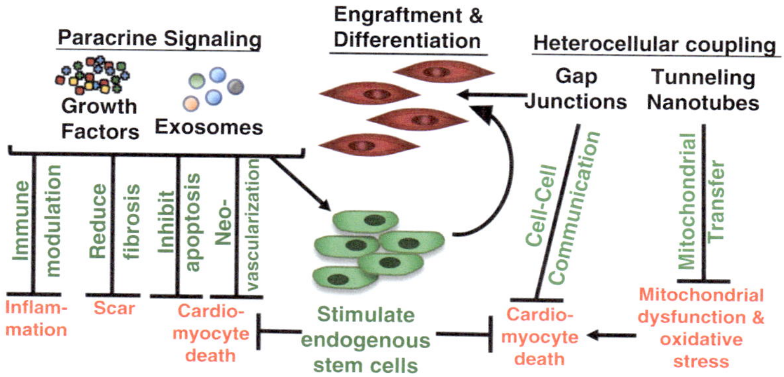

Fig. 5 Mesenchymal stem cells mechanism of action

4 MSCs Preliminary Clinical Outcomes: Acute Myocardial Infarction and Post-ischemic Heart Failure

Given the promising preclinical data on MSCs in IHD, multiple studies have investigated the clinical application of MSCs in humans. In AMI patients, autologous MSCs were first used. Two different trials demonstrated that intracoronary infusion of MSCs (before autologous bone marrow MSCs expansion and after percutaneous coronary intervention) showed better LVEF and ventricular volumes at mid-term follow-up [37, 38]. However, other studies did not find any superiority in the autologous MSCs group in terms of ventricular function improvement in patients with coronary artery disease [39]. This discrepancy might be due to different MSCs injection protocols used. Given the absence of MSCs immunogenicity and the disadvantages of using autologous cells, allogenic MSCs from healthy donors were tested. First clinical experiences show better results in terms of arrhythmias reduction [40], but trials are still ongoing.

Clinical experience with MSCs in ischemic HF has been obtained by means of several studies. Phase I [41] and Phase II studies [42, 43] using MSCs directly injected into the myocardium have demonstrated functional cardiac improvement, reverse remodeling, and improved exercise capacity and quality of life. Other studies have also analyzed MSCs effect after epicardial injection at the time of other surgical interventions (providing a unique opportunity to include cell-based therapies as an adjunct to open surgical procedures), showing an improvement in terms of scar size reduction, perfusion, and contractility [33]. When comparing autologous vs. allogenic MSCs in ischemic HF, both types showed a significant reduction in scar size at 1 year of follow-up as well as a ventricular reverse remodeling [34]. However discordant data are available regarding the dose-dependent effect.

5 Stem Cells Delivery: How and When to Do It

Delivery routes in cardiac cell therapy mainly include thoracotomy injection, system infusion, and imaging guide mini-invasive injection (Fig. 6).

1. *Thoracotomy injection*: Through this access, cells can be delivered in a trans-epicardial intramyocardial fashion directly into the targeted area. Even if this method reduces the cells loss, unfortunately it requires anesthesia and a surgical approach. For this reason, this delivery might be limited to patients undergoing cardiac surgery (e.g., coronary artery bypass grafting). Potential complications are left ventricle perforation, bleeding from the myocardium and unbalanced ventricular motion caused by the uneven distribution of cells after injection.
2. *System infusion*: It includes intracoronary and intravenous injection. Intracoronary has the advantage of increasing the number of cells homing to the ischemia area of the myocardium, while avoiding the damage caused by direct injection in the myocardium. This approach does not require chest opening and can be done at the time of PCI directly [44]. Complications can be cell loss through coronary circulation, and overdose of cell injection that can cause coronary artery occlusion. Intravenous injection is the easiest and the most economical way of infusing stem cells. Even if some researchers argued the real efficacy of this method (primarily due to pulmonary first-pass effect) [45], other studies combining intravenous and intracoronary injection demonstrated improved cardiac function, increased perfusion, and alleviated ventricular remodeling in preclinical ischemia settings [30].
3. *Imaging-guided mini-invasive injection*: This strategy includes trans-endocardial intramyocardial and trans-epicardial intramyocardial injection. These injections are

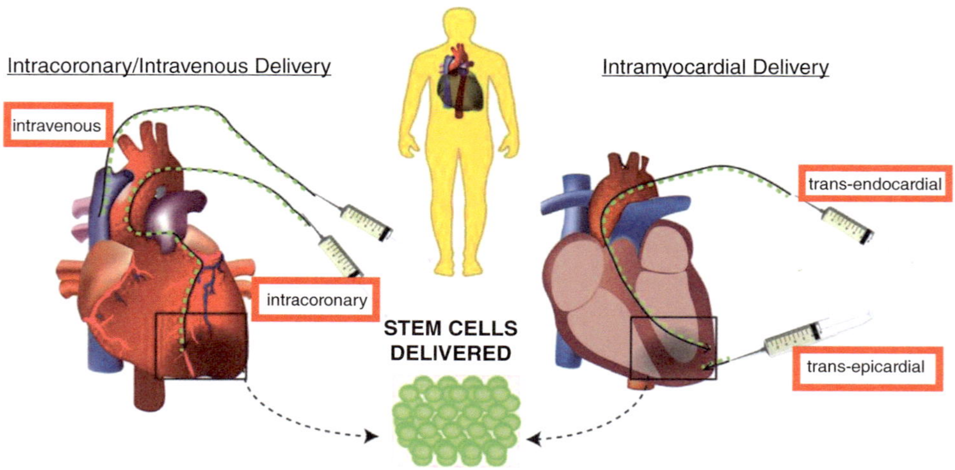

Fig. 6 Stem cells delivery

performed under echo or cardiac magnetic resonance guidance. Advantages are less trauma, fewer complications, and multiple transplantation at different time points [46].

Regarding the optimal timing of cell therapy in AMI, there is evidence that myocardial microenvironment at different time points after infarction has profound influences on stem cells survival, homing, and differentiation [47]. In acute infarct stage, the microenvironment is not conducive to the survival and growth of stem cells because of the overwhelming inflammatory response in the myocardial injury area. It was found that inflammatory reaction peaks at 1–4 days, some cytokines (such as VEGF) which were favorable to stem cells migration reached the peak of secretion at 7 days, and scars began to form at about 14 days after AMI. A recent systematic review found that cardiac function parameters (e.g., diameters, volumes, and LVEF) were significantly improved when stem cells were transplanted between 7 and 10 days after infarction [14]. For chronic IHD, there is no obvious time window problem, so we can select the time when the patients are in good condition (such as no angina attack and general physical activity without discomfort, which denotes that the heart blood supply and heart function are still good), suggesting that the patients' internal environment and myocardial microenvironment are relatively favorable for transplantation, so as to facilitate the survival, homing, and differentiation of implanted cells.

6 Future Perspectives

Current research is oriented toward different new strategies. First, a novel approach is trying to direct MSCs to a cardiopoietic phenotype (by means of a recombinant mix of growth factors, hormones and cytokines which favor the expression of pro-cardiogenic transcription factors). Preclinical and clinical studies are available and have already showed their efficacy and safety [48, 49], but still need to be evaluated in larger cohorts. Analogously, cell combination therapy with different types of stem cells might promote cardiac repair through synergistic interaction [50]. Additional strategies will include: MSC "secretome" including factors within exosomes; bioengineered cellular and acellular matrices and patches that can increase cell/factor retention; repeated injections of stem cells.

References

1. Timmis A, Townsend N, Gale CP, Torbica A, Lettino M, Petersen SE, et al.; European Society of Cardiology. European Society of Cardiology: cardiovascular disease statistics 2019. Eur Heart J. 2020;41(1):12–85. https://doi.org/10.1093/eurheartj/ehz859. Erratum in: Eur Heart J. 2020;41(47):4507. PMID: 31820000.
2. Roth GA, Mensah GA, Johnson CO, Addolorato G, Ammirati E, Baddour LM, et al.; GBD-NHLBI-JACC Global Burden of Cardiovascular Diseases Writing Group. Global Burden of

Cardiovascular Diseases and Risk Factors, 1990–2019: update from the GBD 2019 Study. J Am Coll Cardiol. 2020;76(25):2982–3021. https://doi.org/10.1016/j.jacc.2020.11.010. Erratum in: J Am Coll Cardiol. 2021;77(15):1958–9. PMID: 33309175; PMCID: PMC7755038.

3. Echouffo-Tcheugui JB, Bishu KG, Fonarow GC, Egede LE. Trends in health care expenditure among US adults with heart failure: the Medical Expenditure Panel Survey 2002–2011. Am Heart J. 2017;186:63–72. https://doi.org/10.1016/j.ahj.2017.01.003. Epub 2017 Jan 13. PMID: 28454834; PMCID: PMC5439297
4. Suzuki K, Smolenski RT, Jayakumar J, Murtuza B, Brand NJ, Yacoub MH. Heat shock treatment enhances graft cell survival in skeletal myoblast transplantation to the heart. Circulation. 2000;102(19 Suppl 3):III216–21. https://doi.org/10.1161/01.cir.102.suppl_3.iii-216. PMID: 11082390
5. Kobayashi T, Hamano K, Li TS, Katoh T, Kobayashi S, Matsuzaki M, et al. Enhancement of angiogenesis by the implantation of self bone marrow cells in a rat ischemic heart model. J Surg Res. 2000;89(2):189–95. https://doi.org/10.1006/jsre.2000.5828. PMID: 10729249
6. Kamihata H, Matsubara H, Nishiue T, Fujiyama S, Tsutsumi Y, Ozono R, et al. Implantation of bone marrow mononuclear cells into ischemic myocardium enhances collateral perfusion and regional function via side supply of angioblasts, angiogenic ligands, and cytokines. Circulation. 2001;104(9):1046–52. https://doi.org/10.1161/hc3501.093817. PMID: 11524400
7. Alestalo K, Korpi R, Mäkelä J, Lehtonen S, Mäkelä T, Yannopoulos F, et al. High number of transplanted stem cells improves myocardial recovery after AMI in a porcine model. Scand Cardiovasc J. 2015;49(2):82–94. https://doi.org/10.3109/14017431.2015.1018311. Epub 2015 Mar 18. PMID: 25705991
8. Fuchs S, Baffour R, Zhou YF, Shou M, Pierre A, Tio FO, et al. Transendocardial delivery of autologous bone marrow enhances collateral perfusion and regional function in pigs with chronic experimental myocardial ischemia. J Am Coll Cardiol. 2001;37(6):1726–32. https://doi.org/10.1016/s0735-1097(01)01200-1. PMID: 11345391
9. Waksman R, Fournadjiev J, Baffour R, Pakala R, Hellinga D, Leborgne L, et al. Transepicardial autologous bone marrow-derived mononuclear cell therapy in a porcine model of chronically infarcted myocardium. Cardiovasc Radiat Med. 2004;5(3):125–31. https://doi.org/10.1016/j.carrad.2004.10.001. PMID: 15721847
10. Mathieu M, Bartunek J, El Oumeiri B, Touihri K, Hadad I, Thoma P, et al. Cell therapy with autologous bone marrow mononuclear stem cells is associated with superior cardiac recovery compared with use of nonmodified mesenchymal stem cells in a canine model of chronic myocardial infarction. J Thorac Cardiovasc Surg. 2009;138(3):646–53. https://doi.org/10.1016/j.jtcvs.2008.12.031. Epub 2009 Feb 13. PMID: 19698851
11. Schächinger V, Erbs S, Elsässer A, Haberbosch W, Hambrecht R, Hölschermann H, et al.; REPAIR-AMI Investigators. Improved clinical outcome after intracoronary administration of bone-marrow-derived progenitor cells in acute myocardial infarction: final 1-year results of the REPAIR-AMI trial. Eur Heart J. 2006;27(23):2775–83. https://doi.org/10.1093/eurheartj/ehl388. Epub 2006 Nov 10. PMID: 17098754.
12. Assmus B, Leistner DM, Schächinger V, Erbs S, Elsässer A, Haberbosch W, et al.; REPAIR-AMI Study Group. Long-term clinical outcome after intracoronary application of bone marrow-derived mononuclear cells for acute myocardial infarction: migratory capacity of administered cells determines event-free survival. Eur Heart J. 2014;35(19):1275–83. https://doi.org/10.1093/eurheartj/ehu062. Epub 2014 Feb 25. PMID: 24569031.
13. Traverse JH, Henry TD, Pepine CJ, Willerson JT, Zhao DX, Ellis SG, et al.; Cardiovascular Cell Therapy Research Network (CCTRN). Effect of the use and timing of bone marrow mononuclear cell delivery on left ventricular function after acute myocardial infarction: the TIME randomized trial. JAMA. 2012;308(22):2380–9. https://doi.org/10.1001/jama.2012.28726.

Erratum in: JAMA. 2013;309(4):343. Erratum in: JAMA. 2015;314(1):86. PMID: 23129008; PMCID: PMC3652242.

14. Traverse JH, Henry TD, Ellis SG, Pepine CJ, Willerson JT, Zhao DX, et al.; Cardiovascular Cell Therapy Research Network. Effect of intracoronary delivery of autologous bone marrow mononuclear cells 2 to 3 weeks following acute myocardial infarction on left ventricular function: the LateTIME randomized trial. JAMA. 2011;306(19):2110–9. https://doi.org/10.1001/jama.2011.1670. Epub 2011 Nov 14. PMID: 22084195; PMCID: PMC3600981.
15. Sürder D, Manka R, Moccetti T, Lo Cicero V, Emmert MY, Klersy C, et al. Effect of bone marrow-derived mononuclear cell treatment, early or late after acute myocardial infarction: twelve months CMR and long-term clinical results. Circ Res. 2016;119(3):481–90. https://doi.org/10.1161/CIRCRESAHA.116.308639. Epub 2016 Jun 6. PMID: 27267068
16. Wollert KC, Meyer GP, Müller-Ehmsen J, Tschöpe C, Bonarjee V, Larsen AI, et al. Intracoronary autologous bone marrow cell transfer after myocardial infarction: the BOOST-2 randomised placebo-controlled clinical trial. Eur Heart J. 2017;38(39):2936–43. https://doi.org/10.1093/eurheartj/ehx188. PMID: 28431003
17. Nicolau JC, Furtado RHM, Silva SA, Rochitte CE, Rassi A Jr, Moraes JBMC Jr, et al.; MiHeart/AMI Investigators. Stem-cell therapy in ST-segment elevation myocardial infarction with reduced ejection fraction: a multicenter, double-blind randomized trial. Clin Cardiol. 2018;41(3):392–9. https://doi.org/10.1002/clc.22882. Epub 2018 Mar 22. PMID: 29569254; PMCID: PMC6489870.
18. Xiao C, Zhou S, Liu Y, Hu H. Efficacy and safety of bone marrow cell transplantation for chronic ischemic heart disease: a meta-analysis. Med Sci Monit. 2014;20:1768–77. https://doi.org/10.12659/MSM.892047. PMID: 25270584; PMCID: PMC4199404
19. Garikapati K, Hassan S, Singhvi A, Dania K, Qureshi W. Outcomes of patients with left ventricular diastolic dysfunction in adult hematopoietic stem cell transplantation. Circ Cardiovasc Qual. 2013;6:A72.
20. Babin-Ebell J, Sievers HH, Charitos EI, Klein HM, Jung F, Hellberg AK, et al. Transmyocardial laser revascularization combined with intramyocardial endothelial progenitor cell transplantation in patients with intractable ischemic heart disease ineligible for conventional revascularization: preliminary results in a highly selected small patient cohort. Thorac Cardiovasc Surg. 2010;58(1):11–6. https://doi.org/10.1055/s-0029-1186199. Epub 2010 Jan 13. PMID: 20072970
21. Menasché P, Vanneaux V, Hagège A, Bel A, Cholley B, Cacciapuoti I, et al. Human embryonic stem cell-derived cardiac progenitors for severe heart failure treatment: first clinical case report. Eur Heart J. 2015;36(30):2011–7. https://doi.org/10.1093/eurheartj/ehv189. Epub 2015 May 19. PMID: 25990469
22. Lian Q, Zhang Y, Zhang J, Zhang HK, Wu X, Zhang Y, et al. Functional mesenchymal stem cells derived from human induced pluripotent stem cells attenuate limb ischemia in mice. Circulation. 2010;121(9):1113–23. https://doi.org/10.1161/CIRCULATIONAHA.109.898312. Epub 2010 Feb 22. PMID: 20176987
23. Jung Y, Bauer G, Nolta JA. Concise review: induced pluripotent stem cell-derived mesenchymal stem cells: progress toward safe clinical products. Stem Cells. 2012;30(1):42–7. https://doi.org/10.1002/stem.727. PMID: 21898694; PMCID: PMC3784250
24. Messina E, De Angelis L, Frati G, Morrone S, Chimenti S, Fiordaliso F, et al. Isolation and expansion of adult cardiac stem cells from human and murine heart. Circ Res. 2004;95(9):911–21. https://doi.org/10.1161/01.RES.0000147315.71699.51. Epub 2004 Oct 7. PMID: 15472116
25. Malliaras K, Makkar RR, Smith RR, et al. Intracoronary cardiosphere-derived cells after myocardial infarction: evidence of therapeutic regeneration in the final 1-year results of the CADUCEUS trial (CArdiosphere-Derived aUtologous stem CElls to reverse ventricUlar dySfunction). J Am Coll Cardiol. 2014;63:110–22.

26. Chakravarty T, Makkar RR, Ascheim DD, et al. ALLogeneic heart STem cells to achieve myocardial regeneration (ALLSTAR) trial: rationale and design. Cell Transplant. 2017;26:205–14.
27. Smith RR, Barile L, Cho HC, Leppo MK, Hare JM, Messina E, et al. Regenerative potential of cardiosphere-derived cells expanded from percutaneous endomyocardial biopsy specimens. Circulation. 2007;115(7):896–908. https://doi.org/10.1161/CIRCULATIONAHA.106.655209. Epub 2007 Feb 5. PMID: 17283259
28. Shabbir A, Zisa D, Suzuki G, Lee T. Heart failure therapy mediated by the trophic activities of bone marrow mesenchymal stem cells: a noninvasive therapeutic regimen. Am J Physiol Heart Circ Physiol. 2009;296(6):H1888–97. https://doi.org/10.1152/ajpheart.00186.2009. Epub 2009 Apr 24. PMID: 19395555; PMCID: PMC2716100
29. Vilahur G, Oñate B, Cubedo J, Béjar MT, Arderiu G, Peña E, et al. Allogenic adipose-derived stem cell therapy overcomes ischemia-induced microvessel rarefaction in the myocardium: systems biology study. Stem Cell Res Ther. 2017;8(1):52. https://doi.org/10.1186/s13287-017-0509-2. PMID: 28279225; PMCID: PMC5345145
30. Liu CB, Huang H, Sun P, Ma SZ, Liu AH, Xue J, et al. Human umbilical cord-derived mesenchymal stromal cells improve left ventricular function, perfusion, and remodeling in a porcine model of chronic myocardial ischemia. Stem Cells Transl Med. 2016;5(8):1004–13. https://doi.org/10.5966/sctm.2015-0298. Epub 2016 Jun 22. PMID: 27334487; PMCID: PMC4954453
31. Mayourian J, Cashman TJ, Ceholski DK, Johnson BV, Sachs D, Kaji DA, et al. Experimental and computational insight into human mesenchymal stem cell paracrine signaling and heterocellular coupling effects on cardiac contractility and arrhythmogenicity. Circ Res. 2017;121(4):411–23. https://doi.org/10.1161/CIRCRESAHA.117.310796. Epub 2017 Jun 22. PMID: 28642329; PMCID: PMC5899516
32. Hodgkinson CP, Bareja A, Gomez JA, Dzau VJ. Emerging concepts in paracrine mechanisms in regenerative cardiovascular medicine and biology. Circ Res. 2016;118(1):95–107. https://doi.org/10.1161/CIRCRESAHA.115.305373. PMID: 26837742; PMCID: PMC4874329
33. Karantalis V, DiFede DL, Gerstenblith G, Pham S, Symes J, Zambrano JP, et al. Autologous mesenchymal stem cells produce concordant improvements in regional function, tissue perfusion, and fibrotic burden when administered to patients undergoing coronary artery bypass grafting: the Prospective Randomized Study of Mesenchymal Stem Cell Therapy in Patients Undergoing Cardiac Surgery (PROMETHEUS) trial. Circ Res. 2014;114(8):1302–10. https://doi.org/10.1161/CIRCRESAHA.114.303180. Epub 2014 Feb 24. PMID: 24565698; PMCID: PMC4104798
34. Hare JM, Fishman JE, Gerstenblith G, DiFede Velazquez DL, Zambrano JP, et al. Comparison of allogeneic vs autologous bone marrow–derived mesenchymal stem cells delivered by transendocardial injection in patients with ischemic cardiomyopathy: the POSEIDON randomized trial. JAMA. 2012;308(22):2369–79. https://doi.org/10.1001/jama.2012.25321. Erratum in: JAMA. 2013;310(7):750. George, Richard [added]; Lardo, Albert [added]. PMID: 23117550; PMCID: PMC4762261
35. Bian S, Zhang L, Duan L, Wang X, Min Y, Yu H. Extracellular vesicles derived from human bone marrow mesenchymal stem cells promote angiogenesis in a rat myocardial infarction model. J Mol Med (Berl). 2014;92(4):387–97. https://doi.org/10.1007/s00109-013-1110-5. Epub 2013 Dec 14. PMID: 24337504
36. Liu K, Ji K, Guo L, Wu W, Lu H, Shan P, et al. Mesenchymal stem cells rescue injured endothelial cells in an in vitro ischemia-reperfusion model via tunneling nanotube like structure-mediated mitochondrial transfer. Microvasc Res. 2014;92:10–8. https://doi.org/10.1016/j.mvr.2014.01.008. Epub 2014 Jan 31. PMID: 24486322
37. Chen SL, Fang WW, Ye F, Liu YH, Qian J, Shan SJ, et al. Effect on left ventricular function of intracoronary transplantation of autologous bone marrow mesenchymal stem cell in patients

with acute myocardial infarction. Am J Cardiol. 2004;94(1):92–5. https://doi.org/10.1016/j.amjcard.2004.03.034. PMID: 15219514

38. Lee JW, Lee SH, Youn YJ, Ahn MS, Kim JY, Yoo BS, et al. A randomized, open-label, multicenter trial for the safety and efficacy of adult mesenchymal stem cells after acute myocardial infarction. J Korean Med Sci. 2014;29(1):23–31. https://doi.org/10.3346/jkms.2014.29.1.23. Epub 2013 Dec 26. PMID: 24431901; PMCID: PMC3890472
39. Cogle CR, Wise E, Meacham AM, Zierold C, Traverse JH, Henry TD, et al.; Cardiovascular Cell Therapy Research Network (CCTRN). Detailed analysis of bone marrow from patients with ischemic heart disease and left ventricular dysfunction: BM CD34, CD11b, and clonogenic capacity as biomarkers for clinical outcomes. Circ Res. 2014;115(10):867–74. https://doi.org/10.1161/CIRCRESAHA.115.304353. Epub 2014 Aug 18. PMID: 25136078; PMCID: PMC4358751.
40. Hare JM, Traverse JH, Henry TD, Dib N, Strumpf RK, Schulman SP, et al. A randomized, double-blind, placebo-controlled, dose-escalation study of intravenous adult human mesenchymal stem cells (prochymal) after acute myocardial infarction. J Am Coll Cardiol. 2009;54(24):2277–86. https://doi.org/10.1016/j.jacc.2009.06.055. PMID: 19958962; PMCID: PMC3580848
41. Williams AR, Trachtenberg B, Velazquez DL, McNiece I, Altman P, Rouy D, et al. Intramyocardial stem cell injection in patients with ischemic cardiomyopathy: functional recovery and reverse remodeling. Circ Res. 2011;108(7):792–6. https://doi.org/10.1161/CIRCRESAHA.111.242610. Epub 2011 Mar 17. PMID: 21415390; PMCID: PMC3390160
42. Mathiasen AB, Qayyum AA, Jørgensen E, Helqvist S, Fischer-Nielsen A, Kofoed KF, et al. Bone marrow-derived mesenchymal stromal cell treatment in patients with severe ischaemic heart failure: a randomized placebo-controlled trial (MSC-HF trial). Eur Heart J. 2015;36(27):1744–53. https://doi.org/10.1093/eurheartj/ehv136. Epub 2015 Apr 29. PMID: 25926562
43. Guijarro D, Lebrin M, Lairez O, Bourin P, Piriou N, Pozzo J, et al. Intramyocardial transplantation of mesenchymal stromal cells for chronic myocardial ischemia and impaired left ventricular function: results of the MESAMI 1 pilot trial. Int J Cardiol. 2016;209:258–65. https://doi.org/10.1016/j.ijcard.2016.02.016. Epub 2016 Feb 2. PMID: 26901787
44. Diederichsen AC, Møller JE, Thayssen P, Junker AB, Videbaek L, Saekmose SG, et al. Effect of repeated intracoronary injection of bone marrow cells in patients with ischaemic heart failure the Danish stem cell study—congestive heart failure trial (DanCell-CHF). Eur J Heart Fail. 2008;10(7):661–7. https://doi.org/10.1016/j.ejheart.2008.05.010. Epub 2008 Jun 16. PMID: 18555742
45. Lin L, Gu S, Cheng Y, Ding L. Distribution of adult cardiac stem cells via intravenous cell transplantation in myocardial infarction mouse model. Prog Modern Biomed. 2015;15:7024–7. https://doi.org/10.13241/j.cnki.pmb.2015.36.007.
46. Freyman T, Polin G, Osman H, Crary J, Lu M, Cheng L, et al. A quantitative, randomized study evaluating three methods of mesenchymal stem cell delivery following myocardial infarction. Eur Heart J. 2006;27(9):1114–22. https://doi.org/10.1093/eurheartj/ehi818. Epub 2006 Mar 1. PMID: 16510464
47. Khodayari S, Khodayari H, Amiri AZ, Eslami M, Farhud D, Hescheler J, et al. Inflammatory microenvironment of acute myocardial infarction prevents regeneration of heart with stem cells therapy. Cell Physiol Biochem. 2019;53(5):887–909. https://doi.org/10.33594/000000180. PMID: 31749350
48. Behfar A, Yamada S, Crespo-Diaz R, Nesbitt JJ, Rowe LA, Perez-Terzic C, et al. Guided cardiopoiesis enhances therapeutic benefit of bone marrow human mesenchymal stem cells in chronic myocardial infarction. J Am Coll Cardiol. 2010;56(9):721–34. https://doi.org/10.1016/j.jacc.2010.03.066. PMID: 20723802; PMCID: PMC2932958

49. Bartunek J, Behfar A, Dolatabadi D, Vanderheyden M, Ostojic M, Dens J, et al. Cardiopoietic stem cell therapy in heart failure: the C-CURE (Cardiopoietic stem Cell therapy in heart failURE) multicenter randomized trial with lineage-specified biologics. J Am Coll Cardiol. 2013;61(23):2329–38. https://doi.org/10.1016/j.jacc.2013.02.071. Epub 2013 Apr 10. Erratum in: J Am Coll Cardiol. 2013 Dec 24;62(25):2457-8. PMID: 23583246
50. Bolli R, Hare JM, March KL, Pepine CJ, Willerson JT, Perin EC, et al.; Cardiovascular Cell Therapy Research Network (CCTRN). Rationale and design of the CONCERT-HF Trial (Combination of Mesenchymal and c-kit+ Cardiac Stem Cells As Regenerative Therapy for Heart Failure). Circ Res 2018;122(12):1703–15. https://doi.org/10.1161/CIRCRESAHA.118.312978. Epub 2018 Apr 27. PMID: 29703749; PMCID: PMC5993622.

MIX
Papier aus verantwortungsvollen Quellen
Paper from responsible sources
FSC® C105338

FSC
www.fsc.org

If you have any concerns about our products,
you can contact us on
ProductSafety@springernature.com

In case Publisher is established outside the EU,
the EU authorized representative is:
Springer Nature Customer Service Center GmbH
Europaplatz 3, 69115 Heidelberg, Germany

Printed by Libri Plureos GmbH
in Hamburg, Germany